This book is dedicated to the patients and students
who challenge me daily to learn, listen, and
strive to be a better physician.

For Elsevier

Publisher: *Sarena Wolfaard*
Development Editors: *Claire Wilson, Barbara Simmons*
Project Manager: *Emma Riley*
Designer: *Charles Gray*
Illustration Manager: *Merlyn Harvey*
Illustrator: *Joanna Cameron*

SECOND EDITION

AN OSTEOPATHIC APPROACH TO CHILDREN

THE PERFECT COMPANION TO *PEDIATRIC MANUAL MEDICINE* BY CARREIRO

Jane E Carreiro DO

Osteopathic Physician, Associate Professor and Chair
Department of Osteopathic Manipulative Medicine
University of New England College of Osteopathic Medicine
Biddeford, Maine, USA

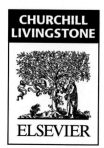

CHURCHILL
LIVINGSTONE

ELSEVIER

Edinburgh London New York Oxford Philadelphia St Louis Sydney Toronto 2009

CHURCHILL
LIVINGSTONE
ELSEVIER

ISBN: 978-0-443-06738-9

British Library Cataloguing in Publication Data
A catalogue record for this book is available from the British Library

Library of Congress Cataloging in Publication Data
A catalog record for this book is available from the Library of Congress

Notice
Neither the Publisher nor the Author assumes any responsibility for any loss or injury and/or damage to persons or property arising out of or related to any use of the material contained in this book. It is the responsibility of the treating practitioner, relying on independent expertise and knowledge of the patient, to determine the best treatment and method of application for the patient.

The Publisher

ELSEVIER your source for books, journals and multimedia in the health sciences
www.elsevierhealth.com

Working together to grow
libraries in developing countries

www.elsevier.com | www.bookaid.org | www.sabre.org

ELSEVIER BOOK AID International Sabre Foundation

The Publisher's policy is to use **paper manufactured from sustainable forests**

Printed in China

Contents

This book is a synthesis of research, study and practice in the science and art of osteopathic medicine as it applies to a pediatric practice. This book emphasizes the contribution of the neuromusculoskeletal system to health and disease, and as an extension of that, focuses on the role of manipulative treatment. However, the art of osteopathic medicine includes the ability to intuit the unspoken, be it emotional, cultural, psychological or spiritual, that holds importance for the patient or family. It is the job of the physician to integrate these subtle and sometimes vague pieces of information which the patient and his or her body are providing, with that which is scientifically known and understood. One type of information does not negate or diminish the value of the other. They dovetail to provide a more complete, a more unified picture of the individual. This book is an attempt to do just that.

This second edition is a composite of information drawn from many and varied sources. The text and references have been updated. The chapter presentation has been reorganized to better reflect ontogeny. Two new chapters have been added to the text, several have been completely rewritten and extended, and new diagrams and photos have been added throughout.

For any clinician, the early foundation of knowledge comes from books, journals, colleagues and teachers, but with time our experiences begin to color what we read and are told. Our patients and their experiences often give us new perspectives. From the tiniest 17-week gestation newborn to the eldest in the ninth decade, our patients' bodies, minds and spirits teach us how to be still, listen and respect the miracle that is Life.

J E Carreiro
December 2007

Acknowledgments

I am so pleased that I was given the opportunity by Elsevier to write a second edition of *An Osteopathic Approach To Children*. Many thanks to Sarena Wolfaard, Emma Riley, and the staff at Elsevier for their help and support with this project.

I would like to thank my colleagues in the Osteopathic Manipulative Medicine department at the University of New England College of Osteopathic Medicine; Stephanie Waecker DO, Ron Mosiello DO, Bill Papura DO, Steve Goldbas DO, Doris Newman DO, John Pelletier DO, Mary Spang and Nancy Goulet who have encouraged and supported this work. Others who have contributed to this process through discussion and analysis include Karen Steele DO, Lisa Gouldsborough DO, Mary Bayno DO, Lisa Milder DO, Hugh Ettlinger DO, and colleagues I have met through the DAAO and DGOM.

I am grateful for support of the administration of the University of New England, College of Osteopathic Medicine, and Boyd Buser DO, now Dean of the Pikeville College of Osteopathic Medicine. The intellectual curiosity, enthusiasm and commitment of the students at the University's College of Osteopathic Medicine continues to be an inspiration for me, as is the dedication, passion, skill and occasional contentiousness of the OPP/Anatomy Fellows who make my job the best in the world.

I especially want to acknowledge the individuals in this text who so selflessly contributed to the Human Anatomy Program at the University of New England. May their sacrifices help us help others.

Finally, my deepest gratitude is reserved for my teachers, students and family who continue to guide, challenge and support me.

The book is arranged in two parts. The first discusses the physiology and development of body systems from the perspective of an osteopathic clinician. The second describes common pediatric pathophysiological processes in those body systems. Several recurring themes are woven throughout the text: the mechanisms by which pathophysiological processes influence each other; the normal changes and adaptations in structure and function that occur throughout childhood and how the changes can be affected by these processes; and a rationale for osteopathic treatment. The presence of somatic dysfunction (see below) may or may not be significant depending upon the clinical context within which it has been found. Somatic dysfunction is discussed from the perspective of the findings in different tissues, i.e. fluid, membranous, articular, osseous and neural findings. Different pathophysiological processes often require different osteopathic approaches, especially in the very young, the very old and the very sick. Although a general overview of osteopathic approaches is presented, specific techniques are not described. Osteopathic treatment is discussed within the context of physiological models: somatovisceral interactions, postural or biomechanical influences, the neuroendocrine-immune system, the respiratory/circulatory system, and the bioenergetic model. Although a discussion of these models is integrated throughout the text, a short synopsis is provided here.

Somatic dysfunction may manifest as a localized area of palpatory change in the muscles and fascia adjacent to the spine. These changes include tissue swelling or edema, increased or decreased temperature, and stiffness or loss of tone. Tissue texture changes represent localized areas of inflammation that can occur in response to direct insult. They may also arise in response to damage or irritation to distal tissues through viscerosomatic reflexes. Viscerosomatic reflexes were first described by osteopaths in the early part of this century. Recent scientific investigation into the mechanism and effects of these interactions has shed new light on the intimate relationship between the musculoskeletal system and the viscera through the sympathetic nervous system. Chapman's reflexes are superficial areas of tissue texture change that have a high correlation with visceral pathology. These pea-sized areas of fibrosis are found on the anterior and posterior torso. The site of location and presence of both anterior and posterior findings suggests a visceral problem (Owen 1963). Chapman's reflexes were first discussed in the early part of the twentieth century by Frank Chapman DO. They are very easily integrated in the general physical exam and provide another tool in developing a differential diagnosis. A general understanding of the viscerosomatic map and Chapman's reflexes can give the clinician clues about what may be causing the patient's symptoms and can provide a pathway for therapeutic approach.

The neuroendocrine immune connection is a term that has been coined to refer to the complicated interdependency between the nervous system, hormone balance and immune function. Basically speaking, the human body maintains internal balance or homeostasis, through rhythmic chemical secretions from the brain (neurotransmitters), immune organs (immunoregulators), and glands (hormones). The chemicals that are secreted interact to stimulate and suppress each other, thus coordinating the internal chemistry of the body. Potentially harmful stimuli from both external and internal sources can alter these rhythmical patterns, thus affecting the homeostasis of the internal body chemistry and creating a *general adaptive response*. Normally, once the stress is removed the adaptive response resolves and homeostasis is re-established. However under long-term or severe stress, the entire physiology of the neuroendocrine immune system can alter, creating a permanent condition of adaptive response. Brain chemistry, immune system function and hormone balance will alter. Not only is this person more susceptible to disease, he or she will have a much harder time adapting to any new stress. Many studies have demonstrated changes in immune cells, hormone levels and nervous system function under stress (McEwan 1987, Ganong 1988, Gold & Goodwin 1988a, b, Keicolt-Glaser & Glaser 1991, Esterling 1992, Sternberg & Chrousos 1992). Stressful stimuli may include psychological and physiological influences. Pain, or nociceptive stimuli, is considered a potent stressor. From an osteopathic perspective, somatic dysfunction or other strains in the patient's body may adversely influence the neuroendocrine immune system.

The postural/biomechanical model views the body as an integration of somatic components. Stresses or imbalances between these components result in increased energy expenditure, changes in joint structure, impediment of neurovascular function and altered metabolism. In very young children biomechanical or postural stresses may influence the development of motor skills, and perhaps even cognitive processes. Furthermore, altered postural mechanics will influence connective tissue and fascia, potentially affecting vascular and lymphatic drainage. These changes can contribute to the accumulation of cellular waste products, altered tissue pH, changes in osmotic pressure, and impediment of oxygen and nutrient delivery. This is important in cases of infection, cardiopulmonary problems, and metabolic diseases such as diabetes. Postural imbalances may also cause irritation to paraspinal tissues, including the articular tissues of the vertebrae. Irritation to these tissues will stimulate somatosympathetic fibers, resulting in sympathetically mediated changes in the involved tissues and potential changes in associated viscera.

The respiratory/circulatory model concerns itself with the maintenance of extracellular and intracellular environments through the unimpeded delivery of oxygen and nutrients and the removal of waste products. The integrity of the respiratory/ circulatory system is influenced by postural changes on a microscopic level through tissue stress and macroscopically through respiratory mechanics. Most of the muscles of the back, thorax, neck and upper extremities play a role in respiratory mechanics. Altered respiratory mechanics can contribute to: tissue congestion and decreased clearance; altered ventilation and increased energy expenditure; and altered lymphatic and venous return pressures. Factors that can affect respiratory mechanics include, but are not limited to, respiratory illnesses, scoliosis, thoracic or abdominal surgery, obesity and postural changes.

The human body requires a balance between energy expenditure and energy supply to maintain homeostasis. Efficient operation of internal body systems conserves energy that can be used to adapt to external stressors such as nutritional deficiencies, trauma, infection, nociceptive stimulation and others. When several stressors occur simultaneously, their influence may become cumulative or synergistic, further compromising the body's ability to maintain homeostasis. Changes in the musculoskeletal system may increase the body's energy requirement. For example, restriction in joint motion because of somatic dysfunction will alter biomechanics and reduce efficiency of motion. It will require more work to use the joint – this increases the metabolic demands placed upon the patient. Now imagine there are many restricted joints, all in the thorax, and the patient is a 4-month-old infant with respiratory syncytial virus. Any process that interferes with local or systemic homeostasis has the potential to increase the body's energy requirements.

In my view these five physiological models interweave to form the fabric of the osteopathic approach. There is one other component that, when added, turns osteopathic approach into osteopathic treatment. That is the relationship between the osteopathic practitioner and the patient. By this I do not mean the personalities – most 2-week olds don't have much personality! I refer to an acknowledgment that must take place between the practitioner and the patient. Though perhaps lacking in conversational skills, even the youngest patient is an individual, a complete human being, with no lesser or no greater bearing in life than the physician. Osteopathic treatment requires two things to be successful – the patient and the practitioner. Osteopaths are not abject healers. We are facilitators. The patient provides the clues that allow us to use our knowledge and skill to facilitate change, but the patient's body, the patient's mechanism has to make that change.

JC, 2008

References

Esterling B 1992 Stress-associated modulation of cellular immunity. In: Willard F H, Patterson M (eds) Nociception and the neuroendocrine-immune connection. American Academy of Osteopathy: 275–294.

Ganong W 1988 The stress response – a dynamic overview. Hosp Prac 23: 155–171.

Gold P, Goodwin F 1988a Clinical and biochemical manifestations of stress: Part I. N Engl J Med 319: 348–353.

Gold P, Goodwin F 1988b Clinical and biochemical manifestations of depression: Part II. N Engl J Med 319: 413–420.

Keicolt-Glaser J K, Glaser R 1991 Stress and immune function in humans. In: Ader R, Felton D L, Cohen N (eds) Psychoneuroimmunology, 2nd edn. Academic Press, San Diego, CA: 849–895.

McEwan B 1987 Glucocorticoid-biogenic amine interactions in relation to mood and behavior. Biochem Pharm 36: 1755–1763.

Owen C 1963 An endocrine interpretation of Chapman's reflexes, 2nd edn. American Academy of Osteopathy, Colorado.

Sternberg E, Chrousos G 1992 The stress response and the regulation of inflammatory disease. Ann Intern Med 117: 854–866.

Chapter One

The nervous system: a clinician's perspective

CHAPTER CONTENTS

INTRODUCTION

In the 4 years since I wrote the introduction to the first edition of this chapter, our understanding of the nervous system has expanded immensely and yet the nervous system remains a vast and complicated subject, which we can only peruse within the confines of this text. This chapter endeavors to provide the reader with a clinician's understanding of some fundamental neurological processes and their potential role in clinical evaluation and management. For more information, readers are directed to the excellent texts and essays referenced at the end of the chapter.

EMBRYOLOGICAL DEVELOPMENT OF THE NERVOUS SYSTEM

The cellular development of the nervous system can be divided into seven stages: proliferation, migration, aggregation, differentiation, synaptogenesis, remodeling and myelination (Kandel et al 2000, Moore 2007). The first three, proliferation, migration and aggregation, happen early in embryological development and are completed at the time of birth. The latter four are not finished at the time of birth; in fact, some of them are just starting and will continue throughout life. Early in gestation, neuronal cells migrate and arrange themselves into clusters based on their functional capabilities. In the primitive brainstem, neuronal cells cluster into nuclei. In the spinal cord, they organize themselves into elongated columns or tracts. The final product of this process is an elongated neural trunk with 41 paired branches, topped by a bulbous crown (Fig. 1.1). We can think of the early embryo as a segmented column with an opening at the most anterior aspect: the anterior neural pore. The most anterior aspect will grow, elongate and turn posteriorly, inferiorly and anteriorly like a ram's horn to form the cortical hemispheres (Fig. 1.2). The remaining columns of neuronal clusters form the primitive spinal cord and the peripheral nerves. It is surrounded by mesodermal cells which will develop into the paired somites of the body. Each somite will cluster around a group of axons from the adjacent neural cells. The somites give rise to all the somatic tissues of the body: skin, muscle, periosteum, fascia, etc. (more on that in Ch. 2). As the somite develops into these tissues, it usually drags its innervation from the adjacent spinal segment. Within the thorax, this arrangement of stacked segmented innervation is readily evident in the dermatomal pattern (Fig. 1.3). However, in the extremities, where the somatic tissue migrated out along the axis of the appendage, the organization is distorted. The stacked arrangement is lost and in its place is left a hodgepodge of overlapping

tissues such that the motor innervation from C3–C4–C5 is found in the diaphragm but the sensory innervation from muscular tissue (the myotome) is found in the trapezius, the sensory innervation from skin (the dermatome) is found over the top of the shoulder and forearm, and the sensory innervation from bone (the sclerotome) is found in the scapula (Fig. 1.4). Irritation of nerve cells in the spinal cord area of C3–C5 could present as pain in the area of the scapula (sclerotome) or in the trapezius (myotome).

MYELINATION

The embryological processes of proliferation, migration and aggregation can be thought of as laying down the paths. You can drive on a road that is not paved, but you have to drive slowly. Paving the road can be compared to myelinating the nerves. Myelination allows the signal to travel very quickly.

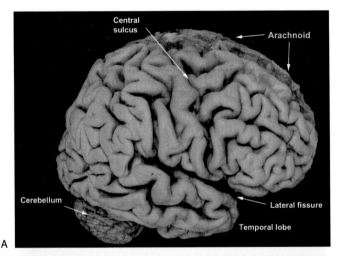

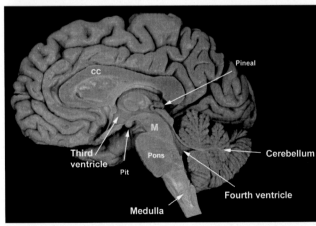

Fig. 1.1 • A posterior view of the brain and spinal cord. The posterior somatic tissues and the osseous structures have been removed from the cranium to the pelvis to reveal the brain, spinal cord and peripheral nerves. *Used with permission of the Willard & Carreiro Collection.*

Fig. 1.2 • (A) Lateral view of the external surface of the brain. The arachnoid has been removed from the surface of the right hemisphere, but is still in place (arrows) on the left. (B) Sagittal section through midline of brain. CC, corpus callosum; M, midbrain; Pit, pituitary stalk. *Used with permission of the Willard & Carreiro Collection.*

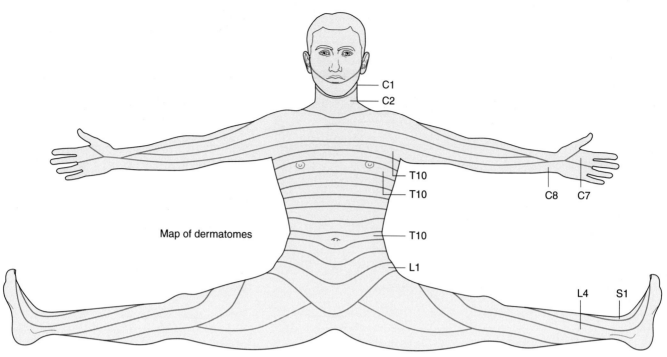

Fig. 1.3 • Map of dermatomes.

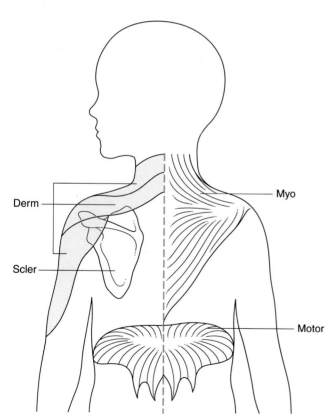

Fig. 1.4 • Schematic diagram depicting the dermatome (Derm), sclerotome (Scler), myotome (Myo) and motor innervation from C3 to C5.

However, a nerve does not need to be myelinated in order to function. In the fully functioning nervous system, pain fibers are very thinly myelinated and their endings are unmyelinated, yet these neurons function appropriately. As might be expected, however, their conduction time is slower than that of more heavily myelinated fibers. The heavily myelinated fibers are called large-calibre fibers, they have rapid conduction times and are involved with proprioceptive input. Because the conduction time on a thinly myelinated fiber is much slower than that of a heavily myelinated fiber, two signals traveling simultaneously on parallel fibers will reach their destinations at different times. If they happen to share a destination, then the signal that arrives first will effectively 'block' the later signal; this is known as the gating phenomenon.

SPINAL REFLEXES

Reflexes can be divided into two categories: spinal reflexes and supraspinal reflexes. Spinal reflexes are segmental and monosynaptic. For example, tapping a patella tendon with a reflex hammer causes the tendon to stretch rapidly, exciting muscle spindles within the quadratus muscle (Fig. 1.5). The signal from the muscle spindle is carried to the spinal cord, where it is relayed through interneurons to the α motor neurons of the ventral horn. The α motor neurons signal extrafusal muscle fibers that cause the quadratus muscle to contract. This is a spinal or stretch reflex.

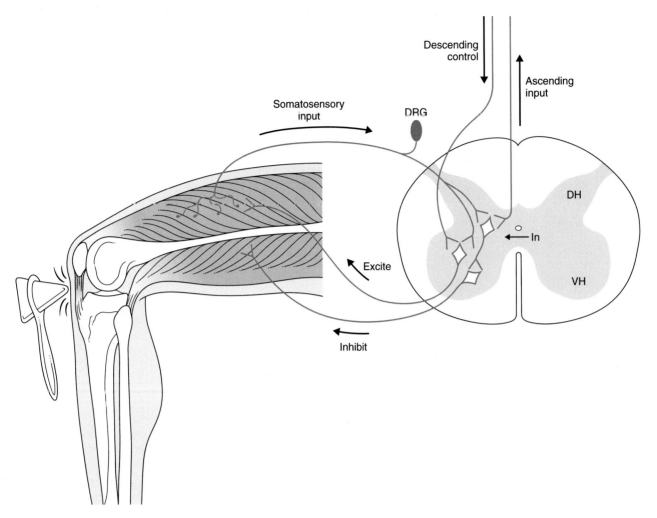

Fig. 1.5 • Schematic diagram of a spinal reflex at the knee. Somatosensory inputs from the stretched muscle spindles of the tendon of the quadratus muscle enter the dorsal horn (DH) via the dorsal root ganglion (DRG). Within the spinal cord, these afferents synapse on interneurons (In), which communicate with motor neurons in the ventral horn (VH). The motor neurons may be involved with excitation or inhibition of α motor neurons in the hamstring muscles. Ascending tracts will carry information from the interneurons to the brain. Descending tracts from the cortex and cerebellum will down-modulate the reflex.

The mature stretch reflex can be broken down into two components: a dynamic stretch reflex, which responds quickly to rapid changes in muscle length, and a weaker static stretch reflex, which continues to maintain contraction of the muscle as long as the stretch force persists. The entire circuit is contained within the spinal cord. The interneuron may also send a signal to the brain to let it know what has happened, but the reflex is not dependent on input from the brain. In fact, input from the brain actually dampens the reflex. As the nervous system matures, myelination in the corticospinal and pyramidal tracts increases, and the spinal reflexes are down-modulated. This process is important for motor control. The ability to execute smooth gross and fine motor activity necessitates modulation of the stretch reflex. Imagine what would happen if you suddenly turned rapidly stretching your patella tendon. Without cortical modulation, the quadratus muscle would quickly contract, destabilizing your posture and balance. Damage to cortical structures involved with motor activity will interfere with the brain's ability to modulate these reflexes. This occurs in spastic cerebral palsy. These children develop increased muscle tone (spasticity) because they cannot properly modulate the stretch reflex. This affects their ability to smoothly execute voluntary movement.

At birth, the spinal reflex has a low threshold for activation and recruits other muscles through a radiate response (Myklebust & Gottlieb 1993). The reflex matures and becomes muscle specific by 6 years (O'Sullivan et al 1991).

SPINAL SEGMENTATION

If you were to look at the neural tube in three dimensions, you would notice that it looks like a smooth, homogeneous tube lacking segmentation. Yet clinically we often speak

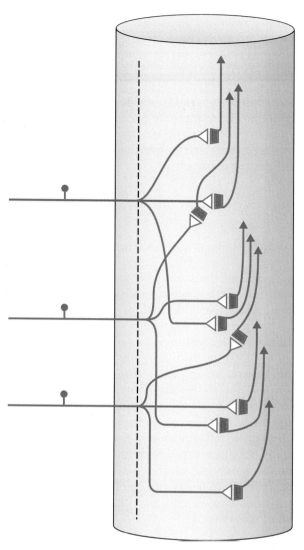

Fig. 1.6 • Schematic diagram depicting segmentation of spinal neurons. Within the spinal cord, axons may travel up or down the cord before synapsing on a cell body.

LOCALIZATION

Dermatomes, myotomes and sclerotomes are areas of sensory innervation associated with a common nerve root. These areas were first described at the turn of the century by Head and are called the 'zones of Head'. A zone of Head represents the summation of the dermatome, myotome and sclerotome patterns which have the same embryological origin, i.e. pattern of innervation. Each of these tissue types has different densities of receptor cell types. Receptors in skin usually respond to light touch, two-point discrimination, temperature and nociception. Receptors in muscle are activated by nociception, stretch and chemical signals. Receptors in bone and periosteum respond to nociception and tend to have higher thresholds for activation than those in the other tissues. A signal coming from a spinal cord level such as T1 will be interpreted by somatosensory cortex as coming from one of the zones of Head. For example, nerve root irritation may present as pain radiating down the extremity in a dermatomal distribution. However, if the pain generator is the disk, the pain may express itself as dull and boring in the sclerotome distribution. Nociceptive stimulation of the tissue in any particular zone will activate cells in the dorsal horn of that area of the spinal cord. In many situations, the same neural cells may receive information from three different kinds of tissue: skin, bone and muscle. This information will be relayed to the brain. Cells in the cortex learn to interpret signals from the spinal cord as coming from specific tissues, based upon the intensity and frequency of the signal and the location of the activated cell. For example, a signal traveling along the anterolateral system (ALS) from the T4 area of the spinal cord may have originated in the shoulder or heart. The signal from T4 is carried by many neurons, some of which will map to specific cells in the somatosensory cortex, and others that are less specific. Cortical cells can recognize the location of the source of the signal by the company it keeps. Cells also 'learn' to associate activity in a certain level of the spinal cord with irritation to a specific tissue. However, if the inciting spinal cord cell or the receiving cortical cell receives input from more than one kind of tissue, the cortex may not be able to differentiate between them. This is one of the mechanisms of referred pain. An irritation or injury to one area of the body is interpreted as coming from a different tissue because the two have a common innervation. Shared innervation is more common between a visceral organ and a somatic tissue than between two somatic tissues. Clinically, we often associate this process with visceral pathology.

Most sensory cells in the spinal cord receiving input from somatic tissue will also receive input from viscera. When the brain receives a signal from that area of the spinal cord, it cannot distinguish between the visceral and somatic tissue. If, during life, the cortex has learned to interpret pain

of segmentation. Conversely, the brainstem and cortex are segmented by chemical boundaries. The boundaries are marked by proteins that form recognition molecules and axons will not grow over these boundaries. These things are absent in the morphology and chemistry of the spinal cord. Axons travel for considerable distances along the spinal cord without barriers, boundaries, or segmentation. Segmentation is artificially enforced upon the spinal cord by the arrangement of the somatic tissues. Somites are collections of mesenchyme positioned along the side of the neural tube; as the axons grow out of the neural tube, they are bunched together by the somites, creating segmentation. However, the central process of the axon splits as it enters the spinal cord and branches up and down the cord to synapse on cell bodies above and below its level of entry (Fig. 1.6). Thus segmentation exists outside the spinal cord.

stimulation from the T4 area as arm or shoulder injury, then when T4 becomes stimulated by myocardial injury, the brain may continue to interpret that signal as shoulder pain. Many incidents of referred pain, such as shoulder irritation with gallbladder disease, and back pain with urinary tract infections, can be accounted for by the convergence patterns of the zones of Head. For most people, the brain is initially exposed to pain signals from somatic rather than visceral tissue. The brain learns to interpret nociceptive signals from most areas of the spinal cord as coming from somatic tissue. Thus symptoms of visceral pathology are referred to the musculoskeletal system. However, when children develop early visceral disease such as reflux, intussusception or surgical correction of congenital heart disease, the brain learns to interpret nociceptive input from those areas of the spinal cord as visceral rather than somatic irritation. Later, when somatic irritation does develop, the child may complain of symptoms similar to those associated with the early visceral pathology.

PRIMARY AFFERENT FIBERS

Afferent fibers are the sensory fibers of the nervous system. For the sake of discussion, we can divide them into two groups. The first group has been called the 'large-calibre afferent system'. It includes the encapsulated, heavily myelinated fibers that are sensitive to very light touch and proprioception. They conduct very quickly and carry information about stretch, pressure and position. This system can be described as being line labeled; that is, a specific sensory organ such as a Pacinian corpuscle on your fingertip would activate only a few cells in the brainstem that would then be connected to a few cells in the cortex. There is a preserved relationship through the whole system that is labeled for that specific Pacinian corpuscle. Consequently, you are able to precisely identify the location of the stimulus. The opposite of this occurs in the group referred to as the 'small-calibre afferent system'. The fibers are small, lightly myelinated or unmyelinated, with slower conduction rates and their nerve endings lack encapsulation. They carry information concerning temperature and pain. Their receptors tend to have a much higher threshold of activation; that is, they require higher levels of stimulation for activation. Often, for the smallest of these fibers, tissue damage needs to occur to activate the receptor. Nociceptive information is obtained through the fibers of the small-calibre system. When this system is activated at a low rate, we may perceive the stimulus as crude touch, whereas when these fibers are firing at a high rate, we interpret that as being pain. This is very different from what happens when the large-calibre system is active. For example, when a Pacinian corpuscle shifts its firing rate, you still perceive it as a Pacinian corpuscle, i.e. you still perceive vibration. However, the 'small-calibre system' works differently. Shifting the firing rate

changes the perception of the stimulus. The interpretation of the same stimulus can change from crude touch to pain. Fibers of the small-calibre afferent system are present in all tissues, both visceral and somatic. In addition to the rate-dependent characteristic of the small-calibre system there are specific fibers with very high thresholds of activation called silent nociceptors. They are more prevalent in the viscera. They can remain quiescent for their entire life until they are exposed to a sufficiently intense stimulus, but once activated they are difficult to turn down.

NEUROGENIC INFLAMMATION

The very small-calibre primary afferent fibers are nociceptors or pain sensors. When activated, their receptor end secretes polypeptides into the tissue. The secreted polypeptides include histamine, bradykinin, substance P, somatostatin, vasoactive intestinal polypeptide and others. These polypeptides comprise a chemical soup that incites a localized inflammatory reaction. The inflammatory compounds are irritating to the primary afferent receptor that secreted them, which causes that receptor to depolarize again and secrete another batch of inflammatory compounds. Consequently, the receptors can become self-stimulating, producing neurogenic stimulation and inflammation. Neurogenic inflammation may be localized to the original site of insult or it may occur at a distal site mediated through converging neurons or spinal facilitation. Neurogenic inflammation may also be initiated through the dorsal horn when two or more neurons converge. This is called a dorsal root reflex.

CONVERGENCE

Convergence occurs when information from two or more primary afferent receptors synapses on a common cell body or group of cells. This can occur through various mechanisms: afferent fibers to different tissues may share the same cell body (McNeill & Burden 1986), two fibers may synapse on the same dorsal horn cell (Cervero & Connell 1984), or information from two primary afferents may converge in the brainstem or cortex (Langhorst et al 1996). In each of these situations, irritation to the primary afferent may be perceived as coming from a different site. As previously described this is a mechanism for referred pain. For example, a cell body may have a bifurcating axon such that a receptor in the heart shares its cell body with a primary afferent in the arm. If the receptor in the heart is activated, it will send a signal to the cell body, which in turn will activate interneurons in the spinal cord. A signal will be sent to the brain, so that the person will perceive that the pain is coming from the heart. Now suppose that the primary afferent in the arm is activated. Its information

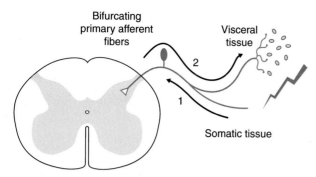

Fig. 1.7 • Schematic diagram of a dorsal root reflex on a bifurcating neuron. (1) Tissue injury stimulates depolarization and signaling to the dorsal horn cells. A retrograde depolarization occurs on the coupled neuron (2) resulting in secretion at the primary afferent ending. *Used with permission of the Willard & Carreiro Collection.*

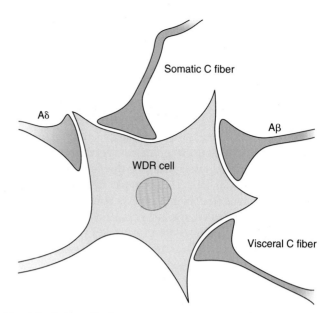

Fig. 1.8 • Schematic diagram of wide dynamic range cell (WDR cell) receiving convergent input from visceral and somatic nociceptors, and various mechanoreceptors (Aδ and Aβ).

will converge onto the same cell body and interneuron. The input to the cortex is coming from the same source. What will determine how the patient perceives the pain? In part this is a learned response. The cortex will interpret the stimulus based upon previous experience and inputs. The same thing can happen to the fibers converging in the brain instead of the spinal cord. In addition to nociception, input from visual, emotional, auditory and other stimuli converge onto common areas of the cortex concerned with interpreting and responding to these stimuli. As with nociceptive input, the interpretation is a learned process. Consequently, convergence can sometimes lead to misinterpretation of the stimulus or pain referral.

From a clinical perspective convergence has several other roles. If a cell body receiving information from multiple converging neurons becomes sensitized it can lose the ability to differentiate the cell type carrying the signal. This is what occurs in patients with acute pain who report changes in sensation although there is no damage to large-calibre fibers or sensory nerves. This can be seen in everything from meniscus and ligament tears to acute low back pain. Convergence also plays a role in neurogenic inflammation. As previously described, when a receptor ending of a primary afferent is activated it will release inflammatory peptides into the local tissue and send a signal to the dorsal horn cell. If that dorsal horn cell is a site of convergence, then activation of the dorsal horn cell can result in retrograde activation of the coupled primary afferent. The coupled afferent neuron responds by secreting inflammatory peptides at its terminal end, producing inflammation in undamaged tissues and irritating its receptor ending (Fig. 1.7).

SPINAL FACILITATION

When nociceptive fibers are activated, they will alter the behavior of neurons in the ventral horn (He et al 1988).

Researchers placed a recording electrode in the appropriate cells of the ventral horn of an anesthetized cat. The cat's knee was then passively flexed and extended. No activity was recorded in the ventral cells. Next, an irritating substance was injected into the cat's knee. Once this quieted down, the cat's knee was again passively flexed and extended. The electrodes in the ventral horn recorded increased activity with this passive movement. This suggested that once the cell population is activated by the knee injection, it develops a lower threshold for subsequent activation. Prior to the injection, passive movement did not activate the cells, but after the injection, the same stimulus turned them on. The state of lowered threshold for activation in a population of cells is termed spinal facilitation. It has been demonstrated that the small-calibre primary afferent fibers are necessary to initiate this type of activity in the spinal cord (Anderson & Winterson 1995). Facilitation is a characteristic of the small-calibre system.

Facilitation occurs and is maintained at the level of the spinal cord. It is not a peripheral process. It occurs when the activity in a pool of interneurons is altered. The interneurons involved with facilitation receive input from many different peripheral tissues: skin, muscle, bone, connective tissue and viscera. They are called wide dynamic range (WDR) cells because they respond to a broad range of stimulation. This convergent input summates on the WDR cell (Fig. 1.8). Consequently, facilitation may be maintained because the same spinal cord cell that received the initial stimulus is now barraged with signals from the soma and viscera affected by the injury. After the injury resolves, the WDR cell continues to receive input from non-nociceptive convergent cells. Although that input may be of normal intensity, it maintains the threshold of activation in the WDR cell.

Fibers of the 'small-calibre afferent system' innervate muscle, joints and skin. When the system is activated it signals the ventral horn, resulting in muscle contraction. When a joint is inflamed, the associated muscles will contract. If the muscle contraction is strong or prolonged, the resultant ischemia activates the small primary afferents. These muscle nociceptors will send input to the same cells that were initially activated by the joint inflammation. There is a summation of activity in the dorsal horn. Spinal facilitation can be sustained because the nociceptive activity from the muscle is driving the dorsal horn, which then drives the ventral horn. This loop may be maintained even if the initial stimulus (the injured joint) is removed. Worse yet, after the tissue has healed, the cell population within the dorsal horn can remain sensitized so that it takes very little input to reinitiate the process. The threshold for activation may be lowered to the extent that non-nociceptive stimuli converging on those same dorsal horn cells can reactivate the patient's symptoms (called hyperalgesia) and the ventral horn response.

For example, a 5-year-old girl developed severe anterior chest wall pain immediately following open-heart surgery for correction of a congenital ventricular septal defect. The surgery was successful without complication. The child's pain was managed with postoperative analgesics for several weeks. She recovered from the surgery and resumed normal activities within an appropriate amount of time. Two years later, this child suddenly began complaining of intense anterior chest wall pain. After extensive work-up the only abnormality found was a mild thoracic scoliosis (less than 10°). The intensity of the pain could not be explained by the mechanical deformation of the thoracic cage. Without entering into a discussion of the potential etiology of the scoliosis, we need to consider the possibility that the perceived intensity of the chest wall pain is due to the fact that neurons responding to the biomechanical stress in the thoracic spine are converging on the same cells that were facilitated as a result of the surgery. The nociceptive input from the thoracic wall tissues injured during the operation facilitated that area of the spinal cord. Now the relatively minor irritation from the scoliosis is being interpreted through the exaggerated perspective of the facilitated neurons. If the scoliosis is addressed such that there is some decrease in the biomechanical strain, the afferent drive on these cells should decrease and the patient's symptoms improve. However, the spinal neurons are still sensitized and the child is at risk for developing similar symptoms again.

Spinal facilitation is one of the mechanisms used to explain chronic pain. Patients with chronic pain will experience exacerbation of the pain with very little irritation. When as practitioners we are faced with patients who repeatedly present with the same complaints, we need to remember the potential role of spinal facilitation in the process. Although we tend to associate the process of spinal facilitation with musculoskeletal tissues, the viscera can be involved. For example, esophageal inflammation may induce spinal facilitation. Once the esophageal problem has resolved, the patient may now have some gastrointestinal sensitivity. The spinal facilitation may also express itself in the somatic tissues of that area. This is frequently the case in children who have severe reflux as infants. This too, is a viscerosomatic reflex. Although gastrointestinal immunity often plays a role in the process, we cannot ignore the neurogenic component (see Chs 6 and 7).

AFFERENT LOAD

Wide dynamic range (WDR) cells receive input from primary afferent fibers in somatic and visceral tissue, and from larger-calibre fibers involved with crude touch. Together these constitute the afferent load on the segment. Once WDR cells have become sensitized they respond to a lower afferent load. Anything that increases the total afferent load, including non-noxious stimuli such as touch or vibration, can activate the WDR. The addition of the input from the non-noxious sensory fibers elevates the afferent load and the activity within the already facilitated neurons, causing them to respond as if they were receiving noxious or nociceptive stimuli. Clinically, non-noxious touch, movement within the permitted range of motion, and tissue loading may be interpreted by the patient as irritating or painful. In its milder forms this is tenderness, in extreme conditions this is allodynia. The afferent load can also include supratentorial influences from the limbic lobe and amygdale determined by emotions and memories.

The process of facilitation can be viewed as a continuum; in the early phase the body can reverse it, but after a certain point it is not reversible. Unfortunately, no one knows where that point is, and it probably differs in patients. One of the goals of treatment is to lower the afferent load being sustained by the patient. Therapeutic modalities that theoretically dampen input into the spinal cord are often used. For example, modalities that decrease muscle spasm, relieve edema and improve oxygen and nutrient delivery are thought to decrease the level of nociceptive drive entering the cord. In addition, because of the convergent nature of sensory input we must also consider other phenomena that may increase the cumulative afferent load such as stress, emotional turmoil, socioeconomic conditions and cultural forces. These may also play a role in the manner in which a person adapts to or compensates for areas of facilitation. In fact some authors will argue that a process similar to facilitation, termed kindling, occurs in the limbic and cortical areas and may play a role in anxiety, depression and other affective disorders.

In some cases lowering the afferent drive involves the phenomenon called gating, which was mentioned previously. Different forms of sensory input from many different tissues converge onto dorsal horn interneurons. When a signal activates a cell, it effectively blocks that cell from responding to concurrent or subsequent stimuli for a period of time. Signals that reach the interneurons first are transmitted to the cortex first. Slower signals go undetected. Modalities such as pressure, light touch and proprioception are all carried on heavily myelinated, rapidly conducting fibers. These signals will arrive at the interneuronal pool before signals from the slower-conducting nociceptive fibers. This means that the nociceptive signal can be gated or masked by the other stimulus. This explains why gentle but firm tactile stimulation or vibration can be used to mask pain, and why gently but firmly rubbing a sick child's back or belly soothes them.

THE CHARACTERISTICS OF DIFFERENT NOCICEPTORS – PAIN

Viscerally driven pain tends to be diffuse, dull, boring, or crushing, while somatic pain is usually sharp, well circumscribed, burning, or pinching. Older children and adolescents with visceral pain will sometimes call it heavy. Sometimes they will say that it's achy, but they will not tell you that it's burning and they cannot localize it to a specific point. They will often use the entire hand rather than one finger to indicate the location of the pain. If the pain is referred, then there will not be any tenderness over the skin or muscles. If abdominal viscera are involved, then deep palpation over the area will produce tenderness. When viscera are irritated the pain initially has the characteristics of visceral pain; however, as the visceral inflammation spreads to the peritoneal tissue, the pain quality becomes more somatic. This explains the clinical course of appendicitis and other acute abdomen conditions.

Initially the appendix is inflamed and the pain is vague, dull and achy. As the appendix stretches and begins to irritate the peritoneum the pain becomes sharp and well localized because the peritoneum is innervated by somatic afferents not visceral afferents. When a visceral pain in the abdomen (diffuse, dull, etc.) takes on a somatic characteristic, we know that the inflammation has spread from the viscera to the connective tissue, i.e. the peritoneum. On physical examination, this is associated with rebound pain. Similarly, when a patient complains of chest pain that is sharp or stabbing, we need to think about musculoskeletal injury. Using the anatomy to understand the characteristics of visceral and somatic pain presentations allows the practitioner to be more precise with his or her differential diagnosis.

In younger children, sensory mapping is immature and inaccurate. Pain patterns can be ill defined and misleading. The best way to assess pain in children is through observation, history and palpation (see Ch. 6). How is the child's behavior different from usual? What postures is he assuming? Does he lay in a fetal position or is he sprawling and unwilling to be moved? Does he want to be held or left alone? Is he eating and drinking? A careful and complete history and physical examination, combined with alert observation of the child's behavior during the examination, will provide many clues to the etiology of the patient's problem.

VISCEROSOMATIC INTEGRATION

Somatic and visceral convergence is primarily achieved through the small-calibre afferent system. Sensory fibers from the viscera and their vascular structures are carried with the autonomic fibers and are called visceral afferents. These fibers enter the spinal cord at the levels of the lateral horn but synapse on cell bodies in the dorsal horn. While somatic sensory fibers are well mapped to cell bodies in the dorsal horn, creating a 'fingerprint' relationship, visceral afferents are less specific. In most cases, visceral afferent fibers converge onto cell bodies receiving somatic input (Garrison et al 1992, Hobbs et al 1992). Consequently, nociceptive input from these visceral fibers may be interpreted as occurring in somatic tissue.

Approximately 5–10% of dorsal root ganglion cells are wired up in such a way that they cannot distinguish between soma and viscera. They have bifurcating axons. This is a very interesting concept, because these neurons are capable of secreting polypeptides. Imagine what would happen if you were to irritate a visceral afferent fiber and produced retrograde conduction into the soma (Fig. 1.9). The somatic tissue would respond to two influences: dorsal horn stimulation would elicit a response in the ventral horn causing muscle spasm, and the local somatic tissue would be exposed to the secreted inflammatory products of the coupled primary afferent. This describes one of the mechanisms behind viscerosomatic reflexes. There are numerous examples of neurogenic inflammation in somatic tissues caused by irritation

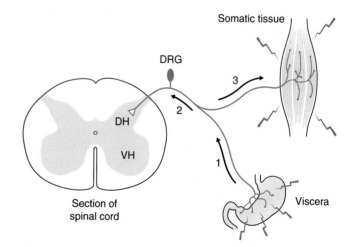

Fig. 1.9 • Schematic diagram depicting retrograde conduction and a viscerosomatic reflex. Initial stimulus from primary afferent in viscera (1) to dorsal horn (2). Activation of the dorsal horn cell stimulates the ventral horn cell, which causes response in muscle (contraction). In addition, retrograde conduction (3) along coupled primary afferent of the muscle. The somatic primary afferent will release proinflammatory substances into undamaged muscle. This is a mechanism for neurogenic inflammation. DH, dorsal horn; VH, ventral horn; DRG, dorsal root ganglion.

to the viscera. The muscle spasm associated with kidney stones, the abdominal wall tension that occurs with gastrointestinal inflammation and the rigidity associated with appendicitis are all examples of this phenomenon. However, there is evidence that the mechanism works in the other direction as well. Somatic irritation may cause changes in visceral tissues.

Aihara et al (1979) demonstrated that viscera respond to nociceptive stimulation of somatic tissue. Intraluminal pressures of the upper gastrointestinal tract were recorded while the abdomen of an anesthetized rat was pinched with a pair of forceps. When the skin over the abdomen was pinched, there was a decrease in peristalsis and an increase in pressure in the gut. Certain areas produced more dramatic changes, with the most significant changes occurring when the medial portion of the abdominal wall was irritated. This area falls into the dermatome range of T5–T9 in a human, the same area that innervates the upper gastrointestinal tract. Aihara et al showed that there was an immediate and very profound inhibition of peristalsis when this area was irritated. If you were to fire a sympathetic volley onto the stomach, what would it do? A sympathetic volley would shut down peristalsis. Essentially, that is what the researcher did. When the rat was pinched, a somatic volley was fired over the small-calibre afferent system into the spinal cord. This activated preganglionic neurons in the spinal cord and shot right back out to the stomach to shut down peristalsis. Once the pinching stopped, the peristalsis returned. This demonstrates that there is a fairly tight coupling between these somatic and visceral tissues, a somatovisceral reflex.

The convergent arrangement of primary afferents also provides an explanation for recurrent symptoms in patients who have been successfully treated for a condition. For example, a child with reflux will soon develop changes in the associated paraspinal muscles. The resultant spasm will irritate primary afferents within the connective tissue and muscle body. These afferents will fire back into the cord to the same cell bodies initially irritated by the reflux. These cell bodies are now receiving stimulation from both the irritated visceral and the irritated somatic tissues. The mother may attempt dietary changes, feeding the baby, sitting up, frequent burps, etc., in an attempt to decrease the extent of the reflux; however, the somatic irritation may cause neurogenic inflammation in the viscera, and the child's symptoms will continue.

VISCEROSOMATIC REFLEXES

Although we have a medial and lateral motor system, viscerosomatic reflexes are represented in only the medial system, the paraspinal or axillary muscles. They do not involve appendicular muscles. In order to understand this, we need to review the topography of the spinal cord. Within

the ventral horn, there are interneurons innervating columns of motor neurons. The lateral columns control the appendicular muscles, and the medial columns control the axillary muscles. The shape of the ventral horn changes as you progress down the spinal cord. The lateral system, the appendicular column, is largest at the brachial plexus and the lumbosacral plexus, sending fibers to muscles of the arms and legs. The axial column runs the length of the cord. Ascending tracts carry sensory information to the brainstem and cortex. The tracts descending from these areas project onto cell bodies of the ventral horn. Projections from the brainstem travel in the medial columns and innervate the axillary muscles. Projections from the cortex travel in the lateral columns to the appendicular muscles. Information from primary afferents activates the reticular formation of the brainstem. Descending input from the reticular formation is strongest in the medial columns where the axillary muscles are represented. To put it another way, pain drives the reticular formation, and the reticular formation drives the axillary muscles. The axillary muscles respond to the increased spinal input with changes in muscle tone. Therefore, changes in tone driven by visceral irritation will be palpable in muscles in the back and the abdomen.

In the clinical setting, changes in the tone of abdominal muscles present as guarding. Guarding is a segmental reflex driven by visceral afferents. Guarding is associated with visceral irritation such as occurs with inflammation or infection. It represents a viscerosomatic reflex. Visceral pathologies commonly associated with guarding include appendicitis and intussusception. Another form of viscerosomatic reflex is found in the paraspinal muscles. These areas of increased muscle tone and vasomotor changes are driven by acute and chronic visceral irritation. Viscerosomatic reflexes in the paraspinal muscles present with changes in tissue texture, alteration in skin temperature and restricted range of motion of the involved joints, the criteria commonly described for somatic dysfunction. The association between focal areas of paraspinal hypertonicity and visceral irritation is well documented in the osteopathic literature (Table 1.1) (Beal & Dvorak 1984, Beal & Morlock 1984, Beal 1985, Beal & Kleiber 1985, Kuchera & Kuchera 1994). These areas can be used to provide diagnostic clues as to what visceral tissue may be involved. Cox et al (1983) has demonstrated the sensitivity and specificity of somatic findings in cardiac disease. This suggests that other areas may also provide reliable information which may be helpful in young children, who are not always clear in their descriptions of pain. Viscerosomatic reflexes can also be driven by spinal facilitation. Primary afferents from diseased or irritated viscera may trigger reflexive paraspinal changes that are then maintained through increased spinal tone. Chapman's reflexes are described as neurolymphatic reflexes. Although their etiology is unclear, there is some empirical evidence in older osteopathic literature that suggests they may provide another toll in the diagnosis of visceral conditions.

Table 1.1 Viscerosomatic reflexes and Chapman's reflexes

Organ	Viscerosomatic reflex level	Chapman's reflexes
Lungs	T2–T5	Anterior 3rd/4th sternocostal Posterior 3rd/4th thoracic spine
Heart	T3–T6	Anterior 2nd sternocostal Posterior 3rd thoracic spine
Upper gastrointestinal tract	T5–T8	
Gastroesophageal junction		Anterior 5th sternocostal Posterior 5th thoracic spine
Liver		Anterior 5th right sternocostal Posterior 5th right thoracic spine
Gall bladder		Anterior 6th right sternocostal Posterior 6th right thoracic spine
Lower gastrointestinal tract	T7–T12	Anterior 8th, 9th, 10th sternocostal Posterior 10th, 11th thoracic spine
Appendix		Right T11
Spleen		Left T7
Kidney	T10–L1	Periumbilical

SOMATOVISCERAL REFLEXES

Studies done by Aihara et al (1979) and Sato (1992) suggest that somatic dysfunction can produce changes in associated viscera through a somatovisceral reflex. This may occur through spinal facilitation or retrograde neurogenic inflammation. When an area of the spinal cord becomes sensitized by visceral pathology, the resultant muscle spasm may sustain retrograde neurogenic inflammation at the viscera. This becomes important in children who experience a visceral pathology at a very young age. There is potential for the symptoms to continue because of persistent somatic dysfunction or through a referred mechanism. For example, a newborn that develops reflux symptoms from a formula sensitivity will often have associated paraspinal changes. The longer the reflux persists, the more likely the child is to develop some degree of spinal facilitation. Once the formula is changed, the spinal irritation from the somatic

dysfunction may continue to drive the symptoms. Alternatively, the child's brain may have learned to interpret signals from that area of spinal cord as irritation to the gastroesophageal junction. Now when a volley of activity enters the cord at that level, regardless of its tissue of origin, the child's brain will interpret it as gastroesophageal irritation.

EMOTIONS

Spinal facilitation is but one of the mechanisms behind chronic and recurring pain presentations. A patient's perception of pain represents the combined influences of visceral and somatic afferent activity, the patient's emotional and psychological states, and his or her memories. The interpretation of afferent input may be influenced by any of these components. Non-noxious and noxious sensory input from somatic and visceral tissues typically summates in the dorsal horn of the spinal cord. As previously discussed the summation effect of afferent activity on a facilitated area can be interpreted as pain. At the locus ceruleus in the midbrain, input from the spinal cord summates with input from the limbic lobe regarding emotions and the patient's psychological state. Spinal cord activity reaching the locus ceruleus may be enhanced or mitigated by the activity in the limbic lobe. A patient's sense of wellbeing and security may influence how he or she interprets and responds to nociceptive activity. Pathways from spinal cord and limbic lobe lead to the amygdala where memory resides. The amygdala can weigh the importance of stimuli based upon previous experiences. This too can affect a patient's interpretation and response to activity in the spinal cord (Fig. 1.10).

Emotions can influence changes in somatovisceral tissue and under certain conditions. Areas of the brain involved with processing emotional stimuli can become facilitated or sensitized. Two areas of cortex contributing to this mechanism are the limbic system and the hypothalamus. The latter is involved with modulating descending control mechanisms on interneurons concerned with autonomic function in the spinal cord. These descending pathways can exert inhibitory or stimulatory influences on efferent activity. The hypothalamus can be considered the regulator of autonomic and somatic responses to emotional states (Iverson et al 2000). Many neuroscientists view emotions as an unconscious process, whereby a stimulus is evaluated as harmful or beneficial, immediately triggering an appropriate response. Feeling is thought to involve a 'conscious reflection of the unconscious appraisal' of the stimulus (Iverson et al 2000). The hypothalamus is involved in the expression of the unconscious process of emotion. This process begins prior to any conscious reflection upon the stimulus (LeDoux 1992). For example, an immediate response to a frightening situation is an increase in heart rate. This reflexive tachycardia is modulated

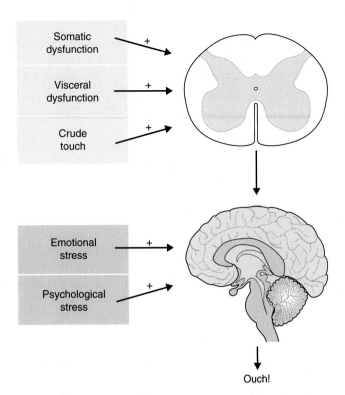

Fig. 1.10 • Schematic diagram depicting the summative effect of somatic and visceral dysfunction, crude touch, emotional stress and psychological stress on the individual's perception of discomfort or pain. *Used with permission of the Willard & Carreiro Collection.*

through signals from the hypothalamus. The hypothalamus influences autonomic and visceral function through synaptic processes and neurohumoral mechanisms.

It is well known that nociceptive stimuli will alter autonomic function (Sato & Swenson 1984, Sato 1992), elevating heart rate and blood pressure and may influence cardiovascular health (Gockel et al 1995a, b). While there is a catecholamine response involved in this reflex, it is delayed (Sato 1992, Budgell et al 1997). The immediate response is neurogenic and occurs via convergent innervation. It has also been shown that non-nociceptive stimulation can affect autonomic parameters (Kurosawa et al 1995). Arterial blood pressure and heart rate were monitored in anesthetized rats while the abdominal wall was gently stroked. Stroking of the ventral surface produced a definite and sustained decrease in both parameters. Stroking the lateral surface produced a smaller and shorter change, and stroking both areas showed the greatest change. This may be due to the gating mechanism or some other yet to be explained phenomenon.

HOMEOSTASIS

The hypothalamus regulates autonomic function in response to visual, auditory, olfactory, emotional, visceral and somatic stimuli (Willard 1993, Kandel et al 2000). It also receives information concerning the internal condition of the body, including glucose and electrolyte levels and temperature. The hypothalamus is concerned with maintaining homeostasis, which is the balance of the body's internal milieu in response to environmental demands. According to Iverson et al (2000), the hypothalamus integrates autonomic and endocrine function with behavior. Most often we think of the hypothalamus as involved in the flight-or-fight response, orchestrating rapid changes in autonomic function to redirect blood flow, prioritize metabolic supply and stimulate immune reactivity. But the hypothalamus is also concerned with general day-to-day, minute-to-minute homeostasis. For example, the hypothalamus receives input from the visual system that it uses to regulate circadian rhythms. It is involved with balancing environmental demands with internal set points (Kandel et al 2000). The hypothalamus modulates water and electrolyte balance, food metabolism, vasomotor tone and a myriad of other homeostatic processes.

The hypothalamus also receives projections from the limbic system, amygdala and prefrontal cortex. These areas are concerned with processing emotional stimuli. Earlier in this chapter, we discussed the mechanism of spinal facilitation, whereby certain conditions can result in a lowered threshold for activation in the interneurons of the spinal cord. This can lead to abnormal response to stimuli. Just as the threshold for activation of spinal interneurons can be lowered, it appears that the same condition can occur in these areas of cortex. This may result in an altered perception or response to a stimulus. Although many of the affective disorders appear to develop under a genetic influence, many investigators think that for a certain population of patients, experiential phenomena may act as inciting events in the process. One or more events summate and alter the individual's response to neurotransmitters that are involved with regulating behavior, sleep, libido, etc. Once the inciting stimulus is removed, the individual continues to have an altered response to similar stimuli. This may explain many conditions seen in adults who were abused or significantly traumatized as children (Lemieux & Coe 1995). It may also explain the withdrawal and flattening affect often seen in children who are in abusive or neglectful situations.

The hypothalamus secretes corticotropin-releasing hormone (CRH) in response to stress (Gold & Goodwin 1988a, b, Li et al 1996). CRH stimulates cortisol release from the adrenal glands. Under normal conditions, there is a negative feedback mechanism whereby the hypothalamus monitors cortisol levels to modulate the secretion of CRH. However, in certain individuals the hypothalamus loses its ability to respond to cortisol, and continues to produce CRH. These individuals often present with symptoms of melancholic depression. Gold & Goodwin (1988a, b) found that elevated levels of CRH are associated with depression. Furthermore, somatic input can trigger this cascade.

Patients with chronic pain exhibit increased cortisol and CRH levels and signs of melancholic depression. Elevated levels of cortisol influence immune and endocrine function, resulting in a stress response or allostatic state (Ganong 1988). As we shall see in subsequent chapters, the factors contributing to allostasis have a role in the pathogenesis of many disease processes (McEwen & Stellar 1993, Seeman et al 1997a, b, McEwen 1998, McEwen & Seeman 1999) (see Ch. 7).

CONCLUSION

The nervous system is a complex organ, which orchestrates interaction between our internal and external worlds. It has great plasticity and, as we shall see, continues to refine and define itself throughout life. However, there are limits to the extent of adaptation that the nervous system can accommodate. We can think of this as its range of motion. When it is pushed beyond these limits, biochemical and physical changes occur which may permanently interfere with our ability to respond appropriately to the world around us. Chronic disease processes can be influenced by early intervention. The role of the musculoskeletal system in these processes should not be underestimated (Gockel et al 1995a, b). Regardless of the etiology, nociceptive input from somatic tissues will contribute to all of the aforementioned mechanisms, increasing the total afferent load on the nervous system and decreasing the ability to respond appropriately to internal and external demands.

References

Aihara Y, Nakamura H, Sato A et al 1979 Neural control of gastric motility with special reference to cutaneo-gastric reflexes. In: Brooks C (ed.) Integrative functions of the autonomic nervous system. Elsevier, New York: 38–49.

Anderson M F, Winterson B J 1995 Properties of peripherally induced persistent hindlimb flexion in rat: involvement of N-methyl-D-aspartate receptors and capsaicin-sensitive afferents. Brain Res 678(1–2): 140–150.

Beal M C 1985 Viscerosomatic reflexes: a review. J Am Osteopath Assoc 85(12): 786–801.

Beal M C, Dvorak J 1984 Palpatory examination of the spine: a comparison of the results of two methods and their relationship to visceral disease. Manual Medicine 1: 25–32.

Beal M C, Morlock JW 1984 Somatic dysfunction associated with pulmonary disease. J Am Osteopath Assoc 84(2): 179–183.

Beal M C, Kleiber G E 1985 Somatic dysfunction as a predictor of coronary artery disease. J Am Osteopath Assoc 85(5): 70–75.

Budgell B, Noda K, Sato A 1997 Innervation of posterior structures in the lumbar spine of the rat. J Manipulative Physiol Ther 20(6): 359–368.

Cervero F, Connell L A 1984 Distribution of somatic and visceral primary afferent fibres within the thoracic spinal cord of the cat. J Comp Neurol 230(1): 88–98.

Cox J M, Gorbis S, Dick L et al 1983 Palpable musculoskeletal findings in coronary artery disease: results of a double blind study. J Am Osteopath Assoc 82: 832–836.

Ganong W 1988 The stress response – a dynamic overview. Hosp Pract 23(6): 155–171.

Garrison D W, Chandler M J, Foreman R D 1992 Viscerosomatic convergence onto feline spinal neurons from esophagus, heart and somatic fields: effects on inflammation. Pain 49: 373–382.

Gockel M, Lindholm H, Vastamaki M et al 1995a Cardiovascular functional disorder and distress among patients with thoracic outlet syndrome. J Hand Surg [Br] 20: 29–33.

Gockel M, Lindholm H, Alaranta H et al 1995b Cardiovascular functional disorder and stress among patients having neck-shoulder symptoms. Ann Rheum Dis 54: 494–497.

Gold P, Goodwin F 1988a Clinical and biochemical manifestations of depression: Part II. N Engl J Med 319(7): 413–420.

Gold P, Goodwin F 1988b Clinical and biochemical manifestations of stress: Part I. N Engl J Med 319(6): 348–353.

He X, Schmidt R F, Schmittner H 1988 Effects of capsaicin on articular afferents of the cat's knee joint. Agents Actions 25(3–4): 222–224.

Hobbs S F, Chandler M J, Bolser D C et al 1992 Segmental organization of visceral and somatic input onto C3–T6 spinothalamic tract cells of the monkey. J Neurophysiol 68(5): 1575–1588.

Iverson S, Kupfermann I, Kandel E R 2000 Emotional states and feelings. In: Kandel E R, Schwartz J H, Jessell T M (eds) Principles of neural science. McGraw-Hill, New York: 982–998.

Kandel E R, Schwart J H, Jessel T M 2000 Principles of neural science, 4th edn. McGraw-Hill, Philadelphia.

Kuchera W A, Kuchera M L 1994 Osteopathic considerations in systemic dysfunction, 2nd edn. Greyden Press, Columbus, OH.

Kurosawa M, Lundeberg T, Agren G et al 1995 Massage-like stroking of the abdomen lowers blood pressure in anesthetized rats: influence of oxytocin. J Auton Nerv Syst 56(1–2): 26–30.

Langhorst P, Schulz B G, Seller H et al 1996 Convergence of visceral and somatic afferents on single neurones in the reticular formation of the lower brain stem in dogs. J Auton Nerv Syst 57(3): 149–157.

LeDoux J E 1992 Brain mechanisms of emotion and emotional learning. Curr Opin Neurobiol 2(2): 191–197.

Lemieux A M, Coe C L 1995 Abuse-related posttraumatic stress disorder: evidence for chronic neuroendocrine activation in women. Psychosom Med 57: 105–115.

Li H Y, Ericsson A, Sawchenko P E 1996 Distinct mechanisms underlie activation of hypothalamic neurosecretory neurons and their medullary catecholaminergic afferents in categorically different stress paradigms. Proc Natl Acad Sci U S A 93(6): 2359–2364.

McEwen B S 1998 Stress, adaptation, and disease. Allostasis and allostatic load. Ann N Y Acad Sci 840: 33–44.

McEwen B S, Stellar E 1993 Stress and the individual. Mechanisms leading to disease. Arch Intern Med 153(18): 2093–2101.

McEwen B S, Seeman T 1999 Protective and damaging effects of mediators of stress.

Elaborating and testing the concepts of allostasis and allostatic load. Ann N Y Acad Sci 896: 30–47.

McNeill D L, Burden H W 1986 Convergence of sensory processes from the heart and left ulnar nerve onto a single afferent perikaryon: a neuroanatomical study in the rat employing fluorescent tracers. Anat Rec 214(4): 441–447.

Moore K L 2007 The developing human, 8th edn. W B Saunders, Philadelphia.

Myklebust B M, Gottlieb G L 1993 Development of the stretch reflex in the newborn: reciprocal excitation and reflex irradiation. Child Dev 64: 1036–1045.

O'Sullivan M C, Eyre J A, Miller S 1991 Radiation of phasic stretch reflex in biceps brachii to muscles of the arm in man and its restriction during development. J Physiol 439: 529–543.

Sato A 1992 The reflex effects of spinal somatic nerve stimulation on visceral function. J Manipulative Physiol Ther 15(1): 57–61.

Sato A, Swenson S 1984 Sympathetic nervous system response to mechanical stress of the spinal column in rats. Journal of Manual Medicine 7(3): 141–147.

Seeman T E, Singer B H, Rowe J W et al 1997a Price of adaptation – allostatic load and its health consequences: MacArthur studies of successful aging. Arch Intern Med 157(19): 2259–2268.

Seeman T E, McEwen B S, Singer B H et al 1997b Increase in urinary cortisol excretion and memory declines: MacArthur studies of successful aging. J Clin Endocrinol Metab 82(8): 2458–2465.

Willard F H 1993 Medical neuroanatomy. Lippincott, Philadelphia.

Further reading

Blanchard C, Blanchard R, Fellous J M et al 2001 The brain decade in debate: III. Neurobiology of emotion. Braz J Med Biol Res 34(3): 283–293.

Bonica J J 1990 The management of pain. Lea and Febiger, Philadelphia.

Donnerer J 1992 Nociception and the neuroendocrine-immune system. In: Willard F H, Patterson M (eds) Nociception and the neuroendocrine-immune connection. American Academy of Osteopathy, IN: 260–273.

Esterling B 1992 Stress-associated modulation of cellular immunity. In: Willard F H, Patterson M (eds) Nociception and the neuroendocrine-immune connection. American Academy of Osteopathy, IN: 275–294.

Gazzaniga M S, LeDoux J E, Wilson D H 1977 Language, praxis, and the right hemisphere: clues to some mechanisms of consciousness. Neurology 27(12): 1144–1147.

Gold P W, Licinio J, Wong M L et al 1995 Corticotropin releasing hormone in the pathophysiology of melancholic and atypical depression and in the mechanism of action of antidepressant drugs. Ann N Y Acad Sci 771: 716–729.

Kandel E R, Schwart J H, Jessel T M 2008 Principles of neural science, 5th edn. McGraw-Hill, Philadelphia.

LeDoux J E 1993 Emotional memory systems in the brain. Behav Brain Res 58(1–2): 69–79.

LeDoux J E 1993 Emotional memory: in search of systems and synapses. Ann N Y Acad Sci 702: 149–157.

LeDoux J E 1994 Emotion, memory and the brain. Sci Am 270(6): 50–57.

LeDoux J E 1995 Emotion: clues from the brain. Annu Rev Psychol 46: 209–235.

LeDoux J E, Muller J 1997 Emotional memory and psychopathology. Philos Trans R Soc Lond B Biol Sci 352(1362): 1719–1726.

Mabry T R, Gold P E, McCarty R 1995 Stress, aging, and memory involvement of peripheral catecholamines. Ann N Y Acad Sci 771: 512–522.

McEwen B S 1997 Hormones as regulators of brain development: life-long effects related to health and disease. Acta Paediatr Suppl 422: 41–44.

McEwen B S 2000 Allostasis and allostatic load: implications for neuropsychopharmacology. Neuropsychopharmacology 22(2): 108–124.

McEwen B S 2000 The neurobiology of stress: from serendipity to clinical relevance. Brain Res 886(1–2): 172–189.

McEwen B S 2000 Allostasis, allostatic load, and the aging nervous system: role of excitatory amino acids and excitotoxity. Neurochem Res 25(9–10): 1219–1231.

McMahon S, Koltzenburg M (eds) 2005 Wall and Melzack's textbook of pain. Churchill Livingstone, Edinburgh.

Morrison J F, Sato A, Sato Y et al 1995 The influence of afferent inputs from skin and viscera on the activity of the bladder and the skeletal muscle surrounding the urethra in the rat. Neurosci Res 23(2): 195–205.

Quirk G J, Armony J L, Repa J C et al 1996 Emotional memory: a search for sites of plasticity. Cold Spring Harb Symp Quant Biol 61: 247–257.

Rogan M T, LeDoux J E 1996 Emotion: systems, cells, synaptic plasticity. Cell 85(4): 469–475.

Saper C B, Iverson S, Frackowiak R 2000 Integration of sensory and motor function. In: Kandel E R, Schwartz J H, Jessell T M (eds) Principles of neuroscience. McGraw-Hill, New York: 349–381.

Sato A 1995 Somatovisceral reflexes. J Manipulative Physiol Ther 18(9): 597–602.

Sato A, Schmidt R F 1973 Somatosympathetic reflexes: afferent fibers, central pathways, discharge characteristics. Physiol Rev 53(4): 916–947.

Schulkin J, McEwen B S, Gold P W 1994 Allostasis, amygdala, and anticipatory angst. Neurosci Biobehav Rev 18(3): 385–396.

Schulkin J, Gold P W, McEwen B S 1998 Induction of corticotropin-releasing hormone gene expression by glucocorticoids: implication for understanding the states of fear and anxiety and allostatic load. Psychoneuroendocrinology 23(3): 219–243.

Seeman T E, McEwen B S, Rowe J W et al 2001 Allostatic load as a marker of cumulative biological risk: MacArthur studies of successful aging. Proc Natl Acad Sci U S A 98(8): 4770–4775.

Sternberg E M, Chrousos G P, Wilder R L et al 1992 The stress response and the regulation of inflammatory disease. Ann Intern Med 117(10): 854–866.

Volpe J J 1995 Neurology of the newborn, 3rd edn. W B Saunders, Philadelphia.

Wall P D, Melzack R 2003 Handbook of pain management. Churchill Livingstone, Edinburgh.

Ward R 1997 Foundations of osteopathic medicine. Williams and Wilkins, Baltimore.

Willard F H, Mokler D J, Morgane P J 1997 Neuroendocrine-immune system and homeostasis. In: Ward R C (ed.) Foundations for osteopathic medicine. Williams and Wilkins, Baltimore: 107–135.

Chapter Two

The musculoskeletal system

2

INTRODUCTION

The musculoskeletal system is the largest system in the body, yet it is often the one which is most taken for granted. At birth it is still a prelude, rather than a miniature of the adult. Many musculoskeletal adaptations and alterations lay ahead for the newborn. This chapter provides an overview of the prenatal and postnatal changes occurring in the primary somatic regions of the body and the factors which influence them.

DEVELOPMENT OF THE MUSCULOSKELETAL SYSTEM

Gestation can be divided into two stages: the embryonic stage and the fetal stage. The embryonic stage commences with fertilization and the subsequent formation of the embryoblast. During the embryonic stage cells undergo proliferation, induction (differentiation) and migration. Proliferation produces the critical cell mass to create an anlage, a group of cells that will respond similarly to the same mechanochemical stimuli. Differentiation of cells occurs through induction, a change in a cell or anlage in response to a biochemical or biomechanical stimulus. Interactive induction occurs when one cell or anlage acts on an adjacent one to produce a third type of cell or anlage. Induction is a molecularly based process that involves homeobox genes. The homeobox genes have patterns of expression that cause a cell to differentiate in a specific way. Groups of cells will differentiate similarly forming a morphogenetic field that possesses the capability to form a specific structure or tissue. Anlages migrate to specific areas in the embryo. The migratory process is not well understood although most cell types leave chemical traces of their migratory path. Upon arriving at the destination further induction, modification, revision and/or apoptosis culminate in the final structure. These processes are at play in the formation of the endoderm, mesoderm and ectoderm layers. They are responsible for the embryonic organization of the notochord and axial skeleton.

In the first week of gestation, there exists a bilaminar disk composed of ectodermal and endodermal layers separated by a basement membrane. In the second week, ectodermal tissue invaginates through a primitive pit in the caudal end of the disk to lie between the ectoderm and endoderm. The tissue elongates in a caudal to cranial direction creating the primitive streak. The cells on either side of the streak differentiate into mesoderm. The cells surrounding the primitive pit form a primitive knot from which will develop the notochord. The notochord will bisect the ectoderm and endoderm, traveling between the two columns of mesoderm in a caudad to cephalad progression. Initially the notochord fuses with the endoderm and a canal or groove develops which soon degrades. Then a second or true notochord forms from the ectoderm. Congenital malformations of the spine that are associated with malformations of the gut are thought to result from interruptions of this process.

The notochord is critical for proper segmentation of the vertebrae, development of the intervertebral disks and bilateral pairing of the spinal ganglion. Maternal lithium ingestion can interfere with notochord development in the embryo. After birth, notochord material persists in the intervertebral disk and stimulates induction and differentiation. Precursors to neuroectodermal cells attach themselves to the basement membrane between the notochord and ectoderm. These cells undergo induction and proliferation, forming the neural plate. The cells change from columnar to apical and the edges of the plate rise, creating the neural groove. This process is repeated until the cresting cells meet, creating the neural tube; failure of the cells to meet results in anencephaly or myelomeningocele, depending upon the location and extent of the defect. The most lateral cells of the developing tube are called the neural crest cells. They will differentiate, proliferate and migrate to form the dorsal root ganglia and the various components of the peripheral nervous system. The neural tube will develop into the cell types of the central nervous system.

Following the appearance of the neural tube, mesodermal cells located along the lateral aspect of the notochord undergo induction to become mesenchymal cells forming three distinct clusters: the medial paraxial columns, the intermediate columns and the peripheral lateral plates. The first of these develop into the axial skeletal components; the second becomes the urogenital system; and the third cluster differentiates into the peritoneal layers of the thorax and abdomen. Development of the somites proceeds cranial to caudal and segmentation is present at 3 weeks' gestation. The medial paraxial columns organize themselves into an epithelial plate of paired somites lining the notochord. Adjacent somites are joined to each other by tight gap junctions. At this stage the somites lie on a basement membrane and are connected to the notochord and neural tube by processes that pass through the basement membrane. Soon after segmentation the somite has six distinct surfaces, each of which will evolve differently depending upon its position along the notochord. The ventromedial surface differentiates into the sclerotome and migrates towards the notochord. These cells are the precursors to the bones, joints and ligaments of the vertebral column. The remainder of the somite is now called the dermomyotome. From these cells, the skeletal muscles and skin will emerge. The cells on the craniomedial surface will give rise to skeletal muscle on the dorsal surface of the body and the epaxial musculature. The cells on the ventrolateral face near the developing limb bud will migrate into the bud to form the skeletal muscles of the limb. Lastly, the cells on the inferior surface become the skeletal muscles of the body flank. Although the majority of the remaining cells will

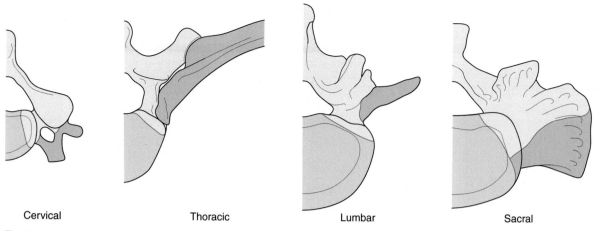

Cervical   Thoracic   Lumbar   Sacral

Fig. 2.1 • Sequential diagram of vertebral development indicating principal morphological parts of the adult. *Used with permission, Williams P (ed.) 1995 Gray's anatomy, 38th edn. Churchill Livingstone, London.*

be precursors to skin and epidermal cells, some will contribute to the skeletal muscle mass as well.

As previously described, the ventromedial surface of the somite differentiates into the sclerotome and migrates towards the notochord. Each sclerotome contains two biochemically different cell types, one which is loosely packed cells that gives rise to the intervertebral disk, and the other, a mass of closely packed cells that will form the neural arch, the pedicle and (in the thorax) the ribs. There is an extracelluar matrix separating the two cell groups. There continues to be some confusion on the origins of the vertebrae and intervertebral disk (this author included). Some authors describe the formation of the intervertebral disk as a sclerotic fissure that splits the somite. Thus each somite differentiates into an intervertebral disk, the inferior surface of the superior vertebrae and the superior surface of the inferior vertebrae (Sensenig 1949, Verbout 1985). However other authors contend that what was previously thought of as a sclerotic fissure is the loosely packed cell mass of the somite (Peacock 2007, Theiler 1988). In this model the sclerotome of a pair of somites form the intervertebral disk, the adjacent vertebra, the transverse, neural and articular processes, and (in the thorax) the rib. This is a very different model of vertebral development.

Congenital malformations arising from interruptions or failures of somite formation include hemivertebrae, when two or more somites fail to separate, and fusion, when a somite fails to form. The vertebral body and neural arch develop through separate induction processes. The sclerotome cells forming the body appear to differentiate in response to influences from the neural tube and notochord, whereas the cells forming the neural arch take their signals from the neural crest. The segmentation of the neural arches is influenced by the development of the spinal ganglia.

Consequently, congenital malformations may occur in the posterior or anterior elements and not necessarily in both simultaneously.

The thoracic vertebrae ossify before those in the lumbar and cervical spines. By 16 weeks' gestation, L5 has begun the process of ossification. The precartilaginous ribs develop from the costal processes of the vertebra arches, bisecting the myotome cells as they extend away from the midline. Initially there is a mesenchymal connection between the developing rib and vertebrae which will differentiate into the ligaments and joint of the costovertebral junction. In the cervical vertebrae the costal process goes on to form the anterior and posterior tubercles (transverse process C1 and C2); in the lumbar vertebrae they become the transverse process, and in the sacrum they are the sacral alar (Fig. 2.1). The sternum develops from two columns of somatopleuric mesenchyme that lie on the ventral surface of the embryo. The condensations migrate towards each other to form the manubrium and the sternal segments. They undergo chondrification in a cranial-caudal direction.

The extremities begin as limb buds derived from mesenchymal cells that migrate laterally from the area around the notochord (Fig. 2.2). The somatopleuric mesenchyme lies on the ventral surface of the developing embryo. It will interact with the paraxial mesenchyme of the notochord to form the limbs. The somatopleuric mesenchyme develops a thickened ridge, the apical ectodermal ridge, at about 26 days' gestation. This is the progress zone, the guiding path for orientation of the skeletal structures in the limb. The progress zone remains until the limb is formed. Soon after, the mesenchymal cells migrate away from the midline, forming the basic architecture of the limb bud. The axis of the developing limb traverses from the center of the base of the bud to the apical ectodermal ridge. Different areas of the bud have different growth

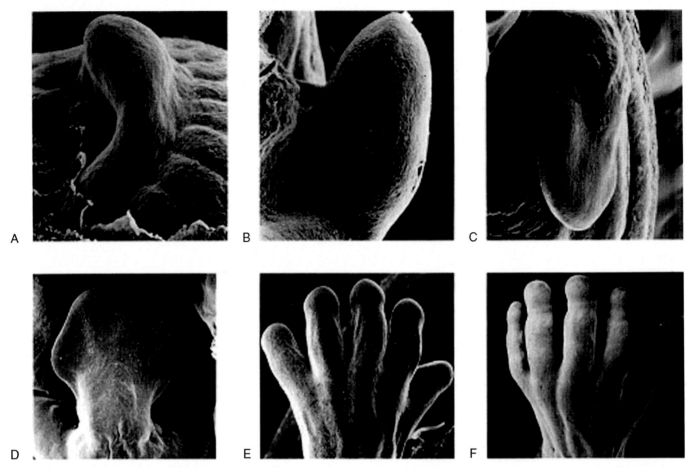

Fig. 2.2 • (A–F) Series of scanning electron micrographs to show the development of the upper limb. (Photographs by P Collins: printed by S Cox, Electron microscopy Unit, Southampton General Hospital.) *Used with permission, Williams P (ed.) 1995 Gray's anatomy, 38th edn. Churchill Livingstone, London.*

rates. As a result the limb bud curves ventrally and rotates. Cartilage first appears at 33 days, following which the neurovascular elements begin to invade the mesenchymal structure. By 38 days the upper extremity has an elbow and digital rays. The cells of the ventrolateral face of the epithelial plate of the somite migrate into the developing limb bud to form the striated muscle. The cells initially migrate en masse surrounded by extracellular fibrils that connect them with other cells. The mass elongates and the leading edge branches out. The cells undergo multiple divisions to form the muscles of the upper and lower extremities. The critical period in limb bud formation is between 4 and 6 weeks of gestation. This is when major abnormalities such as malformations occur. Disruptions in growth and deformation usually occur after the embryonic period in response to some kind of stress.

Myotubules appear at approximately the fifth week of gestation. They are converted to muscle fibers by the 20th week. Innervation of the muscle begins by about the 10th week, with muscle spindles appearing by the 14th week and Golgi tendon organs by the 16th week. This maturation process continues for some time after birth. In term infants, only 20% of the adult muscle fibers are present. At birth, muscles are attached to periosteum, not bone. Over the first 2–3 months of life, the tendinous tissue migrates through the periosteum to establish attachments to the underlying bone.

Joints in the appendicular skeleton differentiate from the mesenchymal tissue through a process called cavitation. Cavitation requires movement. Early intrauterine movements begin in about the seventh week of gestation. These movements act to mold the shape of the articular surfaces. There is hypermobility of the joints in the premature infant. At term, joint mobility is restricted, with a limited range of motion. In fact, the range of motion in any given joint will vary with the child's age. Generally speaking, however, most large joints have full range of motion by 3 years.

Development of the musculoskeletal system is directed and limited by internal and external influences. Internal influences include chemical gradients involving cell-adhesion molecules and surface-adhesion molecules. This appears to be genetically controlled by homeobox genes, as it can occur in in vitro experiments. External influences affecting musculoskeletal tissues include mechanical stressors and movements. Movement of the limb appears to play a role in orientation of the bony trabeculae, attachment of ligaments and tendons, orientation of collagen fibers in connective tissue, and normal skeletal growth.

Congenital abnormalities in the skeletal system arise due to one of the following three processes: malformation, disruption or deformation. Malformation is a failure of differentiation or migration during the embryonic stage. Malformations such as hemivertebrae and hemimelia occur during organogenesis. Interruptions in cell proliferation result in embryonic death or tissue agenesis. Failure of induction also results in agenesis. Abnormal migration results in fusion such as webbed or fused digits. Failure in growth and maturation may result in hypoplasia or cell death. Disruption is a defect in the structural integrity of a tissue that formed normally during the embryonic stage. Disruption is often associated with infection, toxic exposure, metabolic insult or trauma. Deformation of a structure occurs during the fetal or postnatal period in a normally formed structure. Deformation often occurs due to an extrinsic force such as compression on the structure. Deformation is more likely to occur in skeletal structures. In the fetus, extrinsic deformities arise due to uterine lie and reduced intrauterine space. They will typically resolve with conservative treatment.

Wolff's law and mechanical stress

Wolff's law states that mechanical stressors will affect tissue differentiation and growth characteristics of the musculoskeletal tissues. Normal optimal growth requires normal mechanical loads expressed intermittently. Intermittent tension results in chondrogenesis, whereas continuous tension fosters osteogenesis. Normal compression stimulates growth of the epiphyseal plate, while excessive compression retards growth of the plate. In fact, continuous compression results in atrophy of the bone, while intermittent compression stimulates bony growth. Non-perpendicular loads trigger deflected growth and torsional loads lead to rotational growth of the epiphyseal plates.

Muscle forces and gravity are the key sources of mechanical loading on the bones. Any imbalance in these forces or lack of force will alter the growth of the bone and change its growth characteristics. Intermittent loading stimulates collagen synthesis in the affected soft tissues, resulting in increased tissue strength and ability to absorb energy. In the musculoskeletal system, the osteocyte is the cell most responsive to mechanical stress. It is highly sensitive to small changes in fluid pressure. In response to pulsatile fluid pressure waves, the osteocytes will release prostaglandins, which signal osteoclasts to begin bone remodeling (Klein-Nulend et al 1995). Musculoskeletal tissue is most vulnerable to mechanical forces during periods of growth. Although the response is most dramatic during embryological development, it continues during life. This is important to remember when treating children osteopathically. Very often, if a strain pattern can be treated just prior to or during a period of growth, the effects of the treatment will be more dramatic and long lasting.

Although typically applied to discussions of bone, the principle of Wolff's law describes the response of all somatic tissue to applied forces. Somatic tissue will vary in density, length, width and strength in response to the forces applied to it. The determining factors are the consistency or frequency of the load, and the capacity of the tissue to accommodate that load. If a load is too great or applied too quickly the tissue structure may be damaged. However under most conditions, components in bone and connective tissue respond to mechanical forces by remodeling. As previously described, torsional loads will produce rotational growth in bone, while non-perpendicular loads will direct growth away from the load. The fibers of ligaments and tendons will hypertrophy and orient in the appropriate direction to resist stress loading. Alternatively, if inadequate tensile forces are present the orientation of the fibers becomes disorganized and the tissue weakens. The growth potential present in the somatic tissues of the pediatric population provides much greater potential for remodeling than that seen in adults. This is important to remember in terms of both pathology and treatment. Remodeling can occur in bone and connective tissue in response to injury or changes in tissue load. Abnormal stresses placed on bone or connective tissue may have a detrimental effect on growth and function. However removal of abnormal stresses may provide an opportunity for remodeling and correction.

Growth areas and trauma

In the pediatric population there are three types of growth areas associated with most bones. An epiphyseal growth plate located at the proximal and distal ends of the bone adjacent to the metaphysis; an epiphysis or the articular surface; and an apophysis lying beside the diaphysis at the attachment of each tendon. The epiphyseal growth plate and the articular epiphysis are typically hyaline cartilage, while the apophysis is usually fibrocartilage. The differences in histology account for the different tissue responses to stresses. Hyaline cartilage is more vulnerable to loading and compression, whereas fibrocartilage is more vulnerable to tensile forces and shearing. Consequently, stress forces will affect a bone differently depending upon where the forces summate and the nature of the force.

In young athletes repetitive activities may lead to microstresses at the area of greatest vulnerability. With compressive or loading forces the area most at risk is the transitional area between the metaphysis and epiphysis, the epiphyseal growth plate. With tensile or shearing forces, the areas of greatest risk are the transitional area between the insertion of the ligaments and the diaphysis, the apophysis, and the immature Sharkey's fibers of the tendinous insertion. Regardless of the type of stress, repetition results in the development of macrofailures which, if not dealt with, can devolve into microfractures. In bone this produces stress fractures, and in connective tissue it produces sprains, strains and ruptures.

An apophysis is an area of cartilaginous growth at the insertion of a tendon. It will eventually develop into a bony tubercle such as the tibial tubercle or anterior inferior iliac spine. Most apophyses are fibrocartilage and are more vulnerable to tensile forces than the hyaline cartilage found in joints. Apophysitis is an inflammation of the apophysis. From a clinical perspective it can develop when the tensile load on the ligament exceeds the capacity of the periosteum or of the transitional cartilage between the apophysis and the diaphysis. When the periosteum is disrupted the tenoperiosteal fibers pull the periosteum away from the cortical bone, leaving a gap. This is called an enthesopathy. This traumatic rupture of the periosteal-cortical relationship causes an inflammatory response and hypertrophy of the underlying cortical bone, producing an exostosis, or bump. Activity will irritate the exostosis, exacerbating the inflammation and hypertrophy. When the microstress affects the transitional area between the apophysis and the diaphysis a true apophysitis occurs. The difference between an apophysitis and an avulsion fracture is one of severity and clinical-temporal profile. Typically apophysitis develops insidiously while avulsion fractures are more acute. In both cases the area under stress is the cartilaginous junction between the apophysis and the diaphysis. Avulsion fractures are more common in the pediatric population than adults because of the presence of the unossified apophysis.

THE SPINE

Development

All typical vertebrae develop from three primary ossification centers: one for the body and one for each vertebral arch which appear during gestation, and multiple secondary centers which appear sometime after birth. In the past, ossification was thought to proceed in a cephalad to caudal direction; however, more recent studies suggest ossification spreads up and down the spine simultaneously. The body of the vertebra ossifies from a centrum located dorsal to the notochord. The first centrum appears in the lower thoracic and upper lumbar areas. Although there is typically a single centrum, there may be two. Failure of fusion of the two centrums results in a cuneiform vertebra and congenital scoliosis.

At birth, the body and arches are joined by cartilage. During the first year of life, the vertebral arches begin to unite dorsally. At 3 years, the bodies of the cervical vertebrae begin to unite with the arches; the process finishes in the lumbar spine about the sixth year. The periphery of the vertebrae will remain cartilaginous until puberty when the secondary ossification centers appear at the tips of the

Table 2.1 Onset and closure of ossification in various bones

Bone area	Onset of ossification	Closure of ossification
Iliac crest	11–14 years	20 years
Anterior inferior iliac spine	13–15 years	16–18 years
Ischial tuberosity	13–15 years	16–18 years
Acetabulum	Birth	14–16 years
Femoral head	4 months	16–18 years
Greater trochanter	4–6 years	16–17 years
Lesser trochanter	11–12 years	15–16 years
Femoral condyles	Birth	16–18 years
Tibial plateau	Birth	16–20 years
Fibula head	3–4 years	16–20 years
Distal tibia	6 months	17–18 years
Clavicle proximal end	17 years	20 years
Acromial process	14–15 years	18–20 years
Coracoid process	14–15 years	18–20 years
Humeral head	First year	18–20 years
Distal humerus	Various centers 12 months–10 years	14–17 years
Ulnar trochanter	8–10 years	14–17 years
Radial head	3–6 years	14–17 years
Ribs and sternum	First year	25 years

transverse and spinous processes, and around the articular surface of the bodies. These epiphyses will remain until the 25th year (Table 2.1).

The atlas and axis of the cervical spine have a different formation pattern than the remainder of the vertebral column. The somites of the occiput play a role in the early formation of the atlas. Failure of segmentation of the somites of the occiput and C1 result in fusion or occipitalization of C1. Amalgamation of the somites of C1 and C2 forms the dens, the anterior arch of C1, and the odontoid ligaments. In the remainder of the vertebral column the sclerotome cells migrate dorsally to produce the neural arch and then the spinal process. Those cells located more ventrally differentiate into the anlagen of the vertebral body. Centers of chondrification appear as the tissue of the annulus fibrosis condenses and the nucleus pulposus differentiates. By the sixth week of gestation all the precursors of the vertebral components are present. An ossification center appears in each vertebral body, and one or more in each component of the paired neural arch. Ossification begins in the thoracolumbar area and progresses cephalad and caudad. The process of growth and ossification continues after birth. The peripheral and central portions of the vertebrae have different growth characteristics. Whereas vertebral height may be primarily genetically driven, peripheral growth and width are influenced by activity, loading and muscle tone. Spontaneous movements in the embryo stimulate the process of ossification. After birth, the influences of upright posture probably contribute to the process.

Spinal curvatures

Sagittal curves are present throughout the spine and are thought to be a developmental adjustment to the bipedal stance. Sagittal curves have been observed to occur in response to movement as early as 7 weeks' gestation. The flexion position of the embryo results in the primary flexion curves of the thoracic and pelvic areas. The extension or lordotic curves of the cervical and lumbar regions is thought to result from functional muscle development. The cervical lordosis appears early in gestation in response to the development of the dorsal cervical musculature. The lumbar curve also develops quite early although it presents as a lack of flexion posture rather than true extension. During early life the functional changes occurring in the neuromuscular system that allow for the attainment of postural milestones reinforce and exaggerate the sagittal curves.

Muscles of the spine

Three columns of supporting muscles, the iliocostalis, longissimus superficially, and the deep multifidus, travel along the spine from the neck to the sacrum (Fig. 2.3). Although involved in spinal motion, the primary roles of these muscles are in postural stabilization and supporting of the spine. These are long restrictor muscles. Directly on the vertebral column are small segmental muscles spanning one or two segments, the rotatores, interspinales and intertransversarii. These muscles are densely innervated with proprioceptors and directly influence posture and balance strategies. Malformations, deformations and mechanical dysfunction of the spine will affect its proprioceptive mapping and the stabilizing mechanisms. In the infant, this will present as delayed milestones. In the older child, it may present as pain, scoliosis or gait abnormalities.

The thoracolumbar fascia contributes to another myofascial support system spanning from the shoulder across the spinous processes to the contralateral pelvis. Through the latissimus dorsi, the thoracolumbar fascia extends to the arm. The thoracolumbar fascia attaches to the supraspinous

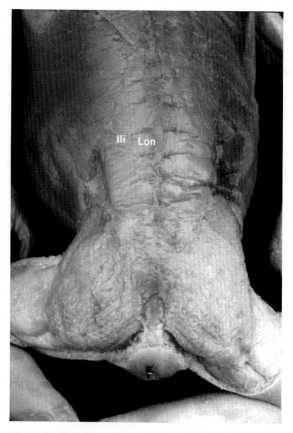

Fig. 2.3 • Posterior view of term neonate. The skin and superficial fascia have been removed. The iliocostalis (Ili) and longissimus (Lon) are labeled. The muscles extend to the sacrum. *Used with permission of the Willard & Carreiro Collection.*

ligaments, the iliac crest and the common raphe. Asymmetrical tension in the latissimus dorsi may influence the position of the vertebra through the thoracolumbar fascia (Fig. 2.4). This relationship may need to be considered in infants who are having difficulty in attaining postural milestones such as sitting or walking. In older children, postural dysfunction from cerebral palsy or other motor dysfunction affecting the upper extremity may compromise posture and balance. In a normal gait pattern, energy generated in the upper extremity and latissimus dorsi can be transferred to the pelvis through the thoracolumbar fascia, decreasing the overall work of ambulation (Vleeming et al 1995). This mechanism is not available to children with motor dysfunction. Consequently, the workload of ambulation is that much greater for them.

At birth many of these relationships are poorly defined. In the newborn the thoracolumbar fascia is a thin velum overlying the erector spinae columns (Fig. 2.5). In a toddler the diamond shape of the thoracolumbar fascia is more evident (Fig. 2.6). The fascia has thickened and is strongly adhered to the spinous processes and supraspinous ligaments. The latissimus dorsi invests into the fascia at its

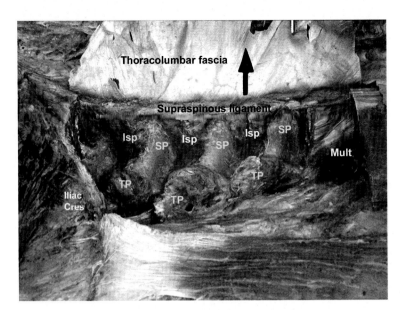

Fig. 2.4 • Dissection of the lumbar spine. The specimen is prone. The thoracolumbar fascia is being lifted away in the direction of the arrow. Its attachment to the supraspinatus ligament can be seen. The spinous processes (SP) and transverse processes (TP) and multifidus (Mult) are labeled. The interspinous (Isp) ligaments lie between the spinous processes. *Used with permission of the Willard & Carreiro Collection.*

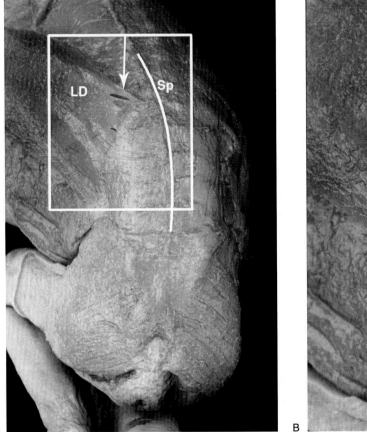

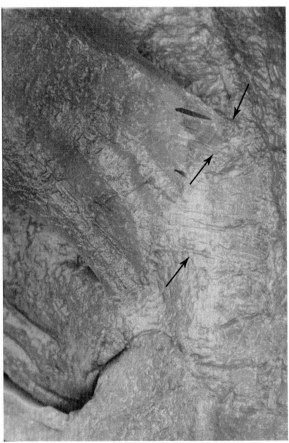

A

B

Fig. 2.5 • Posterior lateral view of term neonate. (A) The latissimus dorsi (LD) muscle is seen as a band of tissue which thins out (white arrow) and attaches at the spine (Sp, white arc). There is no grossly definitive demarcation of muscle and tendon. (B) Close up of area indicated by square in 2.5A. Black arrows point out fascial fibers extending from muscle to spine. *Used with permission of the Willard & Carreiro Collection.*

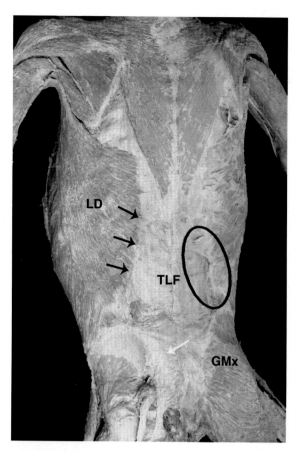

Fig. 2.6 • Posterior view of toddler. The skin and superficial fascias have been removed. The latissimus dorsi (LD) has the well-developed appearance of muscle tissue. The contrast between the muscle fibers and insertion (black arrows) onto the thoracolumbar fascia (TLF) is much more easily seen than in the neonate. The TLF is thickened, as can be seen by the cut edge on the right side of the specimen (black oval). Additionally, the insertion site for the gluteus maximus (GMx) on the right caudal end of the TLF is also identified (white arrow). *Used with permission of the Willard & Carreiro Collection.*

perimeter, and the fascial sheath plainly extends into the pelvis where it provides an insertion for the gluteus maximus muscle.

THE PELVIS

The lumbar spine and pelvis function as a unit for weight-bearing and energy transfer during gait. The ligaments of this area form a support stocking for the lumbar spine and sacrum. The muscular components that attach to this stocking create tension in the ligaments. This has been described as a self-bracing mechanism (Snijders et al 1993). Regardless of which part of the spine is under consideration, certain basic facts must be kept in mind. The anatomy of the various parts is not static. The various tissues of the body are

continually undergoing change. The growing or developing structure is more plastic than in the fully developed one and, because of this, adaptive changes take place more readily.

Development

Depending upon the text one is reading the terms pelvis, pelvis bone, os coxae, hip bone, etc., mean different things. For the purposes of this book the pelvis is composed of two innominate ('without name') bones with a sacrum suspended between them. The innominate bone is actually three bones joined at the acetabulum by a cartilaginous seam, the triradiate cartilage (Fig 2.7). Each of these composite bones, the ileum, ischium and pubic bone, ossifies from its own primary center. There are also five secondary centers scattered amongst the composite bones: one each at the iliac crest, the ischial tuberosity, the anterior superior and inferior iliac spines, the pubic symphysis and the center of the acetabulum.

The first primary ossification center to appear is that of the ileum just superior to the sciatic notch, at approximately 8 weeks' gestation. This will expand anterior and superior, forming the upper rim of the acetabulum and the blade of the ileum. About 4 weeks later the next center appears in the ischial ramus. It will form the inferior-posterior third of the acetabular rim and the remainder of the ischium. The third primary center appears between gestational months 4 and 5 and is located in the superior ramus of the pubic bone. At birth these areas remain distinct and separate, with cartilaginous junctions.

The first primary centers to join are the inferior ramus of the pubic bone and the ischium. This begins to ossify at about 8 years. The secondary centers appear quite a bit later, starting with the os acetabuli in the acetabulum, which appears at about 12 years. The os acetabuli appears between the primary centers of the ilium and pubes. It begins to ossify at 12 years and closes at 18 years, forming the pubic part of the acetabulum. Next the primary centers of the ileum and ischium join at their junction in the triradiate cartilage followed by the pubes and ischium. This process is completed sometime in mid-puberty. The remainder of the secondary centers, the crest of the ileum, the ischial tuberosity, the iliac spines and the pubic tubercle, appear in early puberty and continue to grow until the early twenties. These secondary centers are located at the insertion of long restrictor muscles of the hip and leg and are vulnerable to repetitive microtrauma and overuse. They are the most common sites for apophysitis, avulsion fractures and enthesopathies in young athletes. In most people the composite bones are completely fused by 25 years of age. Throughout life the two pubic bones are joined by a fibrocartilaginous symphysis with an interpubic disk which allows for some movement between the two innominates.

Growth and enlargement of the acetabulum and pelvis occur through appositional growth along the triradiate

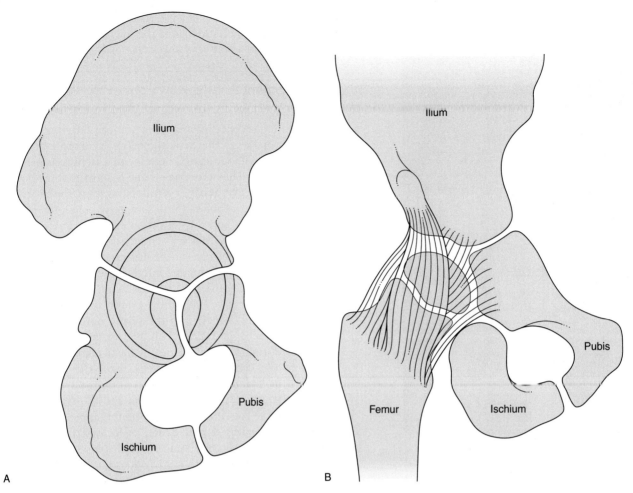

Fig. 2.7 • (A) Schematic diagram depicting the three parts of the innominate bone which comprise the acetabulum. (B) A schematic diagram based upon an X-ray of an infant hip. Note the cartilaginous areas between the parts of the innominate bone. The ischium, ilium and pubic bone are labeled.

cartilage, the iliac crests, the pubic ramus and on the ischial tuberosities. Growth at the triradiate cartilage allows for deepening and expansion of the acetabular cup. The shape of the acetabulum is affected by the relationships of its three components. Furthermore the position and orientation of the femur is influenced by the shape of the acetabulum. This phenomenon may play a role in persistent femoral anteversion.

At birth the sacrum and coccyx are composed of nine segments, five in the sacrum and four in the coccyx (Fig. 2.8). The sacrum is cancellous bone enveloped in a thin layer of compact bone. Like most vertebrae the sacral segments each ossify from three primary centers: one for the body and one for each vertebral arch and a secondary center for each costal element. The centers for the body and vertebral arch appear between 3 and 5 months' gestation and those for the costal (lateral) elements by 8 months. Each costal element unites with its vertebral arch element between 2 and 5 years of life. They unite with the body and each other at 8 years. The articulating surfaces of the body elements of the segments are covered with hyaline cartilage and separated by a fibrocartilaginous

disk. A cartilaginous epiphysis develops between the lateral components of the segments. After puberty epiphyseal centers appear for the bodies, spines, transverse tubercles and the costal elements. The vertebral arches begin to coalesce in a caudal to cephalad direction. At birth, the bodies of the sacral vertebrae are separated by primitive intervertebral disks, which turn to fibrocartilage with aging. The lower two vertebrae become joined by bone at about 18 years. In most people, the process proceeds superiorly so that the segments are all joined at their margins by the third decade. However the interior, the central mass and disk, remain unossified into midlife (McKern & Stewart 1957) and in some people never ossify as evidenced by cadaveric specimens. (Perhaps this may account for the density change many osteopaths describe after treatment of interosseous strains of the sacrum.)

The number of coccygeal segments can vary between three and five. Each segment ossifies from one center. The center for the first segment appears at birth and that for the others is variable. The first segment has a facet joint, which articulates with the sacral apex, while the other segments

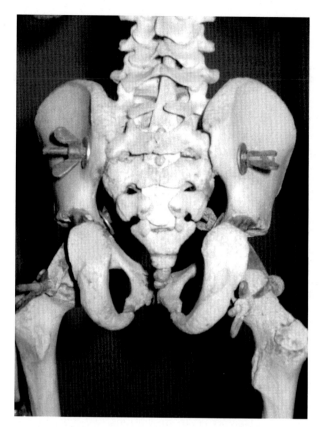

Fig. 2.8 • Posterior view of the pelvis of a young child approximately 4–5 years old. The sacral and coccygeal segments are unfused. There is a spina bifida at S1 and S4. *Used with permission of the Willard & Carreiro Collection.*

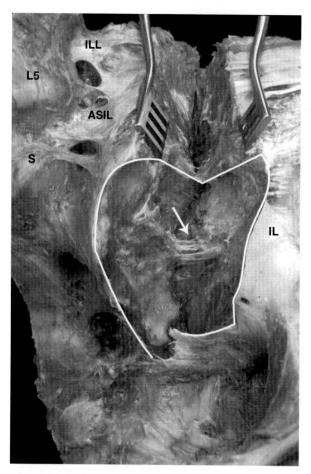

Fig. 2.9 • Anterior superior view into the pelvis with all soft tissue structures and viscera removed. The tissue spreader is positioned to open the sacroiliac joint from its anterior surface. The joint is outlined in white. The intra-articular ligaments can be seen within the joint (white arrow). The fifth lumbar vertebra (L5), sacrum (S), iliolumbar ligament (ILL), anterior sacroiliac ligament (ASIL) and anterior ileum (IL) are labeled. *Used with permission of the Willard & Carreiro Collection.*

are often rudimentary. The sacrococcygeal articulation is a symphysis with a fibrocartilaginous disk and synovium, surrounded by ligaments. The anterior and posterior sacro-coccygeal ligaments extend distally to the tip of the coccyx, forming a stocking around the segments. In children, there are disks between the other coccygeal segments and the articulation between the first and second segments may be synovial. In males, the segments begin to fuse in the third or fourth decade, in females somewhat later. Late in life, the first segment may fuse with the sacrum.

The sacroiliac (SI) joints are synovial joints. They are auricular or C-shaped, with the apex (convex side) facing anteriorly (Fig. 2.9). The sacral surface of the joint is concave and lined with hyaline cartilage. The ilial surface is convex and lined with fibrocartilage. The articular surfaces are smooth at birth. During puberty they begin to roughen with weightbearing and ambulation. This process continues throughout life. The joint capsule of the SI joint is more prominent anteriorly.

The ligamentous complex of the pelvis

The iliolumbar ligament (ILL) extends from the transverse processes of L4 and L5 to the iliac crest. The ligament continues inferiorly along the anterior surface of the sacrum to become the anterior SI ligament. This is one continuous structure (Figs 2.10, 2.11). The ILL limits rotation and side-bending of L4 and L5, and forward motion of L5 on the sacrum. It is sometimes referred to as the suspensory ligament of L5.

Posteriorly the SI joint is stabilized by an SI ligament complex composed of multiple components working synchronistically. Within this complex there is a common raphe separating the multifidus and gluteus maximus muscles. The raphe stretches from the posterior sacroiliac spine (PSIS) to the coccyx. Its anterior border is anchored in the SI joint, while the posterior superior border in an extension of the thoracolumbar fascia (Fig. 2.12). Fibers of the thoracolumbar fascia embed into this ligament complex and transmit influences from the upper extremities into the lumbar spine and pelvis (Vleeming et al 1995). The long posterior SI ligament or long dorsal ligament (LDL) passes

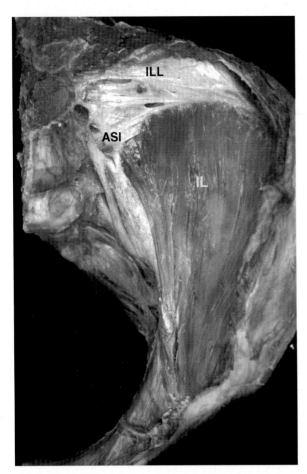

Fig. 2.10 • Superior view looking down into the left side of the pelvis. This is a section through the middle of the sacrum and pelvis, isolating it from the torso at L3, and from the extremities. The pelvic viscera have been removed. The iliacus muscle (IL) is visible along the iliac blade. The iliolumbar ligament (ILL) can be seen to merge with the fibers of the anterior sacroiliac (ASI) ligament. *Used with permission of the Willard & Carreiro Collection.*

counternutation. Thus, this ligament resists nutation of the sacrum (Vleeming et al 1995). The long dorsal and sacrotuberous ligaments play important roles in the stability of the SI joint, guiding and limiting motion on the transverse axis. The sacrospinous ligament extends from the ischial spine to the lateral margin of the sacrum and coccyx (Standring 2004). The anterior aspect of the ligament is continuous with the coccygeus muscle. All of the ligaments of the SI complex carry proprioceptive and nociceptive fibers.

Muscles of the pelvic region

The gluteus maximus muscle is the largest muscle in the body and is most superficial in the pelvic region. It attaches to the posterior surface of the iliac blade, the thoracolumbar fascia, the common raphe, the sacrotuberous ligament, the lateral crest of the sacrum and coccyx, the iliotibial band and the femur (Fig. 2.12). This powerful muscle crosses the SI joint and the hip joint. When it contracts, it compresses the SI joint, contributing to the self-bracing mechanism of the pelvis (Snijders et al 1993). In the back the multifidus firmly attaches to the thoracolumbar fascia, spinous processes, interspinous ligaments and articular capsules of the lumbar vertebrae. It extends into the pelvis, inserting on the PSIS, sacral surface of the ileum and the posterior surface of the sacrum (Fig. 2.13). In dissections, we have found fibers of the multifidus muscle passing under the common raphe to join with the sacrotuberous ligament (Willard et al 1998, Fig. 2.14). The multifidus and gluteus maximus muscles provide a counterforce across the common raphe which further stabilizes the SI joint during loading.

The biceps femoris muscle lies on the posterior lateral aspect of the thigh. It has a long and a short head. The long head plays an important role in pelvic mechanics. Its tendon attaches to the ischial tuberosity and is continuous with the sacrotuberous ligament. Inferiorly, it attaches to the head of the fibula and lateral condyle of the tibia (Standring 2004). The biceps femoris is part of a myofascial chain spanning from the plantar surface of the foot to the sacroiliac joint to the contralateral shoulder.

The piriformis muscle lies on the internal surface of the pelvis. It arises on the anterior surface of the sacrum by three digitations that are attached around the sacral foramina. At times, sacral nerves have been seen to pierce through this muscle as they pass out of the foramina. The muscle also has attachments to the gluteal surface of the ileum near the posterior inferior iliac spine and the capsule of the SI joint, and sometimes from the sacrotuberous ligament. The piriformis muscle leaves the pelvis through the greater sciatic foramen to attach to the greater trochanter of the femur. Contraction of the piriformis rotates the femur laterally, places tension on the SI joint capsule, and pulls the sacrum against the ileum, thereby contributing to the stability of the SI joint.

from the PSIS to the lateral crest of the third and fourth sacral segments. Inferiorly, its fibers may blend with the sacrotuberous ligament (STL). The posterior surface of the long dorsal ligament is an attachment site for the gluteus maximus muscle. Counternutation of the sacrum increases tension in the long dorsal ligament. It is decreased with nutation. Consequently, the long dorsal ligament limits sacral counternutation (Vleeming et al 1995).

The sacrotuberous ligament extends from the inferior lateral angle of the sacrum and to the medial surface of the ischial tuberosity. Its fibers blend with the long dorsal SI ligament (LDL) superiorly and the ligament of the biceps femoris inferiorly. Traction on the biceps femoris tendon will also increase tension in the sacrotuberous ligament. The sacrotuberous ligament connects the sacrum and the ischial tuberosity. Tension in the sacrotuberous ligament increases with nutation of the sacrum and decreases with

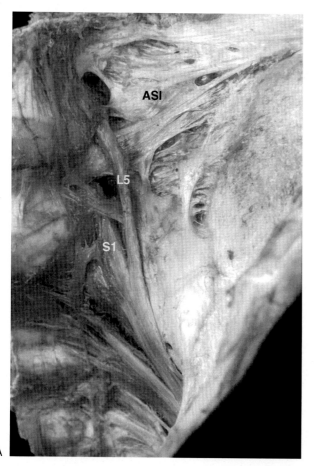
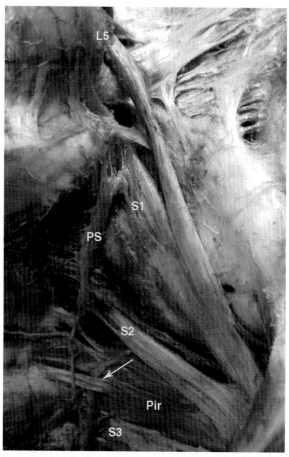

Fig. 2.11 • Same specimen as in Fig. 2.10 but the camera has been moved to present a pure anterior view of the anterior sacroiliac (ASI) joint. (A) The iliacus and piriformis muscles have been removed but the lumbosacral plexus has been left intact. The fibers of the anterior sacroiliac ligament are easily visualized. The L5 and S1 nerves are labeled. Note the proximity of the nerve to the ligament. In 2.11A the S1 nerve passes directly under a section of the ligament. In 2.11B, taken before the piriformis (Pir) was completely removed, nerve fibers from S3 and the pelvic splanchnics (PS) pass between a musculotendinous section and the belly of the muscle (white arrow). *Used with permission of the Willard & Carneiro Collection.*

Self-bracing mechanism of the sacroiliac joints

The SI joints are vulnerable to dislocation from shearing forces, because of their relatively flat surfaces. However, a mechanism of force closure exists between the sacrum and ilia. Muscles crossing the SI joint, such as the gluteus maximus and piriformis, act to compress the joint when they contract. In addition, the biceps femoris below and multifidus above exert forces on the sacrum and its ligaments. Tension in these ligaments pulls the sacrum and ilia together, compressing the SI joint. This mechanism works to stabilize the sacrum against loads. It has been described as the self-locking mechanism (Vleeming et al 1995).

During gait, the ipsilateral sacrum moves into a relative nutation during the swing phases as the contralateral sacrum moves into a relative counternutation. Nutation increases SI joint compression, which prepares the joint for the load of heel strike. The ipsilateral sacrotuberous ligament tenses as nutation increases. Just before heel strike, the biceps femoris becomes active, further increasing tension on the sacrotuberous ligament (Vleeming et al 1995). Consequently, during gait, the sacrum is constantly moving from nutation to counternutation on each side, apparently moving around oblique axes.

The pelvis as related to general body structure and function

The pelvis acts as a unit of function, responding to influences from the lumbar spine and torso above and from the lower extremities below. Biomechanical strains can occur between the pelvis and its surrounding tissues or between the components of the pelvis. The entire pelvic girdle can undergo both side-bending and rotation in relation to the lumbar spine. When the pelvis side-bends and rotates, it causes compensatory changes in the spine which may be responsible for

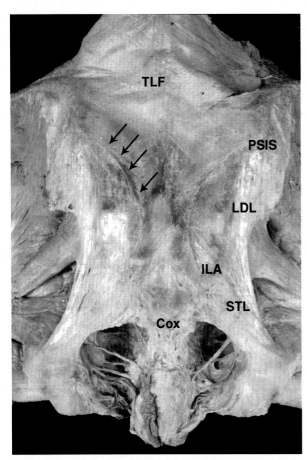

Fig. 2.12 • Posterior view of sacroiliac ligament complex and the common raphe with the specimen flexed forward at the lumbar spine. The gluteal muscles have been removed. The thoracolumbar fascia (TLF), long dorsal ligament (LDL), inferior lateral angle (ILA), sacrotuberous ligament (STL), coccyx (Cox) and posterior sacroiliac spine (PSIS) are labeled. The black arrows indicate the attachment of the gluteus maximus along the common raphe. One can easily visualize the caudal extensions of the TLF merging into the raphe. *Used with permission of the Willard & Carreiro Collection.*

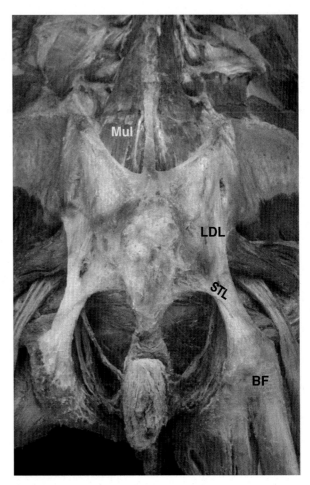

Fig. 2.13 • Posterior view of the sacrum with the common raphe layer partially cut to reveal the multifidus. BF, biceps femoris; LDL, long dorsal sacroiliac ligament; Mul, multifidus muscle; STL, sacrotuberous ligament. *Used with permission of the Willard & Carreiro Collection.*

apparent leg length differences. An isolated strain of an innominate on the sacrum may also result in an apparent leg length difference. In very young children, intraosseous strains involving the components of the innominate, such as the ischia on the ilia, may occur. Generally speaking, intraosseous strains in the innominate occur as a result of severe force or chronic pressure. Intrauterine position and mechanism of delivery are the most likely culprits in infants and toddlers.

Strains in the pelvic tissues, whether intraosseous or interosseous, cause compensatory structural changes which may interfere with the proper respiratory-circulatory function of the body, leading to improper venous and lymphatic drainage. For example, primary dysmenorrhea is thought to be related to congestion of the uterine plexus (Beard et al 1984, 1988a, b). The effects of improper drainage can be felt in any of the tissues of the body, but are particularly easy to palpate in the inguinal area and in the popliteal

fossa. In the young infant, pelvic strains affecting the low-pressure circulatory system may be associated with constipation and straining at bowel movements.

THE LOWER EXTREMITIES

THE HIP

The head of the femur and the acetabulum of the pelvis form the hip joint. The long restrictor muscles of the hip both assist and restrict motion at the hip joint. The hip is intimately related to both abdominal-pelvic function and lower extremity function. It is the major weightbearing structure upon which the pelvis rests. There is direct continuity between the hip and abdominal-pelvic cavities through the fascias and iliopsoas muscles. Abdominal or pelvic disturbance may influence the function of the hip and vice versa. The medial arcuate ligament passes over the proximal

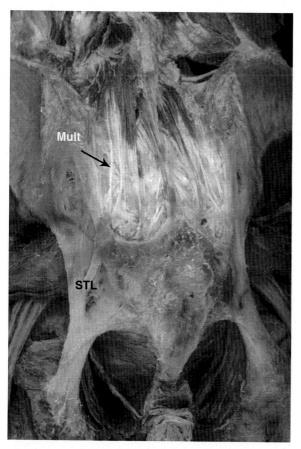

Fig. 2.14 • Posterior view of the sacrum with the common raphe layer removed. The distal fibers of the multifidus (black arrow) can be seen passing under the distal aspect of the raphe to merge with the sacrotuberous ligament (STL). *Used with permission of the Willard & Carreiro Collection.*

fibers of the psoas muscle; hypertrophy, inflammation or spasm in this muscle will affect diaphragm motion. Hip dysfunction may be the result of problems distal to this area as well as to local pathophysiological changes. Hip problems may arise as a secondary compensation to dysfunction in sacropelvic mechanics. Somatic dysfunction of the sacroiliac joint will alter mechanics of the innominate and femur through the piriformis and gluteal muscles as well as the fascial connections. When evaluating and treating any problem of the hip in a non-ambulating child, one must consider the sacroiliac joint, the rotational and medial-lateral mechanics of the innominate, and the long and short restrictors of the hip. These areas all have the potential to impact the hip joint itself. If the child is ambulating then the influences of the knee and foot need to be included as well.

Development

The hip is a ball-and-socket diarthrodial, synovial joint with smooth elastic articular cartilage and sleeve-like capsular ligaments.

In the sixth week of gestation, the primitive mesenchyme of the pelvic girdle undergoes chondrification to form hyaline models that eventually mature as a fusion of the ileum, ischium and pubic bone at a 'Y'-shaped junction in the center of the acetabulum called the triradiate cartilage. Ossification begins in the early part of gestation and completes as late as the 25th year of life. Growth occurring at the epiphysis of the rim of the acetabulum deepens it, and the appositional growth at the triradiate cartilage enlarges the diameter of the cup. The stresses acting upon the triradiate cartilage and the epiphyseal rim determine the morphology of the articular surface of the hip joint and its position. The mechanical relationship between the composite bones and the loading, and tensile forces on the joint, effect the morphology of the acetabulum. Abnormalities or alterations in the loading, tensile or torsional forces between the composite bones of the innominate will increase the risk of acetabular dysplasia or degenerative joint disease.

At birth the acetabulum is rather flat and positioned facing anteriorly. The hip joint is described as being anteverted. It will move to a retroverted, or more posterolateral, position in the child. The shape and position of the hip joint changes in response to growth, weightbearing, muscle enlargement and gait. Concurrent growth at the other epiphyses of the ileum, ischium and pubes expands and remodels the innominate, shifting the position of the acetabulum posterior and lateral. This repositioning is accommodated by and accommodates changes in the femur.

The femur develops from five ossification centers which make their appearance sporadically over the first 14 years of life. One center develops for each of the following: the body, head, greater and lesser trochanter and femoral condyles. At 7 weeks' gestation the first center begins to ossify in the shaft or body of the femur. Ossification extends cephalad and caudad along the long axis. By birth the center that will evolve into the femoral condyles has appeared, followed a year later by the center for the femoral head. The ossification center for the greater trochanter appears at 4 years and that for the lesser trochanter at 14 years (Fig 2.15). After puberty the centers fuse with the body of the femur in the opposite order than they appeared, starting with the lesser trochanter and ending with the condylar parts at 20 years. Changes in the vascular pattern of the head and neck accompany the development of the ossification centers, their growth and eventual fusion with the shaft. As a result the hip has greater risk for complication after trauma or overuse than other joints. Changes occurring with growth also affect the biomechanics of the hip joint. Apophysitis and avulsion fractures are more likely to occur in adolescents in the hip area due to the prevalence of epiphyses and nature of the sporting activities in which this age group participates.

Various authors have reported on the forces acting upon the femur. The key components can be characterized as

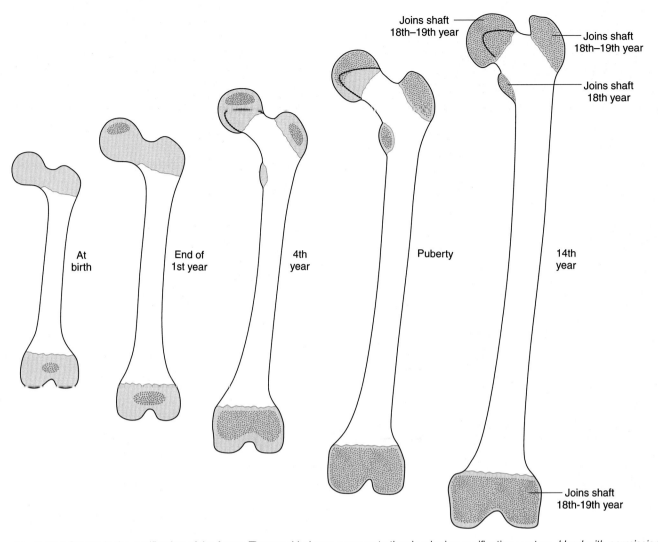

Fig. 2.15 • Stages in the ossification of the femur. The speckled area represents the developing ossification centers. *Used with permission, Williams P (ed.) 1995 Gray's anatomy, 38th edn. Churchill Livingstone, London.*

torsional, compressive and tensile forces. When the child starts to ambulate the hip is placed in an extended position and loaded. This stresses the anterior aspect of the articular capsule where it inserts onto the femoral neck. The resultant mechanical stress produces non-perpendicular and torsional loads on the femoral neck. Non-perpendicular loads deflect growth and torsional loads and cause rotational growth. The two forces act to remold the femoral head and neck into a posterolateral position. Delayed or abnormal weightbearing and ambulation will interfere with this process. Persistent intoeing after 4 years may indicate an anteverted acetabulum. In addition to the anteverted position, the femurs themselves are externally rotated at birth. The resting length of the hip flexor muscles and the external rotator muscles is decreased but the resting tone is increased. As flexor muscle tone in the hip decreases, there is concomitant decrease in the external rotation. With stance, gait and femoral retroversion, tone in the adductors

increases, bringing the femur into a more neutral position so that the patella lies in the frontal plane by the age of 7. Attendant to this mature positioning of the limb is the development of the medial longitudinal arch of the foot. This results due to strengthening and maturation of firing patterns in the anterior and posterior tibialis muscles.

At birth the head and neck of the femur are more anterior in relationship to the femoral condyles than they are in the child. The anteverted position of the newborn and toddler encourages intoeing. Abnormal hip positioning may occur due to a misshapen or malpositioned acetabulum. If the developmental repositioning of the acetabulum is inhibited the femur will persist in an anteverted position. The mechanical forces at play on the femoral neck from the long restrictor muscles and lower leg persist, but the bone may not be able to respond to them appropriately. In some cases persistent hip anteversion is extreme and quite obvious, but more often it is subtle and does not interfere with attaining normal developmental milestones. Children with spasticity affecting the adductor column may have an increase in femoral internal rotation and persistent anteversion. In milder cases of anteversion, compensations develop in the long bones and feet; consequently, anteversion should be considered in the differential diagnosis of lower leg problems. Later in life the abnormal positioning of the hip predisposes the patient to degenerative hip conditions.

Specialized ligaments of the hip

The hip joint has a specialized ligamentous structure which supports the femoral-acetabular articulation. In the erect position, the thigh is extended on the hip and the joint is loaded. These ligaments become very taught, stabilizing the joint, and providing some check to the posterior tilt of the pelvis as a whole. During hip flexion, the joint is unloaded and the ligaments are under slightly less tension. Consequently, femoral head dislocation is more likely to occur when in the flexed position.

There are several ligamentous structures that act to stabilize the hip, provide proprioceptive information for posture and balance, and guide movements of the joint. The capsular ligament surrounds the articulation. It is assisted anteriorly by the iliofemoral ligament (the 'Y' ligament) and posteriorly by the ischiofemoral ligament. The labrum acetabulum is a fibrocartilaginous ring attached along the border of the acetabulum. It serves to deepen the socket and, thus, stabilize the femoroacetabular articulation. The ligamentum teres is a rather short ligament extending from the acetabular notch to the fovea femoris capitis. Functionally, it can be thought of as the fulcrum for movements of the femur in the acetabulum. From a biodynamic point of view, the fulcrum would be the thoracolumbar junction, the neurophysiological origin of the lower extremity. It is important to remember that the artery of the ligamentum teres helps supply the femoral head, assisted by a branch of the obturator artery and/or medial femoral circumflex artery. If the femur is dislocated from the acetabulum, this artery may be compromised, leading to ischemic changes in the femoral head or epiphyseal plate.

The rotator cuff of the hip

The short restrictors or rotators of the hip can be viewed as a rotator cuff, similar to the rotator cuff in the shoulder (Figs 2.16, 2.17). The gluteus medius and minimus attach to the anterior surface of the femoral tubercle and act as abductors and internal (medial) rotators of the femur. Both stabilize the unweighted side of the pelvis during gait. The piriformis, gemelli muscles, obturator muscles and quadratus femoris attach to the posterior surface of the femur. They act as external (lateral) rotators of the thigh. Together, these muscles stabilize and guide movements and position

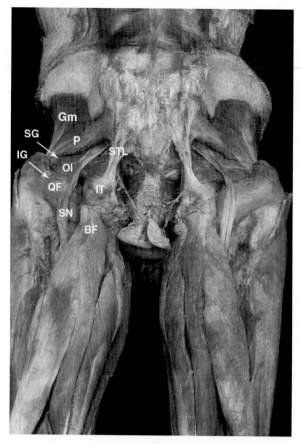

Fig. 2.16 • Posterior view of pelvic and hip dissection. The gluteus maximus and medius have been removed to expose the posterior components of the rotator cuff: the quadratus femoris (QF), piriformis (P), gluteus minimus (Gm), superior gemellus (SG), obturator internus (OI), and inferior gemellus (IG). The sacrotuberous ligament (STL), ischial tuberosity (IT), biceps femoris (BF) and sciatic nerve (SN) are identified. *Used with permission of the Willard & Carreiro Collection.*

of the femoral head in relation to the acetabulum. This needs to be kept in mind when evaluating children with hip clicks. Abnormal tension or tone in any of these muscles will affect the ability of the femur to be stabilized in the acetabulum and will distort the arch of movement of the thigh. This is of special interest in infants and newborns. Abnormal intrauterine position may result in asymmetrical muscle tensions. During passive range of motion testing, instead of an even smooth arc of circumduction, there may be some distortion of movement which could be misinterpreted as ligament laxity. Furthermore, significant muscle tension asymmetries can interfere with normal mechanics at the hip joint and joint development, resulting in delayed or distorted crawling, standing or walking.

Vasculature

The abdominal aorta branches into two common iliac arteries in the upper lumbar region (L4). Each of these divides

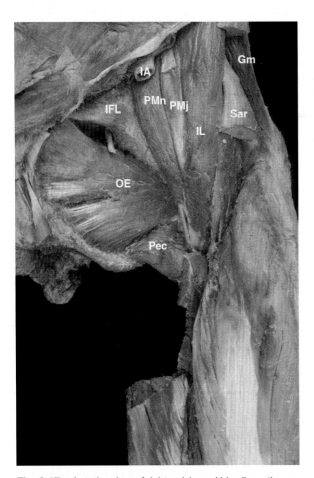

Fig. 2.17 • Anterior view of right pelvic and hip dissection; same specimen as in Fig. 2.16. The sartorius has been cut (Sar). The gluteus minimus (Gm) can be seen laterally. The obturator externus (OE) and pectineus (Pec) are considered the anterior components of the rotator cuff. The iliacus (IL), inguinal artery (IA), psoas major (PMj), psoas minor (PMn) and iliofemoral ligament (IFL) are labeled. *Used with permission of the Willard & Carreiro Collection.*

into an internal iliac artery (supplying the pelvis) and the external iliac artery (supplying the lower extremity). The external iliac artery is renamed the femoral artery as it passes beneath the inguinal ligament, and then the popliteal artery before it branches (below the knee) into anterior and posterior tibial arteries. Arterial supply to the hip joint is multiple, allowing for collateral circulation. Major arterial channels include: the obturator artery, a branch of the internal iliac artery; the medial circumflex femoral artery, a branch of the femoral artery; the lateral circumflex femoral artery, also a branch of the femoral artery; and the superior and inferior gluteal arteries, branches of the internal iliac artery.

Venous drainage of the lower extremity occurs via superficial and deep systems (Fig. 2.18). Venous blood is moved passively through the combined effects of muscle contraction and relaxation, and fascial movements. The veins drain into the inferior vena cava by way of the femoral vein. The veins of the pelvis freely communicate with the valveless venous vertebral plexus, by way of the ascending lumbar veins. In the pelvis, muscle contraction and fascial tensions facilitate venous blood flow but the effects of changing respiratory pressures also help.

Lymph from the lower extremity passes through three sets of nodes, the anterior tibial, the popliteal and some 12–20 inguinal nodes (both superficial and deep). From the inguinal nodes, lymph is transported through the pelvis, in a series of other node networks, to empty into the cisterna chyli at the level of L1/L2. Then it is transported through the thoracic duct to empty into the subclavian vein on the left side. The lymphatics are responsible for the return of fluid, proteins and other particulate matter unable to pass into the venous circulation. The extracellular fluid is returned to the heart through the effects of muscle contraction, intrathoracic pressure gradients (generated through

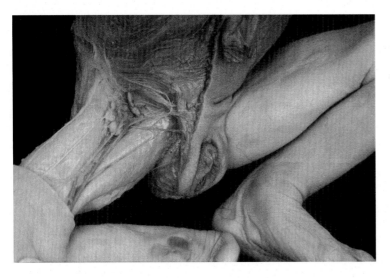

Fig. 2.18 • Anterior view of the left inguinal region in a term neonate. The abductor and quadriceps muscle complexes are exposed. The lymphatic, arterial and venous structures can be seen, including several inguinal lymph nodes. *Used with permission of the Willard & Carreiro Collection.*

the thoracoabdominal pump), pulsations of large arteries and the rhythmic contraction of the intestines. If the lymphatics are not functioning properly, particulate matter and extracellular fluids collect in interstitial spaces.

Nerves

The neural topography of the lower extremity will be clinically significant when evaluating a child with hip problems. Very often, dysfunction in the lower extremity will refer to another joint. For example, hip pathology may refer to the knee and tibia, or into the sacroiliac area, and ankle pain may refer to the hip or knee. It is necessary to understand the structural relationships, since the most common complaint in this area is pain. The physician must differentiate and recognize the significance of pain following myotomes, dermatomes and sclerotomes, from pain generated by a muscle or by a nerve itself. Unfortunately, younger children are not always able to articulate or localize the pain due to the immature mapping mechanisms at the cortical level. Instead they may present with limping, change in activity level, or general irritability. Pain patterns are discussed in Chapter 15.

Biomechanics

The position of the femur will change significantly from birth through adolescence. These changes occur in response to growth, muscle development, weightbearing and gait. In newborns the transverse axis of the femoral head and neck are positioned more anterior in relation to the femoral condyles, than in older children. The femur is said to be in an anteverted position with the angle between the condyles of the femur and its head and neck at 30°. The femur is also externally rotated and the flexor muscles have greater resting tone than the extensors. These factors result in intoeing of the feet in infants and toddlers. When the child starts to ambulate the hip is placed in an extended position and loaded. This stresses the anterior aspect of the articular capsule where it inserts on the femoral neck. This mechanical stress results in non-perpendicular and torsional loads which produce rotational growth of the femoral neck. It is the rotational growth that remolds the femoral head and neck into a retroverted position. If standing or walking is delayed, or connective tissue laxity is present, then remolding may be incomplete.

The head of the femur and the acetabulum of the pelvis form the 'ball and socket' of the hip joint. Movement of the femoral head within the acetabular socket occurs about three axes of motion: flexion and extension occur about a transverse axis; abduction and adduction occur around an anterior-posterior axis; and internal and external rotation occurs about a vertical axis. Circumduction is a combination of the above motions. These motions are accomplished through the activity of long and short restrictor muscles of the hip.

Clinical presentation

Infants and young children with hip dysfunction may present with delayed developmental milestones. Older children may experience a sudden change in activity level. They will walk with a limp or shuffle in an attempt to minimize motion and compensate for improper anatomical weightbearing. If old enough, the child may complain of pain in the area that may be localized, diffuse, constant or remitting. Alternatively, the pain may be referred to the knee or back. Another common symptom in older children is stiffness, decreased range of motion or cramping, especially at night. The pain may improve with activity and be exacerbated when the child rests. For example, young boys may be able to play sports, but at night they are kept awake by the pain. Other complaints include sensory changes such as numbness or tingling, weakness, fatigue, and feeling unstable.

KNEE

The knee is described as a ginglymus or hinge joint, but is really of a much more complicated character. *Gray's Anatomy* (Standring 2004) describes it as three articulations in one, two condyloid joints and one joint between the patella and the femur. From birth to approximately 2 years of age, the tibia has a slight varus (genu varus) angulation in relation to the femur. This is partly a result of developmental muscle imbalances and partly due to the anteverted position of the femur. After age 2, this angulation assumes a valgus position (genu valgus) until the age of 4 or 5. Genu valgus may also be seen in early adolescence when it is thought to be a result of rapid growth. This is usually more pronounced in females due to the greater Q angle.

Development

The patella begins to chondrify at 5 weeks' gestation and its ligament begins to differentiate from the mesenchymal tissue of the anterior femur at 7 weeks. At about the same time, the cruciate ligaments, menisci and joint capsule also form. Rudimentary cartilage lines the surfaces of the tibia, femur and patella by 8 weeks' gestation. Initially the patella, femur and tibia are separated from each other by membranes. By the third month of gestation the knee exists as a cartilaginous structure with adult form. During the early gestational period the patella lies superior to the joint but soon migrates to its appropriate position, dragging the quadriceps tendon with it. An undescended patella is called a patella alta. The primitive quadriceps-patella mechanism is in place and knee flexion can occur by 3 months' gestation. This coincides with internal rotation of the abducted limb bud into a more neutral position with respect to the anterior body surface, thus positioning the patella on the anterior surface of the leg. The intracondylar groove (the trochlear) forms about this same time and spontaneous movements in utero act to remodel the joint surfaces. The condyles of the tibia will ossify from one center that appears at birth. At birth, the patella is a cartilaginous sphere composed of one or two ossification centers. It and the other articular surfaces of the knee will remodel in response to movement and loading, achieving the adult shape by 7 years. By 12 years, the multiple ossification centers of the patella have fused and complete ossification usually occurs by the end of puberty. A bipartite patella occurs when the two ossification centers fail to fuse. In most children the patella is not visible on X-ray until 6 years and then it still appears as cartilaginous. The articular cartilage of the patella is the thickest in the body. Most patellae have three to five facets on the articular surface. These develop in response to movement and tracking in early life and vary considerably in size and shape between patients and even between patient's knees.

The patella is a large sesamoid bone in the tendon of the quadriceps complex (Fig. 2.19). It has five facets on its articular surface. The placement of the patella may follow the developmental position of the femur or the tibia. In femoral anteversion the femur often develops an internal torsion. If the patella aligns itself with the femur it will be medially placed ('squinting' or 'kissing' patella). Conversely the patella may follow the tibia. Then it will appear to be laterally displaced ('grasshopper' knee). A patella positioned superiorly is called patella alta, while one that rides closer to the trochlea is a patella baja. The tibia may develop intraosseous torsion in response to forces in the hip or foot. External or lateral torsion usually occurs in the proximal portion of the bone, resulting in a lateral tibial tubercle. This can increase the stresses acting on the patella tendon during knee flexion and can be a contributing factor in the development of Osgood–Schlatter disease. The tibia may compensate for the lateral torsion by favoring an externally rotated position and limiting internal rotation during flexion. (Internal torsion is more likely to occur in the distal aspect of the tibia in response to over pronation of the forefoot or calcaneus varus.) The position of the patella is also influenced by its myofascial attachments. Incomplete or inadequate insertion of the vastus medialis oblique onto the superior surface of the patella causes the patella to tilt laterally during knee extension. This can increase the compressive forces on the lateral facet and trochlea. Lateral tilt is also the result of a shortened or tight lateral retinaculum.

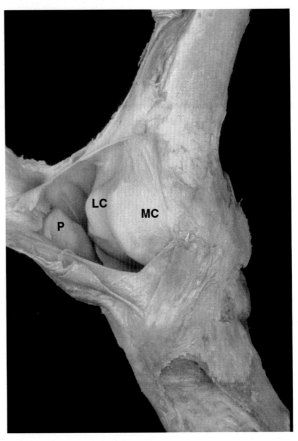

Fig. 2.19 • Medial view of a dissected knee joint. The patella tendon has been cut superiorly and medially to pull the patella away from the joint surface. The articular surfaces of the trochlear, lateral (LC) and medial (MC) condyles and the patella (P) are labeled. *Used with permission of the Willard & Carreiro Collection.*

Ligaments of the knee joint

An articular capsule surrounds the knee joint. It attaches superiorly to the femur above the intracondylar fossa and inferiorly to the condylar margins of the tibia, including the articular margin of the head of the fibula. As a result, fibular dysfunction may present as midline joint pain in the knee. The joint capsule surrounds the patella and attaches to the tibial tubercle. The popliteal tendons pass through defects in the posterior aspect of the capsule. The capsule is innervated by proprioceptive and nociceptive fibers.

Within the joint the anterior and posterior cruciate ligaments guide and limit motion between the femur and the tibia (Fig. 2.20). The anterior cruciate ligament passes from the medial-posterior aspect of the lateral condyle of the femur to the anterior margin of the tibial plateau. It is taut in maximal extension, and limits excessive anterior movement of the tibia relative to the femur. The posterior cruciate ligament attaches to the posterior aspect of the tibial plateau and to the medial condyle of the femur. It is most

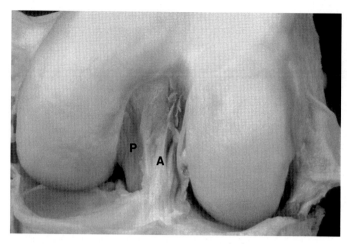

Fig. 2.20 • Close-up of the flexed knee joint. The anterior (A) and posterior (P) cruciate ligaments are identified. *Used with permission of the Willard & Carreiro Collection.*

active in flexion, where it prevents excessive posterior movement of the tibia relative to the femur. The anterior cruciate ligament may be injured in hyperextension traumas to the knee, whereas the posterior cruciate ligament is vulnerable to hyperflexion injuries.

The quadriceps tendon which inserts on the tibial tubercle is home to the large sesamoid bone, the patella. With contraction of the rectus femoris and the vastus lateralis and medialis, the patella travels in the intracondylar groove or trochlear of the femur. The patella ligaments provide stability to the knee in both flexion and extension by limiting posterior movement of the tibia on the femur.

The oblique popliteal ligament is a posterior knee ligament, which passes from the lateral condyle of the femur to the posterior head of the tibia. It lies under the attachments of the medial and lateral gastrocnemius muscle and the semitendinous muscle inserts upon it. The medial collateral ligament connects the medial condyle of the femur to the medial condyle of the tibia and the medial meniscus. Excessive stress on this ligament can be transmitted through to the meniscus and disrupt its integrity. The lateral collateral ligament connects the lateral condyle of the femur to the fibula and bridges over, but does not connect to, the lateral meniscus.

Menisci

The menisci are two horseshoe-shaped rings lying between the tibia and femur. They are present at birth (Fig. 2.21). The menisci increase the articular surface area of the tibia and act as a cushion in weightbearing. The medial meniscus is attached to the articular capsule of the knee and the medial collateral ligament. The lateral meniscus is injured far less than the medial, with a ratio of about eight to one in

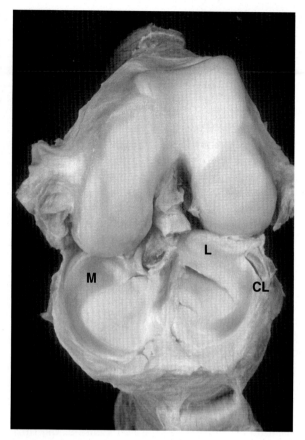

Fig. 2.21 • Anterior view into the knee joint. The cruciate ligaments have been cut and the joint hyperextended to reveal the medial (M) and lateral (L) menisci. The coronary ligament (CL) is also labeled. *Used with permission of the Willard & Carreiro Collection.*

frequency. This is due to three factors: the lateral meniscus is somewhat protected by the head of the fibula; it is firmly attached to the tibia by its coronary ligament; and it is not attached to the lateral collateral ligament. The two menisci are connected anteriorly by the transverse ligament. If it is torn or stretched, the medial or lateral meniscus can be displaced when the knee is stressed. The menisci are primarily avascular. Nutrients and waste products pass through these structures via passive gradients. This makes the menisci more vulnerable to chronic degenerative processes and less able to heal after injury.

Biomechanics

In extension, the anterior cruciate ligaments stabilize the knee and prevent hyperextension. The tibia glides anteriorly under the femur with some external rotation and the patella draws superiorly. The fibrocartilaginous menisci move anteriorly with some deformation of their shape during extension. Through the range of flexion-extension, the menisci move approximately 6 mm (medial meniscus) to 12 mm (lateral meniscus). All of these components are required for normal knee function. Deviations from the physiological norm lead to altered unit loads across the articular surfaces, altered tensile forces in the myofascial elements, and compensations in the knee and associated tissues. This may affect growth patterns and produce microtrauma on myofascial structures.

The tibia and the femur need to adapt to the asymmetry of the menisci and femoral condyles (the medial condyle is larger and longer than the lateral) as the knee flexes and extends. During knee flexion the tibia internally rotates and the femur externally rotates. During extension the opposite occurs. Rotation of the tibia is produced by the action of the hamstrings, the quadriceps and the tibialis muscles. The external rotation of the tibia is sometimes called the screw-home mechanism of the knee. Contraction of the semimembranosus and semitendinosus produces internal rotation of the leg. Contraction of the biceps femoris causes external rotation of the leg and posterior movement of the fibular head. Movement of the tibia can be appreciated by comparing the position of the tibial tuberosity and the middle of the patella in flexion and extension (Fig. 2.22). In extension, the tibial tuberosity will be positioned laterally as compared to the middle of the patella. In flexion, the tibial tuberosity will be positioned directly beneath the midpoint of the patella. Abnormal muscle tensions may exacerbate or impede rotation of the tibia. If, during extension, the tibia does not rotate laterally, then the medial meniscus will be compressed between the femur and tibia. Over time this may lead to meniscus inflammation, medial midline joint pain and eventual meniscus degeneration. Conversely, if the tibia does not medially rotate during flexion, the medial collateral ligament and the posterior cruciate ligament will be subjected to abnormal stretch. Abnormal motion mechanics in the relative positioning of the tibia and femur will increase the load on the menisci, alter tensions on the ligaments and affect resting length of the muscles acting on the knee. Altered mechanics of the tibia also influence ankle and foot mechanics, and vice versa. An internally rotated tibia is often associated with pes planus and excessive supination of the foot. Internal rotation of the tibia may arise from increased tone in the adductor muscles, which limits its external rotation. An externally rotated tibia is typically associated with an over supinated foot or a pes cavus during stance. However, during gait the over supinated foot will compensate by pronating at the subtalar joint and forefoot. Externally rotated tibias are also found with genu varus posture and bowlegs.

Abduction and adduction also occur at the knee and may be compensatory to foot placement, pelvic morphology or myofascial influences among other things. Abduction and adduction are accompanied by glide or translation across the joint. These can also occur when a traumatic force is directed medially or laterally above or below the knee joint.

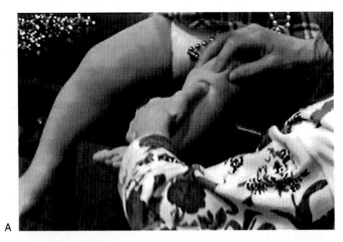

A

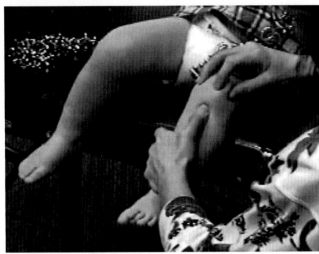

B

Fig. 2.22 • Evaluation of the screw-home mechanism between the tibia and femur. In (A), the child's knee is flexed and the tibial tubercle is in line with the middle of the patella. In (B), the child's knee is extended and the tibia tubercle moves laterally as compared to the same landmark on the patella. This is normal.

At birth, the patella is positioned more laterally and moves to the middle of the knee as the femur moves into retroversion. The patella primarily moves superiorly and inferiorly between the femoral condyles but it may also tilt and rotate in response to muscle forces and pelvic morphology. Instability of the patella is typically associated with excessive tilt or rotation. Abnormal patella tracking leads to increased pressures on the deep cartilaginous surface of the patella facets. The subchondral bone in this area is heavily innervated with primary nociceptors. Continued pressure has the potential to affect the cartilage of the femoral condyles as well, disrupting the proteoglycan molecules and leading to a breakdown in the articular cartilage. The resulting inflammation and surface deformity may exacerbate the tracking problems and cause pain.

Clinical presentation

In children, knee problems present as pain, avoidance of weightbearing or limping. Toddlers with knee pathology may refuse to walk or only ambulate while holding on to something. In this age group distorted knee mechanics may contribute to pes planus, genu valgus, genu varus and genu recavartum. In older children, knee pathology can present as pain in the knee, hip, or ankle. The child may avoid weightbearing and often there is a limp. In this age group biomechanical dysfunction of the knee may also play a role in Osgood–Schlatter syndrome, patella instability, recurrent inversion ankle sprain, plantar fasciitis and iliotibial band syndrome.

FOOT AND ANKLE

In the uterus, the feet are typically supinated and tucked against the thighs. The knees and hips are flexed with tibias crossed and internally rotated. This intrauterine position influences the shape of the long bones of the leg such that congenital torsions and bowing are often present at birth. The shape of the long bones will in turn affect the morphology of the feet, especially the integrity of arches, which are dependent on normal functional relationships in the long restrictor muscles of the ankle and distal leg. The arch arrangement is formed by the bony framework of the foot and supported by the long restrictor muscles of the distal leg, the tibialis anterior and posterior and the peroneus longus. Bony deformities such as tibial torsions can distort the relationship of the soft tissue structures that support the platform upon which the arches are built. This influences foot mechanics.

Development

Ossification of the foot progresses from the hindfoot to the forefoot. The ossification of the talus and calcaneus begins before birth, while the process in the navicular does not begin until 3 years in males and 2 years in females. Except for the calcaneus, each of the bones of the hindfoot ossifies from one center, which appears during the fetal period. The calcaneus has two ossification centers: the first appears during gestation, the second at about 10 years. The second epiphysis fuses with the main bone at about 20 years. The talus will develop a second center that does not join the main body of the bone; this is called an os trigonum. The metatarsal bones each have two ossification centers. Ossification of the body of the second through fifth metatarsals begins in the center during the fetal period and then extends longitudinally towards the ends. The ossification centers for the heads of these metatarsals appear between years 5 and 8, and join the bodies in the twenties. The center for the base of the first metatarsal does not appear until the third year.

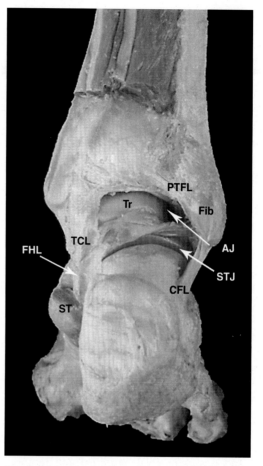

Fig. 2.23 • Posterior view of the right dissected ankle. The plantar flexor muscles have been removed and the posterior fascias and the posterior talofibular ligament have been cut to reveal the trochlear surface of the talus (Tr), the ankle joint (AJ) and the subtalar joint (STJ). The sustentaculum tali (ST) with its groove for the flexor hallucis longus (FHL) and the tibiocalcaneal ligament (TCL) are labeled on the medial side. The fibular (Fib), posterior tibiofibular ligament (PTFL), and the calcaneal fibular ligament (CFL) are labeled on the lateral side. *Used with permission of the Willard & Carreiro Collection.*

Functional anatomy

The talocrural joint or ankle joint is a hinge joint, formed by the articulation of the tibia and fibula with the talus (Fig. 2.23). The tibia and fibula are bound closely, chiefly by the interosseous membrane but also by the anterior and posterior tibiofibular ligaments and the transverse ligament, which is also associated with the talus. The tibia transmits the body weight to the trochlea of the talus. The fibula bears little or no weight. The medial and lateral malleoli form a mortise around the talus that stabilizes the ankle. Medially, the talus is bound to the tibia by the deltoid ligament, which attaches to the malleolus. This ligament also has bands that connect the malleolus with the calcaneus and navicular bone, preventing either forward or backward displacement of the tibia. Laterally, the joint is spanned by the anterior and posterior talofibular ligaments and calcaneofibular ligament. These ligaments serve not only to tie the joint together but also to prevent forward-to-backward displacement of the fibula. The forefoot is composed of the intertarsal, metatarsophalangeal and metacarpophalangeal joints. Gliding movements are permitted by these arthrodial-type joints. Motions of flexion, extension, slight abduction and slight adduction are permitted. The intraphalangeal joints are hinge joints that permit flexion and extension of the toes. The joints and short restrictor muscles of the forefoot are heavily innervated with proprioceptive fibers that play a role in balance and posture.

Neurovascular supply

Sympathetic innervation to the arteries of the leg is derived from L1 to L2. The preganglionic fibers synapse in lumbar ganglia. From here they descend to the leg to influence vasomotor tone. From an osteopathic perspective, one way to increase circulation to the lower extremities is to normalize the thoracolumbar, lumbosacral and pelvic areas, restoring pressure gradients and promoting an increase in venous and lymphatic return.

The veins of the lower extremity may be divided into three groups: superficial, deep and perforating. The superficial veins consist of the great and small saphenous veins and their tributaries, which are situated beneath the skin in the superficial fascia. The deep veins are the venae comitantes to the anterior and posterior tibial, popliteal and femoral arteries and their branches. The perforating veins are communicating vessels that run between the superficial and deep veins. A number of these veins are found particularly in the region of the ankle and the medial side of the lower part of the leg. They possess valves which prevent the flow of blood from the deep to the superficial veins. Within the closed fascial compartments of the lower extremity, the thin-walled, valved venae comitantes are subject to intermittent pressure, both at rest and during exercise. The pulsations of the adjacent arteries help to move the blood up the leg towards the pelvis. The contractions of the muscles within the fascial compartments also facilitate this movement. Superficial veins such as the saphenous lie within the superficial fascia and are not subject to these compressive forces, except near their termination, where they pass through the muscles of the thigh. The valves in the perforating veins prevent the high-pressure venous blood from being forced outward into the low-pressure superficial veins. As the muscles within the closed fascial compartments relax, venous blood is moved from the superficial into the deep veins.

The large veins and major lymphatic channels follow the course of the arteries. Arterial pulsations, altering fascial tensions, and contraction and relaxation of muscle groups during gait, all assist the flow through this low-pressure circulatory system. The most peripheral vessels are at greatest risk for congestion. This may happen after injury or prolonged disuse. With repetitive activity or overuse the circulatory vessels in the deeper compartments may become congested. This usually occurs when repetitive microtrauma on fascia or muscles causes hypertrophy and edema within the muscle or at the periosteal insertion. The subsequent increase in intracompartmental pressure impedes lymphatic and venous drainage through the area. The resultant stasis further increases the compartmental pressure impeding arterial flow. The tissue initially suffers from hypoxia, then ischemia, creating a cascade of tissue damage, edema, congestion and vascular insufficiency. This is the pathophysiology of compartment syndrome.

Arches of the foot

When the body is erect, its weight is transmitted through the foot. Ideally, each foot bears 50% of the body weight, which is distributed evenly across the entire plantar arch. The plantar surface of the foot is covered with dense connective tissue suspended between the calcaneus and the first and fifth metatarsals. In the mature foot, there are four anatomical arches, three of which are functional. Weight is distributed along the functional arches to create a connective tissue pyramid. The arch mechanism is not in place at birth and generally does not develop before the age of 3 years. Deformities of the foot and lower extremity will affect arch development.

The functional arches of the foot are located along the lateral and medial aspects and along the metatarsals (Fig. 2.24). The lateral longitudinal arch is formed by the calcaneus, cuboid and fourth and fifth metatarsals. In most children it is relatively flat during weightbearing but quite flexible. A common finding in this arch is the dropped cuboid. This may result from a direct downward pressure on the cuboid or on the fourth and fifth metatarsals that support the bone anteriorly. Most frequently, the dropped cuboid is secondary to a talocalcaneal dysfunction, in which the talus is anterior and the calcaneus is internally rotated. The descent of the cuboid is often accompanied by lateral rotation of the bone. The lateral longitudinal arch is lowered and the cuboid fails to efficiently support the transverse arch. This can affect the position of the navicular, distorting the plantar vault. There is plantar tenderness and a palpable prominence of the inferomedial angle of the cuboid. Motion restriction at the articulations of the cuboid is usually present.

The medial longitudinal arch is formed by the calcaneus, talus, navicular, cuneiforms and three medial metatarsal bones. This arch acts like a spring, absorbing the natural shocks that come from walking. The navicular is the keystone of this arch and is typically the primary area of dysfunction. When navicular movement is restricted, the weightbearing stress on the medial longitudinal arch is increased and the arch will flatten. A decrease of 3 mm or

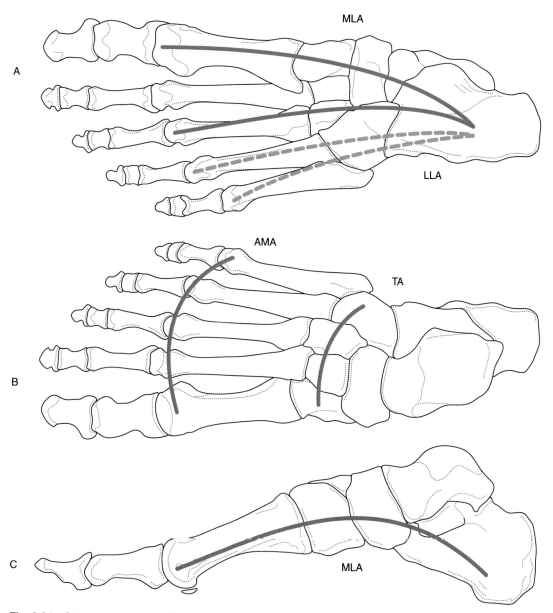

Fig. 2.24 • Schematic diagram of three views of the arches of the foot. (A) Plantar view depicting lateral longitudinal arch (LLA; broken lines) and medial longitudinal arch (MLA; solid lines). (B) Dorsal view showing transverse (TA) and anterior metatarsal (AMA) arches. (C) Medial view showing medial longitudinal arch (MLA).

more in the height of the arch when comparing non-weight-bearing and stance is clinically significant. The navicular dysfunction is further exacerbated by the increased weight load during stance. The cuneiforms and the bases of the first three metatarsals will also flatten. Over time, the plantar fascias are stretched and the supporting muscles are subjected to increased tensile load. This results in venous and lymphatic congestion, impaired trophic flow and irritation to tissues.

The anterior metatarsal arch is formed at the articulations of the metatarsal bones with the phalanges. The first and fifth metatarsals are on a low plane, with the second,

third and fourth being on a higher plane. The metatarsals have no direct muscle attachments; they have a ligamentous mechanism. As the distal ends (heads) of the metatarsals bear weight, the arch flattens. The second metatarsal is the keystone of this arch. During weightbearing, it should lie approximately 9 mm above the ground in the mature foot.

The transverse arch is the fourth arch. It is considered a more rigid arch although there is still flexibility. It is composed of the three cuneiforms and the cuboid. This rigid arch maintains the osseous architecture of the foot, while the more flexible longitudinal and anterior arches support the function of the foot. The intermediate cuneiform is the

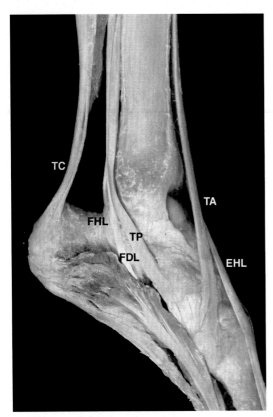

Fig. 2.25 • Ankle dissection with all muscles, fat and fascia around ankle removed to expose the supporting tendons of the arches. Medial view of the dissected ankle. The tibialis anterior (TA) and posterior (TP), the tendocalcaneous (TC), the flexor digitalis longus (FDL), flexor hallucis longus (FHL) and extensor hallucis longus (EHL) are labeled. *Used with permission of the Willard & Carreiro Collection.*

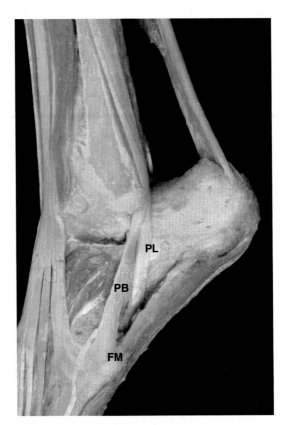

Fig. 2.26 • Ankle dissection with all muscles, fat and fascia around ankle removed to expose the supporting tendons of the arches. Lateral view of the dissected ankle. Peroneus longus (PL) and brevis (PB) and labeled. Peroneus brevis inserts on the lateral tubercle of the fifth metatarsal (FM). *Used with permission of the Willard & Carreiro Collection.*

keystone of this arch, and, along with the second metatarsal, forms the axis of the foot. Dysfunction in the transverse arch typically presents as severe pain with loading.

Tendinous component of the arches

The arches of the foot are supported by a tendinous basket (Figs 2.25, 2.26). The posterior tibialis tendon attaches to the navicular and first cuneiform, and then extends laterally across the plantar surface to attach to the second cuneiform and the second through to fourth metatarsal heads. When the tibialis posterior contracts, the navicular is pulled into a posterior position under the head of the talus. The tendon of the tibialis anterior attaches to the lateral aspect of the navicular. As the foot moves from heel strike to stance the eccentric contraction of the tibialis anterior assists the posterior muscles in distributing the weight load to the medial longitudinal arch. The tendon of the flexor hallucis long courses under the sustentaculum tali and along the plantar aspect of the foot to insert on the base of the distal phalanx of the first metatarsal. During heel strike, it stabilizes the talus and lifts

the anterior aspect of the calcaneus. Dysfunction of this muscle or its mechanical relationships may lead to abnormal weight displacement on the calcaneus.

The tendon of peroneus longus passes in a groove around the lateral edge of the cuboid, and then across the plantar surface of the foot to attach to the first metatarsal and cuneiform bones. This tendon supports the medial and anterior arches. The peroneus brevis attaches to the lateral tubercle of the fifth metatarsal. Mechanical strains of the peroneus muscles or fibula will affect function of the lateral arch. The tendon of the adductor hallicis longus passes from the calcaneus to the phalanx of the first metatarsal. It approximates the two ends of the medial arch. The tendon of the adductor digiti minimus courses laterally from the calcaneus to the proximal phalanx of the fifth digit. It approximates the two ends of the lateral arch. These two structures act as bowstrings for the arches.

The arches as a diaphragm

The fibrous connective tissue arches of the foot function as a diaphragm (Fig. 2.27). With normal gait mechanics,

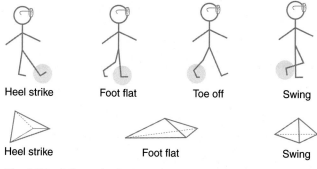

Heel strike   Foot flat   Toe off   Swing

Heel strike   Foot flat   Swing

Fig. 2.27 • Schematic diagram of the diaphragmatic mechanics of the plantar tissues of the foot.

weight forces are initially distributed to the calcaneus and then along the lateral aspect of the foot to pass across the anterior or transverse arch. At full stance, body weight is distributed through three points and dissipated along the arches, similar to a child's pyramidal tent. The connective tissue bands, which are 'slung' between these points, function as the base of the pyramid. The navicular functions as the apex or 'keystone' of the pyramid. This arrangement creates a dynamic, highly adaptable base that can act as both a shock absorber and a stabilizer in gait and stance. During gait, the connective tissue tent alternately flattens with weightbearing and peaks with swing. This flattening-stretching and peaking-relaxing of the plantar connective tissue creates a pumping action which aids in lymphatic and venous flow from the foot. If the structural relationships of the 'tent' are disturbed, the normal mechanics of the foot are affected, in terms of both weight distribution and diaphragmatic activity.

Biomechanics

Movement at the foot and ankle differ during non-weight-bearing and weightbearing postures. In the non-weight-bearing position, inversion, eversion, adduction, abduction, pronation and supination occur between the calcaneus and talus. In the weightbearing posture, the motions of the ankle and tarsal joints are conveniently named and simultaneously described by considering them as foot motions. There are four foot motions. Dorsiflexion, which is also called foot flexion, consists of raising the foot towards the anterior surface of the leg. Most of this motion takes place in the ankle joint. There is also slight motion in the tarsal joints. Plantar flexion, sometimes called foot extension, consists of lowering the foot so that its long axis is in line with that of the leg. Plantar flexion takes place mostly in the ankle joint, but again there is slight motion in the tarsal joints. Eversion occurs when the sole is turned laterally or 'outwards'. Conversely, the sole of the foot is turned medially during inversion. Inversion takes place only in the tarsal joints.

Weight transmission in the foot

The distribution of weight differs during standing and active movement such as walking or running, and it differs in children from adults. The calcaneus is the only bone common to both longitudinal arches. It is also the strongest weightbearing bone of the foot. During quiet stance in the mature foot, much of the body weight is transmitted to the calcaneus from the talus, which lies anterior and superior to the calcaneus. A smaller degree of weight is directed from the talus downwards and forwards to the navicular. The navicular, in turn, transmits weight to the three cuneiform bones with which it articulates. The three cuneiform bones articulate with and transmit weight to the first three metatarsal bones. The cuboid, which lies lateral to the navicular, receives the weight transmitted forwards from the calcaneus and then transmits it to the fourth and fifth metatarsal bones. The five metatarsal bones, which are arranged on different planes, transmit weight to the forward part of the foot.

During mature gait, the weight is transmitted along the foot proximal to distal. At heel strike, weight is transmitted down the leg to the calcaneus. The ankle (the talocrural joint) is flexed, stabilizing the talocalcaneal joint. As the foot moves into the foot flat (or footprint) stage, the talocrural joint passively moves from flexion to a neutral position and the foot meets the ground. Weight is first distributed from the calcaneus through the cuboid and fifth metatarsal, and then, as the foot begins to evert, weight is distributed through the medial arch. At the midstance phase, the weight is distributed medially across the anterior metatarsal arch to the head of the first metatarsal. As the weight approaches the head of the first metatarsal, push-off begins. During gait the foot and ankle absorb the body's weight through plantar flexion and pronation. The actual force across the ankle is approximately 4.5 times body weight when walking and 10 times body weight when running. As the ankle dorsiflexes with loading, the tibia moves anteriorly and internally. The ankle is most vulnerable to injury during plantar flexion and most stable at dorsiflexion.

THE UPPER EXTREMITIES

SHOULDER COMPLEX

The shoulder girdle is a complex structure made up of the glenohumeral joint, the acromioclavicular joint, the sternoclavicular joint and the scapulothoracic joint. Generally, most of the emphasis is placed on the shallow glenoid joint, but most functional problems in the shoulder involve dysfunction in the scapulothoracic joint. Due to the intricate mechanics of the complex, it is almost impossible to have a problem isolated to only one joint. The glenohumeral joint is capable of flexion, extension, internal and external rotation, abduction, adduction and circumduction. Motions at the scapulothoracic joint, including elevation, depression, protraction, retraction, and upward and downward rotation, contribute to the total mobility of the shoulder girdle and, therefore, to the upper extremity. The muscles of the rotator cuff are subjected to tissue stress when the mechanics of the scapulothoracic joint are dysfunctional. Motion of the scapula is dependent on function in the clavicular articulations. Disturbed function in any of those components, which lend support and motion to the unit, will limit the function of the shoulder and of the upper extremity.

Development

By 8 weeks' gestation the components of the shoulder have appeared in their adult-like shape. Over the next 7 months these components will enlarge although many do not mature until the patient is in his or her early twenties. These immature areas are vulnerable to injury from improper or over training. The humeral head ossifies in parts. At birth the diaphysis and metaphysis of the humerus have fused and ossified, but the two ossification centers for the greater tubercle and that of the lesser tubercle do not even appear until after birth. The centers for the greater tubercle appear at 7 months and 3 years and the lesser tubercle at 5 years. These three begin to fuse together between 5 and 7 years but don't complete their ossification until early adulthood. The epiphysis of the humeral head is both intra-articular and extra-articular. It lies inferior to the greater and lesser tubercles and traverses medially to the intra-articular surface. The capsular ligaments cross the epiphysis at its medial end. The glenoid fossa forms from two ossification centers. The upper third of the fossa forms with the base of the coracoid process. The epiphysis appears during the 10th year of life and traverses around the coracoid base and the upper third of the glenoid fossa. It does not begin to close until after puberty. The ossification centers of the acromion process also appear at puberty and fuse by 22 years. The scapula has multiple ossification centers, some of which develop in the embryonic period; others do not appear until after birth. In the embryo, the primary ossification center appears as a chondrification in the mid-cervical area. It undergoes intramembranous ossification and migrates south carrying its sclerotome with it. The peripheral epiphyseal plate located at the inferior perimeter of the scapula appears at the beginning of puberty and closes by 20 years. The coracoid process appears in the first year and its shared epiphysis with the glenoid fossa develops about 9 years later. In adolescence some children will develop a second ossification center at the tip of the coracoid process; this can be a site of inflammation and irritation in young athletes participating in sports using abduction and shoulder flexion. The acromion varies in its development; the first ossification centers appear between 14 and 15 years and close shortly later. Because there are so many ossification centers in the shoulder complex, non-union or failure to

ossify results in various anomalies such as bipartite coracoid, os acromiale, and dysplasia of the glenoid fossa.

There are several structural developments in the shoulder complex during childhood. As with the hip, the humerus moves through a torsional pattern to achieve its adult position. In neonates the humeral head tends to be posteriorly oriented and this decreases in the adult (Cowgill 2007). Although persistent and excessive humeral torsion (retroversion) is found in the throwing arm of high-level athletes, some level of asymmetry appears to be common in most people (Krahl 1976, Cowgill 2007). The mechanism by which normal torsion occurs is unclear, although muscle development probably plays a role. In addition to changes in the orientation of the humeral head, the morphology of the humeral head, scapula and clavicle will also change. At birth the clavicle is rather flat and the acromioclavicular joint is poorly developed. The clavicle also functions as a stabilizer for the first rib and sternum in the young child.

The shoulder girdle

The muscles of the shoulder girdle act as active ligaments, supporting the articulation of the head of the humerus in the glenoid cavity (Figs 2.28, 2.29). They include the supraspinatus, subscapularis, teres minor, infraspinatus and long head of the biceps. The first four of these muscles constitute the rotator cuff. These muscles, their tendons and articular capsule are densely innervated with proprioceptors and play an important role in the development of fine and gross motor control and hand-eye coordination. Other muscles influencing the shoulder include the latissimus dorsi, triceps, levator scapulae, rhomboid, teres major, deltoid and serratus anterior. All except the latter two are thin vellums of tissue in the newborn.

Articular complexes of the shoulder

The shoulder girdle constitutes a multifaceted joint complex between the upper extremity and the thorax. It serves to maintain contact of the upper extremity to the torso while providing a complex three-dimensional range of motion. There are at least five interactive surfaces contributing to this wide range of motion. The scapulohumeral or glenohumeral joint is a true joint with hyaline cartilage lining the oppositional articulatory surfaces. The subdeltoid joint is a physiological joint consisting of two surfaces which slide over each other. The functional joint space is bordered by the deep surface of the deltoid and the superficial and distal surfaces of the supraspinatus, infraspinatus and teres minor muscles. Within this space lies the subdeltoid bursa, which allows the two surfaces to glide over each other. Movement in this joint is intimately related to movement in the scapulohumeral joint. The scapulothoracic joint is also a physiological joint. It influences the quality and range of

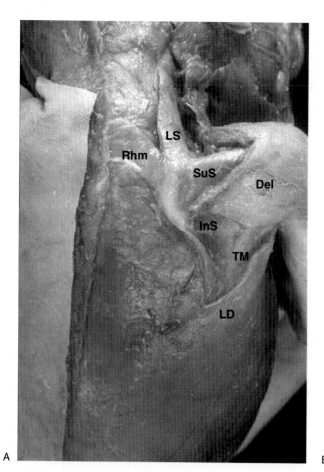
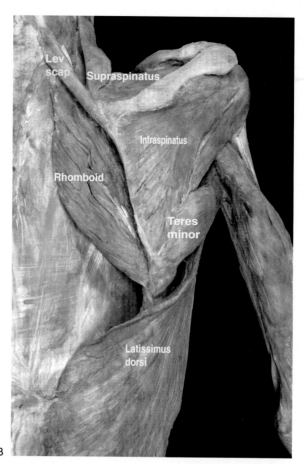

Fig. 2.28 • Posterior view of the shoulder in a term infant (A) and adult (B) with the trapezius muscle removed. Latissimus dorsi (LD), infraspinatus (InS), supraspinatus (SuS), teres minor (TM), rhomboids (Rhm), levator scapulae (LS) and the deltoid (Del) are labeled. The teres and rhomboids are less well defined in the term infant than in the adult. The levator scapulae is relatively larger in the infant. *Used with permission of the Willard & Carreiro Collection.*

motion in all the other joints of the shoulder complex. The scapulothoracic joint consists of two joint spaces. The more superficial space lies between the scapula and serratus anterior muscle. Its borders include the subscapularis muscle posteriorly, and the serratus anterior muscle anteriorly and laterally. The deeper space lies between the thoracic wall and the serratus anterior. During shoulder abduction, the scapular elevates 8–10 cm, rotates 38°, tilts mediolaterally and posteroanteriorly, and swivels around a vertical axis. All of these movements occur within the scapulothoracic joint.

The acromioclavicular joint is made up of the flattened distal head of the clavicle, which fits into the medial aspect of the acromion process of the scapula. The joint has a very limited range of motion and functions to fix the relationship between the clavicle and the scapula. Finally, the sternoclavicular joint represents the only bony articulation between the upper extremity and the thoracic wall. Its motion characteristics are intimately tied to the scapula, such that each clavicular motion requires a movement on the part of the scapula. The clavicle is capable of three types of

motion: elevation–depression, protraction–retraction and rotation. There is 45° of elevation in the clavicle and 15° of depression. The axis of motion is about the costoclavicular ligament, so the clavicular head depresses as the body of the clavicle rises. There is 15° of protraction and 15° of retraction. Again, the axis of rotation is about the costoclavicular ligament, and the clavicular head retracts as the body protracts. Rotation only occurs in a posterior direction, and accompanies flexion and abduction of the upper extremity.

The sternoclavicular articulation is surrounded by dense connective tissue, to which a radial array of ligaments is attached. The sternoclavicular ligament attaches the articular capsule to the sternum on its anterior and posterior surfaces. It is strongest anteriorly. The articular capsule of the sternoclavicular joint completely surrounds and attaches to the articular disk. The disk is thickened superoposteriorly. Two joint spaces surround the disk. The interclavicular ligament represents a bridge between the two clavicular joints. Consequently, displacement or malalignment of one clavicle may affect the other. Suprasternal ossicles can be present

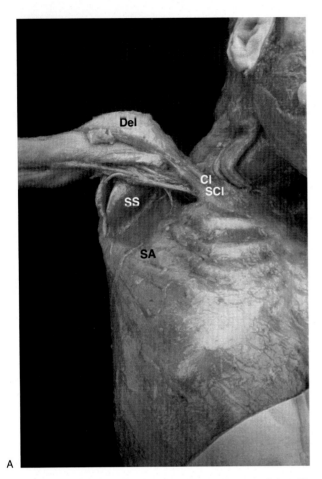 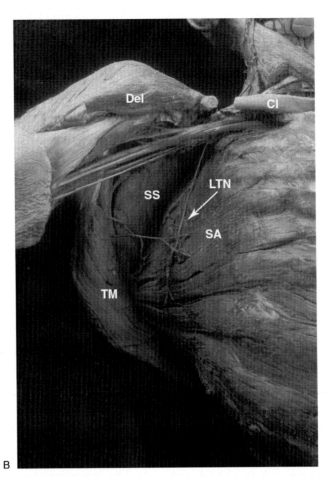

Fig. 2.29 • Anterior dissection of the shoulder in a term infant (A) and in an adult (B). The pectoralis major and minor have been removed, and the clavicle cut in the adult. The subscapularis (SS), serratus anterior (SA), deltoid (Del), clavicle (Cl), teres minor (TM), long thoracic nerve (LTN) and subclavius (SCl) are labeled. *Used with permission of the Willard & Carreiro Collection.*

in this ligament. The costoclavicular ligament has anterior and posterior laminae separated by a bursa. Each tenses at opposite extremes of clavicular axial rotation.

The distal third of the clavicle is flattened along the vertical axis, and the distal end is convex in shape, allowing it to insert into the medial aspect of the acromion. The acromioclavicular joint is completely surrounded by a dense connective tissue capsule. The acromioclavicular ligament represents the thickened superior surface of the joint capsule. A ligament complex passes between the coracoid process and the clavicle. It consists of two parts. The trapezoid portion of the coracoclavicular ligament is the anterolateral ligament between the clavicle and coracoid process. It is horizontal in orientation. The coracoid portion of the ligament is the posteromedial ligament between the clavicle and coracoid process. It is vertical in orientation.

The largest articular joint of the shoulder complex is the glenohumeral joint. The head of the humerus constitutes an irregular sphere, the vertical diameter of which is greater than its posterior diameter. It contains a series of centers of curvature spirally arranged; this increases the stability of the humeral head when the superior portion is in contact with the glenoid cavity. The glenoid cavity is much smaller than the humeral head. It is oriented laterally, anteriorly and superiorly. There is a slightly raised margin. The glenoidal labrum is a fibrocartilaginous rim surrounding the glenoid cavity. This ring effectively deepens the cavity without increasing its diameter. It also increases the traction forces between the glenoid fossa and the head of the humerus (Matsen et al 1991). Lesions of the glenoid labrum represent a source of instability in the glenohumeral joint (Pappas et al 1983). A dense connective tissue capsule attaches to the glenoid cavity outside of the labrum and attaches to the head of the humerus. Its superolateral margin forms a tunnel for the tendon of the long head of the biceps. The external edge of the tunnel thickens to form the transverse humeral ligament. Three thickenings in the anterior wall of the capsule constitute the glenohumeral ligaments (Matsen et al 1991). These ligaments provide support and stability but may become inflamed or irritated by biomechanical dysfunction. The superior glenohumeral ligament becomes tight in adduction and resists inferior translocation. The middle glenohumeral ligament is tightened in external rotation and prevents anterior translocation of the humerus in this position. The inferior glenohumeral ligament becomes tight in abduction, extension and external rotation, and limits anterior-inferior translocation in this position.

Other structures involved in stabilizing the glenohumeral joint include the coracohumeral ligament and bicipital tendon. The coracohumeral ligament is a broad thickening of the superior aspect of the capsule attaching the coracoid root to the greater tubercle of the humerus. The coracohumeral ligament has two bands, a posterior band and an anterior band. The anterior band is tensed during extension, and the posterior band is tensed during flexion. The tendon of the long head of the biceps functions as a ligament to strengthen the anterior portion of the glenohumeral joint capsule. Specifically, the biceps tendon helps diminish the stress placed on the inferior glenohumeral ligament (Rodosky et al 1994). The bicipital tendon contributes to the articular capsule of the humeral head. It originates from the supraglenoid tubercle and the glenoid labrum. It passes distally through the joint space and deep to the articular capsule. Because of its position, when the shoulder is abducted and the biceps contracts, the tendon of the long head compresses the humerus into the glenoid cavity, stabilizing the shoulder. The coracoacromial ligament is a taut band of dense connective tissue stretched between the coronoid process and the acromion. It forms and arches over the glenohumeral joint. It is in a position to impinge on the rotator cuff, especially its lateral band. It has been observed to be abnormally thickened in patients with rotator cuff tears (Soslowsky et al 1994).

Biomechanics

To some extent the shoulder complex has forfeited stability for almost 360° of multiplanar motion, more motion than any other joint in the body. This accomplishment depends upon the coordinated efforts of muscles, tendons and ligaments surrounding the glenohumeral joint and attaching it to the body wall. The various articular complexes of the shoulder are involved in even the most basic movements. Scapula rotation, adduction and elevation accompany most motions of the glenohumeral joint, likewise for rotation, depression and elevation of the clavicle. Consequently, well-orchestrated movement patterns of the upper extremity involve the balanced, coordinated actions of many muscles and joints. We are not born with these movement patterns in place; they develop. There are many changes occurring in the shoulder complex throughout early childhood. These changes are neurological and structural. At birth the motor neuron unit does not lend itself to coordinated muscle contraction due to redundant innervation patterns. As the motor neuron relation matures, such that a single motor

neuron innervates multiple motor neuron junctions, a group of muscle fibers develops the capacity to contract synchronistically. This is the beginning of coordinated movement (see Ch. 9). In fact, adult movement patterns during reaching only begin to appear after 3 years (Konczak & Dichgans 1997). Refinement of proprioceptive mapping further enhances this process. But efficient and effective action requires that the structural relationships of the muscles and joints be optimal for mechanical leveraging. Nowhere is this more important than in the upper extremity, where we have a long lever producing the finest movements in the body.

The muscles of the rotator cuff, the subscapularis, supraspinatus, infraspinatus and teres minor act as dynamic stabilizers of the glenohumeral joint. They stabilize the humeral head into the glenoid fossa as larger muscles such as the trapezius, deltoid and latissimus act on the joint. Contraction of the deltoid abducts and elevates the humerus. The counterforce of the rotator cuff muscles stabilizes the head of the humerus and prevents it from translating cephalad. The combined actions of the deltoid and rotator cuff result in abduction of the humerus. The subscapularis is the anterior stabilizer and is under the greatest strain when the arm is lifted over the head. The supraspinatus, infraspinatus and teres minor muscles act as posterior and superior stabilizers. Together the muscles of the rotator cuff also work in concert with the latissimus dorsi and pectoralis major muscles.

While the muscles of the rotator cuff stabilize and execute actions at the glenohumeral joint, the scapulothoracic and sternoclavicular areas are silent partners whose involvement is necessary for both stabilization and motion. If lacking, inappropriate forces are transferred to the muscles of the rotator cuff and other structures (Mottram 1997). In general, force load is evenly distributed over the muscles of the shoulder complex. However, when one muscle fatigues or strains, the force distribution changes (Jensen et al 2000). Scapular motion in particular plays an important role in rotator cuff function. Restrictions in scapular flare or elevation will change the contractile force, tension, length, and eccentric contractile loads placed on the muscles of the rotator cuff. In many cases it is the pain or injury to the muscles of the rotator cuff that brings the patient in for evaluation. But often a rotator cuff problem represents the accumulation of dysfunction and strain in other components of the shoulder complex.

At birth the range of motion of the shoulder is decreased due to previously mentioned posterior orientation of the humeral head and the functional mechanics in the clavicle. Internal rotation of the humerus is decreased, which affects pronation of the arm and adduction. This affects early movement mechanics. With the advent of structural and functional changes, the range of motion of the shoulder complex increases and the child is able to perfect the precision necessary for mature movement strategies.

ELBOW

The elbow represents the meeting of three separate bones – humerus, radius and ulna – and as such is really a complex of three interconnected joints: the humeroulnar, the humeroradial and the proximal radioulnar. The action of the elbow is described as a hinge, allowing flexion and extension; this action is coupled to rotation, allowing for supination and pronation of the forearm and wrist. These three joints share a common articular capsule, synovial membrane and supporting ligaments. As a unit, they are referred to as the cubital joint. The elbow is much more complex than the simple hinge joint it appears to be. The two forearm bones, the radius and ulna, attach to the humerus in totally different ways. The humeroulnar joint is indeed a true hinge joint, but the humeroradial joint is an arthrodial, or gliding, joint that acts more like an atypical ball-and-socket joint. As a result, the arm is slightly pronated during extension and slightly supinated during flexion.

Development

The elbow complex has primary and secondary ossification centers, some appearing as early as infancy and others not until mid-childhood. All of these centers close in mid-puberty and earlier in girls than boys. Because of the number and variability of growth areas, the elbow is more vulnerable to complicated injury in the pediatric population than the adult. The presence of multiple areas of growth in various phases of maturation in this population results in anatomical and biomechanical differences. The capitellum of the humerus does not begin to appear until the early part of the second year of life and then as a round knob adjacent to the humeral metaphysis rather than the flattened sphere of later life. Early in life the capitellum epiphysis is broader posterior than anterior. The radial head typically begins as a sphere sometime between 3 and 6 years, again earlier in girls than boys, and reaches its adult form and closes by 17 years. The medial epicondyle typically has two ossification centers that appear between 3 and 6 years in girls, and about 2 years later in boys. This is usually the last ossification area to fuse with the shaft of the humerus, sometime around 15–18 years. This area is quite vulnerable to shearing forces and avulsion fractures.

Articular complexes of the elbow

The cubital joint is a complex of three separate joints, humeroradial, humeroulnar and proximal radioulnar, which share a common articular capsule, synovial membrane and supporting ligaments.

The articular capsule is a broad, thin band of dense connective tissue that wraps around the cubital joint. Superiorly, it attaches to the humerus between the medial and lateral epicondyles, extending over the olecranon fossa posteriorly and over the coronoid and radial fossa anteriorly. Its inferior border attaches to the olecranon process of the ulna posteriorly and the annular ligament of the radius anteriorly. Clinically, the capsule divides into four parts: anterior, lateral, posterior and medial (Andrews & Whiteside 1993).

The cubital joint is lined by a synovial membrane which extends superiorly into the coronoid, radial and olecranon fossa and inferiorly under the annular ligament and into the space between the radial head and ulnar. Numerous fat pads surround the synovial membrane. The trochlea is often described as pulley-shaped with a central groove. The capitulum is rather sphere-shaped and flattened and lies laterally to the trochlea. The trochlea will articulate with the ulnar, whereas the capitulum articulates with the radius. The trochlear notch of the ulna corresponds in shape to the trochlea of the humerus.

The proximal surface of the radius is concave, snugly fitting the sphere of the capitulum into its cup. Superior to the joint, the radial fossa of the humerus receives the head of the radius in flexion. The humeroradial articulation is composed of the capitulum of the humerus and the slightly concave saucer-like disk of the radius. In spite of the joint's ball-and-socket structure, it is unable to abduct or adduct because of the annular ligament that encircles the radial head and binds it to the radial notch of the ulna. The radius, with its annular ligament and other ligamentous connections with the ulna, is prevented from moving independently. Adduction and abduction of the forearm is accompanied by a posterior and anterior movement of the radial head.

The humeroulnar articulation exists between the trochlea of the humerus and the trochlear notch of the ulna. The trochlea and the trochlear notch are not perfectly congruent. In full extension, the medial part of the upper olecranon is not in contact with the trochlea, and a corresponding strip on the lateral side loses contact during flexion. As a result, the principal swing (to and fro) of the hinge is accompanied by a screwing motion and conjunct rotation. The ulnar articular surface is a concave hook; the humeral surface, the trochlea, is convex. Superior to the joint, the coronoid fossa receives the coronoid process of the ulna on flexion. A groove separating the capitulum from the trochlea, the capitotrochlear groove, acts as a guide for the movement of the medial aspect of the radial head. The articulation of this joint provides the major stability against varus stress in full extension (55%) and at 90° flexion (75%) (Morrey & An 1983).

The proximal radioulnar joint includes the head of the radius, a cylindrical rim covered in articular cartilage, and the radial notch of the ulna, also covered with articular cartilage. The rim of the radial head fits against the radial notch. The two bones are secured together by the annular ligament and the quadrate ligament. These ligaments can be thought of as extensions of the ridge of the radial notch.

This articulation acts as a ball bearing, allowing limited rotation of the radial head upon the radial notch.

Resistance to valgus stress is divided equally between the anterior capsule, the articulation and the ulnar collateral ligament at full extension of the elbow; at 90° flexion, the task shifts somewhat to the ulnar collateral ligament (Morrey & An 1983). Resistance to varus stress is accomplished primarily by the articulation throughout the range of motion in the elbow. The forearm's major motions of pronation and supination involve the proximal radioulnar joint, the distal radioulnar joint and the intraosseous membrane. Rotation of the radial head upon the radial notch occurs at the superior radioulnar joint within the annular ligament. It is limited by the quadrate ligament. Rotation of the radial head also involves motion at the capitulum-radial joint.

The distal radioulnar joint is a uniaxial pivot joint between the convex distal ulnar head and the concave ulnar notch of the distal radius. The surfaces are enclosed in an articular capsule and held together by an articular disc. Restriction of motion in the joint may prevent the correction of the proximal radioulnar joint or vice versa. The overall shape of the radius has been compared to a crank (Kapandji 1982) which moves around the cylinder of the ulna. The muscles of pronation and supination act to 'wind' and 'unwind' the crank. During movement from pronation to supination, the articular disk of the inferior radioulnar joint literally sweeps across the articular surfaces, so that, in maximal pronation and supination, there is almost subluxation of the ulnar head. At the endpoint of range of motion, the articular disk is relaxed and the interosseous membrane is stretched. In the neutral position, the position of maximal stability, the articular disk has full contact with the articular surfaces, the disk is taut and the interosseous membrane is relaxed. The anterior and posterior ligaments are weak and provide no functional support for the joint. Stability of the articular surfaces of the inferior radioulnar joint is maintained by the interosseous membrane.

The interosseous membrane of the forearm is a thin but strong band of fibrous dense connective tissue that connects the shafts of the radius and ulna. It has been referred to as the middle radioulnar joint. In order for pronation and supination to occur, the radius must rotate around the ulna, effectively pivoting on the capitulum of the humerus. The superior and inferior radioulnar joints are coaxial. Effective movement requires that their respective axes of motion coincide with the fulcrum of pronation and supination, which passes through the heads of the radius and ulna (Kapandji 1982). The fibers of the interosseous membrane of the forearm slant downwards and medially from the interosseous border of the radius to the ulna. The membrane increases the extent of surface area for the attachment of the deep forearm muscles and also serves to connect the bones. It transmits forces from the hand and wrist to the radius and ulna and, then, to the humerus. There are foramina in the membrane for transmission of blood and lymph vessels and nerves. The applied anatomy of this membrane is of great significance to the osteopathic physician, in that arteries, veins, lymphatics and nerves pass through the interosseous membrane in between the anterior and posterior myofascial compartments. Restriction of motion due to proximal or distal dysfunctions can place a torque on the interosseous membrane, resulting in passive congestion in the forearm, wrist and hand. Unless relieved, this passive congestion could lead to dysfunction and eventual pathology such as myofascial contracture, muscle weakness and carpal tunnel syndrome.

Ligaments

The major ligaments of the elbow joint are the ulnar and radial collateral ligaments and the capsular ligament. The annular ligament of the proximal radioulnar joint is also important. These ligaments are very strong, so that trauma to the joint is more likely to fracture bone than tear ligaments. The ligaments also blend with each other and with the fascias of the associated muscles.

The three articulations of the elbow are completely enveloped in an extensive fibrous capsule. This is lined by a synovial membrane which extends into the proximal radioulnar articulation, covers the olecranon, coronoid and radial fossae and lines the annular ligament. Projecting into the joint from behind is a fold of synovial membrane, partly dividing the joint into humeroulnar and humeroradial parts. This fold contains a variable quantity of extrasynovial fat. Between the capsule and the synovial membrane are three other fat pads. The largest is over the olecranon fossa, the second over the coronoid fossa and third over the radial fossa.

The ulnar collateral ligament has three parts: anterior, oblique and inferior. It forms a triangle connecting the medial epicondyle of the humerus to the ridge of the olecranon fossa and to a medial tubercle of the ulnar. This complex provides the major support (55%) against valgus stress at 90° flexion and contributes equally with the articulation and anterior portion of the articulatory capsule at full extension (Morrey & An 1983). The anterior portion is taut throughout the full range of flexion (Regan et al 1991). Damage to this structure results in gross valgus instability of the elbow. The oblique portion of the ligament is contained along the margin of the olecranon fossa and is part of the joint capsule. The posterior portion becomes taut in flexion beyond 60°, but is not that critical to medial stability (Stroyan & Wilk 1993).

The radial collateral ligament is a band of tissue extending from the lateral epicondyle of the humerus to the annular ligament, blending with the extensor attachment of the forearm. This is a complex ligament in which several smaller bands have been described; this entire ligament only provides a small portion of the varus stability at full extension (14%) or at 90° flexion (9%) (Morrey & An 1983).

The annular ligament is a strong band of dense connective tissue which wraps around the radial head and is anchored to the radial notch of the ulna. Its proximal margin is fused with the articular cubital capsule and the radial collateral ligament. Its distal margin circumscribes the neck of the radius, between the head and the biceps tubercle. The inner surface of the annular ligament is lined with cartilage, where it is in contact with the radial head.

Biomechanics

Anatomically, the elbow consists of one joint cavity; however, physiologically, the joint has two distinct functions: flexion-extension and axial rotation (Kapandji 1982). There is generally 135° of flexion and 0–5° of extension at the elbow, and 90° each of supination and pronation.

Flexion and extension occur between the distal end of the humerus and the proximal ends of the ulna and radius. When the forearm is fully extended and the hand supinated, the upper arm and forearm are not in the same line; the forearm is directed somewhat laterally to form, with the upper arm, the 'carrying angle' of about 160° open to the lateral side. The angle is caused partly by the medial edge of the trochlea and partly by the obliquity of the superior articular surfaces of the coronoid process, which is not at right angles to the ulnar shaft. Because of the angles that the humeral and ulnar articulations make with the long axis of the bones, the 'carrying angle' disappears in full flexion. The 'carrying angle' is also masked by pronation of the extended forearm. This arrangement increases the precision with which the hand or anything in the hand can be controlled in full extension of the elbow. The normal carrying angle measures approximately 5° in the male and between 10° and 15° in females. This allows the elbow to fit closely into the depression at the waist. This angle is more noticeable when the hand is carrying something heavy. The muscles that flex the elbow are the brachialis, biceps and brachioradialis. The muscles that extend the elbow are the triceps and anconeus.

Pronation and supination involve two joints which are mechanically linked, the proximal and distal radioulnar joints (Kapandji 1982). The two joints work synchronistically to execute the motions from supination (palm superior and thumb lateral) through neutral rotation (palm medial and thumb superior) to pronation (palm inferior and thumb medial). When these motions are limited to the two radioulnar joints, the hand can turn through an arc of 140–150°. When accompanied by humeral rotation via elbow extension, the arc can increase to nearly 360°. Supination is stronger than pronation. The muscles which supinate the forearm are the supinator and biceps. The muscles which pronate the forearm are the pronator quadratus and pronator teres. Limitation of motion in either direction can be due to dysfunction at either the proximal or distal radioulnar articulations. Supination and pronation can be used to compensate for restriction of the shoulder joint and cervical spine. If the shoulder is limited in internal rotation, excessive pronation may occur. If it is restricted in external rotation, there may be excessive supination.

William Sutherland and other early osteopaths described supination and pronation as a complex motion involving the interosseous membrane of the forearm (Wales 1994). Within this model the radius turns about the ulna suspended from this shared fulcrum. Compression, strain and stress entering the forearm dissipate throughout the interosseous membrane and have the potential to affect its flexibility. Motion mechanics between the ulna and radius are influenced by the tensions and forces within the membrane. Likewise, flow dynamics through the vessels and lymphatics traveling along the membrane are affected by motions of the forearm and strains in the membrane.

Some minor motions of abduction and adduction are allowed at the humeroulnar articulation, with the radial head shifting slightly posteriorly and anteriorly on the capitulum with this motion. There are also minor motions of internal and external rotation at the humeroulnar articulation. Restrictions may occur in any of these motions.

WRIST

The wrist is a complex system composed of many articulations which function as three articular segments: the distal carpal row, the proximal carpal row, and the radioulnar articulation. These segments act as two articular complexes: the midcarpal joint and the radiocarpal joint. There are no direct muscular attachments to the proximal carpal row, so it acts as an intermediary between the radial articulation and the distal carpal row. The proximal row has been described as an intercalated segment, a relatively unattached middle segment of a three-segment linkage (Norkin & Levangie 1992).

Functional anatomy of the wrist

There are two functional joints in the wrist: the radiocarpal joint and the midcarpal joint. During pronation and supination of the distal radioulnar joint, the hand and radius move around the ulna. Wrist flexion and extension, and radial and ulnar deviation, involve intricate movements of the carpal bones. The majority of these movements occur among the bones of the proximal row, with the center of motion located somewhere in the proximal capitate (Nordin & Frankel 1989). Because wrist motion is so complex, the ligaments of the wrist must be able to provide support, allow intricate movement and transmit loads. The palmar ligaments are much thicker than the dorsal ligaments. There are also fewer dorsal ligaments.

The radiocarpal joint is between the radius and the proximal row of carpal bones. The proximal row of carpal bones (scaphoid, lunate and triquetrum) acts as a single convex surface which is cupped within the convex shape of the distal radius and ulna. Functionally for movements of the wrist, the radius and ulna act as a single articular surface. In fact, the ulna does not directly articulate with the carpal bones. It is separated by the triangular fibrocartilage complex, a connective tissue cushion which originates from the lunate fossa of the radius, covers the distal ulna, and inserts into the triquetrum, hamate and fifth metatarsal. It acts as a sling for the distal ulna and a stabilizer for the distal radioulnar joint, absorbing some of the axial load on the radius; so it participates as part of both the distal radioulnar joint and the radiocarpal joint. It has been demonstrated that removal of the triangular fibrocartilage complex results in 95% of the axial load being transferred to the radius and only 5% to the ulna, compared with 60% and 40% (Steinberg & Plancher 1995). The construction of the radioulnar joint favors flexion and ulnar deviation. The ligaments of the radiocarpal joint are described as being palmar extrinsic ligaments, because they originate on the radius and ulna. They can be divided into deep and superficial ligaments.

The palmar radiocarpal ligament has two portions, the radial and ulnar. The radial portion has a deep and superficial component. The superficial component is arranged in a 'V' shape. The deep component consists of three strong bands: the radioscaphocapitate, which supports the waist of the scaphoid; the radiolunate, which supports the lunate; and the radioscapholunate, which acts as a check to scaphoid flexion and extension. These ligaments play important roles in wrist movement by maintaining joint integrity, and checking the movement of joint surfaces. The ulnocarpal complex is composed of the radiotriquetral ligament (the meniscus homolog), the triangular fibrocartilage (the articular disc), the ulnolunate ligament, the ulnar collateral ligament and the dorsal and palmar radioulnar ligaments. The ulnar collateral, which runs between the ulna and the pisiform and triquetrum, provides passive control of frontal plane motion. The ulnocarpal ligament arises from the triangular fibrocartilage complex and attaches to the lunate, the capitate and the triquetrum.

The dorsal radiocarpal ligament is composed of three fascicles which originate on the rim of the radius and insert into the lunate, triquetrum and scaphoid. It is basically a thickening of the articular capsule. It limits wrist flexion and stabilizes the relationship between the lunate and the radius.

The midcarpal joint lies between the proximal and distal rows of carpal bones. It is composed of the scaphoid, lunate and triquetrum proximally, and the trapezium, trapezoid, capitate and hamate distally. The pisiform, which lies in the proximal row, does not participate in the radiocarpal articulation but instead functions as a sesamoid bone of the flexor carpi ulnaris. The midcarpal joint is a functional, rather than an anatomical, joint. The proximal carpal row functions as a 'variable geometric intercalated segment between the distal row and the radius-triangular fibrocartilage' (Steinberg & Plancher 1995). For example, during radial deviation, the scaphoid and lunate palmar flex, while the triquetrum moves proximally. In ulnar deviation, the scaphoid and lunate dorsiflex, while the triquetrum moves distally. The function of the scaphoid varies with motion in the sagittal plane versus the frontal plane. In flexion-extension movements of the wrist, the scaphoid will act as part of the distal row. In ulnar and radial deviation, the scaphoid functions as part of the proximal row. The midcarpal joint is described as a 'condyloid joint with two degrees of freedom' (Norkin & Levangie 1992). The architecture of this joint favors extension over flexion and radial deviation over ulnar deviation. This is opposite to the radiocarpal joint.

The ligaments of the midcarpal joint can be described as intrinsic palmar ligaments. They mainly consist of the deltoid ligaments (Steinberg & Plancher 1995), an inverted 'V'-shaped thickening of connective tissue running from the scaphoid and triquetrum with its apex at the capitate. This structure and the radiolunate-radioscapholunate ligaments form two 'V's, with their apices vertically aligned. Between these two complexes there is an inherently weak area which is filled with synovial fluid, the space of Poirier. The scapholunate and lunotriquetral ligaments form a connective band along the curve of the proximal carpal row. The scapholunate ligament tends to be the most frequently injured ligament in the wrist (Steinberg & Plancher 1995).

Biomechanics

Movement of the wrist occurs around two axes: a transverse axis lying in the frontal plane, around which flexion and extension occur; and an anterior-posterior axis lying in the sagittal plane, around which ulnar and radial deviation occur. The muscular forces which initiate wrist motion act on the distal carpal bones. The majority of motion can be accounted for by passive and active ligamentous forces which govern the mechanics of the carpal bones.

The range of motion in ulnar deviation (adduction) is more than twice that of radial deviation (abduction). Ulnar deviation ranges from 30° to 50°. When the forearm is pronated, ulnar deviation decreases by 25° to 30°. Full flexion and extension will also decrease these ranges. When the wrist moves into ulnar deviation from a neutral position, the distal row moves towards the ulna until checked by the ligaments. The triquetrum glides distally and extends. The hamate moves proximally, causing the proximal row to move radially, until limited by the radial ligaments. Extension of the triquetrum brings the lunate and scaphoid into an extended position, while the distal row palmar flexes (Norkin & Levangie 1992).

Range of motion in radial deviation (abduction) is generally limited to 15°. In full flexion or extension, this range is decreased. During radial deviation from a neutral position, the distal carpal row will move radially upon the proximal row until checked by the ulnar collateral and the ulnocarpal ligaments (Norkin & Levangie 1992). As the space between the trapezoid, scaphoid and radial styloid process narrows, the distal pole of the scaphoid rotates towards the palm. This motion is transmitted across the palmar row through the scapholunate ligament. The triquetrum moves proximally in relation to the hamate. The trapezoid, trapezium and capitate move into a relative extension position.

The range of motion of extension is 85°. Like flexion, it is limited when the forearm is in pronation. Sixty-seven percent of extension takes place at the radiocarpal joint, with 33% occurring at the midcarpal joint (Nordin & Frankel 1989). Extension is initiated at the distal carpal row. In a neutral position, the capitate and scaphoid are closely packed and their ligaments are taut. As the distal carpals glide into extension, the scaphoid moves with them on the relatively fixed lunate and triquetrum. At approximately 45° of extension, the scaphoid and lunate are brought into a close-packed position, so the carpal bones begin to act as a single unit moving on the radius and radioulnar disk (Norkin & Levangie 1992).

Wrist flexion is maximized when the carpal ligaments are relaxed, i.e. the forearm is in a neutral position. Flexion is generally accomplished to 85°. It is estimated that 60% of flexion occurs at the midcarpal joint and 40% at the radiocarpal joint (Nordin & Frankel 1989). Like extension, flexion is initiated at the distal carpal row. As the distal bones

move into a flexed position from neutral, they carry the scaphoid with them. As the ligaments become taut, the lunate and triquetrum follow the scaphoid into extension.

Circumduction is the combination of flexion, extension, abduction and adduction. It occurs about both the anterior-posterior axis and the transverse axis simultaneously.

The muscles of the wrist primarily provide stability for hand motion. They do not act directly on the carpal bones, and nor do they initiate wrist motion. Six muscles have tendons which cross the palmar aspect of the wrist and are capable of creating wrist flexion. Three are primarily wrist flexors, while three are primarily flexors of the digits with secondary effects in the wrist. All the muscles pass under the flexor retinaculum except for the palmaris longus.

CONCLUSION

The axiom 'Children are not just little adults' is well evidenced by the enormous changes undergone by the musculoskeletal system from birth through adulthood. Professionals interested in manual medicine and other 'hands-on' therapies need to be particularly well versed in the changes taking place, their influence on biomechanics, and the potential vulnerabilities created in the patient. Dealing with potential or early problems in the child may prevent chronic issues in the adult.

References

Andrews J R, Whiteside J A 1993 Common elbow problems in the athlete. J Orthop Sports Phys Ther 17: 289–295.

Beard R W, Highman J H, Pearce S et al 1984 Diagnosis of pelvic varicosities in women with chronic pelvic pain. Lancet 2: 946–949.

Beard R W, Reginald P W, Wadsworth J 1988a Clinical features of women with chronic lower abdominal pain and pelvic congestion. BJOG 95: 153–161.

Beard R, Reginald P, Pearce S 1988b Psychological and somatic factors in women with pain due to pelvic congestion. Adv Exp Med Biol 245: 413–421.

Cowgill L W 2007 Humeral torsion revisited: a functional and ontogenetic model for populational variation. Am J Phys Anthropol 134: 472–480.

Jensen B R, Laursen B, Sjogaard G 2000 Aspects of shoulder function in relation to exposure demands and fatigue – a mini review. Clin Biomech 15(Suppl 1): S17–S20.

Kapandji I A 1982 The physiology of the joints. Churchill Livingstone, Edinburgh.

Klein-Nulend J, van der Plas A, Semeins C M et al 1995 Sensitivity of osteocytes to biomechanical stress in vitro. FASEB J 9(5): 441–445.

Konczak J, Dichgans J 1997 The development toward stereotypic arm kinematics during reaching in the first 3 years of life. Exp Brain Res 117: 346–354.

Krahl V E 1976 The phylogeny and ontogeny of humeral torsion. Am J Phys Anthropol 45: 595–599.

Matsen F A, Harryman D T, Sidles J A 1991 Mechanics of glenohumeral instability. Clin Sports Med 10: 783–788.

McKern T W, Stewart T D 1957 Skeletal age changes in young American males, Tech Rep EP 45. Environmental Protection Research Div, Natick, Massachusetts.

Morrey B F, An K N 1983 Articular and ligamentous contributions to the stability

of the elbow joint. Am J Sports Med 11: 315–319.

Mottram S L 1997 Dynamic stability of the scapula. Man Ther 2: 123–131.

Nordin M, Frankel V H 1989 Basic biomechanics of the musculoskeletal system. Lea and Febiger, Philadelphia.

Norkin C C, Levangie P C 1992 Joint structure and function. FA Davis, Philadelphia.

Pappas A D, Goss T P, Kleinman P K 1983 Symptomatic shoulder instability due to lesions of the glenoid labrum. Am J Sports Med 11: 279–288.

Peacock A 2007 Observations on the prenatal development of the intervertebral disc in man. J Anat 85: 260–274.

Regan W D, Korinek B F, An K N 1991 Biomechanical study of ligaments around the elbow joint. Clin Orthop Relat Res 271: 170–179.

Rodosky M W, Harner C D, Fu F H 1994 The role of the long head of the biceps muscle and superior glenoid labrum in anterior stability of the shoulder. Am J Sports Med 22: 121–130.

Sensenig E 1949 The early development of the human vertebral column. Contrib Embryol 33: 21–49.

Snijders C J, Vleeming A, Stoeckart R 1993 Transfer of the lumbarsacral load to iliac bones and legs. Clin Biochem 8: 285–294.

Soslowsky L J, An C H, Carpenter J E 1994 Geometric and mechanical properties or the coracoacromial ligament and their relationship to rotator cuff disease. Clin Orthop Relat Res 304: 10–17.

Standring S (ed.) 2004 Gray's anatomy, 39th edn. Churchill Livingstone, New York.

Steinberg B G, Plancher K D 1995 Clinical anatomy of the wrist and elbow. Clin Sports Med 14: 299–313.

Stroyan M, Wilk K E 1993 The functional anatomy of the elbow complex. J Orthop Sports Phys Ther 17: 279–288.

Theiler K 1988 Vertebral malformations. Adv Anat Embryol Cell Biol 112: 1–99.

Verbout A J 1985 The development of the vertebral column. Adv Anat Embryol Cell Biol 90: 1–122.

Vleeming A, Pool-Goudzwaard A L, Stoeckart R et al 1995 The posterior layer of the thoracolumbar fascia: its function in load transfer from spine to legs. Spine 20: 753–758.

Wales A L 1994 Biomechanics of the forearm. Personal communication.

Willard F H, Carreiro J E, Manko W 1998 The long posterior interosseous ligament and the sacrococcygeal plexus. Third Interdisciplinary World Congress on Low Back and Pelvic Pain.

Further reading

Adams M A, Dolan P 1995 Posture and spinal mechanisms during lifting. In: Vleeming A, Mooney V, Snijders C J, Dorman T (eds) The integrated function of the lumbar spine and sacroiliac joints. European Conference Organ, Rotterdam: 19–28.

Adams M A, Dolan P 1995 Recent advances in lumbar spinal mechanics and their clinical significance. Clin Biochem 10(1): 3–19.

Anetzberger H, Putz R 1996 The scapula: principles of construction and stress. Acta Anat Basel 156(1): 70–80.

Arbuckle J D, McGrouther D A 1995 Measurement of the arc of digital flexion and joint movement ranges. J Hand Surg [Br] 20B(6): 836–840.

Archer I A, Dickson R A 1985 Stature and idiopathic scoliosis. A prospective study. J Bone Joint Surg [Br] 67: 185–188.

Ash H E, Joyce T J, Unsworth A 1996 Biomechanics of the distal upper limb. Curr Orthop 10(1): 25–36.

Beal M C 1982 The sacroiliac problem: review of anatomy, mechanics and diagnosis. J Am Osteopath Assoc 81: 667–679.

Beal M C, Dvorak J 1984 Palpatory examination of the spine: a comparison of the results of two methods and their relationship to visceral disease. Manual Medicine 1: 25–32.

Berthier N E, Clifton R K, McCall D D et al 1999 Proximodistal structure of early reaching in human infants. Exp Brain Res 127(3): 259–269.

Britz G W, Haynor D R, Kuntz C et al 1996 Ulnar nerve entrapment at the elbow: correlation of magnetic resonance imaging, clinical, electrodiagnostic, and intraoperative findings. Neurosurgery 38(3): 458–465.

Browning J E 1990 Mechanically induced pelvic pain and organic dysfunction in a patient without low back pain. J Manipulative Physiol Ther 13: 406–411.

Burnett C, Johnson E 1971 Development of gait in childhood II. Dev Med Child Neurol 13(2): 207–215.

Dandy D J 1996 Chronic patellofemoral instability. J Bone Joint Surg [Br] 78B(2): 328–335.

Dorman T A, Vleeming A 1995 Self-locking of the sacroiliac articulation. Spine 9: 407–418.

Fernandez-Bermejo E, Garcia-Jimenez M A, Fernandez-Palomeque C et al 1993 Adolescent idiopathic scoliosis and joint laxity. Spine 18: 918–922.

Fuss F K, Wagner T F 1996 Biomechanical alterations in the carpal arch and hand muscles after carpal tunnel release: a further approach toward understanding the function of the flexor retinaculum and the cause of postoperative grip weakness. Clin Anat 9(2): 100–108.

Gordon A M, Soechting J F 1995 Use of tactile afferent information in sequential finger movements. Exp Brain Res 107(2): 281–292.

Greenman P E 1990 Clinical aspects of sacroiliac function in walking. Journal of Manual Medicine 5: 125–130.

Greenman P E 1991 Principles of manipulation of the cervical spine. Journal of Manual Medicine 6: 106–113.

Gwinnutt C L 1988 Injury to the axillary nerve. Anaesthesia 43(3): 205–206.

Haggard P, Hutchinson K, Stein J 1995 Patterns of coordinated multi-joint movement. Exp Brain Res 107(2): 254–266.

Hall J E 1996 Three-dimensional effect of the Boston brace on the thoracic spine and rib cage – point of view. Spine 21(1): 64.

Hay M C 1976 Anatomy of the lumbar spine. Med J Aust 1(23): 874–876.

Hollowell J P, Vollmer D G, Wilson C R et al 1996 Biomechanical analysis of thoracolumbar interbody constructs – how important is the endplate? Spine 21(9): 1032–1036.

Horton W C, Holt R T, Muldowny D S 1996 Controversy fusion of L5-S1 in adult scoliosis. Spine 21(21): 2520–2522.

Hutton W C 1990 The forces acting on a lumbar intervertebral joint. Journal of Manual Medicine 5: 66–67.

Johnston R B, Seiler J G, Miller E J et al 1995 The intrinsic and extrinsic ligaments of the wrist. A correlation of collagen typing and histologic appearance. J Hand Surg (Br) 20B(6): 750–754.

Kaigle A M, Holm S H, Hansson T H 1995 Experimental instability in the lumbar spine. Spine 20(4): 421–430.

Kalin P J, Hirsche B E 1987 The origins and function of the interosseous muscles of the foot. J Anat 152: 83–91.

Kindsfater K, Lowe T, Lawellin D et al 1994 Levels of platelet calmodulin for the prediction of progression and severity of adolescent idiopathic scoliosis. J Bone Joint Surg [Am] 76(8): 1186–1192.

Kissling R O 1995 The mobility of the sacro-iliac joint in healthy subjects. In: Vleeming A, Mooney M, Dorman T et al (eds) The integrated function of the lumbar spine and sacroiliac joint. ECO, Rotterdam: 411–422.

Klein P, Mattys S, Rooze M 1996 Moment arm length variations of selected muscles acting on talocrural and subtalar joints during movement: an in vitro study. J Biochem 29(1): 21–30.

Lehman G J, McGill S M 1999 The influence of a chiropractic manipulation on lumbar kinematics and electromyography during simple and complex tasks: a case study. J Manipulative Physiol Ther 22(9): 576–581.

Macintosh J E, Bogduk N 1986 The biomechanics of the lumbar multifidus. Clin Biochem 1: 205–213.

Machida M 1999 Cause of idiopathic scoliosis. Spine 24(24): 2576–2583.

Machida M, Dubousset J, Imamura Y et al 1996 Melatonin – a possible role in pathogenesis of adolescent idiopathic scoliosis. Spine 21(10): 1147–1152.

Machida M, Murai I, Miyashita Y et al 1999 Pathogenesis of idiopathic scoliosis. Experimental study in rats. Spine 24(19): 1985–1989.

Magoun H I S 1973 Idiopathic adolescent spinal scoliosis. DO 13(6).

McGregor A H, McCarthy I D, Hughes S P 1995 Motion characteristics of the lumbar spine in the normal population. Spine 20(22): 2421–2428.

Mitchell F L, Moran P S, Pruzzo N A 1979 An evaluation and treatment manual of osteopathic muscle energy procedures. Mitchell, Moran and Pruzzo, Valley Park, MO.

Mosca V S 1995 Flexible flatfoot and skewfoot. J Bone Joint Surg [Am] 77A(12): 1937–1945.

Moseley L, Smith R, Hunt A et al 1996 Three-dimensional kinematics of the rearfoot during the stance phase of walking in normal young adult males. Clin Biochem 11(1): 39–45.

Oda I, Abumi K, Lü D S et al 1996 Biomechanical role of the posterior elements, costovertebral joints, and rib cage in the stability of the thoracic spine. Spine 21(12): 1423–1429.

Ogon M, Haid C, Krismer M et al 1996 The possibility of creating lordosis and correcting scoliosis simultaneously after partial disc removal – balance lines of lumbar motion segments. Spine 21(21): 2458–2462.

Panjabi M M, White A 1990 Clinical biomechanics of the spine. JB Lippincott, Philadelphia.

Patwardhan A G, Rimkus A, Gavin T M et al 1996 Geometric analysis of coronal decompensation in idiopathic scoliosis. Spine 21(10): 1192–1200.

Perry J 1983 Anatomy and biomechanics of the hindfoot. Clin Orthop Rel Res 177: 9–15.

Pincott J R, Davies J S, Taffs L F 1984 Scoliosis caused by section of dorsal spinal nerve roots. J Bone Joint Surg [Br] 66(1): 27–29.

Pincott J R, Taffs L F 1982 Experimental scoliosis in primates: a neurological cause. J Bone Joint Surg [Br] 64(4): 503–507.

Prasad R, Vettivel S, Isaac B et al 1996 Angle of torsion of the femur and its correlates. Clin Anat 9(2): 109–117.

Raschke U, Chaffin D B 1996 Trunk and hip muscle recruitment in response to external anterior lumbosacral shear and moment loads. Clin Biochem 11(3): 145–152.

Reddy N P, Krouskop T A, Newell P H Jr. 1975 Biomechanics of a lymphatic vessel. Blood Vessels 12: 261–278.

Rupp S, Berninger K, Hopf T 1995 Shoulder problems in high level swimmers – impingement, anterior instability, muscular imbalance? Int J Sports Med 16(8): 557–562.

Scholz J P, Millford J P, McMillan A G 1995 Neuromuscular coordination of squat lifting I: effect of load magnitude. Phys Ther 75(2): 119–132.

Shekelle P G, Coulter I 1997 Cervical spine manipulation: summary report of a systematic review of the literature and a multidisciplinary expert panel. J Spinal Disord 10(3): 223–228.

Stubbs M, Harris M, Solomonow M et al 1998 Ligamento-muscular protective reflex in the lumbar spine of the feline. J Electromyogr Kinesiol 8(4): 197–204.

Sutherland D, Olsen R, Cooper L et al 1980 The development of mature gait. J Bone Joint Surg [Am] 62: 354–363.

Taylor J R, Slinger B S 1980 Scoliosis screening and growth in Western Australian students. Med J Aust 1: 475–478.

Thompson P, Volpe R (eds) 2001 Introduction to podopediatrics. Churchill Livingstone, Edinburgh.

Van Dieën J H, Böke B, Oosterhuis W et al 1996 The influence of torque and velocity on erector spinae muscle fatigue and its relationship to changes of electromyogram spectrum density. Eur J Appl Physiol 72(4): 310–315.

Vleeming A, Snijders C J, Stoeckart R et al 1995 A new light on low back pain: the selflocking mechanism of the sacroiliac joints and its implication for sitting, standing and walking. In: Vleeming A, Mooney V, Snijders C J et al (eds) The integrated function of the lumbar spine and sacroiliac joints. European Conference Organ, Rotterdam: 149–168.

Wu P B, Date E S, Kingery W S 2000 The lumbar multifidus muscle is polysegmentally innervated. Electromyogr Clin Neurophysiol 40(8): 483–485.

Yahia L, Rhalmi S, Newman N et al 1992 Sensory innervation of human thoracolumbar fascia. An immunohistochemical study. Acta Orthop Scand 63(2): 195–197.

Yamada K, Yamamoto H, Nakagawa Y et al 1984 Etiology of idiopathic scoliosis. Clin Orthop Rel Res 184: 50–57.

Chapter Three

Development of the cranium

3

INTRODUCTION

Children have great potential. One of our prime roles as osteopaths is to support that potential through our work with the neuromusculoskeletal system. When you look at a child, you do not know what or who they can be. When you look at an adult, you never know what or who they could have been. You do not know the unmanifested potential that is still dormant, because it has not been or is not supported. In order to begin to look at the hidden potential within each child, we need to come to a rather obvious realization. Children are very different from adults. They are different psychologically, emotionally, spiritually and physiologically. Many tissue structures are very different in children, and as anybody knows who has ever put their hands on a child, the quality of what you palpate, what you sense and what you experience when you are with them is unique. To begin to get an understanding of these differences, we need to look at the adult, because that is the endpoint. That is what the child becomes.

The adult cranium is often viewed as a modified sphere balancing atop a flexible rod. The fact that there are 29 distinct bones joined by harmonic, serrated, beveled and gomphotic sutures is too often forgotten. If all we needed from the head was a protected space for our brain and a soft tissue tube through which to pass food, air and water, why didn't we get just that? Instead, we have a very intricate arrangement of bones, connective tissue and muscles which protect and facilitate the functions of many delicate structures. The 23 bones of the head (excluding the ossicles) started out as many tiny centers of ossification scattered throughout a connective tissue matrix. At birth, many of these bones are in parts and most of them are still cartilaginous. There are six major fontanelles, or soft spots, located between adjoining bones in the vault: bregma at the cranium, these dural structures are described as a series of sickles: the vertically oriented falx cerebri, the two horizontal sickles of the tentorium cerebelli and a small fourth sickle, the falx cerebelli, which is located inferior to the tentorium under the cerebellum. During development, the larger of these intracranial sickles are referred to as dural septa. The falx cerebri is called the median longitudinal septum, and the tentorium cerebelli is referred to as the posterior transverse septum. There is another septum that we will discuss which is often not spoken about in the adult. It is called the anterior transverse septum, and within it lie a tiny venous sinus and the rudimentary lesser wings of the sphenoid.

The layers of the cranium

The adult neurocranium or vault is made of a series of bony plates. If we lifted the vault away and peered into the cranium, we would see a membranous bag, inside which is the brain (Fig. 3.2). This membranous bag is divided by a series of internal partitions, the previously described dural septae. The internal partitions are anchored to the bag, and the bag is anchored to the inside of the bony plates. In fact, the internal partitions and the bag develop from the same tissue and are continuous (Fig. 3.3). These tissues start from one layer of mesenchyme. The mesenchyme will be subdivided into periosteum, bone and dura, and is eventually classified by its divisions. Once we classify it into separate layers, we lose the notion of common origin. We also lose the notion that the bag surrounding the brain is continuous with the dural septae supporting the brain and the periosteum that surrounds the bones. The connective tissues are continuous through the sutures (Fig. 3.4). The bone is formed in the middle of the mesenchymal layer, such that the bone is actually embedded within the layer of mesenchyme. The membrane is continuous across the sutures, and the partitions separating the differing portions of the central nervous system are continuous with the layer surrounding the cranial bones.

Anatomy of the meninges

We can appreciate the continuity of these tissues if we look at the meningeal layers of the cranium at the electron microscopic level (Fig. 3.5). The pial layer is closely adherent to the brain through the glial end-feet. A series of membranous or arachnoid trabeculae extend up from the pia to a membranous arachnoid layer. The cerebrospinal fluid lies within this subarachnoid space. A potential space is usually depicted between the arachnoid and the meningeal dura layer. However, there is actually a transition layer present, in which fibroblasts of the dural layer are woven together with the arachnoid barrier. The dura is described as two layers, inner and outer. The fibroblasts of the inner dura are slightly different at the electron microscopic level in size

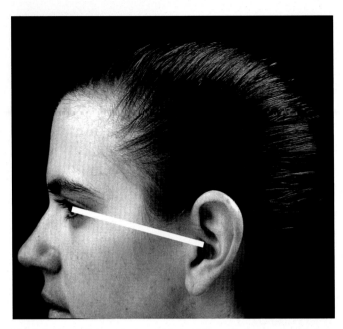

Fig. 3.1 • Lateral view of a human head. The white line represents the position of the median axial stem. *Used with permission of the Willard & Carreiro Collection.*

top of the head, lambda towards the back and a pterion and asterion on each side. In the newborn the sutures between the vault bones are quite plastic and flexible. These characteristics do not change 'overnight' after the child is born. They linger, accommodating growth and development into the early adult years and beyond.

The adult anatomy is our reference point for understanding embryology. Imagine a line that passes along the skull between the eyes and the ears (Fig. 3.1). This line reflects a base or platform, which extends right through the skull. In early development it is called the median axial stem. Everything superior to the line is the vault or neurocranium, the arch that houses the brain. Inferior to the line lie a series of rolled arches, the visceral cranium or face. This base is a major landmark during development. It plays a critical role in the formation of both the neurocranium above and the visceral cranium below. The median axial stem forms a platform to which all the membranous layers of the cranium are attached. All the bones of the cranium develop and are supported in these membranous layers. During development some of the layers will remain membranous and others will become periosteum, but they are all anchored to the median axial stem.

PRENATAL DEVELOPMENT OF THE CRANIUM

The membranes within the cranium are arranged into dural struts or walls that compartmentalize the inner cranial space and provide a support system for the brain. In the adult

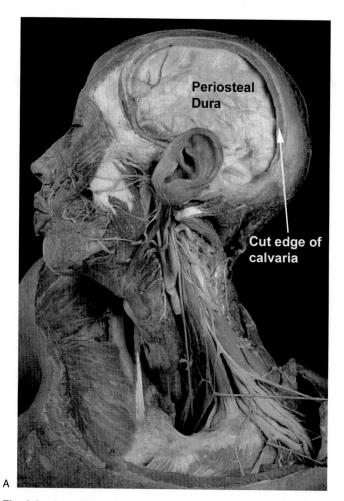

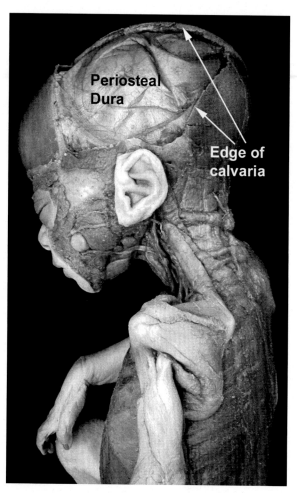

Fig. 3.2 • Adult (A) and neonate (B) view. The parietal bone has been removed in each case to reveal the periosteal dura (internal periosteal layer). *Used with permission of the Willard & Carreiro Collection.*

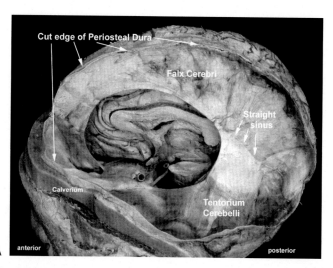

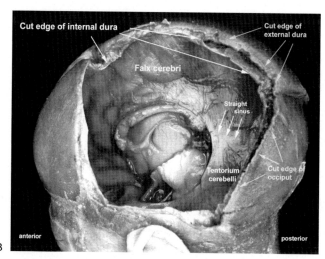

Fig. 3.3 • Adult (A) and neonate (B) specimens. The cranial vault and one hemisphere of cortex have been removed, revealing the continuity of the falx cerebri and tentorium cerebelli. The two layers of dura, external (periosteal) and internal, are indicated by the arrows. This is easier to visualize on the newborn specimen; however, the separation can also be seen on the adult. *Used with permission of the Willard & Carreiro Collection.*

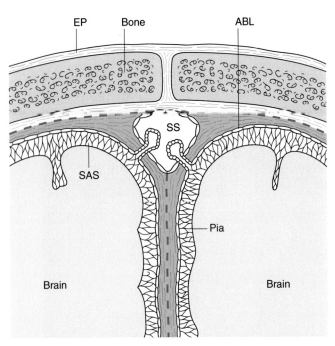

Fig. 3.4 • Schematic diagram depicting the continuity of the intracranial tissues and the external periosteum. SAS, subarachnoid space; EP, external periosteum; SS, sagittal sinus; ABL, arachnoid barrier layer. The light layer beneath the bone represents the internal periosteum, and the darker area represents the internal dura.

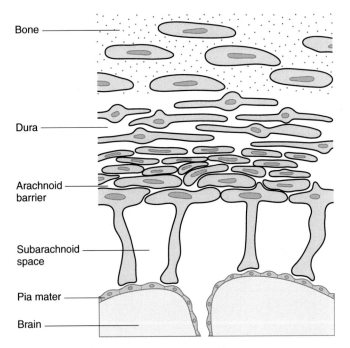

Fig. 3.5 • Schematic diagram of meningeal layers.

and in organelle structure from the fibroblasts of the outer layer, which are periosteal fibroblasts. The connective tissue layers are woven together at the cellular level from the surface of the brain to the cranial bones. It is often assumed,

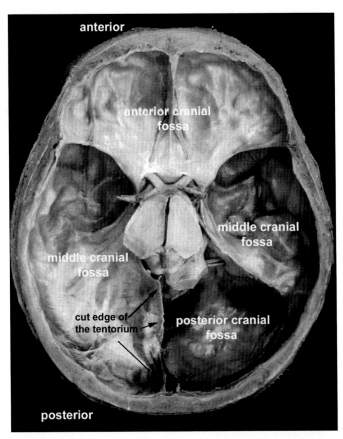

Fig. 3.6 • Superior view looking into the cranium. The cortex has been removed, and the tentorium is still in place on the left side of the specimen. The cerebellum and tentorium have been removed on the right side to visualize the posterior cranial fossa. *Used with permission of the Willard & Carreiro Collection.*

mistakenly, that there is a discontinuity between the arachnoid and dura; however, the tissue layers are continuous. Any space present is pathological. Subarachnoid hemorrhages occur in the trabecular space, tearing through the arachnoid trabeculae. Subdural hemorrhages cleave the transitional zone between the dura and arachnoid. In the cranium, the epidural space is a potential space just below the skull, unlike the true space found in the spine. The fact that there is a continuum of tissue is very important; something influencing the septae intracranially can influence the external tissue and vice versa. The connective tissue and bony structures of the cranium form a continuum differing by cell size and cell number.

If we remove the brain and look into a skull, we can see the 'footprint' of the brain (Fig. 3.6). You might want to ask yourself how it is that something as soft and as delicate as neural tissue, with the consistency of tapioca pudding, could leave a footprint in a hard bony structure. To answer this question, we need to appreciate how soft and delicate these bony structures are as they are forming from mesenchyme.

The struggle between the brain and the heart

Mesenchyme can be thought of as an omnipotent tissue, in that it will develop into what seem to be very different types of tissues. In the cranium, the bones, periosteum and meninges all develop from mesenchyme. Mesenchyme responds differently, depending on the forces that act on it. When it is stretched, it develops into membrane; when it is compressed, it turns to cartilage, and that is basically the place where this all begins. Very early in development, a layer of mesenchyme surrounds the neural tube, which is the primitive brain. As the neural tube begins to elongate and grow, change its shape and move into its adult form, it drags some of the mesenchyme with it. The notochord is an axis or central plate, which extends from one end of the neural tube to the other when the neural tube first forms. The early development of the neural tube is oriented to the notochord. The neural tube overgrows the notochord and bends down in front of it. That growth and bending is driven by the enlargement of the neural tube. The precordial plate (the buccopharyngeal membrane) is positioned anterior superior to the neural tube. Mesoblast cells migrate along the notochord and coalesce around the prechordal plate. These cells are the precursors to the heart and pericardium. As the neural tube expands and the mesoblastic cells multiply, the cardiogenic mesenchyme moves ventral to the notochord (Fig. 3.7). In other words, the heart starts on top of your head and then swings in an arch to come into position in the thorax. When this movement of the heart occurs, mesenchyme is pinned between it and the neural tube. This mesenchyme is under compression as the heart grows below and the brain grows above. In response to the compressive force, the mesenchyme begins to thicken up and form cartilage. As the neural tube expands sideways and the heart widens, this mesenchymal thickening expands laterally. A thickened plate of tissue centered on the notochord and underlying the neural tube is formed. This plate will develop into the primitive basiocciput, basisphenoid and ethmoid, the median axial stem. A portion of this plate will thicken and undergo chondrogenesis around the primitive pituitary. (In the neonate, the remnant of the tip of the notochord is in the body of the sphenoid just inferior to the pituitary.) When the heart finally drops into place in the thorax, the pharyngeal space is formed between it and the mesenchymal plate. Meanwhile, the neural tube is creating a series of bulges as it grows superiorly, posteriorly, inferiorly and anteriorly, like a ram's horns or a 'C'-shaped curl (Fig. 3.8). All of the brain structures are going to be influenced by this C-shaped curl. This is how the ventricles get their C-shaped curl. This is how the hippocampus gets its curl. For example, the temporal lobes, which start out on the anterior aspect of the neural tube, grow through this ram's horn configuration, to end up in the middle cranial fossa.

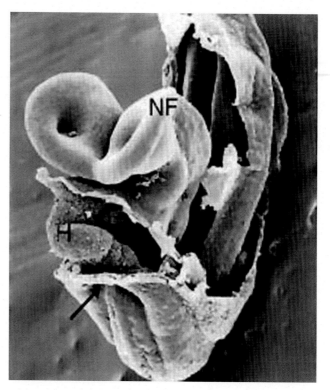

Fig. 3.7 • Ventral view of embryo showing neural fold (NF) and heart (H). The arrow indicates the opening to the foregut. *Used with permission from Williams P (ed.) 1995 Gray's anatomy, 38th edn. Churchill Livingstone, London.*

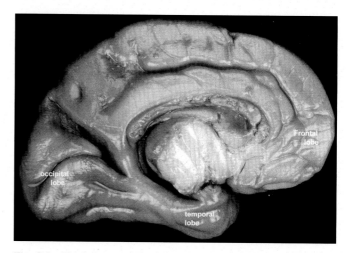

Fig. 3.8 • The left cerebral hemisphere viewed from the medial side. *Used with permission of the Willard & Carreiro Collection.*

The role of mesenchyme

One of the unfortunate things in looking at embryology texts is that they often depict an isolated brain going through a series of bends and folds. But the brain is not isolated; it is bending and folding within a mesenchymal envelope. The brain is attached to the innermost surface of

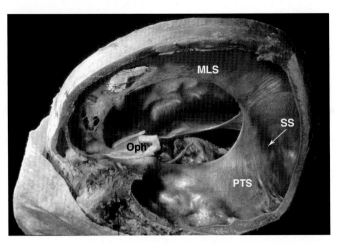

Fig. 3.9 • View from a superior posterior perspective into the adult cranium with the neural tissue removed. The ophthalmic chiasm (Oph) is still in place. The straight sinus (SS) is identified. The dural septa or intracranial membranes are intact. One can see the continuity between the median longitudinal septum (MLS, the adult falx) and the posterior transverse septum (PTS, the adult tentorium). This arrangement was created by the 'C-shaped' movement of the developing neural tube and mimics its silhouette (compare with previous figure). *Used with permission of the Willard & Carreiro Collection.*

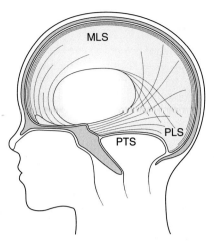

Fig. 3.10 • Schematic diagram of the intracranial dural septae. The median longitudinal (MLS), posterior transverse (PTS) and posterior longitudinal (PLS) septa are labeled. Figure 3.9 is a dissection of the dural septae in the adult. *Adapted from Blechschmidt E, Gasser R 1978 Biokinetics and biodynamics of human differentiation. Charles C Thomas, Springfield.*

the envelope, and as a result its growth will influence the mesenchyme. In fact, the brain is going to create a series of folds and struts inside the mesenchymal envelope that will end up becoming the partitions or dural septae (Figs 3.9, 3.10). As the neural tube differentiates into the brain and spinal cord, the mesenchyme that envelopes the brain also differentiates. It begins to cleave into different layers or zones. But these are not separated layers. Rather, it is the potential of the tissue of these two layers or zones which has changed. The inner zone, the endomeninx, will go on to form the pia and arachnoid. They will be adherent to each other, to the brain and to the outer layer, the ectomeninx. The layer of ectomeninx will be divided by the cranial bone to form an inside layer of inner periosteum and dura, and an outside layer called the external periosteum. This is a very unfortunate choice of terms, because one gets the impression that one layer is to the outside and separate from everything deep to the bone. However, the bone forms in the center of the ectomeninx layer and 'spreads' out, dividing the ectomeninx into two periosteal layers. The inner layer or portion of this periosteal layer specializes into what we eventually call dura.

The biochemical potential of the endomeninx is different from that of the ectomeninx. In a human, the endomeninx does not ossify, while the ectomeninx can ossify in response to appropriate stimuli. The ectomeninx can change in other ways also. Ectomeninx will thicken and form a membrane, which rapidly turns to cartilage when it is compressed. This

cartilage will undergo endochondro-ossification, much like a long bone, except that no periosteal ring will form. The endochondro-ossification process is typified by the mesenchyme that is compressed at the base of the growing brain. This mesenchyme quickly converts to cartilage as the median axial stem. Eventually, it will ossify as the cranial base. Other areas of that same ectomeninx zone of mesenchyme will be stretched. Under the influence of tensile forces, it will thicken up to form a membrane but, instead of converting to cartilage, it will stay membranous until it begins to ossify. This is called intramembranous ossification. The bony plates of the vault will develop in this way, growing towards each other to meet at what will one day be the suture.

The inner dural layer is the layer that does not have the potential to develop into bone. Through the glia, this layer is adherent to the brain and thus influenced by its growth. Mesenchyme has mucoid characteristics; it is rather sticky and closely adherent to the neural tube. Initially, the neural tube is just that, a tube. Then the anterior crests grow superiorly, posteriorly, inferiorly and anteriorly, like a ram's horn. The mucoid layer of mesenchyme that is closely adherent to this neural tube gets dragged along with the developing brain. The effect of that movement is dispersed differently through the mucoid tissue. Cells that are very close to the neural tube become a thin layer of pia closely adherent to the brain tissue. The mesenchymal cells which are further away will also be dragged along, but these cells do not exactly follow all the contours of the brain. Instead, they are influenced by the movement of the developing

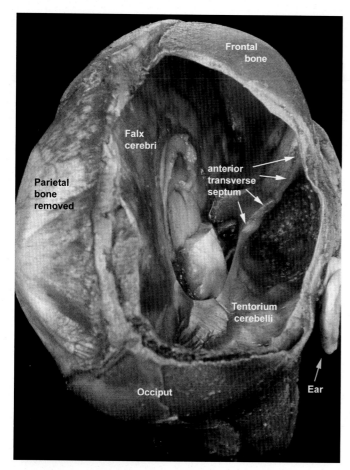

Fig. 3.11 • Posterolateral view taken from behind a neonatal specimen. The right cortical hemisphere has been removed, revealing the middle and anterior cranial fossa. The falx and tentorium are in place. The anterior transverse septum (ATS) would have laid along the plane of the lesser wing of the sphenoid, separating the frontal and temporal lobes. This cartilaginous tissue is where the ATS would have been in the fetus. *Used with permission of the Willard & Carreiro Collection.*

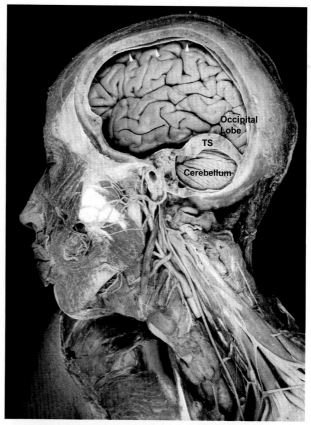

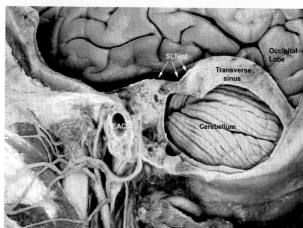

Fig. 3.12 • (A, B) Lateral views of an adult specimen. Parts of the parietal and temporal bone have been removed to reveal the tentorium lying between the occipital lobe and cerebellum. The external wall of the transverse sinus is seen. Arrowheads depict the periosteal dural layer. Transverse sinus (TS): the two layers of the tentorium split; the superior layer (SLTent) is continuous with the periosteum over the superior aspect of the petrous portion.

lobes of the neural tube. There are four lobes on each side of the primitive brain: the cerebellum, occipital, temporal and frontal. As the lobes of the brain move into their adult positions, they compress the mesenchyme between them. The compressed mesenchyme between the lobes is referred to as dural girdles. The temporal lobe meets the frontal lobe anteriorly at the frontotemporal approximation. The mesenchyme between those two lobes will be the anterior transverse septum, which will develop into the inferior wings of the sphenoid (Fig. 3.11). Posteriorly, the occipital lobe grows down to meet the cerebellum which is growing up. Each is covered with mesenchyme. The mesenchyme between these two lobes (occipital and cerebellum) forms the posterior transverse septum. It will become the tentorium cerebelli, within which lies the transverse sinus

(Fig. 3.12). The two cortical hemispheres meet in the midline as they grow up and back. The mesenchyme in the midline will form the corticocortical approximation, which will become the falx cerebri (see Fig. 3.11).

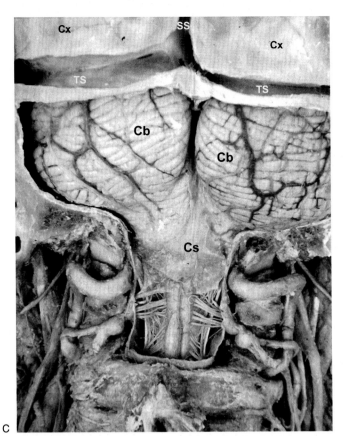

C

Fig. 3.12 • (C) is a posterior view of an adult specimen with the occiput removed; the external wall of the transverse and sagittal sinuses and periosteal dura covering the cerebellum have been dissected away. The spinal cord and exiting nerve roots are visualized. A cisterna magna lies between the cerebellar hemispheres. EAC, external auditory canal; SS, sagittal sinus; TS, transverse sinus; Cb, cerebellum; Cs, cistern; Cx, cortex. *Used with permission of the Willard & Carreiro Collection.*

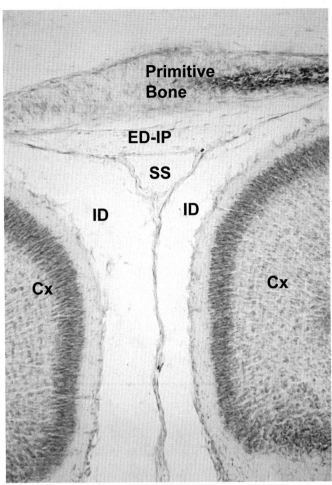

Fig. 3.13 • Sagittal view of a histological tissue section through a developing possum brain (it is similar to the human), depicting the two cortical hemispheres (Cx), and the two layers of internal dura (ID) meeting to form the falx cerebri. The external dura or internal periosteum (ED-IP) can be seen forming the external wall of the sagittal sinus (SS). Primitive bone can be seen developing in the superficial mesenchymal layers. *Used with permission of the Willard & Carreiro Collection.*

Innervation patterns follow the movement of the mesenchyme

The pattern of innervation in the cranial fossa and meninges is derived from the embryological origins of the mesenchyme. The mesenchyme carries its innervation. As the cerebellar bud expands and meets the growing occipital lobe, the mesenchymal layers of each meet to form the posterior transverse septum or the tentorium cerebelli. The inferior layer of the tentorium came from mesenchyme in the lower part of the primitive brainstem. It is innervated by cervical spinal neurons. The superior layer originated in the anterior part of the neural tube. It has trigeminal innervation (specifically, ophthalmic division). This creates a dual innervation in the tentorium. Between the temporal lobe and the frontal lobe, the respective layers of mesenchyme, which are pushed up, will create the anterior dural girdle. It will eventually become the anterior transverse septum, and in the adult it will be the lesser wings of the sphenoid. The

mesenchyme surrounding the temporal and frontal lobes originated in the rostral area. Therefore, this septum is innervated by the trigeminal nerve, as is the falx, whose mesenchyme also carried trigeminal fibers.

The development of the venous sinuses

The venous sinuses are created by the approximations of the lobes of the developing brain. As the cerebral hemispheres enlarge and meet in the midline, the mesenchymal tissue surrounding them approximates in the sagittal plane to form the median longitudinal septum or falx cerebri. Fluid, which is dragged along with the mesenchyme, pools between the two tissue layers as the superior and inferior sagittal sinuses (Fig. 3.13). Posteriorly at the occipital cerebellar approximation, the fluid pools into a

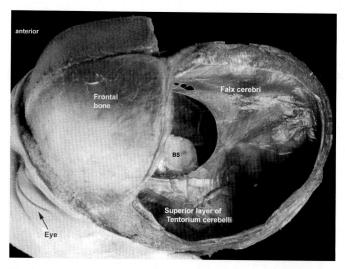

Fig. 3.14 • A newborn cranium viewed from a superior lateral position. Both cortical hemispheres have been removed, with the brainstem (BS) left in place. The continuity between the falx and tentorium is obvious. *Used with permission of the Willard & Carreiro Collection.*

transverse sinus. At the junction of the falx and the tentorium lies the straight sinus. To be precise, the falx and the tentorium do not develop as separate structures. The falx cerebri is swept posteriorly with the growing hemispheres to become the superior layer of the tentorium (Fig. 3.14). The band of mesenchyme, which forms the falx, is attached anteriorly to the cranial base. As it moves backwards, it pulls the crista galli from the cartilaginous base. Meanwhile, the cerebellum grows superiorly with its mesenchymal covering to meet the developing hemispheres. The primitive occipital lobes and cerebellum trap the tentorium cerebelli between them. The mesenchymal layer of the cerebellum contributes the inferior layer, while the mesenchymal layer of the occiput adds the superior layer. Thus, the falx is continuous with the tentorium and the straight sinus pools at the junction between the mesenchyme surrounding the cortex and the mesenchyme surrounding the cerebellum.

The five-pointed star

The dural girdles are thickened membranes and they are less affected by the stresses of the growing neural tube than the mesenchyme that is stretched between them. The dural girdles can be thought of as the ropes of a parachute, and the places in between them as the material of the parachute. The ropes are anchored down below at the thickened mesenchymal plate between the neural tube and the heart. The parachute surrounds the primitive brain. As brain grows, it is going to stretch the parachute, and the dural girdles are going to pull up on the cartilaginous plate to which they are anchored, creating tubercles and mounds in the cranial base: the clinoid processes, the crista galli, the lesser wings of the sphenoid and the apices of the petrous portions of the

temporal bones. This arrangement represents something similar to a five-pointed star superimposed on the base of the cranium (Fig. 3.15). The five-pointed star is described by the two lines of the petrous ridge, the two lines of the anterior transverse septum and the single line through the crista galli and the metopic suture. All of these lines are directed toward the hypophysis, where the notochord ends and the brain development began. When we look at an adult skull, we see a five-pointed star laid down in bones, but it is important to remember that it was not always this hard, brittle cadaveric substance. At birth, it is still a somewhat malleable tissue, vulnerable to stresses and strains. The center of this star sits at the summation of all the developmental forces within the head. It is the fulcrum of all the forces. The sella turcica, with the pituitary inside it, is at the center of the star configuration. The pituitary is covered by a diaphragm of connective tissue which is continuous with the periosteum of the bones around it. This arrangement brings to mind the vulnerability of the pituitary and its vascular stocking, as it sits in the center of the star, with all these developmental forces acting on it from many different directions.

In the condensation of mesenchyme between the brain and the heart, cartilage forms which will begin to ossify in response to the movement of the developing brain. The mesenchymal plate becomes more rigid and acts as an anchor for the dural girdles. The dural girdles create changes in the cranial base as they are stressed, just as a tendon attached to an osseous or cartilaginous structure will eventually form a mound or a tubercle. Lines of force are transmitted through the dural girdles, influencing the structure of the cartilaginous plate and the newly forming bone. The cranial base forms in response to the compressive forces on the mesenchymal anchor and the tensile forces of the dural girdles. Conversely, the vault forms in response to the stretch of the tissue that is being splayed between the dural girdles. The point of maximum stress or stretch between the dural partitions will become the ossification center. As it ossifies, this center becomes rigid. All of the stretch will now occur around that point. The ossification center becomes the hub of the wheel, with the lines of stretch radiating like spokes. Along the lines of stretch, there will be a laying down of bony trabeculae. Initially, the bone will lay down in the area of greatest stress. This will be the ossification center. Then the bone will lay down in a pattern radiating along the lines of stress from this center. These bony trabeculae will cleave the mesenchyme or the ectomeninx into an external and internal periosteum. The ectomeninx does not split; the bone actually develops within the mesenchymal layer. We can almost think of it as a transformation of cell structure within the mesenchyme. There is an accumulation of calcium salt, and a change in cellular make-up and the laying down of bone. The bones of the vault develop within the mesenchymal membrane, cleaving it into two layers: an internal periosteum and an

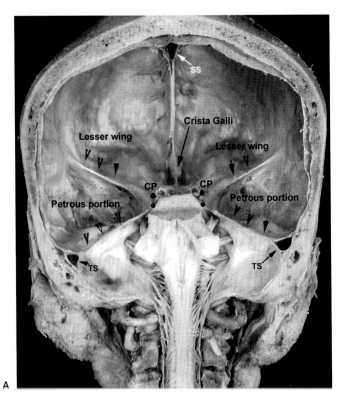 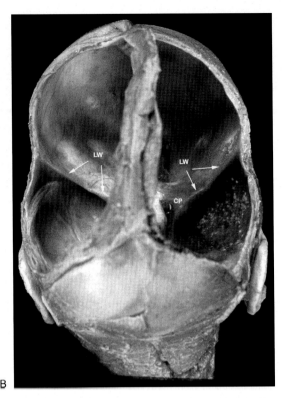

Fig. 3.15 • (A) Posterior view of an adult specimen. The falx, tentorium, cortex and cerebellum have been removed, revealing the five-pointed star arrangement oriented towards the sella turcica and clinoid processes (CP). The cut edge of the transverse (TS) and sagittal (SS) sinuses can be seen. Note the three walls of each sinus. (B) Posterior view of an infant; the occiput and falx are still in place; removal of these structures destroyed the integrity of the view. LW, lesser wing. *Used with permission of the Willard & Carreiro Collection.*

external periosteum. The internal periosteum will go on to differentiate into the outer and inner dura. The developing brain will compress these two layers against the internal surface of the skull but the inner layer remains continuous with intracranial dural septae, the tentorium and falx.

Vault

The vault is composed of a series of squamous bones. The membrane surrounding the brain, and adherent to it, is being deformed as the brain grows inside. By 7 or 8 weeks of gestation, the process of ossification begins and the vault develops directly out of the membrane. This results in a series of plates anchored to the base of the cranium through dural bands, which will go on to form the dural septae. Separate bony plates are suspended in a common membrane (Fig. 3.16). This is a remarkable arrangement, because it allows the membrane to continue to provide housing for the brain at birth while allowing for maximum deformability and plasticity of the structure during the birth process. We tend to think of the periosteal layer on the outside as belonging to bone and unrelated to everything on the inside (known as dura). However, the skull began as a tissue, which was separated into two layers by its biochemical ability to perform osteogenesis. The continuity that exists from the external

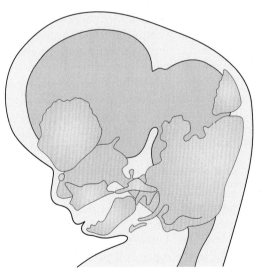

Fig. 3.16 • The bones of the cranial vault develop as plates within the membranous structure of the developing head. *Adapted from Williams P (ed.) 1995 Gray's anatomy, 38th edn. Churchill Livingstone, London, with permission.*

periosteum through the cranial bones, through the internal periosteum, through the meningeal dura, through the arachnoid to the pia and to the brain must not be overlooked. We can think of the bones of the cranial vault as floating in

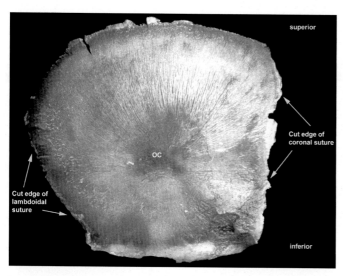

Fig. 3.17 • Right parietal bone from a newborn specimen. The sutures were cut. Radiating lines of development can be seen from the ossification center (OC). *Used with permission of the Willard & Carreiro Collection.*

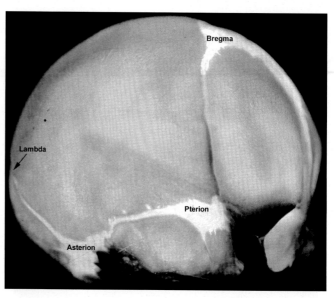

Fig. 3.18 • Transilluminated infant skull viewed from the right. The fontanels are labeled. *Used with permission of the Willard & Carreiro Collection.*

membrane; thus, forces imparted on the cranial vault during the birth process affect the vault as well as the base.

An example of the ossification centers of the vault bones can be seen on the parietal bone of a newborn (Fig. 3.17). The lines of bony development radiate away from this point. There are two ossification centers in the frontal bone, one in each parietal, and two in the occipital squama. The bones are actually osseous plates forming within the mesenchymal membrane. The vault can be thought of as a membrane which has little thickened plates developing in it (this is different from thinking of a series of thickened plates approximating each other in separate membranes). Where the plate has not formed, there is a fontanel. The newborn has six fontanels: one each at bregma and lambda, and two each at asterion and pterion (Fig. 3.18). The fontanel represents the membrane in which the plates are growing. As the plates increase in size, they will approximate at the fontanel. The membrane in which the bony plates of the vault are developing is attached to the cartilaginous cranial base. The vault will adapt to forces transferred from the cranial base and changes in the base will be reflected in the shape of the vault.

In a dissected specimen of a term infant who died intrauterine, the enveloping nature of the cranial membranes is easily appreciated. With the soft tissue removed, the sutures can be seen as areas of thickened membrane where the periosteum and cartilaginous endplate of the bone merge (Fig. 3.19A). When cut, the external periosteum is easily peeled from the surface of the bone, except along the suture, where it merges with the internal tissues (Fig. 3.19B). At the premature suture there is no longer a layer of periosteum overlaying the bone. Rather, there is an area of thickened tissue, similar in consistency to tendon, with no grossly discernible layers. Once the external periosteum is removed, the parietal bone is easily lifted from the internal periosteum (Fig. 3.20), except at the sutures where the tissues are merged into a thickened mass and a small incision needs to be made. The internal dura and the dural septae (in this case the falx cerebri) form a continuous sheet of tissue. This is best viewed in the three walls of the sagittal and transverse sinuses (see Fig. 3.13). The external dura forms the external wall of the sinus; the internal dura from each side forms the lateral walls and continues on as the falx cerebri. This continuity suggests, quite strongly, that changes in the base will contribute to changes in the shape of the vault, and vice versa. This is an important consideration in the treatment of plagiocephaly.

POSTNATAL DEVELOPMENT OF THE CRANIAL BONES

Some bones of the cranium are still in parts at birth. These bones, referred to as composite bones, are the occiput, the sphenoid and the temporal bone. During the first 6 years of life, dramatic changes occur in the cranial base, but changes continue throughout life as well. We are going to focus mostly on what is happening during childhood. In order to get an understanding of this, we need to establish a base around which this is all happening, and that is the median axial stem.

The median axial stem is the center point of the skull. It is organized around the notochord, and in turn the rest of the head organizes around the median axial stem. The imprint of the median axial stem can be seen on the mature human head as a line or a groove that courses between the eyes and the ears (Fig. 3.21). If you were to cut a slice right through that position, you would be cutting directly

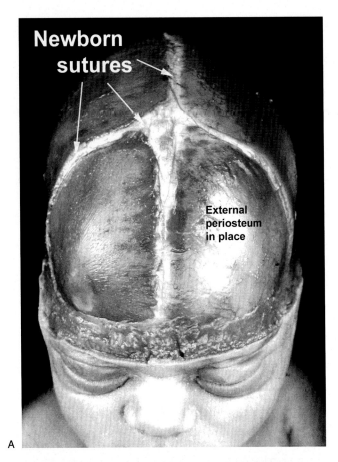

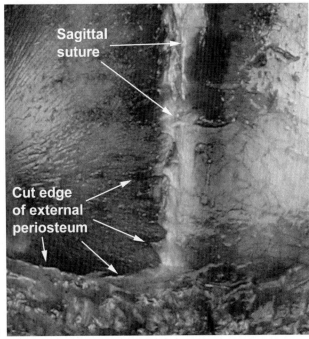

Fig. 3.19 • (A) Anterosuperior view of a neonatal specimen. The external periosteum has been removed from the left frontal bone; it is still in place on the right. The sutures can be seen as thickenings of connective tissue. (B) The close-up view shows the cut edge of the periosteum. *Used with permission of the Willard & Carreiro Collection.*

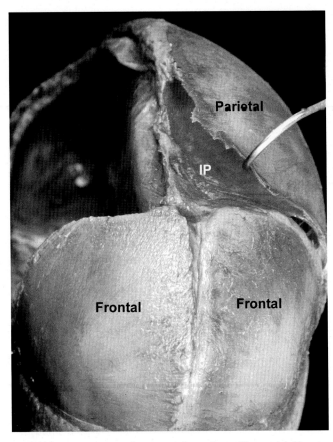

Fig. 3.20 • Anterior view of a neonatal specimen. The parietal bone is lifted from the internal periosteum (IP). As in Figure 3.19, the external periosteum is still covering the right frontal bone. *Used with permission of the Willard & Carreiro Collection.*

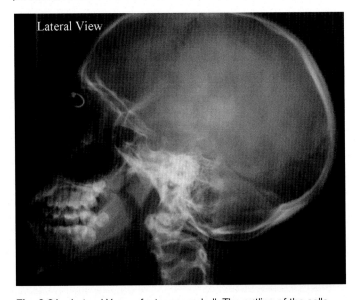

Fig. 3.21 • Lateral X-ray of a teenage skull. The outline of the sella turcica and clinoid processes can be seen. This axis extending anteriorly to the crista galli and posterior through the basiocciput represents the median axial stem. The ring-like structure near the frontal bone is an eyebrow ring. *Used with permission from a teaching file of the UNECOM OMM Department.*

through the basicranium. The median axial stem is composed of three parts. The most rostral part is the ethmoid, posterior to that is the basisphenoid, followed by the basiocciput. The basisphenoid is the portion of the sphenoid that is referred to as 'the body'. The lateral parts of the sphenoid, its greater wings and pterygoid processes are not components of the median axial stem, nor are the lateral masses and squamous portion of the occiput. The median axial stem comprises just the center-pieces which organize directly around the notochord and lie on a line between the orbit and the ear. In the infant, the midline structure and all the parts are separated from each other by cartilage. Forces, distortions or deformations occurring in the lateral components can affect the midline center-piece. Also important in this mechanism are the temporal bones. The temporal bones fit in between the occiput and the sphenoid, acting as a 'buttress' to support the system.

Postnatal changes in the basicranium

In the adult, the basiocciput and basisphenoid are each fused to their respective lateral parts, and this provides stability, support and protection to the central nervous system. Fortunately, these bones are all in parts in the developing child, because there is a tremendous amount of change occurring in the brain. The shape of the intracranial space is going to change considerably over the first 6 years of life, and the base needs to accommodate those changes. The timing of the fusion or ossification between the midline and lateral parts is very important. These are critical periods. Prior to ossification, the structure is quite vulnerable. Forces and stresses may deform the intraosseous as well as interosseous relationships in the cranial base. This may affect cartilaginous, ligamentous and tendinous structures. Many of these connective tissues are located around foramina, so structures exiting through the foramina may be affected. Early in life, many foramina are not well circumscribed. Foramina such as the jugular, lacerum and stylomastoid develop within the cartilage between adjacent bones or composite parts (Fig. 3.22). These foramina may be vulnerable to forces or changes occurring in the developing cranial base.

One important change is the flexion of the basicranium. If we compare the basicranium of an adult with that of an infant, there is a marked difference in the relationship between the sphenoid and occiput. We can create a horizontal reference by drawing a line through the glabella to the inion (Fig. 3.23). A line drawn through the basiocciput transects this horizontal reference. The resultant angle is approximately 31° in the infant and 51° in the adult. There is an additional 20° flexion in the adult median axial stem. This additional flexion is generated over the first 6 years of life. The flexion in the basicranium contributes to the creation

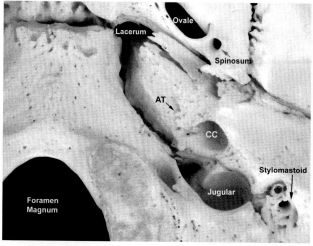

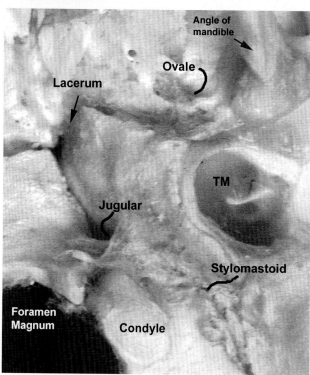

Fig. 3.22 • Inferior views of adult (A) and approximately 2-year-old (B) cranial specimens. The foramina are labeled: CC, carotid canal; AT, auditory tube. Note the position of the tympanic membrane (TM) in the toddler skull. *Used with permission of the Willard & Carreiro Collection.*

of a large space over the top of the larynx, the supralaryngeal space. Adult humans are the only mammals that have this flexed basicranium. The flexion of the basicranium coincides with the development of complex phonemes in our speech which no other primate can generate. These complex phonemes can occur because we are using the supralaryngeal space to shape the air puffs generated by the larynx. Other primates have larynxes and they can generate sound, but they cannot shape it because they do not have this complicated enlarged supralaryngeal space. The supralaryngeal

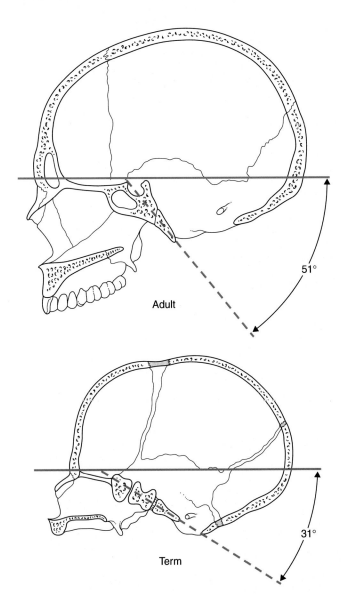

Fig. 3.23 • Diagram depicting changes in the orientation of the median axial stem between term infant and adult. *Used with permission of the Willard & Carreiro Collection.*

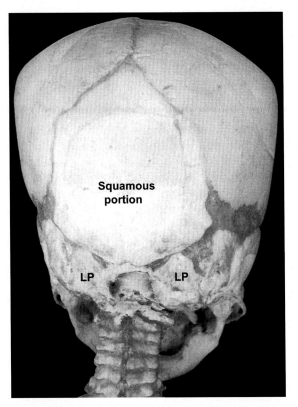

Fig. 3.24 • A posterior view of a specimen of a young child between 5 and 7 years. The lateral parts (LP) or masses and squamous portion are labeled. Note the cartilaginous matrix joining the lateral parts to the occipital squama. This area is vulnerable to compression in occipital-atlantal and condylar dysfunctions, and torsional stress in squamous rotation patterns. *Used with permission of the Willard & Carreiro Collection.*

space and the ability to create complicated, complex phonemes contribute to the way in which we communicate. The flexion of the cranial base results from remodeling of the basicranium due to appositional growth of the bones.

Development of the occiput

At birth, the occipital bone is a composite of four parts: a supraoccipital portion or squamous part, two lateral parts and the basiocciput (Fig. 3.24). The squamous part and lateral parts are joined to each other and the basiocciput by a cartilaginous matrix. Cartilage is deformable. (You may test this hypothesis by pushing on your nose or your ear.) At birth, the condyles are split by a synchondrosis; one-third lies with the basilar process, and two-thirds with the lateral masses.

Deformations in the cartilaginous bridge between the two parts of the condyle will distort its shape and its articular relationship with C1. The condyles are rather marginal in shape at birth because weightbearing has not occurred. Weightbearing affects the shape and size of the condyle and the morphology of its articular surface. The condylar parts will not fuse until about 6 years. At birth, the supraoccipital bone is not fused to the lateral masses (parts) beneath it. This will not occur until 3 years. The junction between the structures is cartilaginous. This allows for growth and expansion of the foramen magnum, but its pliability makes this area vulnerable.

The expansion of the foramen magnum throughout the first 6 years of life is dependent on the fact that the parts of the occiput are not fused. In fact, most of the canals and foramina in the cranium are located between bones or unfused parts of bones. Their shape is not protected by rigid well-developed bone. They are surrounded by cartilage. For example, the jugular canal is formed by the junction of the occiput and the temporal bone, and the hypoglossal canal is formed by the fusion of the parts of the lateral masses (see Fig. 3.22). Changes or deformations occurring within the basiocciput/lateral mass composite may not only affect the shape of the occipital bone but also may affect the shape of the foramina. From a clinical standpoint, that is very important. Nerves and vascular structures do not pass through foramina in isolation. These structures are accompanied by venous plexuses, fascia and fat. The tendon and fascias of the pharyngeal and cervical musculature are attached to the external surface of the occipital bone. Changes in the relationships of adjacent osseous structures will alter the relationships of the soft tissue structures attached to them. This may create compressions or stretch on the nerves and vessels passing in close proximity. Alterations in tissue relationships may impede venous and lymphatic return from the area, leading to tissue congestion and compromising neurotrophic function. Changes in the relation between muscle origin and insertion may affect function.

The squamous portion of the occiput will fuse with the lateral masses by 2–3 years. Prior to that, distortions in the supraoccipital area may affect the relationship between the lateral masses and the occipital squama. If during birth the head meets with resistance as the occiput is pivoting on the pubic symphysis, the supraoccipital bone may rotate slightly, changing the relationship between it and the lateral masses. When this effect is severe enough, the lateral masses may alter their position on the horizontal plane, altering function and proprioception at the craniocervical junction. There is a cartilaginous junction between the lateral mass and the adjacent temporal bone that is also vulnerable to stress. The lateral parts will fuse with the basilar portion at 6 years. During those first 6 years, there is a tremendous amount of change occurring, which is going to affect the angulation at the basiocciput and the relationship between the basiocciput and the lateral parts. Finally, the sphenobasilar junction does not start to fuse until adulthood. Prior to that, there is still cartilage in this area, and at birth it is vulnerable. One can observe the degree of deformation that this area is capable of absorbing by viewing the asymmetry present in many adult cadaveric specimens.

Several changes develop as a result of the muscular attachments to the occiput. The boney tuberosities for these tissues are not present at birth; they develop as a result of maintaining a vertical posture of the head against gravity. During embryological development, we are in a fluid environment. It is not until we start resisting gravity that we begin to develop the paravertebral muscle strength needed to create the tuberosities.

Development of the temporal bone

The occiput is the posterior component of the median axial stem, the sphenoid is anterior, and between the two sit the temporal bones. Both the occiput and sphenoid have lateral components: the lateral angles of the occiput, and the greater wings and pterygoid plates of the sphenoid. Connecting these two wide structures is a thin stem, a cartilaginous rod, the basiocciput. This arrangement

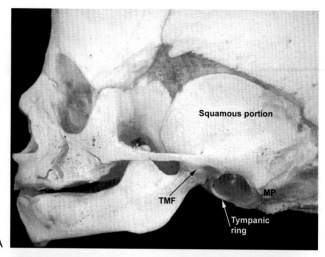

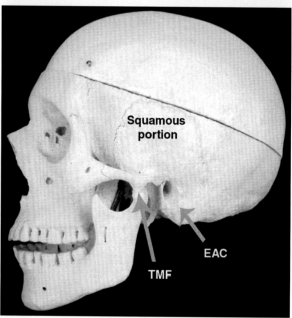

Fig. 3.25 • Lateral view of a newborn early infant (A) and adult (B) specimen depicting the parts of the temporal bone. The undeveloped mastoid process appears as the mastoid portion (MP) in the infant. Note the different orientation of the temporomandibular fossa (TMF) in the two specimens. The tympanic membrane is visible in the external auditory canal (EAC) of the infant skull but not the adult. *Used with permission of the Willard & Carreiro Collection.*

requires a lateral support system to resist twists and torsions. Evolution created a support system in the likeness of the temporal bone, a triangular-shaped bone which snuggles right in between the occiput and the sphenoid, acting like a bolster to prevent deformation within the median axial stem. At birth, the temporal bone is in three parts: the petromastoid part located posteriorly; the squamous part, which includes the zygomatic process of the temporal bone; and the tympanic ring. The temporal bone (Fig. 3.25) has a very complex structure with a complex embryology, both of which contribute to a very complex function. First, through

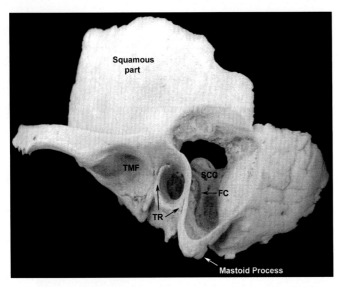

Fig. 3.26 • Lateral view of the temporal bone of a young adult. The central portion has been drilled to reveal semicircular canals (SCC) and canal of the facial nerve (FC). The articulation of the tympanic ring (TR) can be seen lying beside the temporomandibular fossa (TMF). Specimen preparation courtesy of Michael Thomas DO. *Used with permission of the Willard & Carreiro Collection.*

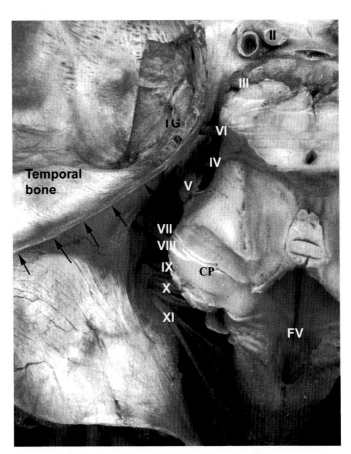

Fig. 3.27 • Posterior view of an adult specimen. The cortex and cerebellum have been removed. The cut edge of the tentorium is indicated by the black arrows. The fourth ventricle (FV) can be seen lying within the brainstem. The cerebellar peduncle (CP) is labeled. Cranial nerves II–IX are depicted. Note the trigeminal ganglion (TG). *Used with of the permission of the Willard & Carreiro Collection.*

its wedge-shaped petrous portion, the temporal bone acts as a buttress for the head. The posterior transverse septum (the tentorium cerebelli) is attached superiorly, the pharyngeal muscles are suspended from the petrous portion inferiorly, and on its lateral side there is a fairly large joint, the temporal mandibular joint, from which the mandible is suspended. Second, in the middle of the petrous portion is the acoustical vestibular organ (Fig. 3.26). This is an organ so delicate it can detect movement of a stereocilia the distance of the diameter of a hydrogen atom. Finally, there are more cranial nerves passing through the temporal bone than through any other bone. Cranial nerves III–XI all have relationships with the temporal bone (Fig. 3.27).

There are several constraints placed upon the growth of the temporal bone. Although it will enlarge and change as the child grows, these changes occur while preserving auditory and vestibular size and function, which are present as early as 23 weeks of gestation. The embryology of the temporal bone is fairly complicated because it develops from a variety of different centers. At birth, there is a petromastoid portion with an annulus and there is a squamous portion with the zygomatic process. The squamous portion develops from membrane, like the cranial vault. It is a typical membranous type of bone, with the ossification centers appearing at 7–8 weeks. The annulus, the tympanic ring, develops from an ossification center at 12 weeks, and the petromastoid portion starts to develop from approximately 20 separate ossification centers at around 16 weeks. The petrous portion initially forms a cartilaginous model and at 16 weeks the ossification centers appear. These centers

are extremely complex. They form around the otocyst, which contains the vestibular-acoustical apparatus. By 20 weeks, the vestibular acoustical organ has reached adult size. As we enter the sixth month of gestation we have in our heads an auditory vestibular apparatus which is as big as it will ever get. In addition, the ossicles, the tympanic membrane and the diameter (but not the length) of the external auditory meatus will also reach adult size prior to birth.

Between birth and the first year, the bulk of the temporal composite will fuse together to form a 'temporal bone'. At birth, we do not have a mastoid process (see Fig. 3.25). It is not until about 2 years of life that we begin to have enough tension in the sternocleidomastoid muscle attached to the bone to form the mastoid process. There are several other features of the temporal bone which have to reach adult size: the labyrinth capsule, middle ear, ossicular chain and length of the tympanic ring. Although the diameter of the ring is of adult size at birth, the ring still needs to develop the long, flared, trumpet-like shape. The flared shape develops during the first 6 years of life. If we compare the inferior

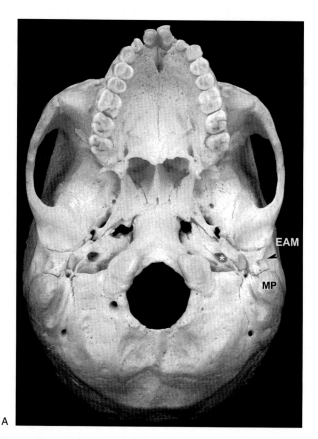 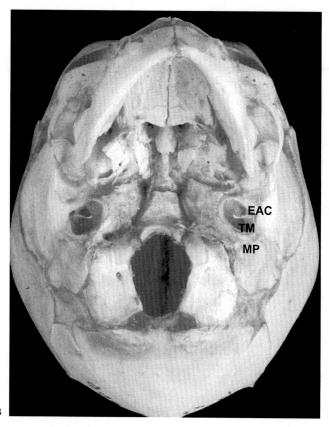

Fig. 3.28 • Comparison between adult (A) and newborn (B) specimens. Inferior view shows the position of the tympanic membrane (TM) on the newborn skull. EAM, external auditory meatus; EAC, external auditory canal; MP, mastoid process. *Used with permission of the Willard & Carreiro Collection.*

views of an adult and infant skull, it can be seen that the external auditory meatus in the infant faces inferiorly, while that of the adult is located in a more sagittal plane (Fig. 3.28). In the first 6 years of life, not only is the temporal bone acting as a buttress, with the pharynx, tentorium and mandible attached to it, but it is also undergoing a complicated remodeling which will shift the external auditory meatus from an inferior position towards the parasagittal plane.

As this happens, the position of the mandibular fossa will also change. At birth it faces somewhat anteriorly, whereas in the adult the fossa is oriented inferiorly. The ramus of the mandible is angled slightly forward in the newborn. That angle will change over the first few years of life as the maxilla grows in length. This changes the axis of rotation for the temporomandibular joint (see Fig. 3.25). Temporal bone remodeling shifts the ears into their sagittal perspective and also remodels the position of the mandibular fossa to account for the growth of the mandible. As the occipital and the sphenoid bones move away from each other, the petrous portion has to elongate to maintain its buttress effect, rotating the external auditory meatus into the sagittal plane. The styloid process will elongate as the muscles attached to it increase in strength and resist the superior

pull of the remodeling temporal bone. The diameter of the tympanic ring is of adult size, but medial to lateral expansion of the meatus will occur. The lateral part of the pharyngeal aponeurosis moves outward, increasing the size of the supralaryngeal space. The flexion of the basicranium coupled with the growth of the petrous portion of the temporal bone also enlarges the supralaryngeal space, contributing to our ability to create complex phonemes of language. Another change which occurs is the encapsulation of the carotid canal. At birth, we do not have a carotid canal. It develops postnatally.

At birth, the petrous portion of the temporal bone has an orientation which is almost horizontal. As the inferior aspect of the petrous portions grows, it swings out laterally, carrying the external auditory meatus with it. This changes the orientation of the carotid canal from being relatively vertical to having a 90° bend in it. The eustachian tubes, which are housed in the petrous portion and exit into the pharynx, are lying on a horizontal plane. As the petrous portion remodels, they will be tipped and take on the oblique angulation present in the adult. All these changes will occur in the first 6 years of life. During this time, there are some important clinical changes as well: the incidence

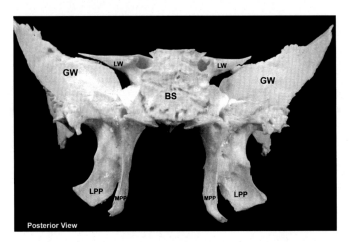

Fig. 3.29 • Posterior view of the sphenoid from an adolescent specimen. Lesser wings (LW), greater wings (GW), basisphenoid (BS), lateral pterygoid process (LPP) and medial pterygoid process (MPP) are depicted. *Used with permission of the Willard & Carreiro Collection.*

of ear infections decreases dramatically in children over 6 years old, and changes in speech occur as the supralaryngeal space takes on an adult geometry. These clinical changes are driven by anatomical development. Consequently, compressive or torsional forces impacting on the squamous or petrous mastoid areas may alter the functional relationships and contribute to otolaryngological conditions in children and adults.

Development of the sphenoid

The occiput is the most posterior aspect of the supportive median axial stem. The temporal bones and the petrous portions act as a stabilizer or buttress. The sphenoid is the anterior component. The sphenoid is a flared bone with a wide lateral expansion, balanced on a narrow medial stem (Fig. 3.29). During gestation, the center of the sphenoid or basisphenoid is in two parts, the presphenoid and the postsphenoid, which fuse at about 8 months. (This does not occur in children with Down's syndrome.) The area of fusion lies around the sphenoid sinus. In the postnatal period, the term 'basisphenoid' refers to the body and lesser wing composite, whereas the term 'alisphenoid' refers to the greater wing pterygoid plate composite. There are three parts of the sphenoid present at birth: two alisphenoids and a basisphenoid. They will go through some significant changes during the first few years of life which will affect the shape of the eyes, the anterior cranial fossa, the middle cranial fossa and the pharynx.

Like the temporal bone, the sphenoid has a fairly complicated role in stabilizing the skull. That role is reflected in its anatomy and very complicated embryology. The sphenoid is situated at the convergence points for a variety of different structures. It is at the convergence between the forebrain and the midbrain, the area where the pituitary develops. It is also at the endpoint of the notochord, which is once again where the pituitary develops. It is at the center of the convergence of all the dural septae; the five-pointed star comes together in the body of the sphenoid (see Fig. 3.15). Cranial nerves I–VI converge at the sphenoid. Below the cranial base, the sphenoid is the convergence of the three major cavities involved in the visceral cranium: the optic cavities, the nasal cavity and the pharyngeal cavity. Thus the sphenoid is at the center of the development of the head; it is the area around which the head organizes and forms during development.

An ossification center develops in the lesser wing at 9 weeks. By 16 weeks, about the same time as the temporal bone starts ossification, an ossification center develops in the postsphenoid. At 8 weeks, the ossification center for the greater wing appears in cartilage but the structure will grow out through the membrane, much like the other squamous bones. The pterygoid plates begin their ossification in and around this same 8–9-week period. Each plate initially develops as a medial and lateral lamina, which remain separate until about the sixth month of gestation, when they fuse together to form a pterygoid plate attached to the bottom of each greater wing. At birth, the sphenoid does not have the same appearance as it will have in the adult. The two lesser wings are connected by a small amount of cartilage and membrane (Bosma 1986). Each lesser wing is attached to the body, while the greater wing is attached to the pterygoid plate (Fig. 3.30). The hamulus, a small process at the inferior end of the medial pterygoid plate, appears to start ossification around 3 months. The tendon of the tensor veli palatini muscle bends around the hamulus, which improves the leverage of the muscle. The postsphenoid will fuse to the presphenoid at around 8 months of gestation.

In their first year, the two lesser wings will fuse, forming a plane or bridge (Fig. 3.31). Passing beneath this area on either side are cranial nerves III, IV, VI and the ophthalmic division of V. As the sphenoid grows, its rostral caudal axis expands, moving the attachment of the falx anterior away from the lesser wings. Meanwhile, the lesser wings are being pulled laterally by the anterior transverse septum. Over the first year or so, these components of the bone fuse together while maintaining the patency of the many foramina which traverse through them. The closing of the lesser wings of the sphenoid, which occurs in that first year of life, bridges the gap between the sides of the anterior transverse septa. At birth, the falx attaches to the area where this bridge will develop, creating a continuity between the anterior and posterior transverse septa, so that the falx is a sickle between the anterior and posterior transverse septa and is directly attached to them. During the first year of life, this bridge between the lesser wings expands, pushing the attachment

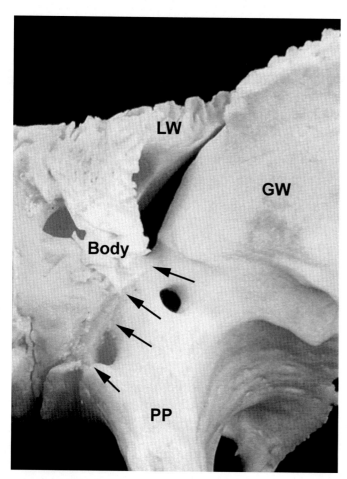

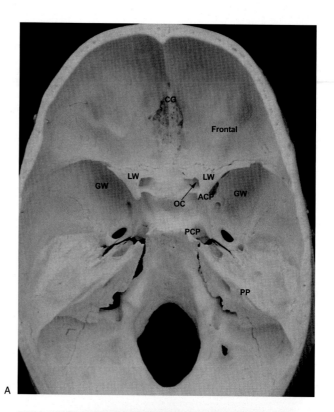

Fig. 3.30 • Magnified anterior view of the right side of the sphenoid. The articulation between the greater wing (GW), pterygoid (PP) part and the body/lesser wing (LW) unit is indicated by the black arrows. *Used with permission of the Willard & Carreiro Collection.*

of the falx (the neonatal crista galli) anteriorly, away from the anterior transverse septum. Recall that in an adult cranium the crista galli is anterior to the lesser wings of the sphenoid, while in the newborn these structures lie on the same plane. As a result, some of the motion characteristics of the anterior cranium will differ between a newborn and older child. This change in position also reflects a change in the forces working in the anterior cranial fossa.

The oral nasopharynx is another area where tremendous change occurs. The orbits come together with the nasopharynx and the oral pharynx. To maintain the patency of this area, the pterygoid plates acquire a 'U' shape, with the nasopharynx in between. However, this is not the condition at birth. In the newborn, the pterygoid plates are short and somewhat horizontally positioned, which compresses the pharynx under the basicranium and proportionately decreases the size of the oral and nasal cavities when compared with a child. The size of the space is further compromised because the infant tongue is larger and the mucosa lining the oral-nasopharynx is thicker. Fortunately

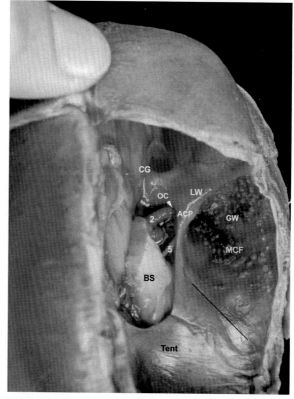

Fig. 3.31 • View of the cranial fossa in an adult (A) and slightly posterolateral view of the neonate (B). There is a bridge of bone between the lesser wings (LW) in the adult. Compare the position of the crista galli (CG) and the optic canal (OC) in the adult and newborn. *Used with permission of the Willard & Carreiro Collection.*

these factors increase the effectiveness of the tongue during suckling. In the infant, the tongue works on an anterior-posterior axis, which requires a small compressed space to create suction. However, it is harder to maintain patency in a narrow space. Consequently, the infant is at risk for maintaining patency of the airway, especially if the musculature is weak or innervation is immature. As the child grows, the maxilla elongate, the mandible acquires its adult configuration, and the pterygoid plates drop down into the U-shaped relationship. Combined with the flexion of the basicranium, these changes expand the face, open the oronasopharyngeal cavity, and facilitate the production of complicated speech.

CONCLUSION

There are many changes which will occur in the anatomy of the infant head during the first 6 years of life. These changes represent alterations in the forces and biomechanics within the growing child. Any osteopath wishing to treat children needs to consider the changes and variations present in their patient's anatomy. It is my hope that this description will give the reader a picture of the dynamics occurring during pediatric growth and development, and will emphasize to the practitioner that children are not simply little adults.

Reference

Bosma J F 1986 Anatomy of the infant head, 1st edn. Johns Hopkins University Press, Baltimore.

Further reading

Blechschmidt E, Gasser R 1978 Biokinetics and biodynamics of human differentiation. Charles C Thomas, Springfield.

Bluestone C D, Klein J O 1995 Otitis media in infants and children. W B Saunders, Philadelphia: 39–54.

Bluestone C D, Klein J O 1995 Otitis media in infants and children. W B Saunders, Philadelphia: 5–16.

Bosma J F 1973 4th symposium on oral sensation and perception. Prologue to the symposium. Symp Oral Sens Percept (4): 3–8.

Bosma J F 1975 Introduction to the symposium. In: Bosma J F, Showacre J (eds) Development of upper respiratory anatomy and function. National Institutes of Health, Bethesda, MD: 5–49.

Bosma J F 1985 Postnatal ontogeny of performances of the pharynx, larynx, and mouth. Am Rev Respir Dis 131(5): S10–S15.

Bosma J F, Bartner H 1993 Ligaments of the larynx and the adjacent pharynx and esophagus. Dysphagia 8(1): 23–28.

Bosma J F, Showacre J (eds) 1975 Symposium on development of upper respiratory anatomy and function: implications for sudden infant death syndrome. National Institutes of Health, Bethesda, MD.

Donner M W, Bosma J F, Robertson D L 1985 Anatomy and physiology of the pharynx. Gastrointest Radiol 10(3): 196–212.

Geurkink N 1983 Nasal anatomy, physiology, and function. J Allergy Clin Immunol 72: 123–128.

Graves G O, Edwards L F 1944 The eustachian tube. Arch Otolaryngol 39(5): 359–397.

Proctor B 1967 Embryology and anatomy of the eustachian tube. Acta Otolaryngol 86: 51–62.

Rood S R, Doyle W J 1978 Morphology of the tensor veli palatini, tensor tympani, and dilatator tubae muscles. Ann Otol 87: 202–210.

Rubesin S E, Jessurun J, Robertson D et al 1987 Lines of the pharynx. Radiographics 7(2): 217–237.

Standring S (ed) 2004 Gray's anatomy, 39th edn. Churchill Livingstone, New York.

Chapter Four

The cardiovascular system

INTRODUCTION

The primordial heart develops from a bulb of mesenchyme located on the most cephalad portion of the neural tube. At approximately 8 days of gestation, the embryo bends its head and drops the primitive heart into the area which will one day be the throat. Over the next several days this primitive heart tissue migrates into the thoracic region as the neural tube moves up and away (Bleschmidt & Gasser 1978). Thus begins the never-ending struggle between the heart and the head. A very interesting discussion, however, in this chapter we will limit ourselves to the functional and developmental anatomy of the cardiovascular system and its clinical implications. The cardiovascular system can be viewed as a transport system for blood, nutrients, waste products and immune cells. There are two primary components: a high-pressure system composed of the heart and arterial vasculature; and a low-pressure system that includes the venous and lymphatic systems. We will discuss the structure and function of these pressure systems separately and review their interaction.

DEVELOPMENT

Sometime around day 19 of gestation, vasculogenesis in the thoracic region leads to the formation of the endocardial tubes, which then fuse at approximately 21 days and the heart begins to beat. During the next 6 weeks the tube will fold, septate and develop involutions that will evolve into the septa, valves and sinuses of the mature heart (bu-Issa & Kirby 2007). Interruptions or interference with any of these processes will result in congenital cardiovascular defects.

The heart's main function is the propulsion of blood into the systemic vascular system. Its ability to do this at any given stage of development is influenced by different factors. The cells of the myocardium are called myocytes.

The structure and biochemistry of the myocytes change as the heart matures (Bernstein 2000). During gestation, the heart increases in size due to the increased myocyte division; this is also referred to as hyperplasia. After birth, the heart grows due to enlargement of the myocyte size. This is called hypertrophy. Throughout the remainder of a person's life, these two processes continue to operate in response to cardiac demand and pathological mechanisms.

The characteristics of contraction and relaxation of myocardial tissue change as the heart develops. In the fetus the channels for depolarization and repolarization of the myocytes are immature. The immature sodium–potassium pumps impede cell depolarization. In addition, calcium ions are removed more slowly from the contractile organ, delaying muscle relaxation. Because of these factors the contractile force of the fetal heart is impeded; in order to meet elevated cardiac demands the rate rather than the force of contraction is increased. At birth, the depolarization–repolarization mechanism remains somewhat immature. Clinically, this is especially important in the infant or young child with cardiac disease or increased cardiac demand. The inability of the immature heart to meet the escalated demands may lead to cardiac failure or end-organ hypoxia.

ANATOMY

The heart sits upon the central tendon of the diaphragm. The pericardium extends inferiorly and inserts onto the superior diaphragmatic fascia (Fig. 4.1). Some authors have referred to these insertions as the pericardial diaphragmatic ligaments; however, they are more like thickened bands of fascia. The pericardium has two components: a fibrous pericardium and a serosal pericardium. The fibrous pericardium loosely clothes the heart, attaching to the central tendon of the diaphragm. Superiorly, the fibrous pericardium is continuous with the pretracheal fascia and the adventitia of the great vessels (i.e. the aorta, superior vena cava, right and left pulmonary arteries and the four pulmonary veins). It attaches to the cricoid cartilage and acts as the posterior supporting sheath or sling for the thyroid gland. Superior and inferior sternopericardial ligaments attach the anterior surface of the fibrous pericardium to the sternum, which is cartilaginous and remains in five parts until some time between puberty and middle age.

The serosal pericardium is a closed sac within the fibrous pericardium. It consists of two layers. The visceral layer, called the epicardium, covers the heart and great vessels

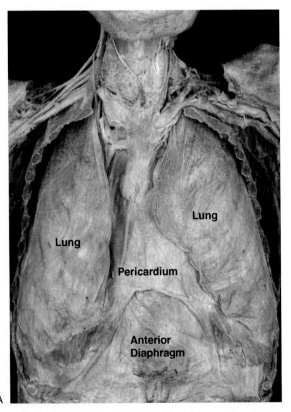
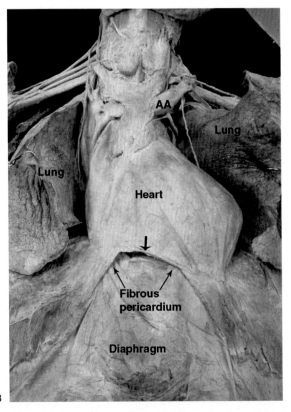

Fig. 4.1 • Anterior view of thoracic dissection. (A) The sternum and rib cage have been removed to reveal the lungs positioned over the heart. The pericardium is visible. (B) Close-up view. The lungs have been lifted laterally to expose the heart. The space inferior to the heart indicated by the thickened black arrow is a dissection artifact. The thin black arrows indicate the periphery of the fibrous pericardium as it inserts onto the superior fascia of the diaphragm. AA, aortic arch. *Used with permission of the Willard & Carreiro Collection.*

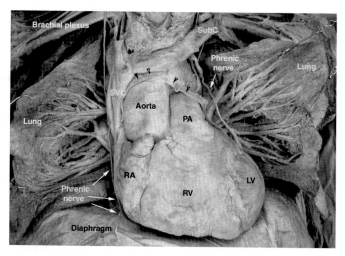

Fig. 4.2 • Anterior view of dissection of the heart and lungs. The pulmonary vasculature is exposed. The chambers and vessels of the heart are labeled: aorta, pulmonary artery (PA), superior vena cava (SVC), left subclavian vein (SubC), right atrium (RA), right ventricle (RV), left ventricle (LV). The phrenic nerves can be seen passing along the lateral aspects of the heart. Note the close proximity. This proximity accounts for phrenic nerve damage due to myocardial cooling during cardiac surgery. The small black arrowheads indicate the superior cut edge of the parietal pericardium. *Used with permission of the Willard & Carreiro Collection.*

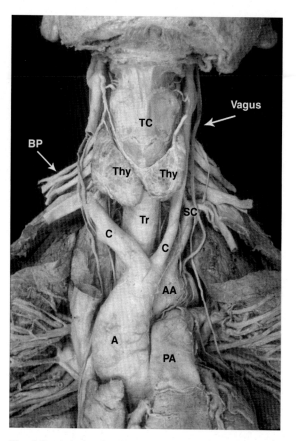

Fig. 4.3 • Anterior view into mediastinum and deep cervical space. The great vessels and their branches are labeled: aorta (A), aortic arch (AA), pulmonary artery (PA), carotids (C), subclavian (SC). The vagus, trachea (Tr), thyroid glands (Thy), thyroid cartilage (TC) and cut edge of the brachial plexus (BP) are identified. *Used with permission of the Willard & Carreiro Collection.*

and is reflected back onto the parietal layer, which lines the interior of the fibrous pericardium. The parietal pericardium is continuous with the tunica adventitia of the great vessels (the aorta, vena cavae and pulmonary vessels) (Fig. 4.2). Between the two layers of the serosal pericardium is a narrow space, the pericardial cavity. Within this pericardial space, fluid may accumulate due to trauma, inflammation or infection. If the volume is significant enough, the heart may be compressed, resulting in cardiac tamponade. This is a critical condition wherein the heart cannot pump due to the excess fluid pressure surrounding it, even though the electrical activity through the myocardial muscle is normal. The parietal and fibrous pericardia are adhered to each other. At the inferior aspect of the heart the fibrous pericardium inserts onto the superficial fascia of the diaphragm and the parietal pericardium pulls away to lie under the heart between the heart and the central tendon of the diaphragm.

The normal perinatal heart has four chambers situated asymmetrically in relationship to the sternum. The right ventricle is positioned most anteriorly, book-ended by the left ventricle and right atrium. The left atrium sits more posteriorly. The great vessels rise from the heart into the deep inferior aspect of the neck, suspended by the deep cervical fascias (Fig. 4.3). Branches of the aorta supply the myocardial muscle as coronary vessels. The right and left coronary arteries branch from the aorta close to its origin. The left coronary divides into the left anterior descending and left circumflex arteries (Fig. 4.4). The left anterior descending artery travels in the

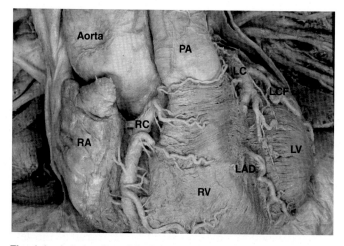

Fig. 4.4 • Anterior view of the heart exposing the coronary arteries. The right coronary (RC) artery traverses through the atrioventricular groove. The left coronary (LC) artery branches into the left circumflex (LCF) and left anterior descending (LAD) arteries. The right atrium (RA), right ventricle (RV), left ventricle (LV), aorta and pulmonary artery (PA) are labeled. *Used with permission of the Willard & Carreiro Collection.*

intraventricular groove, and supplies the right and left ventricles and the intraventricular septal wall. The left circumflex artery passes posteriorly, supplying the left atrium. The right coronary artery travels in the atrioventricular groove and supplies the right atrium and right ventricle. The myocardial vessels fill and perfuse the myocardium during diastole when the heart is relaxed. This is very important. As cardiac rate and contractility increase, the length of diastole shortens and myocardial perfusion time is compromised, putting the heart at risk for ischemia. This is a factor in exercise-induced cardiac ischemia and acute cardiac failure.

THE TRANSITION FROM FETAL TO NEONATAL CIRCULATION

Circulation in the fetal heart occurs in a parallel circuit. Blood cells and plasma flow into either the right or left ventricle, but not through each of them. Oxygenated blood enters the fetal circulation via the placenta, where gas exchange occurs (Fig. 4.5). Oxygenated blood traveling through the umbilical vein passes either to the fetal liver or into the inferior vena cava via the ductus venosus. In the inferior vena cava oxygenated blood mixes with deoxygenated blood from the lower extremities and pelvis. This mixed blood enters the right atrium and crosses through the foramen ovale into the left atrium driven by the flow characteristics of this area. It then flows through the left ventricle to the ascending aorta. Blood returning from the head and upper body flows through the superior vena cava into the right atrium, where it will pass via the tricuspid valve into the right ventricle. From the right ventricle, this blood enters the pulmonary artery and is shunted through the ductus arteriosus because of the high resistance of the pulmonary vasculature. From the ductus arteriosus it enters the descending aorta to perfuse the lower extremities, abdomen and pelvis before entering the umbilical arteries. Thus, during gestation the head and upper body receive blood with a higher oxygenation level than do the lower body.

After birth, the vascular resistance in the pulmonary tree decreases in response to the increased partial pressure of arterial oxygen (PaO_2), decreased lung fluid and decreased alveoli surface tensions (see discussion in Ch. 5). This results in movement of blood through the tricuspid valve rather than the ductus arteriosus. At the same time, systemic peripheral resistance (afterload) increases, so that systemic resistance is greater than pulmonary resistance. As a result, flow through the ductus arteriosus reverses and eventually declines. The increased blood volume and resultant pressures in the left atrium act to close the foramen ovale. Initial closure of the foramen ovale and ductus arteriosus is functional, not hormonal. In a healthy term newborn, the ductus arteriosus is closed within 18 hours from birth. Closure of the foramen ovale takes up to 3 months and in some individuals it never completely closes (Bernstein 2000).

THE CARDIAC CYCLE

The postnatal heart can be viewed as four pumps: the two atria and the two ventricles. Contraction of each of these chambers should result in the forward propulsion of blood. Normal contraction and relaxation of the heart occurs in a sequential manner with the atria contracting prior to the ventricles. This delayed sequencing facilitates the flow of blood from the high pressure of the contracting atrium into the lower pressure of the relaxed ventricle. One complete sequence of contraction and relaxation of the atria and ventricles is called a cardiac cycle. The cardiac cycle is divided into two parts: the diastolic and the systolic periods. The diastolic period consists of the time when the ventricles are relaxed and can fill with blood. This is also the period when the coronary vessels can perfuse the myocardium. The systolic period is the time during which the ventricles contract, ejecting blood into the pulmonary artery and aorta. The atrioventricular (AV) valves close in response to elevated pressure in the ventricles during systole. This allows the atria to fill with blood from the vena cava and pulmonary veins. At the end of systole, the intraventricular pressures drop as the ventricles relax and the elevated pressure in the atria causes the AV valves to open. Blood flows from the atria into the relaxed ventricles. This marks the beginning of the diastolic period. Once the atria are emptied, blood will continue to flow directly from the vena cava and pulmonary vessels through the AV valves and into the ventricles. In the last stage of diastole the atria contract and further fill the ventricles. Contraction of the ventricles marks the beginning of systole. As previously described, at the onset of ventricular contraction the AV valve closes. Continued contraction propels the blood forwards through the arterial system – this is the cardiac ejection period and this completes the cardiac cycle. The cardiac cycle is represented electrically by the electrocardiogram (ECG). Normal electrical conduction through the myocardial tissue is necessary for optimal cardiac function. Nevertheless, abnormalities of cardiac function may exist in the presence of normal electrical activity.

CARDIAC FUNCTION

Cardiac function is the ability of the heart to meet the metabolic demands of the body. The delivery of oxygenated blood and removal of cellular waste products is fundamental to life. Oxygen demand will increase as a result of elevated metabolic need. This can occur with stress, disease and physical exertion. There are two methods by which the body can meet elevated oxygen demand: increase the oxygen levels in the alveoli so that the blood has a higher saturation level; or increase the rate of perfusion to the tissues so that

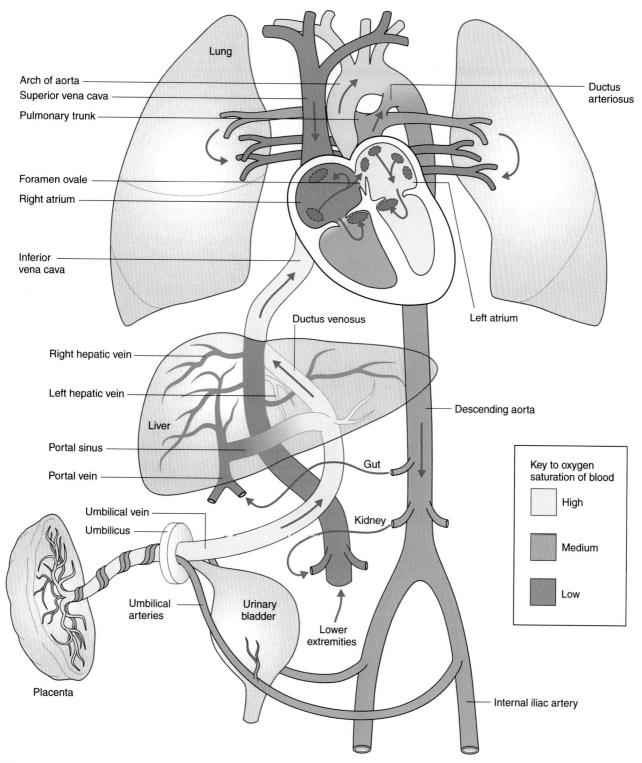

Fig. 4.5 • Schematic diagram of blood flow pathways in utero.

the blood circulates through the tissue more often. The first response manifests as increased respiratory rate, increased respiratory volume or prolonged inhalation phase of respiration. The second response presents as increased heart rate or stroke volume. The stroke volume is the volume of blood ejected from the ventricle during systole. It is affected by the force of the ventricular contraction and the volume of blood filling the ventricle. In the mature heart, stroke volume can be increased to meet the demands of the body. However, the immature sodium–potassium pumps of the neonatal heart impede contractile force.

Cardiac function is affected by filling volume (preload), vascular resistance (afterload) and myocardial contractility. Preload is the volume of blood entering the chambers of the heart. Restrictive cardiomyopathies, valvular stenosis, valvular insufficiency and venous atresia will decrease preload. Afterload is the force against which the heart must contract to move the blood into circulation. Afterload is regulated by the muscle tone in the blood vessels and their ability to distend to accommodate blood flow. Cardiac function is expressed as cardiac output – the volume of blood circulated through the lungs and into the aorta. Effective and synchronized contraction of the myocardium and the filling volume of the atria and ventricles influence cardiac output.

Cardiac function can be measured directly by cardiac catheterization. A catheter is passed into the right and left sides of the heart via a large peripheral vessel. Hemodynamic parameters and vascular resistance can be accurately measured. This is one of the most important tools for evaluating cardiac function and is considered the gold standard by most practitioners. An indirect means of measuring cardiac output is the thermodilution method. A catheter with a thermal sensitive tip (Swan–Ganz catheter) is placed in the pulmonary artery. Normal saline solution is injected into the vena cava, resulting in a change in the temperature of the blood. The resultant change in temperature at the site of the catheter (pulmonary artery) can be used to calculate the cardiac output. In addition, a wedge can be used to measure pulmonary capillary wedge pressure, which is another indicator of cardiac function. A small balloon at the tip of the catheter is inflated within the distal end of the pulmonary artery. A pressure sensor on the tip of the balloon can measure the pressure in the pulmonary vasculature. Other methods of measuring cardiac function include echocardiology and exercise testing. ECG provides information concerning the conduction of electrical activity through the heart. Magnetic resonance imaging (MRI) can be used either in static or dynamic mode to provide information about cardiac structure and function.

CONGENITAL HEART DISEASE

Congenital cardiac abnormalities are the most common etiology of cardiac disease in the pediatric population. The causes, however, are unclear. There is some evidence that genetic, environmental, teratogenic and maternal influences may have a role (Crawford et al 1988, Gillum 1994). Congenital cardiac disease can be classified as cyanotic heart disease and acyanotic heart disease. Pathologists and clinicians use this terminology slightly differently. Pediatricians and other clinicians classify these conditions based on whether the child's presenting symptom is cyanosis or something else. Pathologists define congenital cyanotic heart disease as an abnormality involving a shunt, and acyanotic heart disease as one involving obstruction. Although there is much similarity between the two definitions, we will use the clinical rather than pathological terminology.

Cyanotic heart disease occurs when inadequately oxygenated blood enters the systemic circulation and the metabolic demands of the tissues are not met. Conversely, in acyanotic heart disease the blood entering the systemic system is adequately oxygenated, but the volume or rate of flow is significantly decreased. Eventually, cyanosis may develop in patients with acyanotic heart disease but it is usually a secondary complication of the initial abnormality.

Cyanotic heart disease

Cyanotic heart disease is characterized by abnormal communication between chambers and/or within the cardiac system. The pathology can be further divided into early-onset cyanosis and late-onset cyanosis. Early cyanosis presents when there is a right-to-left shunt within the cardiac circulation such that the pulmonary system is bypassed and deoxygenated blood is sent into the body. In other words the blood moves from the right side of the heart to the left side without entering the pulmonary circulation. This is akin to in utero circulation. The magnitude of the defect will determine the extent and rapidity of onset of the symptoms. Tetralogy of Fallot, transposition of the great vessels, tricuspid atresia and persistence of the truncus arteriosus are all forms of early-onset cyanotic heart disease. In each of these cases, right-to-left shunting is present and clinical signs often appear soon after birth. These congenital forms of cyanotic heart disease require surgical correction. For the latter three, surgery is usually performed soon after diagnosis, the risk of delay being greater than the risks associated with the procedure. In cases of tetralogy of Fallot with mild cyanosis, surgery may be delayed for a short time.

Although relatively uncommon, tetralogy of Fallot is the most common form of cyanotic heart disease in children (approximately 6% of patients). It involves four abnormalities. There is a defect in the intraventricular septum, atresia of the pulmonary artery, displacement of the aorta onto the intraventricular defect and hypertrophy of the right ventricle (this last characteristic is secondary to the altered hemodynamics within the heart). Children with this condition have a greater incidence of associated extracardiac abnormalities. In tetralogy of Fallot, blood entering the right ventricle is shunted into the left ventricle and/or the overriding aorta. The extent of the symptoms will depend on the severity of the atresia of the pulmonary artery. As resistance in the pulmonary trunk increases, more blood will move towards the lower-pressure intraventricular septum or aorta. Cyanosis usually occurs with activity such as crying or feeding. If the defects are small and pressures balanced, the symptoms may not present until the child is a toddler and cardiac demand increases with walking activities. In these cases the parents often report that the child squats when playing, then gets up and continues the activity for a few moments before squatting again. The squat increases peripheral resistance in the lower extremities, shunting blood towards more vital organs.

Another example of congenital cyanotic heart disease is transposition of the great vessels. The aorta is attached to the right ventricle and the pulmonary artery to the left. Prior to birth, oxygenated blood can pass through the ductus arteriosus, but after birth this arrangement is incompatible with life. These children usually have an atrial septal defect (ASD), patent foramen ovale and patent ductus arteriosus (PDA). Once the ductus closes, these children develop severe cyanosis. Prior to modernization of cardiac surgery repairs, 90% of children with transposition died in the first year of life.

A third form of congenital cyanotic heart disease is truncus arteriosus, which occurs when the pulmonary and aortic vessels fail to separate so that both right and left ventricles feed into the same structure. Cyanosis occurs relatively early in life. Surgical correction is necessary at an early age. Lastly, atresia of the tricuspid valve presents with early cyanosis and, again, as with the other conditions, early surgical correction is required.

In cyanotic heart disease the volume of blood perfusing the tissues may be adequate but the concentration of oxygen being carried by that blood is not. In other words with a right-to-left shunt, the effort of the left ventricle to meet the needs of the body is undermined by the fact that the total blood volume delivered into circulation has a less than optimal oxygen saturation level. As the metabolic demands of the tissues increase, the left ventricle will have to compensate by increasing stroke volume and rate. If the ventricle is unable to meet the demands placed on it, the tissue will become hypoxic and all the complications of chronic hypoxia will develop. This manifests as signs of compromised end-organ perfusion such as digital clubbing and renal failure.

Acyanotic heart disease

Although it typically presents later, acyanotic heart disease can be just as detrimental to the health of a child as its cyanotic counterpart. Acyanotic heart disease typically involves a congenital left-to-right shunt. Oxygenated blood is moved back into the pulmonary circulation and the overall volume of blood sent to the systemic circulation decreases. During the neonatal period left-to-right shunts are usually silent. This is probably because right-sided pressures are still high, thus limiting left-to-right flow, and the neonate has relatively low oxygen demands. During the first months of life the extensive remodeling of the pulmonary alveoli and capillaries decreases pulmonary resistance. Pressures on the right side of the heart become lower than those on the left and as a result the left-to-right shunt is exacerbated. The heart will compensate for this situation by increasing cardiac output through greater stroke volume and rate of contraction. Eventually however, the persistent back flow into the right side of the heart can elevate right-sided pressures and produce right ventricular hypertrophy and pulmonary hypertension. Now the pressures in the right side of the heart exceed those of the left, pushing the blood from the right side to the left, bypassing the pulmonary circulation. By the time acyanotic heart disease becomes symptomatic, permanent damage to the cardiopulmonary system may have already occurred. Nevertheless, some forms of acyanotic heart disease can persist for many years without complications. This generally occurs when there are small defects that do not compromise pulmonary vascular resistance.

The most common forms of acyanotic heart disease include ventricular septal defect (VSD), ASD and PDA. Of the three, VSDs are the most common, as well as being the most common congenital cardiac abnormality, full stop. VSD is usually associated with a harsh, widely transmitted, holosystolic murmur along the left parasternal area. The intensity of the murmur will vary depending on the size of the defect and the intracardiac pressures. VSDs can vary in size and location, ranging from small fenestrations to complete absence of the septal wall. They may occur in the membranous portion of the septum or the muscular portion. Approximately 30–70% of defects close spontaneously during the first 3 years. Defects of the muscular portion appear to have a greater incidence of spontaneous closure; however, the size of the defect and the pressure within the pulmonary circulation are greater factors in the natural course of VSD than location. Small VSDs may be well tolerated throughout life without adverse sequelae. However, evidence of right-to-left shunting or pulmonary hypertension necessitates prompt medical response.

Small ASDs, less than 1 cm, tend to be tolerated and are often asymptomatic. Larger ones are at risk for developing right-to-left flow. The evolution of ASDs is influenced by the compliance of the ventricle and valves. Restrictive or obstructive pathology of the left-sided structures will facilitate the left-to-right shunt. Restrictive pathologies affecting the right ventricle, tricuspid or pulmonic valves will facilitate right-to-left shunt.

PDA occurs when the ductus arteriosus fails to close in the postnatal period. This may be due to prematurity, abnormal response to prostaglandins, persistent hypoxia or intrauterine exposure to certain viruses. A patent ductus results in left-to-right blood shunting from the aorta back to the pulmonary artery. PDA is associated with a harsh, rumbling machine-like murmur heard throughout the cardiac cycle in the second and third costal interspaces on the left. There is increased load on the ventricle and pulses may be bounding. Eventually, pressure within the pulmonary vasculature rises and hypertension ensues. A right-to-left shunt develops. In cases of PDA without any complicating factors, immediate closure is recommended. This can usually be accomplished with the administration of indometacin, which suppresses prostaglandin synthesis. Pharmacological treatment provides a low-risk treatment option but when necessary surgical correction can be performed.

In acyanotic heart disease, the blood is oxygenated but the total blood volume being distributed to the tissues is decreased. Tissue perfusion with the available oxygenated blood needs to be maximized. The ability of oxygen to diffuse to tissues is influenced by the pH of the tissue and the fluid pressures within the interstitium. Tissue edema increases interstitial pressure and may impede oxygen diffusion. The low-pressure circulatory system, the venous and lymphatic structures all have an important role in maintaining fluid pressures within the interstitium. Factors that may affect fluid movement through the interstitium include venous stasis, fascial restriction, limb immobility, lymphedema, impeded muscle pumping and lymph vessel dysfunction.

THE LOW-PRESSURE CIRCULATORY SYSTEM

Within the osteopathic concept the venous and lymphatic systems comprise the low-pressure circulatory system of the body. This system is responsible for maintaining homeostasis within the cellular milieu through the removal of cellular waste, foreign particulate matter, inflammatory products, and fluid and particles that have extravasated from blood vessels. In addition, the ability of oxygen to diffuse to tissues is affected by the pH of the tissue and the fluid pressures within the interstitium, both of which are influenced by lymphatic function. Terminal lymphatic endings absorb most of the fluid that extravasates from blood vessels. Although some variability exists between different tissue types, terminal lymphatics are essentially single cell lymphatic capillary beds. Anchoring filaments extend from each cell into the surrounding interstitium. Movement of the interstitium, whether by arterial pulsation, respiration or gross motion, moves the anchoring filaments. This in turn influences the relative positions of the endothelial cells. Fluid and particles flow into the terminal lymphatic ending via the resultant interruptions in the endothelial wall of the lymphatic capillary. Once fluid and particles enter the terminal lymphatic, they are moved forward via external forces such muscle and fascial motion, pulsation of adjacent arteries and respiratory movements. Semilunar valves scattered along the collecting lymphatic vessels prevent retrograde flow. When the contents enter the lymphatic trunk, they are propelled forward by sympathetically mediated smooth muscle contractions in the wall of the trunk.

Within the osteopathic concept, the functions of the low-pressure circulatory system and the respiratory system are closely entwined and described by the respiratory-circulatory model of structure–function relationships. Several studies support the concept of a role for the respiratory system in proper function of the low-pressure circulatory system. Two patterns of pressure fluctuation are observed in lymphatic capillaries: rhythmic low-amplitude waves with a frequency identical to respiratory movements of the thorax; and spontaneous non-rhythmic, low-frequency waves with a higher amplitude. The prevalence of waves synchronous with respiration is identical in patients with lymphedema and controls, whereas the low-frequency waves have a higher prevalence in the lymphedema patients than in the controls (Wen et al 1994). The hypothesis is advanced that in primary lymphedema a considerable amount of lymphatic fluid is removed by lymphatic pathways with small calibre and high resistance, resulting in microvascular hypertension. This in turn enhances the contractions of the few preserved large proximal lymphatic collectors. The latter mechanism could explain the increased prevalence of spontaneous microlymphatic pressure fluctuations with high amplitude and low frequency (Wen et al 1994).

Fluids within the lymphatic vessels are moved via external massage, inherent peristalsis or alternating pressure gradients. External massage is responsible for movement of fluids in the veins and large lymphatic channels of the extremities. The contractions of surrounding muscles and movements of fascias act to compress the vessels. One-way valves direct the fluid towards the proximal end of the limb and away from capillaries. Peristaltic movement is present in the larger lymphatic vessels, but movement through the smaller lymphatic channels of the extremities relies on the same mechanisms as movement through small veins. Within the pelvic, abdominal and thoracic basins, external massage cannot account for fluid movement. Pressure gradients aid lymphatic and venous return in these areas. Numerous lacunae on the abdominal surface of the diaphragm absorb fluid from the abdominal cavity. Their rate of uptake increases with diaphragm contraction. The removal of fluid within the alveolar space is accomplished through the pulmonary lymphatics. The pressures and movements associated with respiration account for over 50% of lymph movement in the thorax. Respiratory excursion must be sufficient to generate the needed pressures for lymph and venous return, especially when infection or inflammation is present. This becomes particularly important in the very young child, who lacks mature respiratory function, and the very sick child, who may not be able to meet the increased metabolic demands of the tissues.

Factors affecting blood movement in the main vessels of the venous system, and the changes in pressure and flow values in the vena cava, portal and hepatic veins, have been simultaneously recorded and related to the phases of the respiratory cycle (Rabinovici & Navot 1980). Although the experiments were done in rabbits, they do provide interesting information. There appears to be an asymmetrical pressure gradient in the vena cava centered around the diaphragm, with larger pressure differences in the thoracic segment, no pressure gradient in the portal vein and a sharp gradient at the caval end of the hepatic veins. Fluctuations in flow were noted during the respiratory cycle. Portal, hepatic and abdominal caval pressures were positive although unequally distributed. Pressures in the vena cava above the diaphragm were predominantly negative. The distribution of opposite pressure and flow values within these vessels and their integration during the respiratory cycle suggest that, in the process of venous return, each component and each segment fulfills simultaneously different functions coordinated by respiration and cardiac activity (Rabinovici & Navot 1980). Maximal pressure and flow values in the portal and hepatic veins were concomitant with the lowest values in the vena cava and closely related to respiration. During Valsalva maneuver, portal pressure was doubled, and during coughing it increased fourfold (Burcharth & Bertheussen 1979). According to Franzeck et al (1996) mean lymphatic capillary pressure is significantly higher during sitting than when lying down. In the supine position, venous pressure and lymphatic pressure are virtually the same; however, during sitting, lymphatic pressure rises more than venous pressure. This may be increased by the discontinuous fluid column in the lymphatic system and enhanced orthostatic contractile activity of lymphatic collectors and precollectors. Spontaneous low-frequency pressure fluctuations occurred in 89% of recordings during sitting, which was significantly higher than in the supine position. This suggests the presence of enhanced intrinsic contractile activity of lymph precollectors and collectors in the dependent position. This mechanism is primarily responsible for the propulsion of lymph from the periphery to the thoracic duct during quiet sitting, when extrinsic pumping by the calf muscles is not active (Franzeck et al 1996).

Positive end-expiratory pressure (PEEP) is the pressure within the airway at the end of the exhalation phase, and can be used to determine the residual volume of the lungs. PEEP is an important component of ventilatory support. It can improve oxygenation by increasing functional residual capacity, improving ventilation–perfusion matching and increasing pulmonary compliance. Its use is especially important in cases of respiratory distress due to prematurity and near-drowning. However, there can be complications. The pressures needed to maintain PEEP can increase vascular resistance in the lung, decrease cardiac filling and cause pulmonary interstitial emphysema. According to Brienza et al (1995), total venous return decreases with PEEP. The liver probably has an important role in this response, either through the development of an increase in venous resistance, or through an increase in the venous back pressure at the outflow end of the liver. As a result, the administration of PEEP can decrease oxygen delivery, and increase tissue edema through venous and lymphatic stasis, both of which increase cardiac workload. In addition, the rate of hepatic arterial flow is selectively decreased by the application of PEEP (Brienza et al 1995). This has the potential to affect the hepatic metabolic process involved with bilirubin breakdown and glucose supply. The latter could prove especially important in a sick infant with increased metabolic demands.

CLINICAL DIFFERENCES IN CHILDREN

The hallmarks of a cardiac examination are cardiac rate, rhythm, sound and blood pressure. What is considered normal for each of these parameters will change from birth through puberty. Understanding these changes can help in clinical diagnosis. The rate of cardiac contraction will vary throughout the first decade due to changes in muscle contractility and sodium–potassium pumps (Table 4.1). In general the heart rate increases in children with fever, severe anemia, hypoxia, hyperthyroidism, myocarditis and Kawasaki's syndrome. Tachycardia is defined as a rate of 150–200 beats per minute (bpm) in infants and 100–150 bpm in older children. Congestive heart failure will evolve in infants if tachycardia lasts over 24 hours. In children, bradycardia may be associated with severe systemic disease, acidosis, increased intracranial pressure, hypothyroidism and anorexia nervosa. In neonates, bradycardia associated with asphyxia is a sign of compromised function and the child's prognosis is guarded.

Table 4.1 Range and average heart rate in children

Age	Range of heart rate (bpm)	Heart rate average (bpm)
Newborn	70–190	125
1st year	80–160	120
2nd year	80–130	110
4th year	80–120	110
6th year	75–120	115
8th year	70–110	90
10th year	70–110	90

Cardiac rhythm is the second component of the cardiac exam that is different in children. In children less than 3 years of age, sinus arrhythmia can be a normal finding. The pulse rate increases during inspiration and decreases during expiration. Dropped beats or premature contractions may also be present. These findings are asymptomatic. Coarctation of the aorta is associated with absent or weak femoral pulses. Simultaneous palpation of the radial and femoral pulse may demonstrate a slight delay in femoral pulse wave. Pulsus paradoxes is a decrease or disappearance of the arterial pulse during inspiration. It is associated with severe asthma, increased intrapericardial pressure, pneumothorax and pleural effusion.

As with adults, cardiac sounds in children, particularly murmurs, are described by their direction of transmission, the quality, pitch, intensity, duration and timing in relation to the cardiac cycle. The quality may be blowing, rumbling or raspy. The intensity of the murmur ranges from grade 1 which is barely audible to grade 5 which can be heard without a stethoscope, and grade 6 which is a palpable thrill. The intensity and quality of the murmur is affected by the volume of flow through the space. Murmurs can be intensified by an increase in cardiac output such as occurs with fever, exercise, anxiety or anemia. Murmurs may disappear during vigorous crying episodes. Murmurs may be systolic or presystolic. Those that last through the entire cycle are called holosystolic and are often due to an organic lesion. VSDs are usually accompanied by a grade 3/4 harsh, widely transmitted, holosystolic murmur along the left parasternal area. PDA has a harsh, rumbling, machine-like murmur heard throughout the cardiac cycle in the second and third left interspaces. Mitral insufficiency typically presents as a grade 3 or lower, high-pitched, holosystolic murmur, best heard at the apical region during expiration. Aortic stenosis produces a harsh, very loud, systolic-ejection murmur with a crescendo-decrescendo pattern best heard in the second right costal interspace. Aortic clicks and a systolic thrill are common.

The fourth component of the cardiac examination is blood pressure. Blood pressure will vary in children based on the child's height percentile and gender (Table 4.2). In general, blood pressure in girls is higher than boys by approximately 5 mmHg. The reason for this is unclear.

Table 4.2 Blood pressure (mmHg) in children

Age (years)	Male	Female
1	94/50–102/55	97/53–104/56
5	104/65–112/69	107/65–109/69
8	107/71–116/78	112/74–118/78
10	110/73–119/78	116/77–122/80
14	120/76–128/80	123/81–130/85
17	132/85–140/89	126/83–132/86

Other components of a cardiovascular examination include pulse, viscerosomatic reflexes, capillary filling time and signs of chronic hypoxia. Pulses should be present and equal bilaterally in all four extremities. Coarctation of the aorta is associated with absent or weak femoral pulses. There may also be a delay in the femoral pulse when compared to the radial pulse. Paraspinal muscle spasm in the T3 through T6 area can be a viscerosomatic reflex from an injured or stressed myocardium. Delayed capillary filling time may be a sign of anemia or compromised flow. In children with chronic heart disease clubbing of the fingers or toes may be present. More often, however, one will see delays in growth and development. As a result, cardiovascular disease needs to be considered in any child with failure to thrive, small stature, congenital osseous defects or developmental delay.

CONCLUSION

The cardiovascular system undergoes tremendous structural change during the first few days of life and functional changes persist throughout the first year. While surgery and pharmacological therapy are the treatment of choice for congenital cardiac disease, a whole patient approach incorporates those modalities that can facilitate and support optimal cardiopulmonary function prior to, during, and following definitive treatment.

References

Bernstein D 2000 The cardiovascular system. In: Behran R E, Kliegman R M, Jenson H B et al (eds) Textbook of pediatrics. W B Saunders, Philadelphia: 427–429.

Bleschmidt E, Gasser R 1978 Blood vessels. Biokinetics and biodynamics of human differentiation. Charles C Thomas, Springfield: 80–87.

Brienza N, Revelly J P, Ayuse T et al 1995 Effects of PEEP on liver arterial and venous blood flows. Am J Respir Crit Care Med 152: 504–510.

bu-Issa R, Kirby M L 2007 Heart field: from mesoderm to heart tube. Annu Rev Cell Dev Biol 23: 45–68.

Burcharth F, Bertheussen K 1979 The influence of posture, Valsalva manoeuvre and coughing on portal hypertension in cirrhosis. Scand J Clin Lab Invest 39: 665–669.

Crawford D C, Chita S K, Allan L D 1988 Prenatal detection of congenital heart disease: factors affecting obstetric management and survival. Am J Obstet Gynecol 159: 352–356.

Franzeck U K, Fischer M, Costanzo U et al 1996 Effect of postural changes on human lymphatic capillary pressure of the skin. J Physiol Lond 494: 595–600.

Gillum R F 1994 Epidemiology of congenital heart disease in the United States. Am Heart J 127: 919–927.

Rabinovici N, Navot N 1980 The relationship between respiration, pressure and flow distribution in the vena cava and portal and hepatic

veins. Surg Gynecol Obstet 151: 753–763.

Wen S, Dörffler-Melly J, Herrig I et al 1994 Fluctuation of skin lymphatic capillary pressure in controls and in patients with primary lymphedema. Int J Microcirc Clin Exp 14: 139–143.

Chapter Five

5

The respiratory system

INTRODUCTION

Maturation of the respiratory system in humans progresses through three main phases: development of the structures and their physical relationships, adaptation to the postnatal environment and dimensional growth in proportion to the growth of the individual. Although the first two phases begin in utero, they all continue after birth. The most basic function of the respiratory apparatus is the exchange of gases. The invaginated architecture of the alveolar spaces provides maximum surface area for gas exchange, while limiting the evaporation of heat and water. Pulmonary surfactant, which coats the alveolar walls, decreases the surface tension and prevents adhesion. The respiratory muscles and the rib cage function as a mechanical pump, which can generate large and very rapid changes in ventilatory volume when needed. The respiratory apparatus of the newborn and infant differs from that of the adult in more than just size. The configuration of the terminal air spaces, the biochemical milieu and positional relationships of the respiratory tissues, and the physiology of the respiratory muscles, will undergo significant change during the first few years of life before finally obtaining their adult form.

EMBRYOLOGICAL DEVELOPMENT

At 4 weeks' gestation, the primitive trachea first appears as an outpouching from the ventral wall of the foregut. It divides into two mainstem bronchi, which branch into bronchial buds, from which secondary buds will arise. The bronchial buds are surrounded by a vascular plexus, which originates from the embryonic aorta. These vessels are derived from mesenchyme, as are all the supporting structures of the lungs. Division of the secondary bronchial buds continues through the 26th to 28th weeks of gestation.

During these latter weeks, the lung enters into a saccular period. The terminal airways, which consist of a thin epithelium, begin to widen. Their internal surfaces develop ridges and folds. Each fold contains a double capillary layer with a thin basement membrane separating it from the potential air space. This process, called septation, continues at a rapid rate, producing many alveoli by the 32nd week of gestation. The timing and progression of alveolar septation are influenced by thyroid hormone and glucocorticoids, which, respectively, stimulate and inhibit this process.

Physical stimulation of alveolar development is provided by the accumulation of fetal lung fluid and the action of respiratory muscles in utero. If the lungs or chest are compressed, as can occur with diaphragmatic hernias or oligohydramnios, alveolarization is arrested, resulting in pulmonary hypoplasia. Spinal cord lesions that adversely affect respiratory muscle activity will also inhibit alveolarization.

TRANSITION FROM FETAL TO NEONATAL RESPIRATION

In utero the lung has a secretory role with fluid-filled alveoli sacs surrounded by stiff, non-compliant arterioles. The vascular resistance of the pulmonary circulation is greater than that of the systemic circulation. Because the flow of blood occurs across the path of least resistance, blood bypasses the high-resistance lung fields by shunting via the ductus arteriosus to the aorta and into systemic circulation. Within the heart, pressures in the right ventricle exceed those in the left. Blood flows through the foramen ovale from the right atrium to the left atrium, driven by the pressure gradient created by the alignment of the inferior vena cava with the foramen ovale (Fig. 5.1). The transition from fetal to neonatal life necessitates that the pulmonary circulatory pressures drop below those of the systemic circulation and that the lung changes from a secretory organ to one of gas exchange.

During gestation, fetal oxygen levels are relatively low. As a result, fetal pulmonary circulation is constricted and pulmonary vascular resistance is high. At birth, the first breaths create an air–fluid interface in the alveoli and expand the lung. Surfactant acts to decrease the surface tension within the alveolar spaces. Without surfactant, the alveolar walls would collapse and gas exchange would be impossible. Once the alveolar spaces fill with air, the pressures within the pulmonary capillaries decrease. This is partly due to the increased partial pressure of arterial oxygen (PaO_2), which cause arteriolar resistance to diminish. Consequently, the overall vascular resistance within the lung becomes less than that in the systemic circulation. This allows fetal lung fluid within the alveoli to be slowly absorbed into the venous and lymphatics channels. The mechanics of breathing assist fluid drainage from the alveoli, as do changes in intrathoracic pressures. Alterations of intra-abdominal and intrathoracic pressures

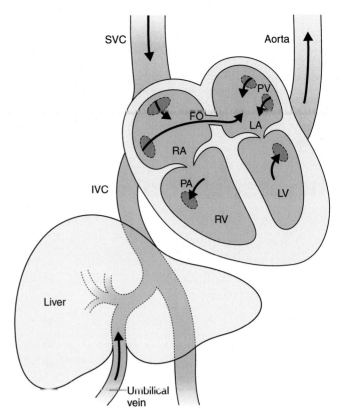

Fig. 5.1 • Schematic diagram depicting direction of blood flow through the fetal heart. Blood flows easily from the inferior vena cava (IVC) through the foramen ovale (FO) to the left atrium (LA), due to the alignment of the IVC and FO. PA, pulmonary artery; SVC, superior vena cava; PV, pulmonary vein; RA, right atrium; LV, left ventricle.

assist lymphatic drainage from the lungs. When the movement of fetal lung fluid from the alveoli is hampered, a condition known as transient tachypnea of the newborn (TNN), or respiratory distress syndrome type II, may develop.

During the first day of life, fluid volume within the alveoli decreases and air volume within the lung increases. Both act to increase PaO_2 and decrease the vascular resistance within the pulmonary tree. As a result blood will flow towards the low-resistance pulmonary system rather than passing through the ductus arteriosus or foramen ovale. The decreased volume of flow, increased concentration of oxygen and altered fetal prostaglandin levels all lead to closure of the ductus towards the end of the first day of life. It is important to remember that the newborn pulmonary vasculature retains its thick musculature during the early newborn period. The smooth muscle of the vascular walls will constrict under hypoxic or acidotic conditions, which may lead to the development of pulmonary hypertension. If this occurs the increased resistance in the lung can raise the pressure in the right ventricle to a higher level than that of the left and 're-open' the still functional foramen ovale.

The neonatal lung differs from that of the adult, and even child, in the number, size and topography of the alveoli.

At birth, the alveoli have a double capillary network, which subsequently fuses, creating a single system. During the first 18 months of life, the alveoli will continue the process of septation that began in utero. Arteries, veins and capillaries accompany alveoli as they fold, branch and lengthen. During this time there is a disproportionate increase in surface area inside the lungs when compared with the enlargement of the lung itself. Throughout the first 3 years of life, the number of alveoli increases from 20 million to 200 million (O'Brodovich & Haddad 2001). Once the respiratory tree has developed, the process of septation slows. A second phase of pulmonary growth begins, and while new alveoli may still form, growth primarily affects alveoli volume and capillary space in proportion to somatic growth. This second phase continues through adolescence, increasing the dimensions of the alveoli fourfold (O'Brodovich & Haddad 2001). Factors such as height, level of activity and level of oxygen exposure (altitude) all influence the ultimate size and configuration of the lung fields.

SURFACTANT

There is a natural tendency for the lungs to recoil. This results from two factors: the numerous elastin fibers scattered throughout the lung parenchyma that stretch during inhalation and contract as the lung deflates; and the surface tension of the fluid coating the alveoli walls. The elastic fibers account for one-third of the lungs' recoil tendency, while the surface tension accounts for the remaining two-thirds. These factors are partially countered by the intrapleural pressure, which remains negative, at about 24 mmHg (Guyton 1996). However, the intrapleural pressures alone would be unable to prevent atelectasis and collapse in the absence of pulmonary surfactant. Surfactant is a lipoprotein substance that is secreted into the alveolar space. It acts to decrease the surface tension at the air–fluid interface. In the absence of surfactant, intrapleural pressures would need to be maintained at 220–230 mmHg to counteract the surface tensions in the alveoli and small airways. When surfactant production or function is impaired, respiratory distress develops.

Surfactant is primarily secreted into the alveolar subspace by type II granular pneumocytes. During the respiratory cycle, surfactant is absorbed into the alveolar fluid, forming a hydrophobic lipid monolayer over the film of alveolar fluid. The lipid component acts to decrease the surface tension by interfering with attraction between the molecules of the fluid. The delivery and absorption of the phospholipids is dependent on the protein component of surfactant. There are at least four types of surfactant protein (and probably more) responsible for increasing the rate of delivery of phospholipids, the formation of tubular myelin (a repository for intermediate surfactant), and the reuptake and recycling of surfactant. In addition to decreasing surface tension within the alveoli, surfactant has a role in maintaining the patency of small airways, preventing leakage of fluid from the interstitium and assisting in host defense mechanisms (Griese 1992, Mason & Lewis 2000), such as increasing phagocytic activity in pulmonary macrophages (Arnon et al 1993, Bellanti & Zeligs 1995).

Surfactant is first present at about 24 weeks of gestation, but levels are insufficient to support ventilation. Mature levels of surfactant are normally present after 35 weeks of gestation (Kliegman 1996). In the presence of diminished surfactant, the alveoli collapse and atelectasis develops. This is the initiating mechanism for hyaline membrane disease (see Ch. 13). Hyaline membrane disease or neonatal respiratory distress syndrome type I, as it is sometimes called, is the most common complication of prematurity and is due to insufficient surfactant production. Fetal lungs do not begin to produce sufficient levels of surfactant until the third trimester and infants born before sufficient levels are present often experience neonatal respiratory distress (NRD). As a result, infants of early gestational age and/or low birthweight have increased risk of NRD. The sequelae of NRD will vary, depending on the extent of hypoxia and damage to the lungs. Complications include atelectasis, microhemorrhage, inflammation, pulmonary hypertension and hyaline membrane formation. NRD increases the long-term risk for bronchopulmonary dysplasia, intraventricular hemorrhage, retinopathy and brain damage. Surfactant production is adversely influenced by prematurity, hypoxia, genetic abnormalities, cold stress and multi-fetal pregnancy. There also appears to be an association between decreased levels of surfactant and cesarean section (Kliegman 1996). Surfactant production is stimulated by the presence of thyroid hormone and glucocorticoids. Delayed maturation of surfactant production is seen in infants of mothers with diabetes and hypothyroidism, although the mechanisms are unclear (Murray & Nadel 2000).

THE FIRST BREATH

The first breath occurs in response to many factors, including increased carbon dioxide, decreased oxygen and pH, decrease in body temperature and alteration in hemodynamics (Haddad & Perez Fontain 1996a–c). The first breath occurs due to a forceful contraction of respiratory muscles. Ideally, it should occur after the infant is completely delivered. A first breath taken while the infant's torso is still in the mother's vaginal canal is met with the resistance of the surrounding maternal tissues and is ineffective. As one would expect, these children have somatic dysfunction in the thorax, ribs and diaphragm, as well as the scalene muscles and cranial base. Often these children have irritability and/or reflux, which develop soon after birth. Under normal conditions the first breath is long and accompanied by increased pulmonary pressures that overcome the surface and viscous forces within the alveoli. Infants lacking the strength or coordination to generate the forces needed to inflate the alveoli will have delayed onset of normal breathing mechanics, even if surfactant levels are mature. The functional residual capacity established with the first breath is built upon with each subsequent breath as, over the next few hours, the lung physiology changes. The first breath is the most difficult, with each subsequent breath becoming more effective and less strenuous. Accordingly, it takes over 40 min for near-normal lung compliance to develop (Murray & Nadel 2000).

Osteopathic observation of 1600 neonates immediately after birth demonstrated the presence of a functional fulcrum in the deep tissues at the level of T3–T4 on the right (Carreiro 1994). Because this fulcrum was only observed in newborns who attempted spontaneous breathing, it is assumed to be associated with the transition to air breathing. This thoracic fulcrum was ill-defined in newborns older than 25 weeks who had respiratory complications. In addition, tissue strains at the area of this fulcrum have also been found in older children with chronic respiratory disease (chart review and physician survey).

BREATHING: RESPIRATORY CONTROL

Respiratory control is under a negative feedback system. Chemoreceptors and mechanoreceptors in the larynx and upper airways respond to stretch, temperature and chemical stimuli. Information from sensors in the larynx and upper respiratory tree travels along the superior laryngeal and vagus nerves to the brainstem. This information is relayed to centers in the brainstem and medulla that control the timing and activity of all the muscles of respiration, including the intercostal muscles and diaphragm. The carotid bodies sense oxygen levels. Signals from the carotid bodies travel along the carotid sinus nerves. Information from the tissues of the airways and the carotid bodies is compared in the central nervous system. It may be integrated with information concerning the emotional state of the individual or level of stress to influence breathing (Chow et al 1986). However, afferent information is not necessary for respiration to occur. In animal models phrenic nerve activity can be detected after removal of the brainstem and spinal cord, although it is slower than would be considered normal (Haddad & Perez Fontain 1996a–c). It is hypothesized that pulmonary chemotactic receptors have a role in respiratory control in this situation.

Afferent input from lung parenchyma is primarily from rapidly adapting C fibers and slowly adapting stretch fibers. The slowly adapting fibers are located in bronchial smooth muscle and are triggered by increases in lung volume or pressure. Stimulation of slowly adapting fibers can trigger bronchodilation, tachycardia, decreased blood pressure and/or respiratory

inhibition. Alternatively, the rapidly adapting C fibers respond to mechanical and chemical irritation, resulting in bronchospasm and cough. In general, the neonate is much more sensitive to afferent input than the adult. Laryngeal reflexes triggered by aspiration or stimulation of laryngeal chemoreceptors will inhibit respiration in the infant; this is the Hering-Breuer reflex (Haddad & Perez Fontain 1996a–c). Hypoglycemia and anemia in the neonate will also adversely affect respiration. Hypoxia will decrease ventilatory effort in the neonate, in contrast to the adult, in whom it will cause an increase. The overall ventilatory response to increased levels of carbon dioxide in the infant and newborn is also diminished, when compared with the adult.

BREATHING: THE VENTILATORY PUMP IN THE INFANT AND YOUNG CHILD

Coordinated interaction between respiratory muscle groups is necessary for effective ventilation. All respiratory muscles are skeletal in nature and the pattern of skeletal muscle innervation changes during postnatal development. At birth, motor units may overlap, such that a given muscle fiber is innervated by more than one axon. By adulthood, the motor units have matured and remodeled, so that each muscle fiber or group of muscle fibers will be innervated by a single axon. This maturation and remodeling process occurs in response to various stimuli, and represents an activity-dependent mechanism. The neuromuscular junction and synaptic cleft will also undergo changes. For example, infant acetylcholine receptors differ from those of the adult and acetylcholinesterase activity is decreased in infants. This makes infants susceptible to neuromuscular transmission failure during rapidly repeated stimulation, such as tachypnea. In addition, the sarcoplasmic reticulum within the muscle fiber is poorly developed in the newborn, which increases the contraction and relaxation times of the muscle.

The respiratory muscles of the infant labor under an increased workload created by the structural characteristics of the infant chest. The pliability of the rib cage and thorax in the newborn is necessary for passage through the vaginal canal. After birth, however, it becomes something of a detriment. In the adult, the functional residual capacity (FRC) of the lung is maintained through a balance between the recoil tendency of the lung and the resistance of the stiff rib cage. FRC is the volume of air left in the lung at the end of a normal exhalation. The presence of FRC provides a supply of oxygen to alveolar capillaries and a repository for carbon dioxide between the respiratory phases. FRC is important for maximizing gas exchange and hemoglobin saturation. As FRC falls, hemoglobin saturation falls and hypoxemia develops. Because the newborn's rib cage offers no resistance to the recoil properties of the lung, FRC must be maintained through active work (Wohl 2000). The muscles of inhalation sustain some contractile tone at all times to prevent the chest wall from collapsing. This significantly increases the work of breathing in the infant. During rapid eye movement (REM) sleep, infants do not maintain inhalation tone and typically exhibit chest wall retractions even during quiet breathing. When the respiratory system is stressed, as may occur with infection, atelectasis, pulmonary edema and obstructive processes, FRC is compromised, placing the infant at increased risk for hypoxemia. As previously described, the skeletal muscles of newborns possess immature neuromuscular junctions, and fatigue quickly under increased workloads. Clinically, positive end-expiratory pressure (PEEP) can be used to assist infants and newborns in maintaining FRC when respiration is compromised. The ability of the infant to passively maintain FRC is not established until the end of the first year (Collin et al 1989), when rib cage compliance begins to decrease due to ossification. The ossification of the rib cage and sternum continues through the first 25 years of life (Wohl 2000).

THE RESPIRATORY TREE

There are three anatomical components to the respiratory tree: the upper airway that extends from the nose to the thoracic inlet, the middle airway that extends from the thoracic inlet to the main stem bronchi and the lower airway from the main stem bronchus to the alveoli. From the trachea through the bronchial tree to the labyrinth of the alveoli, the narrow airways of newborns and infants are vulnerable to congestion, inflammation and edema. Even under normal conditions, their small airways have greater resistance than that found in older children. Increased airway resistance causes air flow turbulence which impedes air movement and gas exchange. Increased airway resistance may present clinically as stridor, grunting or wheezing depending on the level of involvement. In the adult, constant tone is present in the upper airways so that during inhalation this section expands and during exhalation it narrows but maintains patency. In the newborn and infant, the upper airway expands with normal inhalation, but under stress the airway can collapse if the negative intrathoracic pressures supersede the relatively weak pharyngeal musculature. Collapse may also occur as a result of an obstructive process in the upper airway such as laryngotracheobronchitis, atresia or abscess. This typically presents as inspiratory stridor. Obstruction in the lower airway, such as occurs with asthma, will present as expiratory wheezing.

MUSCLES OF RESPIRATION

Inhalation requires that the forces of lung recoil, chest wall elasticity and airway resistance be overcome. This is the work of the diaphragm and muscles of respiration. The most obvious muscles of respiration are the diaphragm and intercostals; however, there are two other muscle groups that also have respiration as a primary function. These are the scalene muscles of the neck and the quadratus lumborum muscles of the back. Each of these muscle groups acts to stabilize the rib cage during active contraction of the diaphragm. Without them, the mechanical efficiency of the thoracic cage would be undermined. Within the osteopathic concept, the importance of the pelvic diaphragm in respiration cannot be overlooked. In concert with abdominal and thoracic muscles, the tissues of the pelvis act to generate intra-abdominal pressures that facilitate ventilation and generate flow gradients in the low-pressure circulatory system. There are also numerous accessory muscles of respiration, ranging from retrosternal muscles to hip flexors. These are called upon during times of respiratory distress to assist the primary muscles in their function. The extent to which an individual uses accessory respiratory muscles can be used as a rough assessment of the degree of respiratory distress. However, this is less the case in the very young child, where, as we shall see, the mechanics of normal respiration differ significantly from those of an adult.

In infants, the muscle sequencing for inhalation differs from that of the adult. The genioglossus muscle contracts, moving the tongue anteriorly. This opens the posterior pharyngeal space. The vocal cords abduct, decreasing laryngeal resistance. Then the scalenes, intercostals and diaphragm engage. During REM sleep, the intercostal muscles are inhibited in the infant, so that the chest wall becomes very compliant. With each inspiration, the anterior chest wall collapses as the abdomen protrudes. This is readily observed in a sleeping baby. Compliance of the anterior chest wall increases the workload of respiration, potentially leading to muscle fatigue (Haddad & Mellins 1984, Haddad & Perez Fontain 1996a–c).

The scalene–intercostal–oblique muscles: a functional unit

The intercostal muscles are arranged in three layers, with their fibers perpendicular to the ribs (Fig. 5.2). Embryologically, they are formed as the diaphragm etches down the inner surface of the thorax and the primitive rib cartilage condenses. The external intercostal muscles are involved in inhalation. The internal intercostal muscles are involved in exhalation. The function of each muscle group has to do with the sequencing of contraction rather than the orientation of the muscle fibers. According to De Troyer and Estenne (1988), elevation of the first rib by the scalene muscles establishes an anchor against which the contracting intercostal muscles may act. If the first rib is elevated when the intercostal muscle contracts, it will draw the second rib superiorly, and then the third and so on. Conversely, if the lower ribs are pulled down and prevented from

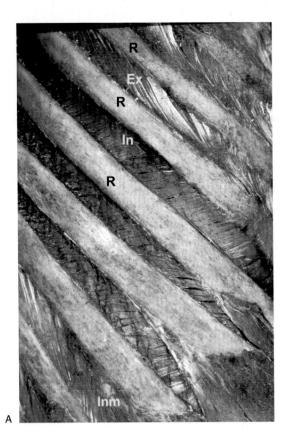
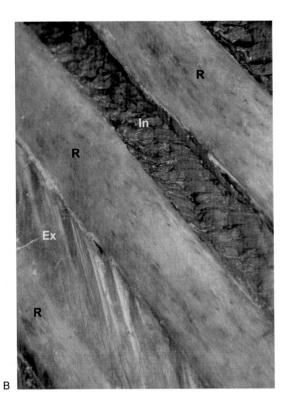

Fig. 5.2 • Distant (A) and close-up (B) views of the intercostal muscles of an adult specimen. Note the different orientation of the muscle fibers. R, rib; Ex, external intercostal; In, internal intercostal; Inm, innermost intercostal. *Used with permission of the Willard & Carreiro Collection.*

moving, then contraction of the intercostal muscles would draw the adjacent rib inferiorly. The external intercostals contract during inhalation after the scalene muscles have raised the first rib. They contract sequentially from a rostral to caudal position, lifting the ribs, increasing the intrathoracic space and creating a negative intrathoracic pressure. Consequently, the external intercostals act as muscles of inhalation. After the abdominus oblique and quadratus muscles have fixed the lower ribs, the internal intercostals contract sequentially from the bottom upwards, drawing the ribs inferiorly, which decreases the intrathoracic space and increases intrathoracic pressure. Thus the internal intercostal muscles are involved with exhalation. The innermost intercostal muscles can be divided functionally into the parasternal muscles involved with inhalation, and the transversus thoracic and subcostal muscles involved with forced or late exhalation. The thoracic cage in the infant and neonate tends to be splayed laterally and the ribs oriented horizontally. The adult configuration will not be reached until about 10 years of age (Openshaw et al 1984). This alters the biomechanical efficiency of the intercostal muscles, forcing the child to engage accessory muscles.

The diaphragm

The diaphragm is actually a continuation of the innermost intercostal muscles. It forms around a thin aponeurosis, called the central tendon. The ventral portion of the diaphragm develops from septum transversum mesenchyme and attaches the diaphragm to the anterior abdominal wall. The central portion develops from splanchnopleuric mesenchyme (which also coats the pleuroperitoneal membrane). The lateral portion of the diaphragm develops from somatopleuric mesenchyme. Somatomyocytes from C3–C5 migrate into the lateral portion carrying the innervating neurons of the diaphragm. Once the plate of the diaphragm is formed, it descends so that the posterior portion migrates to the level of T12–L1.

The central tendon lies immediately below the pericardium, with which it is partially blended (Fig. 5.3). It is trifoliate in shape. The anterior leaf is shaped like an equilateral triangle, with the apex towards the xiphoid process. The right and left folia are tongue-shaped and curve laterally and backwards. The left is slightly narrower. The central area of the tendon has four diagonal bands fanning out from a thickened node in front of the esophagus and left of the vena cava.

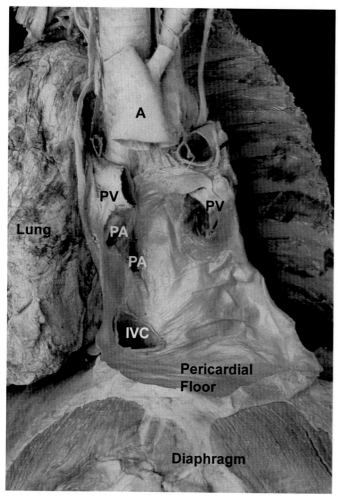

Fig. 5.3 • This is a view into the deep mediastinum of an adult specimen. The anterior chest wall has been removed, the pericardium has been opened and the heart removed. The posterior wall of the visceral pericardium is displayed. The great vessels are labeled: A, aorta; PV, pulmonary vein; PA, pulmonary artery; IVC, inferior vena cava. The superior vena cava has been removed. The floor of the pericardial sac rests upon the central tendon of the diaphragm. Other attachments between the pericardium and diaphragm can also be seen. *Used with permission of the Willard & Carreiro Collection.*

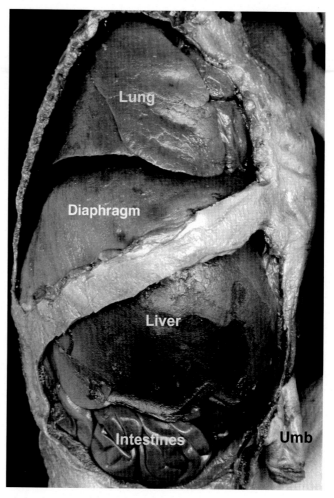

Fig. 5.4 • Right-sided, anterolateral view of a newborn specimen. The rib cage and lateral abdominal wall have been removed to expose the intrathoracic and intra-abdominal contents. The diaphragm can be seen draped over the liver. Its peripheral attachment to the lower ribs has been left in place. Umb, umbilicus. *Used with permission of the Willard & Carreiro Collection.*

The fibers of the diaphragm radiate out from the central tendon. The posterior muscular fibers are much longer than the anterior, extending into the lower thoracic area. This arrangement gives the diaphragm a butterfly shape. The butterfly is draped over the abdominal contents, attaching to the surrounding osseous structures at its periphery (Fig. 5.4). The sternal part of the muscle arises from two fleshy slips off the back of the xiphoid process. The costal part arises from the internal surfaces of the lower six costal cartilages and their adjoining ribs on each side. It interdigitates with the transversus abdominis muscle. The lumbar part arises from two aponeurotic arches, the medial and lateral arcuate ligaments, and from the two crura attached to the lumbar vertebrae.

The crura of the diaphragm are tendinous attachments that blend with the anterior longitudinal ligament (Fig. 5.5). When the diaphragm contracts, the crura will exert a force on their vertebral attachments. This accounts for some of the vertebral motion observed with respiration. According to early osteopathic teaching (A Wales, personal communication, 1989), the influence of the crura upon the anterior longitudinal ligament rocks the vertebra and connective tissue structures of the posterior thoracic wall. Passing through these tissues are prevertebral lymphatics, veins and the sympathetic trunks (Fig. 5.6). The gentle rocking of the vertebrae and surrounding tissues has been described by early osteopaths as a passive pump mechanism which influences fluid movement through Batson's plexus and other structures of the low-pressure circulatory system. Thus the movements generated through the anterior ligament via its

An Osteopathic Approach to Children

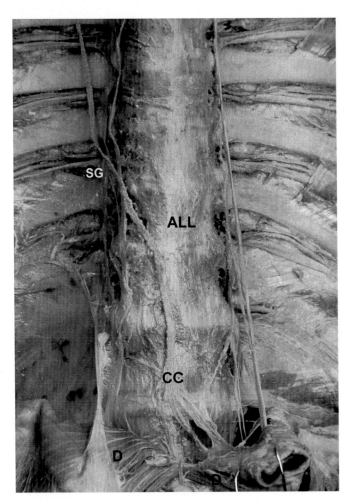

Fig. 5.5 • View of the posterior wall of the thorax. The vertebral column is in the middle of the photograph. The great vessels have been removed and the esophagus has been pulled forward. The posterior aspect of the diaphragm (D) can be seen. Sympathetic chain ganglia (SG) run along the heads of the ribs. ALL, anterior longitudinal ligament; CC, cisterna chyle. *Used with permission of the Willard & Carreiro Collection.*

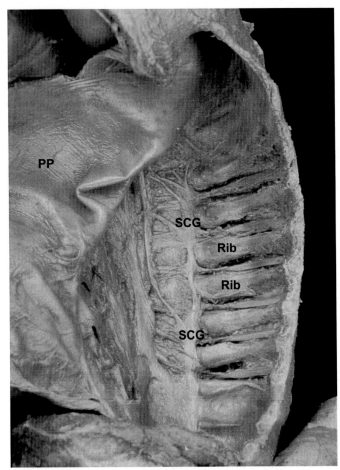

Fig. 5.6 • Posterior thoracic wall of a newborn specimen viewed from a slightly lateral perspective. The rib cage has been cut and the left side is displayed. The parietal pleura (PP) has been lifted away to reveal the ribs and sympathetic chain ganglia (SCG). *Used with permission of the Willard & Carreiro Collection.*

connections to the diaphragmatic crura act to promote fluid homeostasis and trophic function within structures surrounding the spine.

The right crus is broader and longer than the left. It arises from the anterolateral surfaces of the bodies of the upper three lumbar vertebrae. The left crus arises from the anterolateral portion of the bodies of the upper two lumbar vertebrae. The medial tendinous margins of the crura meet in the midline to form the median arcuate ligament, an arch across the front of the aorta at the level of the thoracolumbar disk. Andrew Taylor Still metaphorically referred to this relationship in his 'goat and the boulder' analogies (A Wales, personal communication, 1990). Compression or narrowing of this arch will affect flow in the aorta, increasing afterload on the heart. The medial arcuate ligament is continuous medially with the lateral margin of the crus and

is attached to the side of the body of the first or second lumbar vertebra. Laterally, it is fixed to the front of the transverse process of T12 and arches over the psoas muscle (Fig. 5.7). Abnormal tensions in this ligament may irritate the psoas muscle, resulting in pain and spasm. Conversely psoas spasm may influence diaphragmatic mechanics. Infants will present with a tendency to keep the hips flexed and act irritably when they are extended for nappy changing. The lateral arcuate ligament is a thickened band of fascia extending from the anterior aspect of the transverse process of the first lumbar vertebra to the lower margin of the 12th rib near its midpoint. It arches across the upper part of the quadratus lumborum muscle. The iliohypogastric and ilioinguinal nerves pass under the lateral arcuate ligament (Fig. 5.8). Besides affecting respiratory excursion, malpositioning of the 12th rib may create abnormal tensions in the lateral arcuate ligament, resulting in irritation of the iliohypogastric or ilioinguinal nerves. In the older child

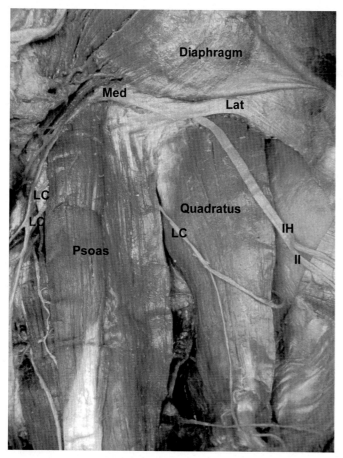

Fig. 5.7 • The medial (Med) and lateral (Lat) arcuate ligaments of the left side of the body. The diaphragm has been lifted. The psoas and quadratus are visible, as are branches of the lateral cutaneous nerve (LC) passing under the medial arcuate ligament. The relation between the iliohypogastric nerve (IH), ilioinguinal nerve (II) and lateral arcuate ligament is also evident. *Used with permission of the Willard & Carreiro Collection.*

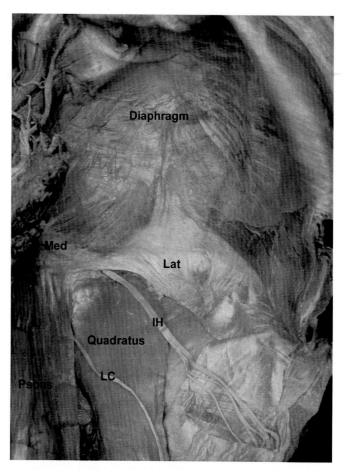

Fig. 5.8 • In this photograph the diaphragm has been stretched so that the full architecture of the lateral arcuate ligament (Lat) can be appreciated. The lateral cutaneous (LC) and iliohypogastric (IH) nerves are also labeled. Med, medial arcuate ligament. *Used with permission of the Willard & Carreiro Collection.*

or young athlete, this may present as paresthesias or radiating pain over the anterior aspect of the thigh and groin with running activities.

Functional anatomy of the diaphragm

When laid out on a flat surface and viewed from above, the diaphragm resembles a butterfly with the central tendon lying between the two wings. It drapes over the abdominal contents, attaching to the upper portion of the lower six ribs anterolaterally, the first three lumbar vertebrae posteriorly and the sternum anteriorly. The costal portion drapes down over the abdominal viscera and attaches to the lower ribs. Consequently, the diaphragm is superior to its attachments. This creates a 'zone of apposition' (Fig. 5.9) in which the costal fibers are oriented cranially. The zone of apposition represents about 30% of the total surface of the rib cage in an erect adult, although in the very

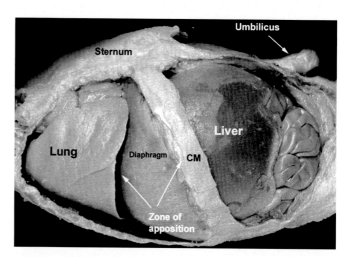

Fig. 5.9 • A lateral view of a newborn specimen. The lateral rib cage and abdominal wall have been excised to reveal the viscera. The zone of apposition is indicated by the arrows. CM, costal margin. *Used with permission of the Willard & Carreiro Collection.*

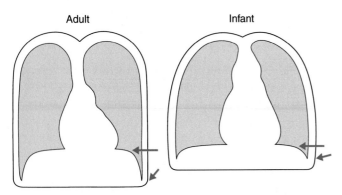

Adult   **Infant**

Fig. 5.10 • Schematic diagram comparing the zones of apposition in the newborn and adult.

young child the proportion is considerably less (Fig. 5.10). In the toddler and older child, as in the adult, the abdominal viscera act as a piston resisting the compressive forces of the descending dome. The diaphragm uses this resistance to lift the ribs and expand the size of the rib cage. As the diaphragm muscle contracts during inhalation, the muscle fibers shorten, the zone of apposition decreases and the dome of the diaphragm descends (De Troyer & Estenne 1988). This creates negative pressure within the thoracic cage and decreases pleural pressure. At the same time, the intra-abdominal pressure increases, causing an outward motion of the anterior abdominal wall. The abdominal muscles must resist this motion in order to maximize diaphragmatic work. Newborn infants and young children lack sufficient muscle coordination to engage the abdominal muscles against the diaphragm. This compromises the efficiency of diaphragmatic breathing. Consequently, infants and young children must rely on abdominal breathing, which involves using the abdominal muscles to facilitate diaphragm descent. The result is shallower and faster respiration, which increases the overall work of breathing. Once the anatomical relationships have attained a more adult configuration, average respiratory rate decreases and tidal volumes increase.

In addition to the less efficient configuration of the zone of apposition, newborns also need to overcome the negative contribution of chest wall compliancy during respiration. In a non-compliant chest wall, the work of the descending diaphragm against the resistant rib cage increases the intrathoracic volume. However, the compliant thoracic cage of the infant may be overcome by the force of the descending diaphragm and distort inwardly, decreasing the intrathoracic volume. In order to maintain tidal volume, the diaphragm needs to increase its descent proportionately to the inward movement of the rib cage. This is not an easy feat, especially during times of increased respiratory demand as may occur in infection or with other respiratory disease. The newborn will often resort to increasing ventilatory rate to compensate for the decreased volume. This soon leads to

muscle fatigue, dehydration and respiratory distress. Even under relatively normal conditions, the neonatal respiratory system may be compromised by somatic dysfunction.

The muscles of the oropharynx

In newborns, the pharyngeal muscles are of particular importance in respiratory function. The muscles of the pharynx form a tube anchored posteriorly to the pharyngeal raphe, and suspended from the inferior surfaces of the sphenoid and petrous portions of the temporal bones. The inferior portion is more flexible and narrow than the superior (Bosma 1986). This tubular structure forms the nasopharynx and supralaryngeal space. Its patency is necessary for the unobstructed movement of gases into and out of the lungs. Like the chest wall during inhalation, the upper airway must also resist the negative intrathoracic pressure created by the descending diaphragm. If the walls of the pharynx come into contact with each other, the resulting surface tension will draw them together and the tube will collapse. The presence of a cough reflex in children and adults protects them from the collapse of the tube. Irritation to the walls of the pharynx triggers a cough reflex, which inhibits diaphragmatic contraction and generates a forceful exhalation that opens the pharyngeal tube. However, the cough reflex is not present in newborns and premature infants. Consequently, if the walls of the pharynx begin to come into contact with each other, there is nothing to stop their progress. Continued diaphragmatic activity will draw the pharyngeal walls closer and collapse the airway. This is thought to be one of the mechanisms of apnea in the newborn (Bosma 1986). The area between the posterior pharyngeal wall, the soft palate and the genioglossus muscle is most often involved. Adding to this situation is the fact that the tone in the pharyngeal and oral muscles relaxes during sleep. Studies investigating the effect of posture on muscle tone and activity have shown that tone in the genioglossus muscle changes in response to the position of the head and neck. Flexion of the neck tends to increase the pliability of the pharynx and narrows its lumen (Thach & Stark 1979), contributing to the risk of collapse. Studies have also shown that the workload demand on the pharyngeal muscles to maintain patency against diaphragm contraction is increased in cervical flexion (Bosma 1986). There is an increase in the incidence of apnea in infants who sleep in the prone position (Willinger et al 1994), a position in which the baby tends to tuck the chin and flex the neck.

Apneic episodes in any child deserve a comprehensive medical evaluation. Findings on osteopathic evaluation often include restrictions at the craniocervical junction and condylar area, and interosseous strains in the cranial base. Dysfunction of the previously described neonatal respiratory fulcrum at T3–T4 is rarely found in children with apnea (physician and practitioner survey). Most adults and infants experience some type of respiratory pause during sleep. These are usually very brief and are followed by a return to normal breathing activity. When accompanied by cyanosis or when they occur in the very young or premature, the pauses are of greater significance. Undiagnosed illness, congenital abnormalities, immature function of the respiratory tract, and cardiovascular and central nervous system pathology must all be considered.

The abdominal muscles

The primary muscles of exhalation are the abdominal muscles, although they do show some activity during inhalation, when they contract to stabilize the abdominal piston. The rectus and transverse abdominis and the oblique muscles are engaged during exhalation, contracting against the abdominal contents and increasing intra-abdominal pressure. The increased abdominal pressure forces the diaphragm cephalad. Concurrently, the lower ribs (10th–12th) are pulled inferiorly and stabilized by the rectus and oblique muscles. Once this has occurred, then the sequential contraction of the internal intercostals pulls the remaining ribs inferiorly as the diaphragm rises. In conjunction with the natural recoil of the lungs the intrathoracic volume decreases and intrathoracic pressure increases, forcing air out of the lungs. Rapid and forceful contraction of the abdominal and intercostal muscles results in forced exhalation and/or cough.

OTHER IMPORTANT ANATOMICAL RELATIONSHIPS OF THE THORAX

The cardiac plateau of the diaphragm is positioned more to the left than the right, and upon it rests the pericardium and its contents (Fig. 5.11). Laterally, the diaphragm has two domes or cupolas; the right is higher and broader, and covers the liver. The diaphragm and liver are in close contact. As the diaphragm descends, the liver is moved inferiorly. In conditions of hepatic inflammation, the diaphragm may become irritated, resulting in referred pain to the right shoulder via afferents in the phrenic nerve. There may also be splinting of normal diaphragmatic contractions which causes decreased ventilatory volumes.

Motor supply to the diaphragm is through the phrenic nerve. The right crus is innervated by both left and right phrenic nerves. Although all motor supply is carried in the phrenic nerve, the crural portion of the diaphragm contracts slightly before the costal portion. Sensation is carried from the peripheral part of the muscle fibers via the lower six or seven intercostal nerves.

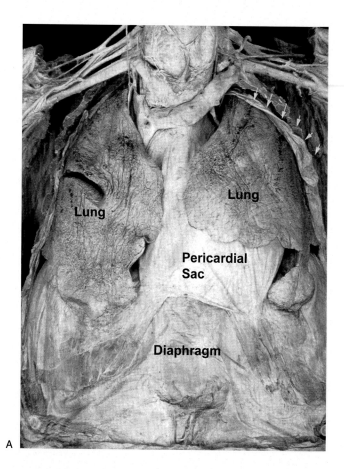

A

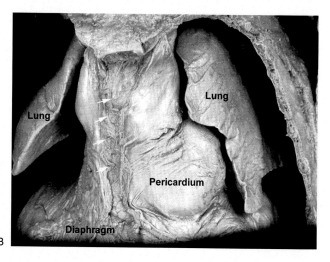

B

Fig. 5.11 • An adult (A) and newborn (B) specimen are presented for comparison. A complete anterior thoracotomy has been done to reveal the intrathoracic viscera. The newborn view is slightly lateral to the midline. Note the roughness of the mediastinal tissues where the sternum was attached (white arrowheads, newborn specimen). The thymus is the large structure perched on top of the heart. The pericardial sac displays continuity with the superior surface of the diaphragm, which is more prominent in the newborn than in the adult. The white arrows in the adult specimen mark the cut edge of the pleural sac. *Used with permission of the Willard & Carreiro Collection.*

APERTURES IN THE DIAPHRAGM

The aortic aperture is the lowest and most posterior, at the level of the 12th thoracic vertebra and the thoracolumbar intervertebral disk, slightly to the left of the midline. It is an osseous-aponeurotic opening defined by the diaphragmatic crura laterally, the diaphragm muscle anteriorly and the vertebrae posteriorly. When the diaphragm is flattened or the crura tight, this space and the contents passing through it may be restricted (Still's goat and the boulder). Occasionally, some tendinous fibers from the medial aspect of the crura pass behind the aorta. Accompanying the aorta are the azygos and hemiazygos veins, and lymphatic trunks draining the lower posterior thoracic wall.

The esophageal aperture is located at the level of the T10 vertebra. It is superior, anterior and to the left of the aortic aperture. The esophagus, gastric nerves, esophageal branches of the left gastric vessels and some lymphatic vessels pass through this space. The aperture has an oblique shape. Fibers from the medial part of the right crus cross the midline, encircle the esophagus and form a chimney for the terminal portion (Fig. 5.12). The innermost fibers are arranged circumferentially, and the outermost in a vertical direction. This arrangement is capable of exerting a radial pressure on the esophagus. As the diaphragm descends during inhalation, the fibers around the esophagus contract and the esophagus is compressed. This prevents gastrointestinal contents from refluxing into the thoracic esophagus during respiration. Abnormalities in diaphragm mechanics may interfere with this process and result in symptoms of reflux and spitting up. Even in a normal situation, the decreased vertical excursion of the infant diaphragm compromises the ability of the diaphragm to compress the esophagus and prevent reflux. (This is made evident on your shoulder when a baby is overfed.) Although there is no direct continuity between the esophageal wall and the muscle forming the aperture, the fascia on the inferior surface of the diaphragm extends upwards to form a flat cone which blends with the wall of the esophagus, 2–3 cm above the gastroesophageal junction. Some elastic fibers carried within this fascia penetrate into the esophageal submucosa to form the phrenoesophageal ligament. This connects the esophagus with the diaphragm while allowing some freedom of movement during swallowing and respiration. It also limits upward displacement of the diaphragm.

The venal caval aperture lies at the level of the eighth and ninth thoracic vertebrae. It is quadrilateral-shaped and located between the right leaf and the central area of the tendon. The margins are aponeurotic. The vena cava, which passes through this aperture, adheres to the margin of the opening. During inhalation, the fibers forming this aperture contract and the opening widens. This allows venous blood to flow into the heart, enhanced by the negative

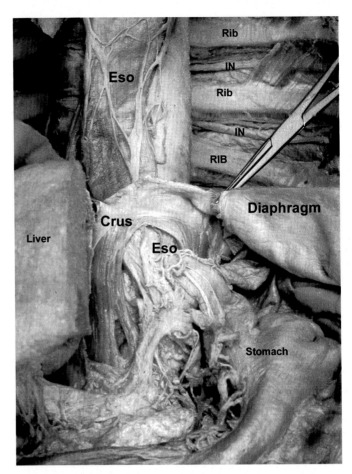

Fig. 5.12 • Anterior view of the thorax at the level of the diaphragmatic crura. The liver has been resected and the diaphragm cut and lifted to reveal the crus. The esophagus (Eso) can be seen passing through the hiatus. The ribs and intercostal nerves (IN) are labeled. *Used with permission of the Willard & Carreiro Collection.*

intrathoracic pressure. Branches of the right phrenic nerve also traverse this space.

THE SECRETORY ROLE OF THE RESPIRATORY TREE

The pulmonary system is one of the few places in the body where the internal milieu is directly exposed to substances in the environment. This, combined with the fact that all the blood of the body is continuously filtered through the lungs, means that the immune system can receive information about antigenic substances entering the respiratory tree. In the newborn and infant, the lung, along with the gastrointestinal tract, is one of the foremost priming sites for immune activity.

The airways of the lungs are blanketed by a viscoelastic mucus which traps contaminants and antigens entering the bronchial tree. Pulmonary mucus is primarily composed of water, with a small amount of lipids, proteins and minerals. Secretory IgA is the major immunoglobulin in the bronchial mucus. In combination with IgG and IgM, it will opsonize particulate antigens and participate in complement fixation. Lysozymes are also secreted into the airways. These enzymes have a bacteriolytic function which is effective against *Streptococcus pneumoniae* and certain types of fungi.

Mucus secretion is stimulated to the same extent by sympathetic and parasympathetic activity (Gallagher et al 1975). Mucus secretion represents the efferent loop of a reflex pathway. Similar to the mechanisms discussed in Chapter 1, there is a certain amount of convergence occurring between visceral tissues, a viscerovisceral reflex. In the lung this is probably mediated through the vagus nerve. Irritation of gastric mucosa will stimulate mucus production in the lungs (German et al 1982). This is probably the result of neurogenic inflammation. When irritated, primary afferents in the lungs secrete substance P, tachykinins, vasoactive intestinal polypeptide and other substances. These substances act on epithelial cells, smooth muscles and glands within the walls of airways, causing increased production of mucus and lysozymes, vasodilation and smooth muscle contraction.

Mucus containing waste products and contaminants is cleared from the lungs via the mucociliary transport system. The cilia of the respiratory tract act to move the mucus secretions towards the glottis, where they will be swallowed. There is some suggestion that mucociliary clearance is slower in the infant than in the adult (Wanner et al 1996). Impairment of this transport system will adversely affect the individual's health. These children usually present with chronic cough productive of thick mucus. The level of hypoxia and hypercapnia will be proportional to the severity of the involvement. Genetic abnormalities in the mucociliary system are rare and usually picked up when the child is young. Certain viruses, especially influenza, attach to the cilia and paralyze them, rendering transport ineffective. This leads to increased inflammation and compromised gas exchange. Bronchiectasis, secondary to NRD or meconium aspiration, is associated with impaired ciliary function. Children with severe asthma may also have a component of ciliary dysfunction. Mucociliary transport dysfunction is present in children with cystic fibrosis.

THE IMMUNE SYSTEM OF THE LUNG

Bronchial lymphoid tissue is scattered along the larger airways and some blood vessels of children and adolescents. It does not appear in healthy adult lungs (Tschernig & Pabst 2000). There is some controversy as to whether bronchus-associated lymphoid tissue (BALT) is present at birth or if it develops in response to antigenic stimulation (Hiller et al 1998). The BALT is part of the mucosal-associated lymphoid tissue (MALT) system. It is a localized collection of lymphocytes, analogous to Peyer's patches of the gut. These collections of lymphocytes are covered by modified epithelium with microvilli rather than cilia. The majority of the cells in these collections are B cells or cells without markers. There is some controversy concerning the function of BALT, although most researchers suspect that it probably has a role in establishing early immune function. Macrophages move into and out of the air spaces from the BALT. B lymphocytes, macrophages, mast cells and T cells appear to communicate between the lymphoid populations of mucosal tissues. For example, in patients with asthma, activated lymphocytes have been shown to circulate between the mucosal tissues of lungs, salivary glands and gut (Lamblin et al 2000). This communication is thought to have a role in skin and respiratory manifestations of food allergies (Oehling et al 1997). While BALT is not found in healthy adults, it is present in adults with certain diseases such as rheumatoid arthritis, lymphoma, chronic respiratory infection and asthma. Although BALT is present in children who have died of sudden infant death syndrome (SIDS), its frequency and intensity match those of control patients (Tschernig et al 1995).

Along with the immunoglobulins already mentioned, the lung houses many other immune cells. The lymph nodes, bronchoalveolar space and interstitial tissues contain various types of T cells, natural killer (NK) cells, macrophages and B cells. Within the lung, these components of the immune system are in an environment where they are continuously exposed to antigenic substances and can function as primers and initiators of immune responses.

THE LYMPHATIC SYSTEM OF THE LUNG

The lymphatic system of the lung is extensive and has a role in maintaining fluid balance within the air spaces of the respiratory tree. The terminal lymphatics are located in the loose connective tissue and peribronchovascular spaces of the lung (O'Brodovich & Haddad 2001, Standring 2004). They extend as far as the bronchioles, but not into the alveolar walls. Although there is an inherent pump mechanism present in the larger lymphatics, passage of fluids into the terminal lymphatic capillaries is assisted by ventilatory pressures and movement of the surrounding fluid. This becomes especially important when an inflammatory response is generated. The single-layer epithelial cell walls of the terminal lymphatic will collapse under the pressure of the interstitial fluid, rendering them useless. The valves close and fluid is unable to pass into the lumen. Likewise, from an osteopathic viewpoint, tissue restrictions affecting the collecting or proximal lymphatic will create a backup of fluid into the terminal lymphatic which also closes the epithelial valves. In either case, the mechanics of breathing assist in creating fluctuations in the fluid and cells surrounding the lymphatic vessel, generating a pump mechanism through the anchoring filaments. This is especially important in infectious processes, chronic diseases with inflammatory components such as asthma and obstructive lung disease, and diseases with mucociliary transport defects such as cystic fibrosis.

Most of the collecting lymphatics of the lungs drain into the thoracic duct, and those of the upper right lung drain directly into the right subclavian vein and internal jugular vein.

INNERVATION OF THE RESPIRATORY SYSTEM

The lung is innervated by afferent and efferent fibers. Although there are some sensory fibers arising from slowly adapting stretch receptors, the bulk of afferent information comes from small-calibre primary afferents, the C fibers. These visceral afferents travel with the vagus nerve to the medulla. Efferent activity is modulated through the sympathetic and parasympathetic systems to influence smooth muscle and secretory glands. In addition to the above, the lung also contains neuroepithelial bodies which store serotonin, dopamine, norepinephrine, calcitonin and leu-enkephalin. However, their role is still not well understood.

Smooth muscle bands in the submucosal layer line the airways of the intrapulmonary bronchial tree to the level of the alveolar duct. They receive sympathetic and parasympathetic innervation. During quiet breathing, a small amount of dynamic tone is maintained in these bronchial muscles, to resist collapse. This is primarily modulated through the vagus. Changes in autonomic activity or inflammation will alter the tone of the muscle. Inflammation or increased parasympathetic drive results in muscle contraction and bronchospasm. This is the pathogenesis for reactive airways disease and asthma. The airways of infants and children tend to be more reactive to histamine and methylcholine than those of adults (Wohl 2000). This is mirrored in the clinical propensity for children to develop bronchospasm in response to inflammation from cold and viral infections. Bronchial smooth muscle also has an increased response to acetylcholine in children due to the lack of mature degrading enzymes (Panitch et al 1993).

The pulmonary vasculature in the newborn has a much higher tone than in the adult. This tone is probably modulated through the activity of numerous α-adrenergic receptors of large vessels. These same α-adrenergic receptors have considerably less influence in adult pulmonary vasculature, for when they are blocked there is no appreciable change in vasomotor tone (Silove & Grover 1968). The higher tone in neonatal pulmonary vasculature is also due to the thickened smooth muscle layer. During development, vasoconstriction of the pulmonary bed occurs in response to hypoxia and acts to shunt blood away from the unventilated lung, via the foramen ovale and ductus arteriosus. This reflex is still present at birth. In adults, the reflex is used to correct for ventilation–perfusion mismatch. However, because the vascular smooth muscle is considerably thicker and tone considerably higher in newborns and infants, the risk of developing pulmonary hypertension in response to the reflex is increased. In addition, local changes in vascular tone may be mediated through substances with constrictive and/or dilatory effects which appear in response to tissue injury or inflammation. Tissue response to these substances may be enhanced through blockade of β-adrenergic receptors. All in all, the role of the sympathetic and parasympathetic nervous systems in the control of pulmonary vascular tone in infants is poorly understood (Malik et al 2000).

As alluded to earlier, the pattern of innervation of the muscles of respiration in the newborn differs from that in the adult. Most muscle fibers receive polyneural innervation; that is, the axons of two or more motor neurons synapse on the same fiber. The reverse is true in the adult, where the axons of a motor neuron will synapse on more than one muscle fiber, but each muscle fiber receives only one axon. Thus, synchronized contraction of a group of muscle fibers is controlled by a single motor neuron, whereas in the newborn and infant muscle, contraction is often uncoordinated and random. Adding to this problem is the fact that immature sarcoplasmic reticulum increases the contraction and relaxation times of muscle. Furthermore, as previously described, neuromuscular junctional folds, postsynaptic membranes and some neurotransmitter receptors must undergo significant change to reach the adult form. This means that the muscles of respiration, particularly the diaphragm, are at increased risk of neuromuscular transmission failure at high frequencies of stimulation (Haddad & Perez Fontain 1996a–c). This makes decreasing the work of breathing through optimizing mechanical efficiency of the respiratory muscles all the more important in infants and young children with pulmonary disease.

CONCLUSION

Optimal function of the respiratory–circulatory system is a major tenet in osteopathic philosophy. On first evidence, this appears obvious: what healthcare philosophy wouldn't recognize the necessity of oxygen to life? But the osteopathic philosophy delves deeper, recognizing the role the low-pressure circulatory system plays in maintaining the interstitial milieu, stabilizing pH, and promoting an optimum extracellular environment for intercellular function. The osteopath sees in each breath the workings of the complex respiratory system all the way down to its most basic component, the mitochondria, the seat of primary respiration. In the newborn and infant, optimal gas exchange through the pulmonary system is dependent upon

neurological, biochemical, hormonal and mechanical influences. Many of these same forces continue to play a role in the child and adult. Supporting these processes and removing any impediment to proper respiratory–circulatory function is always a goal of a treatment plan, regardless of the patient's actual diagnosis. The appropriate movement and exchange of gases and fluids is fundamental to the osteopathic approach.

References

Arnon S, Grigg J, Silverman M 1993 Association between pulmonary and gastric inflammatory cells on the first day of life in preterm infants. Pediatr Pulmonol 16(1): 59–61.

Bellanti J A, Zeligs B J 1995 Developmental aspects of pulmonary defenses in children. Pediatr Pulmonol (Suppl 11): 79–80.

Bosma J F 1986 Anatomy of the infant head, 1st edn. Johns Hopkins University Press, Baltimore.

Carreiro J E 1994 Osteopathic findings in 1600 newborns. Paper presentation, American Academy of Osteopathy, March.

Chow C M, Winder C, Read D J 1986 Influences of endogenous dopamine on carotid body discharge and ventilation. J Appl Physiol 60(2): 370–375.

Collin A A, Wohl M E, Mead J 1989 Transition from dynamically maintained to relaxed end-expiratory volume in human infants. J Appl Physiol 74: 2107.

De Troyer A, Estenne M 1988 Functional anatomy of respiratory muscles. Clin Chest Med 9(2): 175–193.

Gallagher J T, Kent P W, Passatore M et al 1975 The composition of tracheal mucus and the nervous control of its secretion in the cat. Proc R Soc Lond B Biol Sci 192: 49–76.

German V F, Corrales R, Ueki I F 1982 Reflex stimulation of tracheal submucosa gland secretion by gastric irritation in cats. J Appl Physiol 52: 1153–1155.

Griese M 1992 Pulmonary surfactant and the immune system. Monatsschr Kinderheilkd 140(1): 57–61.

Guyton A C 1996 Textbook of medical physiology, 9th edn. W B Saunders, Philadelphia.

Haddad G G, Mellins R B 1984 Hypoxia and respiratory control in early life. Annu Rev Physiol 46: 629–643.

Haddad G G, Perez Fontain J J 1996a Regulation of respiration. In: Behrman R E,

Kliegman R M, Jenson H B (eds) Nelson's textbook of pediatrics. W B Saunders, Philadelphia.

Haddad G G, Perez Fontain J J 1996b Development of the respiratory system. In: Behrman R E, Kliegman R M, Jenson H B (eds) Nelson's textbook of pediatrics. W B Saunders, Philadelphia.

Haddad G G, Perez Fontain J J 1996c Congenital abnormalities. In: Behrman R E, Kliegman R M, Jenson H B (eds) Nelson's textbook of pediatrics. W B Saunders, Philadelphia.

Hiller A S, Tschernig T, Kleemann W J et al 1998 Bronchus-associated lymphoid tissue (BALT) and larynx-associated lymphoid tissue (LALT) are found at different frequencies in children, adolescents and adults. Scand J Immunol 47(2): 159–162.

Kliegman R 1996 Respiratory tract disorders. In: Behrman R E, Kliegman R M, Jenson H B (eds) Nelson's textbook of pediatrics. W B Saunders, Philadelphia.

Lamblin C, Saelens T, Bergoin C et al 2000 The common mucosal immune system in respiratory disease. Rev Mal Respir 17(5): 941–946.

Malik A B, Vogel S V, Minshall R D et al 2000 Pulmonary circulation and regulation of fluid balance. In: Murray J, Nadel J (eds) Textbook of respiratory medicine. W B Saunders, Philadelphia: 119–154.

Mason R, Lewis J 2000 Pulmonary surfactant. In: Murray J, Nadel J (eds) Textbook of respiratory medicine. W B Saunders, Philadelphia.

Murray J, Nadel J (eds) 2000 Textbook of respiratory medicine. W B Saunders, Philadelphia.

O'Brodovich H M, Haddad G G 2001 The functional basis of respiratory pathology and disease. In: Chernick V, Boat T (eds) Kendig's disorders of the respiratory tract in children. W B Saunders, Philadelphia: 27–73.

Oehling A, Fernandez M, Cordoba H et al 1997 Skin manifestations and immunological parameters in childhood food allergy. J Invest Allergy Clin Immunol 7(3): 155–159.

Openshaw P, Edwards S, Helms P 1984 Changes in rib cage geometry in childhood. Thorax 39(8): 624–627.

Panitch H B, Wolfson M R, Shaffer T H 1993 Epithelial modulation of preterm airway smooth muscle contraction. J Appl Physiol 74(3): 1437–1443.

Silove E D, Grover R F 1968 Effects of alpha adrenergic blockade and tissue catecholamine depletion on pulmonary vascular responses to hypoxia. J Clin Invest 47: 274–285.

Standring S 2004 Gray's anatomy, 39th edn. Churchill Livingstone, New York.

Thach B T, Stark A R 1979 Spontaneous neck flexion and airway obstruction during apneic spells in preterm infants. J Pediatr 94(2): 275–281.

Tschernig T, Pabst R 2000 Bronchus-associated lymphoid tissue (BALT) is not present in the normal adult lung but in different diseases. Pathobiology 68(1): 1–8.

Tschernig T, Kleemann W J, Pabst R 1995 Bronchus-associated lymphoid tissue (BALT) in the lungs of children who had died from sudden infant death syndrome and other causes. Thorax 50(6): 658–660.

Wanner A, Salathé M, O'Riordan T G 1996 Mucociliary clearance in the airways. Am J Respir Crit Care Med 154(6 Pt1): 1868–1902.

Willinger M, Hoffman H J, Hartford R B 1994 Infant sleep position and risk of sudden infant death syndrome: report of meeting held January 13 and 14, 1994. Pediatrics 93: 814–819.

Wohl M E 2000 Developmental physiology of the respiratory system. In: Chernick V, Boat T (eds) Kendig's disorders of the respiratory tract in children. W B Saunders, Philadelphia: 19–27.

Further reading

Burcharth F, Bertheussen K 1979 The influence of posture, Valsalva manoeuvre and coughing on portal hypertension in cirrhosis. Scand J Clin Lab Invest 39: 665–669.

Chernick V, Boat T (eds) 2001 Kendig's disorders of the respiratory tract in children. W B Saunders, Philadelphia.

De Troyer A, Legrand A 1995 Inhomogeneous activation of the parasternal intercostals during breathing. J Appl Physiol 79(1): 55–62.

De Troyer A, Peche R, Yernault J C et al 1994 Neck muscle activity in patients with severe chronic obstructive pulmonary disease. Am J Respir Crit Care Med 150: 41–47.

Fischer M, Franzeck U K, Herrig I et al 1996 Flow velocity of single lymphatic capillaries in human skin. Am J Physiol 270(1 Pt 2): H358–363.

Franzeck U, Fischer M, Costanzo U et al 1996 Effect of postural changes on human lymphatic capillary pressure of the skin. J Physiol 494: 595–600.

Gandevia S C, Leeper J B, McKenzie D K, De Troyer A 1996 Discharge frequencies of parasternal intercostal and scalene motor units during breathing in normal and COPD subjects. Am J Respir Crit Care Med 153: 622–628.

Hoffmann U, Uckay I, Fischer M et al 1995 Simultaneous assessment of muscle and skin blood fluxes with the laser-Doppler technique. Int J Microcirc Clin Exp 15(2): 53.

Moore K L, Persaud T V N 1993 The developing human, 5th edn. W B Saunders, Philadelphia.

Wen S, Dorffler-Melly J, Herrig I et al 1994 Fluctuation of skin lymphatic capillary pressure in controls and in patients with primary lymphedema. Int J Microcirc Clin Exp 14(3): 139–143.

Wendell-Smith C P, Wilson P M 1991 The vulva, vagina and urethra and the musculature of the pelvic floor. In: Philipp E, Setchell M, Ginsburg J (eds) Scientific foundations of obstetrics and gynaecology. Butterworth-Heinemann, Oxford: 84–100.

Zaugg-Vesti B, Dorffler-Melly J, Spiegel M et al 1993 Lymphatic capillary pressure in patients with primary lymphedema. Microvasc Res 46(2): 128–134.

Chapter Six

The gastrointestinal system

6

CHAPTER CONTENTS

INTRODUCTION

The gastrointestinal (GI) tract, from mouth to anus, is the single largest area of the human body exposed to the environment. While its primary role is the digestion and absorption of nutrients, the GI tract is also involved with endocrine and immune mechanisms. At birth, these functions are rudimentary at best. Weaning to solid foods represents the first major maturation milestone in the postnatal gut. The ability to digest and extract nutrient materials from solid foods is a multifaceted process, involving motor, secretory, immune, endocrine and absorptive mechanisms. Because gut function is a complicated and age-dependent activity, a myriad of factors may influence it. The development and presentation of diseases of the gut will also vary with its level of maturation. An obvious example is frequent spitting up. While this may be a normal occurrence in very young infants, it would not be viewed with the same complacency in an adolescent. The diagnosis and treatment of GI disorders in children is best served by an understanding of each of the various functions of the GI tract, their developmental sequence and the possible pathologies which may affect them. This chapter will provide a basis for understanding normal GI function. Common problems will be discussed in Chapter 14.

DEVELOPMENTAL ANATOMY

A thorough discussion of the development and anatomy of the GI tract can be found in Moore (2007) and Standring (2004).

The human gut begins as a 4 mm tube in the fourth week of gestation, and will reach a length of 400 cm by term. The mature gut is primarily visceral smooth muscle, except for the terminal ends, the proximal esophagus and anus, where striated muscle allows for voluntary control. The primitive gut forms as an infolding of the embryonic disk. Very early

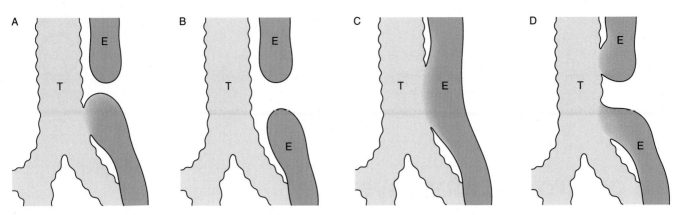

Fig. 6.1 • Schematic of the four most common types of congenital tracheoesophageal deformity. T, trachea; E, esophagus. (A) is the most common, at approximately 85%. There is a fistula between the trachea and distal esophagus, with complete upper esophageal atresia. Types (B) and (C) are fairly equal in occurrence, between 5% and 10%. There is no fistula in type (B) and no atresia in type (C). Type (D) is the rarest.

in gestation, the midgut and its mesenteries elongate and protrude into the umbilical celom. Then, at 6 weeks, the gut begins a process of rotation and migration which concludes by the 20th week of gestation with the gut oriented in the adult position. Many abnormalities in this process are survivable but may result in a host of congenital disorders, ranging from volvulus to malrotations, and hernia to omphalocele. Early on, the pancreas, liver and gallbladder develop as buds off the embryonic gut. Their positions and gross morphology will change over the next several weeks. By 6 weeks, the liver is involved in hemopoiesis and by 9 weeks it accounts for 10% of the fetal weight (Moore 2007).

During the early weeks of gestation, the GI tract is composed of multiple layers of simple epithelium. By the end of the first trimester, the lumen of the esophagus has recanalized and is lined with ciliated epithelium, the small intestine is lined with columnar epithelium and villi, and muscle layers have begun to appear throughout the length of the gut. The muscle layers have a role in coordinating effective gut motility.

The esophagus develops early in fetal life, when the primitive foregut separates into the trachea and esophagus. This is a complex process, and there are several congenital abnormalities which may result if all does not go according to plan. Incomplete separation of the esophagus and trachea may result in esophageal atresia and/or tracheoesophageal fistula (Fig. 6.1). These may or may not occur together. If a fistula is present, then food and secretions may pass into the trachea, resulting in choking and asphyxia. The esophagus is approximately 10 cm long in the term infant, and will grow at a rate of 6 mm a year until reaching its adult length of 32–50 cm (Boyle 1992, Pelot 1995). The primary role of the esophagus is the transmission of food from the pharynx to the stomach. The esophagus has a functional sphincter located at each end. Normally, the esophagus is in a collapsed, relaxed state and the two sphincters are contracted. The upper esophageal sphincter is composed of

the cricopharyngeal muscle and is present by 32 weeks of gestation. The lower sphincter is a functionally competent area of the distal esophagus, measuring 3–4 cm in the adult, which is capable of contracting and generating forces which resist backflow from the stomach (Boyle 1992, Pelot 1995, Milla 1996). The existence of discrete sphincter muscle tissue is controversial; however, the presence of a functional sphincter is beyond question (see Ch. 14).

The surface area of the mature GI tract approximates 300 times its length. This is accomplished through the presence of valvulae conniventes, villi and microvilli, primarily in the small intestines (Weaver 1996). These modifications begin developing in the duodenum, jejunum and ileum around the ninth week of gestation. Villus formation proceeds craniocaudally, and by 16 weeks extends the length of the intestine (Weaver 1996). Crypts and microvilli appear between 10 and 12 weeks, further increasing intraluminal surface area. The morphology and concentration of the villi vary between the three parts of the small intestine. The most densely populated area is the jejunum. Here the villi are long and thin. Fewer villi are present in the duodenum and ileum. The villi are short and blocky in the duodenum and more pyramidal in the ileum. Between the villi lie the crypts of Lieberkühn, the site of stem cell activity and location of endocrine cells, which secrete regulatory polypeptides.

The viscera of the GI system are suspended and enveloped in a thin serous membrane called the peritoneum. This arrangement evolves through a series of complex embryological events, but suffice it to say that the embryological gut begins development inside the primitive peritoneum and then, through a process of outgrowth, rotations and reductions, ends up being suspended from and within the peritoneal tissue (Moore 2007). To picture this in its mature form, one can think of the peritoneum as a sack within the abdominal cavity. Some abdominal viscera, such as the liver and stomach, have pushed into the posterior wall of the

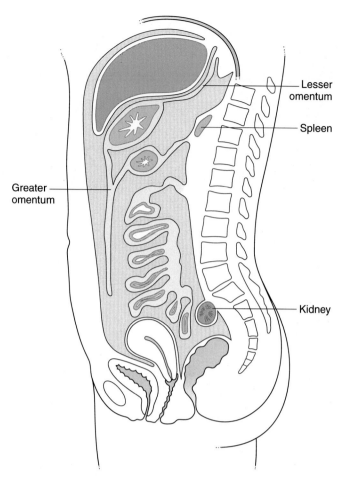

Fig. 6.2 • Schematic diagram depicting the distribution of dorsal mesenteries. The intraperitoneal space is outlined by the central shaded area. The greater and lesser omentum are labeled. Note that the kidney and spleen lie dorsal to the peritoneum and are not enveloped by them.

sack to be covered by a thin layer of the membrane called visceral peritoneum. These organs are considered intraperitoneal. Other organs, such as the kidneys and pancreas, lie against the posterior abdominal wall, outside the peritoneum, and these organs are called retroperitoneal (Fig. 6.2).

A series of dorsal mesenteries suspend the viscera from the posterior abdominal wall. These doubled layers of peritoneal membrane are continuous with the peritoneum enveloping the organs. Two of these mesenteries are called omental folds. The greater omentum is suspended from the inferior aspect of the stomach and superior surface of the transverse colon. It doubles up on itself to form a blanket of mesentery which overlies the gastrointestinal tract (Fig. 6.3A). Where the greater omentum doubles up on itself, it creates an omental bursa between the stomach and colon. Superiorly, the layers of the greater omentum are continuous with the peritoneum of the stomach and duodenum.

Inferiorly, they merge with the transverse mesocolon. The lesser omentum is suspended from the undersurface of the diaphragm between the lobes of the liver, to the stomach. It is a double layer of peritoneum which splits upon reaching the stomach to engulf the organ (Fig. 6.3B). The omenta contain fat, blood vessels, nerves and lymphoid cells, particularly macrophages. In cases of infection or injury, the greater omentum will often wall off the involved area, protecting the rest of the viscera. As a result, many surgeons refer to the omentum as the Band-Aid of the gut.

The two other dorsal mesenteries suspend the remainder of the small intestine and the sigmoid colon from the posterior abdominal wall. In both cases, the organs are enveloped in peritoneum and the mesenteries carry blood vessels, nerves, lymphatic channels and nodes. The ascending and descending colon are retroperitoneal.

HISTOLOGICAL ANATOMY

While the entirety of the GI tract is composed of three layers, the muscularis mucosa, the submucosa and the mucosa, there are variations throughout. In fact, the gross and histological morphology of each region of the GI tract change according to its function. For example, the esophagus is adapted solely for the passage of food, and no digestion or absorption take place in this organ. Consequently, its lumen is a smooth tube lined with ciliated epithelium without secretory glands. Contrast this with the stomach, which is concerned with dissolving large food particles. The interior of the stomach is covered by gastric pits containing mucous cells, chief cells and parietal cells. The entire gastric mucosa, including the pits, is lined with simple columnar secretory epithelium. Parietal cells in the gastric mucosa secrete hydrogen ions and chloride to acidify the stomach. This is necessary for proper functioning of the potent gastric enzyme pepsin, which is secreted by the chief cells. The mucosal surface of the stomach is protected from this highly acidic environment by a mucous layer secreted by the neck cells. Inhibition of the secretory activity of the neck cells may result in gastritis and ulceration.

The small intestine is primarily involved with the breakdown, digestion and absorption of foodstuffs. Here is an organ peppered with cells involved in secretory and immunoregulatory processes. The mucosal surface is organized into crypts and valvulae conniventes (infoldings), the latter of which are topped by villi. The villi are covered with a brush border of microvilli involved with absorption. The mucosa itself is composed of numerous and varied secretory cells, some of which are involved with hydrolysis of ingested proteins, fats and carbohydrates, and some of which play a role in the transepithelial movement of these substances. Mucosal cells are also involved with immune regulatory processes, including antigen recognition.

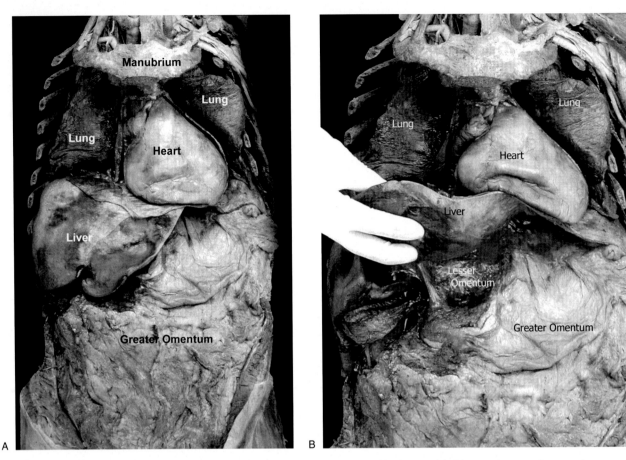

Fig. 6.3 • (A) Dissection showing anterior view of the thoracic and abdominal cavities in an adult. The greater omentum can be seen completely covering the abdominal viscera. (B) Close-up of the same dissection; the liver is being lifted to reveal the lesser omentum. *Used with permission of the Willard & Carreiro collection.*

Most water and ions are absorbed in the large intestine, where the chyme is concentrated and readied for excretion. The proximal portion of the colon is the main site of absorption, while the distal portion provides storage of fecal matter. The primary villi of the colon begin appearing by about the 13th week of gestation. Subsequently, these split into secondary villi and develop a brush border at about the same time that crypts begin to form (Schmitz 1996, Moore 2007). The development of this mucosal arrangement proceeds distal to proximal and is completed by 16 weeks of gestation. The presence of digestive enzymes correlates with development of the villi and brush border of the colon. However, there are no villi in the adult colon, and digestive enzymes are absent. Consequently, the colon of premature infants does not function like that of the term baby or adult. During the latter part of the second trimester and early third trimester, the colon looks like the small intestine, in both morphology and function, which is reflected in its capacity for absorption and digestion. Thus, in the premature infant, the colon may play a role in nutrient delivery. Maturation of the colon involves regression of the villi and secretory cells. The

process of regression begins some time after 25–28 weeks of gestation and is completed by birth. Levels of digestive enzymes decrease as the villi disappear. In the mature colon, chloride, sodium and bicarbonate are exchanged across the gut wall, creating an osmotic gradient which draws water out of the chyme. Colonic bacteria produce vitamins K and B_{12}, thiamine and riboflavin, all of which are also absorbed. The preterm gut lacks many of these capabilities, and some, like vitamin production, are not present until long after birth.

VASCULAR SUPPLY

Anatomically speaking, the GI tract can be divided into three parts: the foregut, midgut and hindgut. The foregut is composed of the oropharynx, esophagus, stomach and proximal duodenum. The liver, gallbladder, biliary ductal system and pancreas develop from the primitive foregut and share vascular and neurological characteristics with it. The midgut is defined as the remainder of the small intestine, along with the cecum, appendix, and ascending and transverse colon.

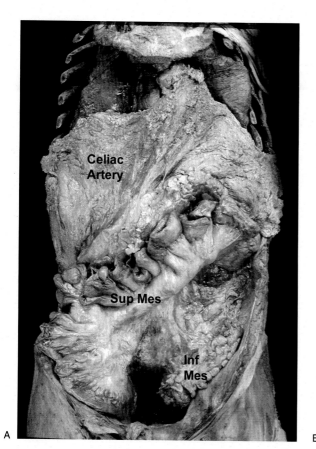 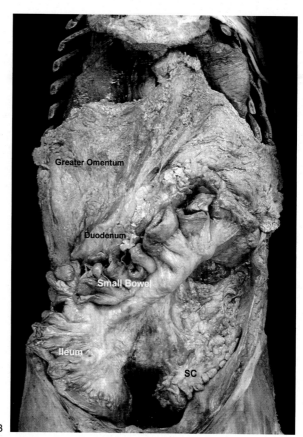

Fig. 6.4 • (A, B) The same dissection. In (A), the regional anatomy of the viscera is labeled according to the arterial supply. In (B), the actual anatomical structures are indicated. *Used with permission of the Willard & Carreiro collection.*

The descending and sigmoid colon and the rectum make up the hindgut. Although anatomical variations exist, generally speaking each of these areas has a distinct blood supply which can be traced back to one of the ventral branches of the abdominal aorta: the celiac, superior mesenteric or inferior mesenteric arteries (Fig. 6.4).

The celiac trunk, with its primary and secondary branches, supplies the foregut between the distal esophagus and proximal duodenum. While the duodenum also uses the splenic vessels for venous drainage routes, the distal esophagus and stomach drain primarily through the portal system. Consequently, esophageal and gastric varicosities may develop secondary to portal hypertension. The midgut receives its arterial supply from a vascular arcade representing the anastomoses of the superior mesenteric artery with its branches: the right and left colic and the ileocolic arteries. The hindgut, including the splenic flexure, descending and sigmoid colon and rectum, is supplied by the inferior mesenteric artery and its branches. Thus, the three ventral aortic trunks supply the length of the GI tract, with frequent anastomoses between their primary and secondary branches. This vascular arrangement accounts for the general success of most surgical procedures in the gut, whereby relatively large sections can be removed without significant complications. The vascular arrangement also explains the rapid spread of infection and cancer through this system.

Nutrients and water are carried from the gut lumen via the vasculature and lymphatics of the GI tract. These desirable substances are frequently accompanied by less desirable materials. Bacteria, antigens and unwanted particulate matter need to be filtered from the blood before it enters systemic circulation. This is accomplished by the reticuloendothelial cells of the liver. Venous blood from the gut, spleen and pancreas enters the portal circulation. In the sinusoids of the liver, reticuloendothelial and hepatic cells absorb many of the water-soluble nutrients for storage. The reticuloendothelial cells also remove potentially harmful substances (Guyton 1996). (The lymphatics of the GI tract drain through a series of channels and nodes which will be discussed later in this chapter.)

The gut receives more than 10% of the total cardiac output per cycle, with the majority of this volume perfusing the microcirculation of the mucosal layer, and the remainder flowing to the submucosa and muscularis mucosa (Tepperman & Jacobson 1981). The intestinal villi house a dense network of arterioles, venules and capillaries. This dense capillary network lies in the lamina propria just below the basement membrane of the luminal epithelium (Fig. 6.5). The capillary

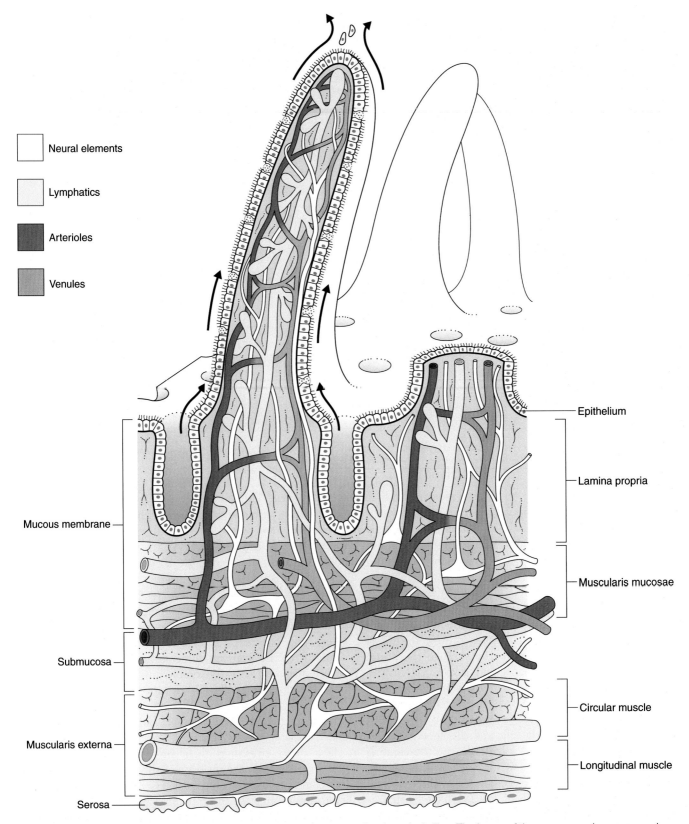

Legend:
- Neural elements
- Lymphatics
- Arterioles
- Venules

Labels: Epithelium, Lamina propria, Muscularis mucosae, Circular muscle, Longitudinal muscle, Mucous membrane, Submucosa, Muscularis externa, Serosa

Fig. 6.5 • This diagram from *Gray's anatomy* depicts the microanatomy of an intestinal villus. The layers of the mucosa, submucosa and muscularis are labeled. *Used with permission from Williams P (ed.) 1995 Gray's anatomy, 38th edn. Churchill Livingstone, New York.*

walls are heavily fenestrated with diaphragm openings that control the transport of molecules into the general circulation (Clark & Miller 1992, Standring 2004).

REGULATION OF HEMODYNAMICS

A mechanism of vascular autoregulation exists throughout the gut which compensates for normal systemic fluctuations in blood flow and oxygen delivery. This ensures that oxygen delivery and waste removal within the gut are maintained within fairly constant parameters. This is necessary, because the high metabolic rate and turnover of GI tissues make them particularly susceptible to hypoxic injury. Vascular autoregulation of blood flow, blood pressure and oxygen delivery exists in the stomach, small intestine and colon and occurs in response to tissue demand (Crissinger & Granger 1995). Blood flow increases during the postprandial period, when digestion, motility, secretion and absorption are high, and decreases during the fasting period. Autoregulation appears to occur through several mechanisms, including vasoactive peptides, proinflammatory substances and reflexive smooth muscle response to hypoxia (Crissinger & Granger 1995, Guyton 1996). One example of vascular autoregulation is the modulation of vascular tone by certain peptides released during digestion. Cholecystokinin, vasoactive intestinal polypeptide (VIP), gastrin and secretin are all digestive hormones which can stimulate dilation of local blood vessels in the surface of the gut lumen. Another example of locally controlled vascular tone occurs when secretory glands involved with digestion concurrently release the vasodilators bradykinin and kallidin into the gut wall. A third example involves a reflex whereby vascular smooth muscle relaxes in response to decreased oxygen levels, thereby decreasing vascular resistance and increasing blood flow. Other mechanisms exist and have been presented in numerous texts (Tepperman & Jacobson 1981, Crissinger & Granger 1995, Guyton 1996). The autoregulatory reflex is influenced by input from autonomic fibers. Parasympathetic stimulation increases blood flow to the stomach and lower colon, but this may be a result of the concurrent increase in secretory activity in the glands of these tissues. Sympathetic activity affects the entire gut, causing vasoconstriction of the arterioles. However, autoregulatory mechanisms, primarily mediated through the ischemic reflex, will overcome this situation in a matter of minutes, restoring GI blood flow to an appropriate level (Crissinger & Granger 1995, Guyton 1996).

The microcirculation of the intestinal villi differs from that of the larger vessels in the gut, due to the presence of a countercurrent arrangement of arterioles and venules (Fig. 6.6). Because of the close proximity of these vessels, oxygen can diffuse directly from the arterial to the venous compartment without disseminating to the surrounding

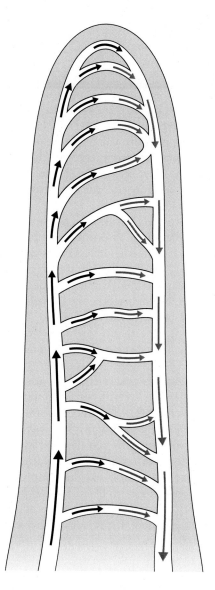

Fig. 6.6 • Schematic diagram depicting the countercurrent vascular flow in the intestinal villi. Arterial flow is represented by the dark arrows, while venous flow is represented by the lighter arrows.

cells. Up to 80% of oxygen in the villous plexus may be unavailable to tissues because of this arrangement (Guyton 1996). As a consequence, the villi are quite vulnerable to changes in oxygen delivery, and the villous tips may become ischemic and die (Lanciault & Jacobson 1976). In the term neonate, the autoregulatory mechanisms are not well established and they may even be absent in the premature infant (Nowicki & Miller 1988, Crissinger & Granger 1995), yet the metabolic activity of these tissues exceeds that of the adult. This further increases the vulnerability of the intestinal villi, which may undergo ischemic injury because of fetal distress during the latter part of pregnancy or during labor and delivery. Depending on the extent of the ischemia, the tissue may lose its absorptive capabilities, or become vulnerable to digestive enzymes, leading to further complications (Tepperman & Jacobson 1981, Crissinger & Granger 1995). Under conditions of severe or extensive injury, the newborn may develop necrotizing enterocolitis, a condition where the involved area becomes necrotic and infected (Israel 1996). In chronic diseases of the gut or other systems, where the oxygen supply to villous cells is compromised, the villous tips or entire villi may be blunted, resulting in decreased absorption from the gut lumen (Crissinger & Granger 1995, Guyton 1996). This may be the pathogenesis of growth delay in children with chronic disease.

The delivery of nutrients to body tissues is dependent on the coordinated efforts of digestion, absorption and blood flow. Circulation within the intestine is influenced by many factors. First and foremost, cardiovascular status must be maintained, with adequate hemodynamic function to deliver blood to the gut. Just as importantly, the concentration of oxygen in the blood needs to be sufficient to meet the needs of cells in the gut. The tissues of the GI tract have a high metabolic rate and are vulnerable to ischemia, especially in the neonate. The existence of an autoregulatory escape phenomenon ensures that blood flow to the gut remains fairly constant in the face of normal systemic fluctuations (Clark & Miller 1992). The mechanism for this phenomenon is not well established, but it involves the autonomic and enteric nervous systems and humeral influences. For example, digestive hormones such as glucagon and cholecystokinin increase intestinal blood flow, and gastrin creates the same response in gastric blood vessels. Not only will the antiregulatory process respond to the acute influences of the neural and humoral mechanisms, it will also respond to chronic influences. This relationship needs to be considered in functional bowel disease and stress-associated changes in gut function. Empirically, many clinicians note that adults with functional gut disorders describe stressful lives and childhoods. Does chronic stress in the young infant also contribute to this phenomenon? And how can we therapeutically intervene?

During digestion, the metabolic rate of many mucosal cells increases, raising oxygen demand and creating a relative hypoxia. This stimulates the release of proinflammatory substances such as histamine, bradykinin, VIP and prostaglandins, which are all vasodilators. Though it is recognized that the integrity of GI circulation is dependent upon many factors, the extent of their influence and ability to interact in the newborn is poorly understood. Premature infants and newborns appear to be vulnerable to gut ischemia. Neonates experiencing perinatal hypoxia frequently have associated GI complications, including malabsorption, diarrhea and, in the extreme case, ischemic necrosis. These are often the result of injury due to poor tissue perfusion (Clark & Miller 1992). Congenital abnormalities affecting oxygen-carrying capacity or delivery are liable to produce hypoxia in the gut.

Respiratory diseases or complications which alter ventilation or perfusion in very young infants and children may lead to chronic hypoxia of the vulnerable intestinal tract. Likewise, premature infants requiring prolonged ventilation or supplemental oxygen may be susceptible to gut hypoxia.

ANATOMY OF GUT LYMPHATICS

The lymphatic vessels of the small and large intestine begin as lacteals, distended blind appendages extending into the villus (see Fig. 6.5). There is usually one lacteal per villus, and infrequently two. The lacteal traverses the length of the villus to empty into a lymphatic plexus in the lamina propria (Standring 2004). Within the mucosal and submucosal layers, the lymphatics merge and are joined by vessels draining lymph follicles to form a dense plexus which travels in the submucosal layer. Lymphatics draining the muscularis mucosa anastomose into a plexus which travels between the circular and longitudinal layers of the gut. Both of these plexuses eventually empty into collecting vessels and the mesenteric nodes. The collecting lymphatic vessels follow the course of the mesenteric arteries, with lymph nodes positioned along the way. The first group of nodes lies near the juncture between the terminal arteries and the arterioles entering the intestine. The second group is positioned along primary mesenteric branches forming the arterial arcade. The last and largest group of nodes lies beside the superior mesenteric artery. Vessels collecting lymph from the proximal jejunum to the anal canal will drain into the thoracic duct.

The villous lacteals are exposed to substances passing through the gut lumen. Nutrients, water and less desirable substances enter the lymphatic system through the lacteal. Fluid that escapes into the peritoneal cavity is primarily removed by lymphatic stomata lining the undersurface of the diaphragm. These lymphatic lacunae lie between muscle fibers of the diaphragm. They are covered with a thin layer of lymphatic endothelium, a fenestrated elastic membrane and the mesothelial cells of the peritoneum (Negrini et al 1991, Abu-Hijleh et al 1995). The shape of the stomata is affected by diaphragm motion during respiration. Changes in diaphragm tension affect the muscular and tendinous portions of the stomata differently, resulting in alternating shapes of the lymphatic valves, which can then act as a pump (Negrini et al 1991, Abu-Hijleh et al 1995).

MOTILITY

Before the GI tract can undertake the processes of digestion and absorption, it has to be able to move foodstuffs from the oropharynx to and through the anus. This requires organized motor activity modulated by mechanisms which are intrinsic and extrinsic to the gut. Effective motor activity of the GI tract is dependent on proper function of the enteric nervous system, the smooth muscle layers, and the hormonal environment (Milla 1996). Major changes in patterns of motor activity occur during the latter half of the third trimester and into the first several months of post-uterine life. For example, although peristaltic motions can be observed at 26 weeks of gestation (Weaver 1996), they lack organization and strength. Furthermore, adult patterns of motor activity in the gut are normally absent in children even several months after birth (Milla 1996). This probably represents immaturity in the aforementioned modulating mechanisms.

The pattern of motor activity and muscle organization varies along the length of the mature gut, a reflection of the diverse function of different areas. The proximal esophagus, within a couple of centimeters of the pharyngeal esophageal junction, is primarily striated muscle, which, when mature, allows for voluntary swallowing. The middle portion of the esophagus is a mixture of striated and smooth muscle, while the distal third, like the remainder of the gut, is solely smooth muscle under control of the enteric nervous system.

The mature gut has three layers of smooth muscle arranged in oblique, circular and longitudinal sheets. Smooth muscle begins to appear in the gut between 8 and 10 weeks of gestation as a sheet of outer circular muscle, and by 12 weeks the longitudinal layer appears. It is unclear when the innermost layers develop (Milla 1996, Standring 2004, Moore 2007). However, as the layers develop and mature, the force, frequency and efficacy of contraction improve until adult function is reached prior to the end of the first year of life. The layers of smooth muscle are arranged slightly differently along the course of the GI tract. In the stomach, the oblique, circular and longitudinal layers are present but the circular layer is not continuous over the lesser curvature (Standring 2004). In the small intestine, the circular layer is thickened and the longitudinal layer is thinned. This arrangement is most prominent in the jejunum. In the large intestine, the longitudinal layer is structured into three bands called taeniae coli, which are thought to pucker the colon wall into haustrations (Standring 2004). The variation in smooth muscle organization probably accounts for the slightly different patterns of motility seen throughout the gut.

Movements of the gut represent the summation of neurological, hormonal and inherent mechanisms. There are two types of movement: mixing and peristalsis. Mixing is accomplished by localized contractions of gut segments. Peristalsis is a wave of contraction which moves along the gut, pushing the luminal contents before it. Within each muscle layer of the gut, the muscle fibers are connected by gap junctions, effectively converting the muscle layer into a syncytium across which action potentials are freely dispersed. The cell membrane of visceral smooth muscle undergoes spontaneous rhythmic depolarization and repolarization as sodium and calcium ions are transported across the cell membrane. This is called electrical control activity (ECA), and results in a slow-wave rhythm of membrane potential. The capacity for visceral smooth muscle to self-stimulate can result in a self-generated action potential. When the potential of the ECA, or slow wave, reaches 235 mV, an action potential develops and spreads through the visceral smooth muscle via gap junctions, resulting in muscle contraction (for complete discussion, see Guyton 1996). This mechanism of excitability is primarily responsible for the rhythmic contractions which act to mix the foodstuffs with digestive secretions. Smooth muscle contraction generated by slow waves or the ECA is called rhythmic contraction, the frequency of which varies throughout the mature gut. The smooth muscle of the stomach has an ECA of 3 cycles/min, while in the duodenum the rate is 12 cycles/min (Foulk 1954, Milla 1996). Slow waves in the large colon are inconsistent and the rate is quite variable (Huizinga et al 1985). Studies have demonstrated that the rate or frequency of ECA increases with gestational age (Milla 1996). Maturation of the ECA occurs through changes in activity and control of the ion pumps and channels of the cell membrane.

In addition to rhythmic contractions, the GI tract also displays tonic contractions which can last minutes to hours and account for peristalsis. Peristalsis propels the bolus of foodstuffs along the length of the gut. The intensity of the tonic contractions of peristalsis may vary within any given segment and between the segments of the GI tract. Tonic contractions can be generated electrically, hormonally, ionically or by certain substances which act as toxins to the gut, such as bacteria. For many years, the slow-wave activity of gut smooth muscle was thought to act as a pacemaker for peristalsis. However, lying within the smooth muscle layers are the interstitial cells of Cajal, which are now thought to be the primary pacemakers of peristalsis. Various studies (Gershon 1999) have found that these cells influence the electrical slow-wave activity of smooth muscle, although the mechanism by which this occurs is unknown. The ontogeny of these cells is still poorly understood, but their appearance and maturation is probably related to increased frequency of intestinal contraction. Normal fasting intestinal peristalsis has a cyclical pattern. This cycle time increases with gestational maturation (Milla 1996). For example, in premature infants of 30 weeks' gestation, the length of the intestinal cycle is 10–13 min. By term, the newborn's peristaltic cycle lasts 40–45 min. As the cycle increases, there is more time for digestion and absorption of nutrients, and gut efficiency improves.

PATTERNS OF INNERVATION

Although the activities of the GI tract are modulated through hormonal, immune and neurological inputs, the enteric nervous system retains primary control of normal function. There are two plexuses of ganglionated fibers in the enteric nervous system: the myenteric or Auerbach's plexus, and the submucosal or Meissner's plexus. Auerbach's plexus lies between the circular and longitudinal layers of the muscularis externa, while Meissner's plexus is located in the submucosal layer. These plexuses first appear during the ninth and 13th gestational weeks, respectively (Weaver 1996). Neurons in Auerbach's plexus are involved with gut movements and mediating enzyme output (Gershon 1999), while those of Meissner's plexus moderate blood flow and secretory gland activity (Guyton 1996) and appear to influence the myenteric plexus. The neurons of Meissner's plexus communicate with those of Auerbach's plexus and are thought to be sensitive to serotonin (Gershon 1999). Neurons of Meissner's plexus receive afferent input from stretch receptors located in the gut wall and input from various sensors in the gut lumen. Under normal conditions, the myenteric and submucosal plexuses orchestrate fasting peristaltic activity in the gut. These plexuses may be influenced by various extrinsic factors, such as the autonomic nervous system, polypeptide hormones and immune regulators (Ritchie et al 1980, Bueno 1985, Gershon 1999).

Specialized cells such as chromaffin, osmiophilic and acidophilic cells are located in the epithelial lining of the gut. They secrete endocrine and paracrine substances which influence nerve endings of the enteric nervous system, smooth muscle fibers in the gut wall and vasculature, and local epithelial cells. Many of these same substances also act as neurotransmitters in the enteric and central nervous system and can be found in the secretory granules of their neurons (Scott 1996). This suggests interplay between humoral and neural systems in maintaining gut motility. Absence of ganglion cells in Meissner's and Auerbach's plexus results in obstructive constipation with resulting megacolon (Wyllie 2000).

Postganglionic parasympathetic fibers lie with the submucosal and myenteric plexuses. Parasympathetic input is primarily through the vagus, although its fiber content is 50–90% afferent. The esophagus, stomach, gallbladder, small intestine and proximal colon are innervated by the vagus. Parasympathetic fibers from the sacrum supply the remainder of the gut. Sympathetic innervation arises from the thoracic and upper lumbar cord. Innervation to the gastroesophageal junction is generally thought to arise from T4 to T6, to the stomach from T6 to T7, to the intestine from T7 to T10, and to the colon from T12 to L1 (Willard 1997). This pattern of segmental innervation gives rise to the viscerosomatic reflexes discussed in Chapter 1 (Beal 1985) (Table 6.1). Parasympathetic and sympathetic fibers innervating the GI tract have a strong influence on its function. However, the enteric nervous system can function quite normally without input from the autonomic nervous system, as is seen in patients with vagotomy and mesenteric ablation (Thompson et al 1982, Gershon 1999).

Parasympathetic stimulation is generally thought to increase peristalsis and secretory activity, and sympathetic

Table 6.1 Chart of most common viscerosomatic reflexes

Viscera and/or problem	Segmental reflex
Thyroid	C7 and C8
Bronchus	T2–T4
Lung	T2–T5
Pleura	T1–T11, same level
Heart	T2–T5, left
Stomach	T5–T9, left
Duodenum	T7–T10, right
Gallbladder	T9, right
Liver	T5–T9, right
Pancreas	T6–T9, both
Kidney, ureters	T10–T12, same side
Ovaries and tubes	T12, L1, same side
Adrenals	T10–T11, same side
Appendix	T11–T12, ribs right
Uterus	L4 and L5, both
Bladder and prostate	L3–L5
Colon	L1–L5, ascending right, descending left
Rectum	L4–L5
Fallopian tubes	T11–T12, L1

stimulation slows gut motility and digestive mechanisms. However, it must be remembered that autonomic fibers have stimulatory and inhibitory influences, depending on their target tissue. In general, gut responses to central nervous system influences through the parasympathetic and sympathetic nervous systems tend to have a shorter duration but greater intensity than those orchestrated by the enteric nervous system. This also supports the idea that the enteric nervous system is probably the most potent modulator of the three (Guyton 1996).

Interestingly enough, sleep has an influence on gut motility, and there appears to be a diurnal pattern to the fasting peristaltic cycle (Ritchie et al 1980, Ruckebusch 1986). Studies have demonstrated a simultaneous increase in the length of the sleep cycle and cycle of peristalsis. In other words, as the infant begins to sleep for longer periods of time, the peristaltic cycle is also increasing. The transit time through the GI tract lengthens, which provides more time for digestion and absorption. In addition, changes in the electroencephalogram, specifically the development of α cortical activity (Ruckebusch 1986, Milla 1996), also correlate with the appearance of a prolonged peristaltic cycle. Existing research suggests that the maturation of GI function is in large part a product of developmental changes in the central and enteric nervous systems after birth (Milla 1996).

REGULATORY PEPTIDES

The human GI tract is littered with cells which secrete regulatory proteins involved with gut development and function, immune regulation, hormonal processes and neural mechanisms. Populations of secretory cells are located in the mucosal layer and distributed from the mouth to the rectum. These cells appear early in gestation, as the crypts and villi are developing in the small intestine, and begin functioning shortly thereafter (Milla 1996, Moore 2007). Their secretory products, the regulatory peptides, first appear between 6 and 16 weeks of gestation and reach significant levels by 20 weeks (Murphy & Aynsley-Green 1996). The proteins secreted by these cells may be classified as neurotransmitters, hormones or immune regulators. Although the mechanisms are not well understood, these peptides are involved with cell growth and differentiation, gut motility, and food digestion and absorption. Interestingly, many of these same peptides are also found in the developing lung, and although definitive evidence is lacking, there is some suggestion that they play a role in the development of both organs during gestation (Murphy & Aynsley-Green 1996).

Regulatory peptides and gut growth

Throughout life, the GI tract is exposed to a myriad of substances, some of which are beneficial and some which are not. This may have special implications in the intestines, where food travels more slowly and most absorption takes place. The cells within the mucosal surface of the small and large intestines have a high rate of turnover. As cells become dysfunctional or die off, they are sloughed from the gut wall and replaced by cells from within the crypts of Lieberkühn. Undifferentiated precursor cells line these intestinal crypts. The cells migrate along the walls of the crypts towards the surface of the gut lumen. They differentiate and mature as they do so (Murphy & Aynsley-Green 1996). In this way, the mucosa of the lumen is continuously being turned over and replenished with new cells. Researchers have identified three polypeptides involved with the modulation of this obviously complicated and well-organized process: epidermal growth factor (EGF), transforming growth factor (TGF) and insulin-like growth factor (IGF). EGF is the longest known and most well researched of these peptides. It is present in amniotic fluid by the second trimester and

is produced by salivary glands, Brunner's glands in the duodenum and Paneth's cells in the small intestine (Murphy & Aynsley-Green 1996). EGF is present in breast milk and colostrum (Murphy & Aynsley-Green 1996). When EGF binds to receptors on cells in the gastric glands, mucosa of the small intestine, and the liver, it induces cell proliferation. In this way, EGF may influence secretion and cell proliferation. EGF also appears to play a role in healing ulcers in the gut (Wright et al 1990).

Another group of polypeptides involved with cell proliferation are the transforming growth factors (TGF-α, TGF-β, etc.). The TGFs can be found in embryonic and adult tissue. Members of this family of polypeptides can induce or suppress cell differentiation, proliferation and chemotaxis (Murphy & Aynsley-Green 1996). TGF-β is thought to control migration and maturation of intestinal crypt stem cells (Barnard et al 1993). Consequently, they may be involved with tissue repair after injury, as well as cell growth. A third modulator of gut growth and maintenance is IGF. Levels of this peptide are increased by growth hormone from the anterior pituitary gland and exposure to nutrients in the gut. IGF has been shown to stimulate normal brush border development in the jejunum (Murphy & Aynsley-Green 1996).

Regulatory peptides and digestion

Effective gut function involves the breakdown of food into ever smaller units, until nutrients can be extracted and transported across the gut wall into the awaiting blood vessels. This is a well-orchestrated event, engaging many players. The quality and speed of movement of food through the tract is of the utmost importance. When food moves too quickly, there is little time for appropriate digestion and absorption, and the patient has diarrhea. When food moves too slowly, cells are exposed to waste products for an extended period, there is increased gas build-up, bloating, pain, constipation and even nausea. Food breakdown is initiated in the mouth through maceration by the tongue and teeth, and the secretion of enzymes and mucus which lubricate and digest. In the stomach, gastrin is the substance responsible for stimulating the secretion of the gastric acids: pepsin and hydrochloric acid. Gastrin is secreted by gastrin cells or G cells located in the antrum of the stomach and proximal duodenum. Gastrin is released by a local nerve reflex in response to the actual distention of the stomach and the presence of certain chemicals called secretagogues, found in some proteins, alcohol and caffeine (Guyton 1996). As a point of information for the reader, there are to date four types of gastrin discussed in most GI literature; big big gastrin, big gastrin, little gastrin and mini gastrin, named for their size (Murphy & Aynsley-Green 1996). The primary effect of gastrin is the production of gastric acid; however, gastrin also stimulates contraction of the lower esophageal sphincter and gastric smooth muscle, inhibits contraction of the sphincter of Oddi, increases gastric blood flow, releases histamine, and acts as a neurotransmitter (Castell & Harris 1970, Murphy & Aynsley-Green 1996). As previously stated, the effect of gastrin on the secretion of pepsin and hydrochloric acid outlasts the effect produced by vagal stimulation, although the intensity is less. According to Guyton (1996), acids are secreted at a rate of 500 ml/h following vagal stimulation and 200 ml/h in response to gastrin; however, the gastrin response continues for several hours, while the vagal response is much more acute (Guyton 1996). In addition, histamine also stimulates gastric acid secretion and is a suspected precursor to the influence of gastrin. Histamine is not a polypeptide. It is a neurotransmitter and a mediator of inflammation. Histamine is released by primary afferent nociceptors in response to tissue damage. It most probably plays a role in the development and maintenance of gastritis and ulcer disease.

Once food has passed through the stomach, the remainder of the gut needs to ready itself to complete the job. One substance which plays a role in this process is VIP, which is a type of neurotransmitter found in the gut and the brain. Elevated levels of VIP have been shown to increase the movement of fluid into the gut lumen, decrease the secretion of pepsin and hydrochloric acid from the stomach, stimulate glycogenolysis, and relax smooth muscle of the gut and vasculature (Murphy & Aynsley-Green 1996). High levels of this substance have been found in patients with Crohn's disease (O'Morain et al 1984). VIP also has proinflammatory properties and can be released by small-calibre nociceptor fibers. Somatostatin is another regulatory peptide that can act as a proinflammatory substance. It too is a modulator of GI function, and is found in the brain, spinal cord and D cells of the GI tract. Levels of somatostatin are significantly elevated in the fetus and newborn but decrease by maturity (Murphy & Aynsley-Green 1996). Somatostatin is classified as a neurotransmitter and paracrine substance (paracrine substances are secreted and act on local target tissues). Somatostatin inhibits the release of other secretory substances such as pepsin and gastric acid. It appears to impair intestinal absorption, and increased levels of this peptide result in steatorrhea. Somatostatin also inhibits growth hormone, thyroid-stimulating hormone (TSH), insulin, motilin and calcitonin. Neurotensin is similar to somatostatin in that it appears to inhibit gastric function and gut motility. In addition, elevated levels of neurotensin will stimulate the pancreas to increase bicarbonate production. This peptide is found in the small intestine, the hypothalamus and basal ganglia. It is released from the ileum in response to food ingestion.

Motilin is secreted by cells of the duodenum and jejunum in response to gastric distention. This polypeptide stimulates gastric motility, increasing transit times through the stomach and proximal small intestine. It is inhibited by somatostatin. Levels of motilin are lower in preterm infants and neonates than in adults, and appear to rise in response to enteric feeding in infants greater than 33 weeks' gestation (Lucas et al 1980a–c).

As can be seen, many of the regulatory peptides of the gut are multifunctional, demonstrating hormonal, neurotransmitter and immune regulator properties. Two other substances found in the nervous system and GI tract fall within this group: cholecystokinin and substance P. Cholecystokinin acts as a proinflammatory peptide, neurotransmitter and hormone. Although the mechanisms are not well understood, it appears to have a role in altering postsynaptic membranes, pancreatic enzyme secretion, contraction of gallbladder wall, and the release of bile (Murphy & Aynsley-Green 1996). Substance P is found within neurons of the enteric nervous system and fibers of the autonomic nervous system innervating the pancreas. Substance P affects smooth muscle, resulting in vasodilation of blood vessels and increased contractions of the gut wall. In response to elevated levels of substance P, the pancreas decreases insulin and increases glucagon secretion, and increases gut levels of amylase and bicarbonate. Substance P also has natriuretic and diuretic properties. In the central nervous system, this peptide is involved with pain perception, and decreased levels are seen with some movement disorders (Kandel et al 2000). Interestingly, there are areas of the gut with reduced substance P in Chagas' disease and Hirschsprung's disease, both of which involve localized abnormalities of the enteric nervous system (Long et al 1980, Murphy & Aynsley-Green 1996).

PANCREATIC FUNCTION

The pancreas secretes several substances involved with digestion, absorption and energy homeostasis. Enzymes produced by the pancreas which are involved with protein digestion include trypsin, chymotrypsin and carboxypolypeptidase. Carbohydrate digestion is dependent on pancreatic amylase, while fats are broken down by pancreatic lipase, cholesterol lipase and phospholipase. Pancreatic polypeptide is a regulatory peptide involved with gallbladder function and protein and fat metabolism. Bicarbonate is an ion secreted by the pancreas to neutralize acidity in the intestine. This helps to protect the intestinal mucosa and aids in some of the absorptive processes. Bicarbonate secretion in the preterm and newborn infant is decreased when compared with the adult. It is unclear when adult levels are reached. The pancreas releases bicarbonate in response to secretin. Secretin, a polypeptide in the proximal intestine, is released when acid chyme enters the duodenum.

In general, pancreatic activity is depressed in children when compared to adults. For example, pancreatic amylase activity necessary for the breakdown of carbohydrates is extremely low in normal newborns and remains so for several weeks after birth (Schmitz 1996). Undigested saccharides increase the osmotic gradient in the feces, which then retain water. As a result, stools are loose and watery in the premature infant and neonate. With increase in amylase activity, the stool takes on the typical pudding-like consistency of the infant. To some extent, maturation of pancreatic activity in the premature infant may be influenced by the type of carbohydrate the child ingests. Higher levels of amylase have been found in preterm infants receiving starch-rich formulae, while higher levels of trypsin and lipase were found in those receiving a glucose-rich formula (Hadorn 1968, Zoppi et al 1972, Werlin 1992, 1996). Other enzymes involved with digestion, such as chymotrypsin, trypsin and carboxypeptidase, have also been reported at decreased levels in newborns (Lebenthal & Lee 1980). There is some discrepancy, between the various studies published, regarding actual enzyme levels and their pattern of maturation in premature neonates, term newborns and infants. However, one thing is clear: the newborn infant and premature infant do have a certain level of pancreatic insufficiency when compared with the adult. Furthermore, secretion of some enzymes, such as amylase, has still not reached adult levels in the young teenager (Werlin 1996). Consequently, infants and children can digest and absorb fats, proteins and carbohydrates, but perhaps not with the same efficiency as adults.

The two substances for which the pancreas is most famous are glucagon and insulin. These are both endocrine substances in that they can affect target tissues at distant sites. Glucagon is a polypeptide secreted by the α cells of Langerhans. It is released into the portal circulation, where it triggers glycogenolysis and gluconeogenesis in the liver. Conversely, insulin produced in the β cells of Langerhans enhances glucose transport across cell membranes, promotes uptake and storage of glucose in the liver, and facilitates uptake into muscle. Insulin is secreted by the pancreas in the postprandial period. In the liver, glucose is converted to glycogen through a phosphorylation process involving insulin. Insulin also facilitates the transport of glucose into the cells of resting muscle, where it can be stored as glycogen, although it is more often quickly metabolized for energy (Guyton 1996).

Insulin and glucagon are responsible for maintaining energy homeostasis throughout the gut and the entire body. In the immediate postprandial period, the gut is exposed to large concentrations of glucose and lipid. Changes in vascular tone result in increased vascular permeability and blood flow in vessels within the gut wall. Nutrients, water and ions are more easily absorbed and delivered to distant tissues. However, a mechanism needs to be in place to sustain energy levels between feedings. This is accomplished through the interaction of glucagon and insulin. In response to elevated plasma glucose levels, the pancreas secretes insulin, which promotes storage. When glucose levels fall, glucagon is released to stimulate glycogenolysis in the liver, thus providing an energy source to the tissues of the body.

One of the first steps in the transition to extrauterine glucose homeostasis appears to involve cutting the umbilical cord. There is a sudden increase in circulating catecholamines which stimulates a rise in glucagon in some newborn mammals (Gajwer 1977) and is thought to do the same in humans. A concomitant increase in plasma epinephrine levels during labor acts to stimulate hepatic gluconeogenesis (Padbury & Ogta 1992). Nevertheless, during the first few hours of birth, plasma glucose levels fall by 40–50%, then return to normal levels over the next 2 days (Padbury & Ogta 1992). In premature infants, imprecise control of gluconeogenesis often results in hypoglycemia. In combination with poor oral intake, this may lead to severely decreased levels of plasma, glucose which, in this population, will have cardiac, respiratory and neurological sequelae. Signs of hypoglycemia in the neonatal period include, but are not limited to, apnea, cyanosis, jitteriness, hypotonia, tachypnea, hypothermia and tremors (Cowett 1992). Hypoglycemia may also result from hyperinsulinism. Elevated levels of neonatal insulin are most commonly seen with maternal diabetes, Rh incompatibility, hemolytic disease of the newborn, and as a consequence of exchange transfusion. Even in the term newborn, glucose homeostasis can be affected by hypoxia, cold stress and sepsis leading to hypoglycemia. In fact, signs of hypoglycemia – listlessness, pallor and sweating – are often present in older infants with serious infection.

ACTIVATION OF GUT FUNCTION

By 16 weeks, the fetus can swallow and will ingest amniotic fluid, which is then transported through the GI tract. Initially, the volume ingested is fairly low, at 2–7 ml/day, increasing to 16 ml/day towards the end of the second trimester, and reaching 450 ml/day at term (Milla 1996). Amniotic fluid is a product of the dialysis of maternal and fetal plasma. The fetal gut is exposed to a fairly constant flow of amniotic fluid from 16 weeks to birth. Substances present in the amniotic fluid are thought to play a role in the development of GI structure and function (Milla 1996). Likewise, fetal ingestion plays a role in maintaining appropriate intrauterine volumes of amniotic fluid. For example, an insufficient level of amniotic fluid during gestation is associated with atresia of the GI tract.

In term newborns, mature gut function appears to be stimulated by the first feedings. In fact, there is some evidence that, in neonates, levels of certain regulatory peptides in the gut are influenced by the presence or absence of breast milk in the diet (Lucas et al 1978, 1980a–c, Lucas & Bloom 1986). During pregnancy, the GI tract of the developing fetus is exposed to simple proteins through the ingestion of amniotic fluid which it is able to digest and absorb. However, when enteral feeding is initiated, lactose, fat, higher concentrations of proteins and microscopic organisms are introduced into the gut lumen. Developmental changes in gut function and structure have been observed in various mammals in association with postnatal feeding or the lack thereof (Murphy & Aynsley-Green 1996). In term newborns, the activity of many gut enzymes is enhanced or triggered by the first enteral feedings. This may be a response to peptides, hormones and neurotransmitters present in milk. For example, there are high levels of EGF, prostaglandin E, neurotensin, melatonin, calcitonin, TSH, thyrotropin-releasing hormone (TRH), adrenocorticotropic hormone (ACTH), and other hormones in breast milk (Lucas et al 1980a–c, Milla 1996, Murphy & Aynsley-Green 1996). As previously discussed, many of these are involved with growth and function of the GI tract.

The actual presence of food in the gut lumen may also trigger responses from secretory cells within the mucosa. It is known that enterochromaffin cells release serotonin in response to distention of the gut lumen (Gershon 1999), and G cells release gastrin (Guyton 1996). Plasma levels of gastrin and enteroglucagon (glucagon secreted by intestinal cells) increase during the first 4 days of life in infants (Rodgers et al 1978), and research on humans and other mammals suggests that this is in response to the ingestion of milk (Litchenberger & Johnson 1974, Von Berger et al 1976, Aynsley-Green et al 1979). Breast milk has been found to increase blood glucose levels and concentrations of insulin, growth hormone, gastrin and enteroglucagon in full-term infants, making *it* the drink of choice for this population. Conversely, premature infants do not experience the same immediate response to the first feed. However, Lucas has shown that with subsequent bolus feeds there are elevations in gut hormone levels in premature infants. Furthermore, as feeds continue, there are changes in the responses of many other substances, including gastrin, glucose, insulin and growth hormone (Lucas et al 1980a–c, 1981a, b, 1982a, b). Studies comparing the response of term infants to breast milk and formula concluded that insulin and growth hormone were significantly increased in the formula-fed babies when compared with breastfed infants of the same age. Altered levels of motilin and neurotensin were also present in the formula-fed babies when compared with breastfed infants (Lucas et al 1980a–c, 1981a, b, Murphy & Aynsley-Green 1996). Moreover, infants continue to have differences in gut hormone response to formula versus breast milk until at least 9 months after birth (Murphy & Aynsley-Green 1996). The altered concentrations of peptides responsible for digestion, absorption and motility of the gut may provide an explanation for the apparent anecdotal increase in the incidence of colic in children who are formula-fed.

Markedly elevated levels of gastrin are present in the umbilical cord blood of infants delivered vaginally as compared to those delivered via cesarean section. It has been suggested that this may be a response to vagal stimulation, because the levels rapidly decrease to normal neonatal levels within hours after birth (Lucas et al 1979, 1980a–c, Murphy & Aynsley-Green 1996). Furthermore, elevated levels of motilin, VIP, glucagon and neurotensin are seen in the cord blood of infants who have experienced fetal distress (Lucas et al 1979, 1980a–c). Elevated levels of motilin may account for the intrauterine passage of meconium in stressed babies. The elevated glucagon levels are particularly important, in that they will often lead to rebound hypoglycemia shortly after birth. It goes without saying that these factors and their implications should come to mind when taking the labor and delivery history from parents.

DIGESTION AND ABSORPTION

Food entering the mouth begins to be digested through the work of the teeth, the tongue and the salivary glands. These contents are then passed through the esophagus into the stomach. Within the stomach, further breakdown will take place under the influence of hydrochloric acid, but it is not until the food enters the intestinal tract that it feels the full onslaught of digestive enzymes. Once in the intestine, the next step in breakdown of proteins, carbohydrates and fats involves enzymes secreted by the pancreas in response to vagal stimulation and the presence of secretin (a regulatory peptide) and cholecystokinin. Pancreatic secretions ready these basic dietary components for exposure to mucosal enzymes. It is the enzymes of the brush border and epithelial cells which complete the final step in the process of digestion and prime the nutrient for absorption across the gut wall.

All carbohydrates are hydrolyzed into lactose, sucrose or maltodextrins through a process involving enzymes from the salivary glands, stomach and pancreas. Once in this form, they can be taken up by cells in the brush border of the intestine, where they are further hydrolyzed by lactase, sucrase, maltase or α-dextrinase into glucose, fructose or galactose, and transported across the intestinal mucosa by a carrier protein. This transportation pathway is coupled to movement of sodium ions across the gut wall. Glucose enters the portal and systemic circulation, where, under the influence of insulin, it will be stored or used up as an energy source by the tissues of the body. The ability to transport glucose across the gut wall is present at 11 weeks of gestation, though at slow rates. Transport capacity increases throughout gestation and into the postnatal period, but at 1 year after birth, it is still approximately one-fourth to one-fifth that of an adult (Schmitz 1996). It is unclear when infant rates reach those of the adult. The increased rate of glucose transport appears to be related to increases in the density of transport sites (Schmitz 1996). The maturation of the fructose and galactose systems is unclear, although fructose is carried by a carrier protein not coupled to sodium ions. Galactose is transported by the same carrier protein as glucose.

Compared to carbohydrates, the digestion of proteins is a much more complicated process. Dietary proteins are primarily digested in the stomach and proximal small intestine. After mastication, pepsin in the gastric lumen splits the proteins into proteoses, peptones and large polypeptides. The pancreatic enzymes trypsin, chymotrypsin and carboxypeptidase further digest the peptides. Peptidases in the brush border then hydrolyze the peptides into amino acids, which are absorbed. Alternatively, very small soluble proteins may be directly absorbed into cells and then broken down to amino acids by peptidases in the cytoplasm (Schmitz 1996). The concentration and activity of the different brush border peptidases vary immensely during development. Some reach adult levels and function early in gestation, while others still show variation from the norm at the time of birth. Movement of dietary amino acids and peptides across the gut wall occurs through two mechanisms, one of which involves sodium ion transfer and another which does not. These systems are present and functioning by 20 weeks of gestation, although not at adult levels.

The first step in fat digestion involves emulsification by bile salts secreted by the liver. The bile salts decrease the surface tension of the fat globules, while the rhythmic movements of the intestine break them apart. Then the pancreatic enzyme lipase, with some minor assistance from enteric lipase, splits the fat into monoglycerides and fatty acids. The bile salts then form micelles with the monoglycerides and ferry them to the brush border. Free fatty acids and monoglycerides diffuse across the brush border and plasma membrane. Once they are inside the endothelial cell, the endoplasmic reticulum combines the fatty acids and monoglycerides to reform triglycerides. The triglycerides aggregate with phospholipids and cholesterol and, in combination with apolipoprotein, form a chylomicron. Chylomicrons are exocytosed from the cell into the lymph system, via which they enter the systemic circulation. Concentrations of the different types of apolipoprotein appear at various stages of development, and their precise ontogeny in humans is not well understood.

THE GUT WALL AS A PROTECTIVE BARRIER

The activity and concentration of the transport systems and digestive enzymes of the gut show some differences in the newborn and premature infant when compared with the adult. However, the contrast between these two groups is

much greater when one looks at the overall level of permeability of the infant gut wall. In adults, the gut mucosa forms a protective barrier between ingested samples of the external world and the well-orchestrated homeostasis of the body. Premature and term newborns show increased permeability to macromolecules. Plasma levels of small protein and carbohydrate molecules, such as α-lactalbumin, β-lactalbumin, lactulose, mannitol and rhamnose, are higher in premature infants than in term infants, and higher in term neonates than in adults. Maturation of gut permeability appears to be stimulated by feeding, with a more rapid response occurring in breastfed babies than in those fed formula. Interestingly, baby mammals, which receive passive immunity from colostrum and maternal milk, also exhibit increased gut permeability during the early part of life, whereas the gut wall exhibits more mature barrier activity in the newborns of species not relying on passive immunity (Schmitz 1996).

The human gut is exposed to an immeasurable number of antigens throughout life. As we age, many become familiar, but new antigens are always popping up. A mechanism has to be in place to protect the GI tract, and through it the body, from ingested substances which might be harmful. This task is accomplished in several ways. Breast milk supplies many immunological substances to the newborn GI tract. Secretory immunoglobulin A protects the infant from microbial infection and is present in breast milk and colostrum. Special forms of enzymes, glycoproteins and oligosaccharides also act as antibacterial and antiparasitic agents. These factors also provide a measure of protection against ingested substances which might be irritating to the gut.

Mucus secreted by stem cells in the gut wall lubricates chyme for easy passage and coats the lining of the lumen with a layer of viscoelastic gel, composed of water, mucin, electrolytes, immunoglobulins, glycoproteins, peptides and phospholipids. Protective factors from breast milk are also incorporated if available. The mucus performs several functions. It binds to pathological antigens, enterotoxins, bacteria, viruses and parasites, preventing colonization of the gut wall. It acts as a solvent to lubricate and remove unwanted substances. It provides a barrier and contributes to impenetrability of the gut wall. The mucous layer also contains immunoglobulins, which can respond as necessary. It is unclear whether mucus from the neonatal gut differs from that in the adult in humans, but differences do exist in other mammals (Sherman & Litchtman 1996).

As has been previously mentioned, the cells of the mucosal layer undergo rapid turnover and are replaced approximately every 5 days by cells migrating up the walls of the crypts of Lieberkühn. This allows for the rapid replacement of diseased or damaged tissue. Cell death and sloughing are well controlled through an apoptotic process. Other factors contributing to gut protection include gastric acid production, gut transit time, and mature cell receptor expression. Many bacterial toxins cause GI disruption by binding to cell receptors. The ability of many ingested pathogens to actually infect the host is often related to the affinity of host receptor cells for the enterotoxin produced by the pathogen, and this can vary with age. For example, receptor cells of young infants and children have a higher affinity for botulism toxin than those of the adult. Consequently, one needs to avoid giving honey to this age group. The enterotoxins of *Escherichia coli* and *Vibrio cholera* also bind more easily to the immature receptors of the infant, making them more susceptible. Conversely, *Clostridium difficile* appears to have a more difficult time binding to immature receptors (Sherman & Litchtman 1996) and is less often a problem in this age group.

IMMUNE FUNCTION OF THE GUT MUCOSA

Early in life, the gut and lung are the sites where immune recognition begins. The immature immune system learns to identify and respond to antigens as they are carried into these organ systems. An intricate scheme of antigen identification, recognition and response is carried out by the GI immune system. As a result, the gut has been described as the largest lymphoid organ in the body, teeming with populations of lymphoid and myeloid cells (Blumberg & Stenson 1995, MacDonald & Spencer 1996). There is a whirlwind of activity happening through the labor of the cells of the gut mucosa having to do with antigen processing, and humoral and cellular immunity. This work is carried out through the gut-associated lymphoid tissue (GALT), localized collections of immune cells scattered throughout the mucosal layer of the GI tract. The GALT interacts with lymphoid tissue in the lung, breast, skin and genitourinary tract as part of the mucosal-associated lymphoid tissue (MALT) complex. This allows for rapid transmission of immunity and antigenic information between these systems. For example, in the adult female, B cells stimulated in the gut migrate from Peyer's patches to the breast, where they secrete IgA into colostrum and breast milk (MacDonald & Spencer 1996).

Several modifications exist in the GALT to facilitate the acquisition of cellular and humoral immunity. In the small intestine, the GALT is composed of three types of lymphoid tissue which differ in structure and cellular components. Although interaction takes place between the three, each has a different ontogeny and microenvironment. Peyer's patches are the most ordered of the three types, composed of organized aggregates of T and B cells lying within the lamina propria of the small intestine. The second compartment is a layer of lamina propria cells, composed primarily of IgA and IgM-secreting plasma cells, along with B cells, T cells, natural killer cells, mast cells and phagocytes. Finally, there is a more sparse population of T cells and lymphocytes lying between the columnar epithelial cells of the villi, called human intraepithelial lymphocytes (HILs). Peyer's patches have been described as the afferent limb of GALT, and the plasma-secreting cells of the lamina propria as the efferent limb (Blumberg & Stenson 1995).

T and B cells located in Peyer's patches are sensitive to antigen and mitogen. Both cell types communicate with MALT. When stimulated, B cells differentiate into plasma cells that synthesize and secrete antibody. When T cells are stimulated, they differentiate into various types of T effector cells, which are capable of damaging target tissue, inducing or inhibiting antibody synthesis from B cells, and inciting other T cell differentiation. Overlying Peyer's patches is a specialized cuboidal epithelium containing M cells (microfold cells), which act to separate the lymphoid tissue from the intestinal lumen. Rather than the well-developed microvilli of the columnar cells, M cells contain many vesicles which are pinocytotic and capable of sampling antigen from the gut lumen and delivering it to the underlying B and T cells (Silverstein & Lukes 1962, Owen & Jones 1974, Owen 1977, MacDonald & Spencer 1996). M cells first appear at approximately 17 weeks of gestation and lymphocytes at 19 weeks. After birth, Peyer's patches undergo excessive growth and development in response to antigen exposure (MacDonald & Spencer 1996). The B cells of Peyer's patches react to antigen present in ingested substances by proliferating and migrating to the thoracic duct, from which they can enter the systemic circulation (Losonsky & Ogra 1992). In the adult, the B cells of Peyer's patches tend to generate a higher proportion of IgA-secreting lymphoblasts, which circulate to other mucosal-associated tissue to provide immunity in the mouth and pharynx, respiratory tract, kidneys and reproductive organs. Furthermore, IgA lymphoblasts produced in the gut travel to the breast, where they are excreted in breast milk to provide immunity for the suckling infant. At birth, there are no IgA-generating cells present in Peyer's patches. The neonate primarily receives IgA through the breast milk. IgA plasma cells begin to appear by 2 weeks and will increase in number until reaching adult levels by 2 years (Perkkio & Savvilahti 1980). IgA plasma cell proliferation appears to be influenced by milk ingestion (Knox 1986).

In the adult, lymphoid cells in the lamina propria include T and B cells, plasma cells, phagocytes and mast cells, with the majority being IgA-secreting plasma cells. However, because Peyer's patches of the neonate do not produce IgA-secreting plasma cells, there is no IgA in their lamina propria. By 12 days, both IgA and IgM appear, but IgM predominates for the first few months. The most abundant cell types present in the neonatal lamina propria are T cell lymphocytes expressing the HLA-DR, the CD4 and CD45 antigens. These play a role in cytolytic and immune memory activities. IgA is particularly important in the gut, where it is expressed as a specialized secretory immunoglobulin capable of withstanding degradation by digestive enzymes. Secretory IgA prevents binding of bacteria to the mucosal surface of the gut, blocks absorption of toxic antigens, and has antiviral activity (Blumberg & Stenson 1995, Guyton 1996, MacDonald & Spencer 1996).

Intraepithelial lymphocytes (IELs) express a limited number of T cell receptors for antigens. Although they appear to be involved with acute response to local injury or damage of the cells of the gut wall, their primary function may involve monitoring epithelial cells for cytological abnormalities. The extreme rate of proliferation and turnover of gut epithelial cells increases the chance of replication defects and dysplasia. The IELs are capable of destroying dysplastic cells, based on the expression of specific surface antigens (Blumberg & Stenson 1995). IELs may provide the immediate local response which can then be backed up by activity in the lamina propria or Peyer's patches.

MECONIUM

Meconium is a collection of secretions and desquamated cells from the digestive tract, and waste products from ingested amniotic fluid. It begins to appear towards the beginning of the second trimester and accumulates in the colon until birth. Meconium is usually passed in the first 24 h after birth, and should be passed within 48 h (Stoll & Kliegman 2000).

Failure to pass meconium may be due to intestinal obstruction including atresia, an imperforated anus, Hirschsprung's disease and meconium plug. Meconium plugs occur when the meconium has a lower than normal water content and cannot be passed. They can lead to ulceration and peritonitis if not treated successfully. Meconium may also be passed in the uterus during times of fetal distress. Under normal conditions, meconium is not passed before birth. Intrauterine exposure is probable if the neonate exhibits meconium staining, a greenish discoloration which generally occurs in the nails of the hands and feet when the fetus is exposed to meconium for a prolonged period of time. Meconium is toxic to the respiratory tract, and aspiration is a serious complication of premature passage of meconium. At-risk neonates are suctioned immediately after delivery before any respiratory activity can occur. The vocal cords are visualized for staining, and intubation with deep suction is carried out if needed.

CONCLUSION

The GI system is a large and complex organ involved with nutritive delivery, waste excretion and immune recognition. Many of these processes are poorly developed at birth and mature over weeks to years. Consequently, the gut and its many functions can be vulnerable to injury in the formative years. Prevention, diagnosis and treatment of GI dysfunction depend on a good understanding of these processes and their development.

References

Abu-Hijleh M F, Habbal O A, Moqattash S T 1995 The role of the diaphragm in lymphatic absorption from the peritoneal cavity. J Anat 186: 453–467.

Aynsley-Green A, Lucas A, Bloom S R 1979 The effect of feeds of differing composition on entero-insular hormone secretion in the first hours of life in human neonates. Acta Paediatr Scand 68(2): 265–270.

Barnard J, Warwick G, Gold L 1993 Localization of transforming growth factor beta isoform in the normal murine small intestine and colon. Gastroenterology 105: 667–673.

Beal M C 1985 Viscerosomatic reflexes: a review. J Am Osteopath Soc 85(12): 786–801.

Blumberg R S, Stenson W F 2003 The immune system and gastrointestinal inflammation. In: Yamada T (ed) Textbook of gastroenterology. W B Saunders, Philadelphia.

Boyle J 1992 Motility of the upper gastrointestinal tract in the fetus and neonate. In: Polin R, Fox W (eds) Fetal and neonatal physiology. W B Saunders, Philadelphia.

Bueno L 1985 Central control of intestinal motility by prostaglandins: a mediation of the action of several peptides in rats and dogs. Gastroenterology 88: 1888–1894.

Castell D, Harris L 1970 Hormonal control of gastroesophageal sphincter strength. N Engl J Med 282: 886–890.

Clark D, Miller M 1992 Development of the gastrointestinal circulation in the fetus and newborn. In: Polin R, Fox W (eds) Fetal and neonatal physiology. W B Saunders, Philadelphia.

Cowett R M 1992 Hypoglycemia and hyperglycemia in the newborn. In: Polin R, Fox W (eds) Fetal and neonatal physiology. W B Saunders, Philadelphia.

Crissinger K, Granger D N 2003 Gastrointestinal blood flow. In: Yamada T (ed) Textbook of gastroenterology. Lippincott, Philadelphia: 498–521.

Foulk W T 1954 Gastroenterology 26: 601–611.

Gajwer L 1977 Possible mechanisms and significance of the neonatal surge in glucagon secretion: studies in newborn lambs. Pediatr Res 11: 883.

Gershon M D 1999 The enteric nervous system; a second brain. Hospital Practice 34: 31–52.

Guyton A C 1996 Textbook of medical physiology, 9th edn. W B Saunders, Philadelphia.

Hadorn B 1968 Quantitative assessment of exocrine pancreatic function in infants and children. J Pediatr 73: 39–50.

Huizinga J D, Stern H S, Chow E et al 1985 Electrophysiologic control of motility in the human colon. Gastroenterology 88(2): 500–511.

Israel E 1996 Necrotizing enterocolitis. In: Walker W A, Durie P R, Hamilton J R et al (eds) Pediatric gastrointestinal disease, vol 1. Mosby, St Louis: 750–761.

Kandel E R, Schwart J H, Jessel T M 2000 Principles of neural science, 4th edn. McGraw-Hill, Philadelphia.

Knox W 1986 Restricted feeding and human intestinal plasma cell development. Arch Dis Child 61: 744–749.

Lanciault G, Jacobson E 1976 The gastro-intestinal circulation. Gastroenterology 71: 851–873.

Lebenthal E, Lee P 1980 Development of functional response in human exocrine pancreas. Pediatrics 66: 556–560.

Litchenberger L, Johnson L 1974 Gastrin in the ontogenic development of the small intestine. Am J Physiol 277: 390–395.

Long R G, Bishop A E, Barnes A J et al 1980 Neural and hormonal peptides in rectal biopsy specimens from patients with Chagas' disease and chronic autonomic failure. Lancet 1(8168 Pt 1): 559–562.

Losonsky G, Ogra P 1992 Immunology of the breast and host immunity. In: Polin R, Fox W (eds) Fetal and neonatal physiology. W B Saunders, Philadelphia.

Lucas A, Bloom S 1986 Gut hormones and 'minimal enteral feeding'. Acta Paediatr Scand 75: 719–723.

Lucas A, Bloom S, Aynsley-Green A 1978 Metabolic and endocrine events at the time of the first feed of human milk in preterm and term infants. Arch Dis Child 53: 731–736.

Lucas A, Bloom S, Aynsley-Green A 1979 Gut hormones in fetal distress. Lancet ii: 718.

Lucas A, Bloom S, Aynsley-Green A 1980a Development of gut hormone responses to feeding in neonates. Arch Dis Child 55: 678–682.

Lucas A, Sarson D L, Bloom S R et al 1980b Developmental aspects of gastric inhibitory polypeptide (GIP) and its possible role in the enteroinsular axis in neonates. Acta Paediatr Scand 69(3): 321–325.

Lucas A, Adrian T E, Christofides N et al 1980c Plasma motilin, gastrin and enteroglucagon and enteral feeding in the human newborn. Arch Dis Child 55(9): 673–677.

Lucas A, Boyes S, Bloom S R et al 1981a Metabolic and endocrine responses to a milk feed in six-day-old term infants: differences between breast and cow's milk formula feeding. Acta Paediatr Scand 70(2): 195–200.

Lucas A, Aynsley-Green A, Blackburn A M et al 1981b Plasma neurotensin in term and preterm neonates. Acta Paediatr Scand 70(2): 201–206.

Lucas A, Bloom S, Aynsley-Green A 1982a Plasma vasoactive intestinal peptide (VIP) in the neonate. Acta Paediatr Scand 71: 71–74.

Lucas A, Bloom S, Aynsley-Green A 1982b Postnatal surges in gut hormones in term and preterm neonates. Biol Neonate 41 (1–2): 63–67.

MacDonald T T, Spencer J 1996 The ontogeny of the mucosal immune system. In: Walker W A, Durie P R, Hamilton J R et al (eds) Pediatric gastrointestinal disease. Mosby, St Louis: 115–126.

Milla P J 1996 The ontogeny of intestinal motor activity. In: Walker W A, Durie P R, Hamilton J R et al (eds) Pediatric gastrointestinal disease. Mosby, St Louis: 31–41.

Moore K L 2007 The developing human, 8th edn. W B Saunders, Philadelphia.

Murphy M, Aynsley-Green A 1996 Regulatory peptides of the gastrointestinal tract in early life. In: Walker W A, Durie P R, Hamilton J R et al (eds) Pediatric gastro-intestinal disease. Mosby, St Louis: 43–70.

Negrini D, Mukenge S, Del Fabbro M et al 1991 Distribution of diaphragmatic lymphatic stomata. J Appl Physiol 70(4): 1544–1549.

Nowicki P, Miller C 1988 Autoregulation in the developing postnatal intestinal circulation. Am J Physiol 254: G189–G193.

O'Morain C, Bishop A E, McGregor G P et al 1984 Vasoactive intestinal peptide concentrations and immunocytochemical studies in rectal biopsies from patients with inflammatory bowel disease. Gut 25(1): 57–61.

Owen R L 1977 Sequential uptake of horseradish peroxidase by lymphoid follicle epithelium of Peyer's patches in the normal unobstructed mouse intestine: an ultrastructure study. Gastroenterology 72(3): 440–451.

Owen R L, Jones A L 1974 Epithelial cell specialization within human Peyer's patches: an ultrastructure study of intestinal lymphoid follicles. Gastroenterology 66: 189–203.

Padbury J F, Ogta E S 1992 Glucose metabolism during transition to postnatal life. In: Polin R, Fox W (eds) Fetal and neonatal physiology. W B Saunders, Philadelphia.

Pelot D 1995 Anatomy, anomalies and physiology of the esophagus. In: Haubrich W, Schaffner F, Berk J (eds) Bockus gastroenterology. W B Saunders, Philadelphia: 397–410.

Perkkio M, Savvilahti E 1980 Time of appearance of immunoglobulin-containing cells in the mucosa of the neonatal intestine. Pediatr Res 14: 953–957.

Ritchie H, Thompson D, Wingate D 1980 Diurnal variation in human jejunal fasting motor activity. J Physiol 304: 54.

Rodgers B M, Dix P M, Talbert J L et al 1978 Fasting and post-prandial serum gastrin in normal human neonates. J Pediatr Surg 13: 13–16.

Ruckebusch Y 1986 Development of digestive motor patterns during perinatal life: mechanisms and significance. J Pediatr Gastroenterol Nutr 5(4): 523–536.

Schmitz J 1996 Digestive and absorptive function. In: Walker W A, Durie P R, Hamilton J R et al (eds) Pediatric gastrointestinal disease. Mosby, St Louis: 263–279.

Scott R 1996 Motility disorders. In: Walker W A, Durie P R, Hamilton J R et al (eds) Pediatric gastrointestinal disease. Mosby, St Louis: 936–954.

Sherman P M, Litchtman S 1996 Mucosal barrier function and colonization of the gut. In: Walker W A, Durie P R, Hamilton J R et al (eds) Pediatric gastrointestinal disease. Mosby, St Louis: 103–114.

Silverstein A M, Lukes R J 1962 Fetal response to antigenic stimulus. 1. Plasmacellular and lymphoid reactions in the human fetus to intrauterine infection. Lab Invest 11: 918–932.

Standring S (ed) 2004 Gray's anatomy, 39th edn. Churchill Livingstone, New York.

Stoll B J, Kliegman R M 2000 The newborn infant. In: Behrman R E, Kliegman R M, Jensen H (eds) Nelson's textbook of pediatrics. W B Saunders, Philadelphia: 454–460.

Tepperman B, Jacobson E 1981 Mesenteric circulation. In: Johnson L (ed) Physiology of the gastrointestinal tract. Raven Press, New York: 1317–1336.

Thompson D, Ritchie H, Wingate D 1982 Patterns of small intestinal motility in duodenal ulcer patients before and after vagotomy. Gut 23: 517–523.

Von Berger L, Henrichs I, Raptis S et al 1976 Gastrin concentrations in plasma of the neonate at birth and after first feeding. Pediatrics 58: 264–267.

Weaver L T 1996 Anatomy and embryology. In: Walker W A, Durie P R, Hamilton J R et al (eds) Pediatric gastrointestinal disease. Mosby, St Louis: 9–30.

Werlin S 1992 Exocrine pancreas. In: Polin R, Fox W (eds) Fetal and neonatal physiology. W B Saunders, Philadelphia.

Werlin S 1996 Development of the exocrine pancreas. In: Walker W A, Durie P R, Hamilton J R et al (eds) Pediatric gastrointestinal disease. Mosby, St Louis: 143–161.

Willard F H 1997 The autonomic nervous system. In: Ward R (ed) Foundations for osteopathic medicine. Williams & Wilkins, Baltimore: 53–83.

Wright N A, Pike C, Elia G 1990 Induction of a novel epidermal growth factor secreting cell lineage by mucosal ulceration in human gastrointestinal stem cells. Nature 343(6253): 82–85.

Wyllie R 2000 Congenital aganglionic megacolon. In: Behrman R E, Kliegman R M, Jenson H B (eds) Nelson textbook of pediatrics. W B Saunders, Philadelphia: 1139–1141.

Zoppi G, Andreotti G, Pajno-Ferrara E et al 1972 Exocrine pancreatic function in premature and full term infants. Pediatr Res 6: 880–886.

Further reading

Bernbaum J C, Pereira G R, Watkins J B et al 1983 Non-nutritive sucking during gavage feeding enhances growth and maturation in premature infants. Pediatrics 71: 41–45.

Daniel E, Berezin I 1992 Interstitial cells of Cajal: are they major players in control of gastrointestinal motility? J Gastrointest Motility 4: 1–24.

Guyton A C, Hall J E 2005 Textbook of medical physiology, 11th edn. W B Saunders, Philadelphia.

Kagnoff M F 1981 Immunology of the digestive system. In: Johnson L (ed) Physiology of the gastrointestinal tract, vol II. Raven Press, New York: 1337–1359.

Kleinman R E, Sanderson I R, Goulet O et al (eds) 2008 Pediatric gastrointestinal disease. B C Decker, Ontario, Canada.

Menard D, Arsenault P, Pothier P 1988 Biologic effects of epidermal growth factor in human fetal jejunum. Gastroenterology 94: 656–663.

Padbury J F, Ludlow J K, Ervin M G et al 1987 Thresholds for physiological effects of plasma catecholamines in fetal sheep. Am J Physiol 252(4 Pt 1): E530–537.

Walker W A, Durie P R, Hamilton J R et al (eds) 1996 Pediatric gastrointestinal disease, vols I and II, 2nd edn. Mosby, St Louis.

Weaver L T 1992 Breast and gut: the interaction of lactating mammary function and neonatal gastrointestinal function. Proc Nutr Soc 51: 155–163.

7

Nociception and the neuroendocrine immune system

INTRODUCTION

The primary role of the nervous, endocrine and immune systems is to maintain a dynamic homeostasis between the various cells, fluids and tissues of the body. Although traditionally they are viewed as three separate systems, the extent of interdependence between them makes the boundaries almost nonexistent. Chemicals which have traditionally been viewed as neurotransmitters can influence endocrine and immune cells, while hormones and inflammatory substances can act as neurotransmitters. The neuroendocrine immune system has a key role in the body's response to stress. It influences homeostatic rhythms and colors the way an individual compensates and responds to disease and dysfunction (Fig. 7.1). Each of the components of the neuroendocrine immune system learns its role and its relationship to the others as a result of exposures and experiences gained throughout life. At birth, these connections and relationships are often primitive at best, and the organ systems themselves are immature. Many important factors contributing to health mechanisms, such as baseline levels of activity, patterns of response and thresholds for activation, will be established during the early years of life. If distorted, each of these phenomena can alter the body's ability to successfully adapt to the demands placed on it, thus undermining the individual's general state of health.

THE BIG PICTURE

Homeostasis is a term coined by Walter Cannon in 1932. It refers to the tendency of the body to move towards stability. Allostasis is a dynamic process whereby subtle and not so subtle adaptations occur in the biochemistry and physiology of our internal world, to allow us to function optimally in our environment. Allostasis involves changes in the immune, endocrine and nervous systems in response

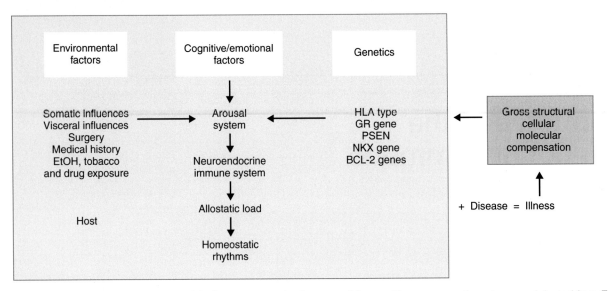

Fig. 7.1 • Schematic representation of the host response to disease and the resulting compensatory changes. *Adapted from Ed Stiles DO.*

to short-term or long-term stress. The physiological cost of these changes is called the allostatic load (McEwen & Stellar 1993, McEwen 1997, Karlamangla et al 2002, McEwen & Dhabar 2002).

Osteopathic philosophy has long recognized the importance of homeostasis for optimum health and the cost of compensation, although the term allostasis has only recently been coined (McEwen & Stellar 1993). The body is self-regulating and self-healing in the face of disease processes. Adequate function of body systems depends on circulatory mechanisms, and neurologic, immune and endocrine influences. The goal of osteopathic treatment is to remove any impediments to these mechanisms, facilitate the homeostatic processes of the body and, in contemporary language, to decrease allostatic load.

ALLOSTATIC LOAD

Allostasis describes the general adaptive response of the body to prolonged, chronic or significant stress. Stress can occur in any condition which requires adaptation and change. Allostasis is mediated through neurotransmitters, hormones and immune components. In the short term these changes typically have beneficial effects for the individual. However when the body is exposed to these substances for a prolonged period of time physiological changes occur which may be detrimental to the overall state of wellbeing. This is called the general adaptive response (McEwen & Stellar 1993). McEwen and Stellar (1993) described a method of measuring dysregulation of multiple physiological systems to establish a score, the allostatic load, which could be used as a predicator of health and wellness. The components of the allostatic load measured by McEwen include: 12-h

overnight urinary excretions of cortisol, norepinephrine and epinephrine; serum dehydroepiandrosterone sulfate (DHEAS) level; systolic and diastolic blood pressure; waist-to-hip circumference ratio; serum high-density lipoprotein (HDL) cholesterol level, total serum cholesterol to HDL cholesterol level; and glycosylated hemoglobin level. Each component of the allostatic load measurement is related to demise or dysfunction in a system. For example, elevated cortisol increases the resistance of insulin receptors. Chronically elevated cortisol is associated with insulin resistant diabetes and hyperlipidemia. It also interferes with interleukin and other immune components, affecting immune function. Chronically elevated norepinephrine and epinephrine is associated with atherosclerosis and cancer. Decreased levels of DHEAS can also be related to cardiovascular health. It has been shown that an individual's allostatic load can accumulate over one's lifetime (Karlamangla et al 2002). Elevated allostatic load is associated with cognitive decline, cardiovascular disease, and mortality (Karlamangla et al 2002). It may be also related to the development of autoimmune disease (McEwen & Dhabar 2002), changes in brain morphology and psychiatric disease.

WHAT KIND OF INPUT AFFECTS HOMEOSTASIS?

Homeostasis is influenced by all manner of inputs. Light influences the normal rhythmic production and release of chemicals that control the diurnal rhythms of our bodies. Emotional stimuli affect homeostatic mechanisms through the limbic system and the hypothalamus. Visceral and somatic inputs play a role via primary afferent fibers. In this chapter we will focus on the influence of visceral and somatic systems.

To briefly review, the sensory portion of the nervous system can be divided into two groups, which we will call the A afferent and B afferent systems. Fibers of the A afferent system are large-calibre, heavily myelinated fibers with rapid conduction times. They have encapsulated nerve endings with a low threshold for activation. The A afferent system is responsible for carrying information concerning crude touch and proprioception. Fibers of the B afferent system are small-calibre and lightly myelinated, with slow conduction times. The nerve endings of the small-calibre afferent system are usually unencapsulated and have neurosecretory properties. They have a high threshold for activation and some are actually silent. The small-calibre afferent system carries information concerning pain, temperature and light touch. And, as we shall see, it can influence the regulation of homeostatic mechanisms of the body.

The small-calibre afferent system is a nociceptive system, relaying information about noxious stimuli to the spinal cord and brain. Our body will respond to this input through changes in the motor and autonomic systems. We may or may not have a conscious appreciation of the nociceptive stimulus, depending on the intensity of the signal. When a nociceptive stimulus is of sufficient intensity to reach conscious proportions, our brain interprets the signal as pain. The quality of the pain we experience is determined by the type and quantity of receptors located in the injured tissue. Some tissues have mostly low-threshold receptors, so pain is duller. Other tissues have high-threshold, fast-conducting receptors, so the pain is sharp. The pathway that the afferent information takes to the cortex will also affect the quality of the pain experienced.

Two types of fibers in the small-calibre afferent system are the A-δ and C fibers. A-δ fibers carry both non-noxious and noxious information. The information enters the dorsal horn of the spinal cord, crosses at the anterior white commissure, and travels through the anterior lateral system to the lateral thalamus and on to the somatosensory cortex. Stimulation of A-δ fibers produces sensations of well-localized irritation, or sharp pain. We are able to rapidly localize the stimulus.

Nociceptive information traveling through C fibers enters the dorsal horn and ascends through the anterior lateral system to the brainstem, the medial thalamus, prefrontal cortex and anterior cingulate cortex. Stimulation of C fibers produces poorly localized discomfort or generalized pain, often described as a deep, throbbing or pulsating pain. For example, if you were to cut your finger on a very sharp knife, the immediate sensation would be a burning, sharp, well-localized pain over the area of the injury. This would soon be followed by a deep, throbbing ache extending over a much larger part of the finger. The first sensation is carried by the A-δ fibers, and the second by C fibers.

Small-calibre afferent fibers follow the vasculature throughout the visceral organs and somatic tissues. A-δ and C fibers can also be found in muscle, joint, ligament, tendon, periosteum and virtually all connective tissues. Within the nervous system, fibers of this afferent system are primarily found traveling with the blood vessels, although there is some evidence that dura contains a scant population of proprioceptive and C fibers.

PROCESSING AND INTERPRETATION OF NOCICEPTION

Nociceptive information from both A-δ and C fibers passes to higher centers via five ascending pathways: the spinothalamic, spinoreticular, spinomesencephalic, cervicothalamic and spinohypothalamic tracts. The spinothalamic, cervicothalamic and spinoreticular tracts terminate in the thalamus and are involved with the perception of pain. The spinoreticular tract also sends fibers to the reticular formation, an area involved in modulating autonomic processes. The spinomesencephalic tract also projects to the reticular formation, as well as the amygdala, and is probably involved with the affective component of pain (Basbaum & Jessell 2000). The spinohypothalamic tract projects directly to supraspinal centers to mediate neuroendocrine and cardiovascular responses (Basbaum & Jessell 2000).

Thalamic nuclei process and relay nociceptive information to the higher centers of the cortex. Cortical centers are involved with the interpretation of pain based on prior experience and the context in which the stimulus occurs (Basbaum & Jessell 2000). Areas of the brain concerned with emotion and autonomic function, such as the limbic system and insular cortex, also have a role in this process (Craig et al 1994, 1996, Basbaum & Jessell 2000). Consequently, the perception of a nociceptive stimulus as pain may be coupled with both an emotional and a physiological response. It has been shown that these areas are altered under the influence of chronic stimulation, resulting in an altered perception of the stimulus.

The reticular formation is another major site receiving nociceptive information. Its fibers extend to the medulla, pons and midbrain, exerting a strong influence on autonomic function and the maintenance of homeostasis. Directly and indirectly, the reticular formation orchestrates control over visceral, cardiovascular, respiratory and secretory motor activity. The locus ceruleus is located directly cephalad to the reticular formation. This small cluster of cells has diffuse projections branching throughout the cortex, thalamus, hypothalamus and brainstem. Through the reticular formation, nociceptive information from the spinal cord can indirectly influence the locus ceruleus. The locus ceruleus is a secretory center. It does not have synaptic connections with cells and it secretes neurotransmitter through widely splayed projections (Fig. 7.2). Consequently, its neurotransmitter is able to reach a large area of cells. The locus ceruleus is very sensitive to external stimuli: visual, acoustical, somatic and visceral. When stimulated, it responds by producing vigilance, arousal and concern for the environment. It has

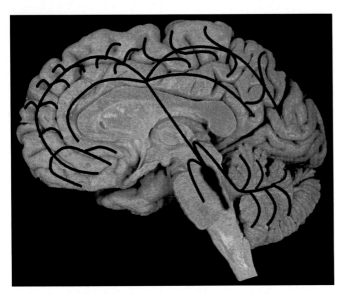

Fig. 7.2 • Sagittal section of a human brain. The area of the reticular formation lies within the brainstem and is depicted in gray. The arousal system lays at the most cephalad portion. The tracts radiating from the top of the column throughout the cortex and cerebellum indicate the extensive projections from the arousal system throughout the brain. *Used with permission of the Willard & Carreiro Collection.*

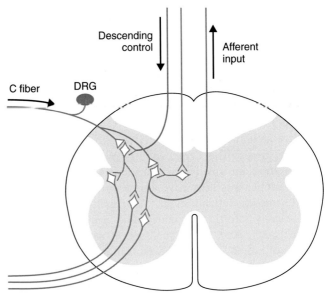

Fig. 7.3 • Schematic diagram illustrating descending control from the hypothalamus and limbic system to spinal cord interneurons. DRG, dorsal root ganglion.

sometimes been called the behavioral inhibition system, because it keeps us out of trouble.

PAIN CONTROL

Under normal circumstances, there are two mechanisms by which our bodies can suppress painful sensations: a descending mechanism, which is initiated in the hypothalamus, and a spinal mechanism, which occurs within the involved neurological segment. The descending mechanism is composed of pathways from the hypothalamus and limbic system which act on cells in the dorsal horn (Fig. 7.3). The hypothalamus has projections to the periaqueductal gray matter surrounding the third ventricle and cerebral aqueduct in the midbrain. The hypothalamus stimulates the periaqueductal gray matter to secrete endorphins and opioids, which act on cells in the nucleus raphe that carry serotonin. Serotonin stimulates enkephalinergic fibers in the spinal cord to shut off the synaptic cells in the dorsal horn. Enkephalinergic fibers will also dampen the signal being carried on postsynaptic nociceptive fibers. In this way, descending pathways can completely shut off pain. However, these pathways can act in both directions, turning the nociceptive signal down or turning it up.

The second mechanism for pain control occurs at the level of the spinal cord and is referred to as the gate control theory (Fig. 7.4). This mechanism was briefly introduced in Chapter 1. Both large- and small-calibre afferent fibers project onto interneurons. Since large-calibre afferents are fast-conducting, their signal will reach the interneuron before

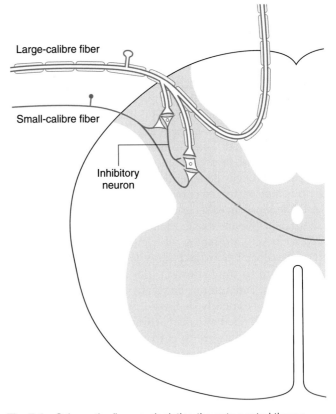

Fig. 7.4 • Schematic diagram depicting the gate control theory. A stimulus from the large-calibre fiber activates the inhibitory neuron, which then dampens the signal coming from the small-calibre fiber. Although both fibers synapse on the same interneuron, activity in the large-calibre fiber gates the signal from the small-calibre fiber.

the signal from the small-calibre afferent system. When the large-calibre afferent signal reaches the interneuron, inhibitory neurons, which are thought to be enkephalinergic, are stimulated. These inhibitory neurons dampen the nociceptive signal from the small-calibre afferent system. For example, when you bang your head on the cupboard door, rubbing it makes it feel better. The small-calibre afferent signal, the pain, is muted by the large-calibre afferent signal, the pressure. Transcutaneous nerve stimulation (TENS) units work on the gated control principle. However, this segmental system is not capable of completely shutting off pain.

SENSITIZATION OF PRIMARY AFFERENT NEURONS

We perceive acute pain when a primary afferent is activated. There are several types of primary afferent fibers involved with nociception, with different requirements for activation. One type of nociceptor has a particularly high threshold for activation and is called a silent nociceptor. Although silent nociceptors are usually quiescent, once activated they can become sensitized to various chemicals and evolve into a chronic source of pain.

All primary afferent neurons involved with nociception have receptors for bradykinins, prostaglandins and other proinflammatory substances. When injured, they may become sensitized to catecholamines as well. Fibers of the sympathetic nervous system release norepinephrine and prostaglandins for modulation of autonomic activities. Sympathetic discharge which triggers vasodilation will also cause the release of bradykinins. Consequently, nociceptive primary afferent neurons may read normal levels of sympathetic output as an irritant. When primary afferents are sensitized, they will respond to even low levels of sympathetic activity. Repeated stimulation of the primary afferent may lower the threshold of activity of the neuron even further. Once primary afferent neurons become sensitized, the noxious stimuli can be removed but the pain can continue because the neuron is now responding to non-noxious stimuli. The sensitized primary afferents will interpret non-painful stimuli as pain. This produces the clinical symptom of hyperesthesia.

As discussed in earlier chapters, primary afferent neurons from both visceral and somatic tissue enter the dorsal horn to synapse on interneurons. These interneurons receive input from the A-δ and C fibers of the small-calibre afferent system and the A-δ fibers of the large-calibre afferent system. They are called wide dynamic range (WDR) cells, because they can respond to the various levels of activity carried by primary afferent fibers. WDR cells receive polymodal input from A-β, C and A-δ fibers. Information from joints, muscle, skin and viscera converge onto these cells (Fig. 7.5). The response properties of WDR cells change with the nature of the stimulus. WDR cells are capable of long-term changes

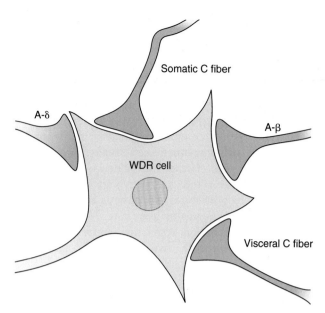

Fig. 7.5 • Wide dynamic range neurons (WDR cells) receive input from many sources.

which are stimulus driven. For example, the summation of input from all the aforementioned primary afferent neurons can lower the threshold of activity in the WDR cells and in the surrounding cells. N-methyl-D-aspartate (NMDA) channels located on WDR cells are usually closed. Under tonic primary afferent firing, these channels are opened and there is an influx of calcium into the cell. This sensitizes the cell, lowering its threshold for activation. Lowering the threshold of the interneuronal pool creates a facilitated segment, or spinal facilitation (see Ch. 1). Altered activity in the interneuronal pool can occur in the lateral, dorsal and ventral horn cells. Tonic primary afferent activity may be from noxious, thermal, electrical or chemical stimuli.

Facilitation represents increased activity in the interneuronal pool. Clinically, it presents as changes in visceral function, somatic muscle tone, vasomotor tone and fluid balance. Signs or symptoms of hyperalgesia and inflammation often accompany these changes. Early osteopaths described the osteopathic lesion as an area of tissue texture changes, asymmetry, restricted range of motion and tenderness. These are all signs of spinal facilitation.

WDR cell axons project into the ventral horn and the lateral horn of the sympathetic nervous system, and cross the midline to join the anterolateral system. Information from WDR cells will ascend through the anterolateral system (ALS) to the reticular formation, thalamus, and finally cortex.

NOCICEPTION, STRESS AND ALLOSTATIC LOAD

Nociceptive information ascending through the ALS will indirectly stimulate activity in the locus ceruleus via the reticular formation. Projections from the locus ceruleus pass to the cortex, thalamus, hypothalamus and brainstem. The hypothalamus is particularly important. It responds to stimulation from the locus ceruleus by increasing neural efferent activity to the sympathetic fibers and increasing neurohumoral activity to the anterior pituitary gland.

The hypothalamus modulates activity in the sympathetic nervous system through complex projections to the brainstem, spinal cord and sympathetic cell bodies in the lateral horn of the spinal cord. Under the influence of norepinephrine from the locus ceruleus, the hypothalamus releases norepinephrine, which increases sympathetic activity. In this way the hypothalamus regulates heart rate, blood pressure, gastrointestinal (GI) function, respiration, and vascular tone. Through the sympathetics, the hypothalamus also influences the immune system. The sympathetic fibers follow blood vessels into all lymphoid organs, lymph nodes, the thymus, bone marrow, tonsils and lamina propria of the gut. These fibers branch out and surround T cells, many of which have receptors for norepinephrine (Fig. 7.6). When the locus ceruleus increases secretion of norepinephrine in response to nociceptive stimuli, the hypothalamus responds by turning up sympathetic activity, and sympathetic fibers release norepinephrine. Norepinephrine increases the rate of T cell differentiation but decreases the rate of cell division. This means that the immune system can react quickly to many different types of antigens; however, because the rate of cell division is dampened, the response cannot be maintained. This is useful in stressful conditions, because it gives the body the necessary artillery to combat a broad range of insults while conserving energy for other processes. Because the hypothalamus responds to all forms of stimuli, this immune response is not limited to nociceptive stress. Whether the stress is physical (pain) or emotional (fear/anger), the immune system can be primed to instantly respond, but its ability to mount an effective response is compromised.

The hypothalamus also exerts influences through a neurohemal system. This system involves the anterior pituitary gland and, consequently, the endocrine system. The hypothalamus produces and secretes hypophysiotropic hormones into a dense capillary network extending from the base of the hypothalamus to the anterior pituitary (Fig. 7.7). These hormones influence the production and release of hormones from the anterior pituitary. One of these hormones, corticotropin-releasing hormone (CTRH), triggers an increased release of adrenocorticotropic hormone (ACTH) from the anterior pituitary. ACTH, in turn, stimulates release of glucocorticoids from the adrenal gland. Normally, there is a balance between

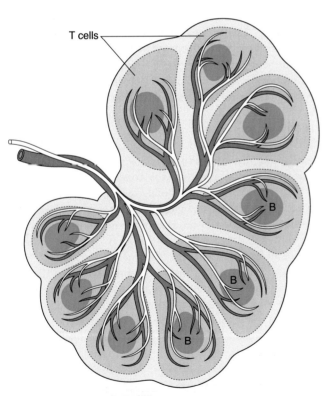

Fig. 7.6 • Schematic diagram of a lymph node. Sympathetic fibers follow the arterial supply into the node and are distributed throughout the B and T cells. *Adapted from Williams P (ed.) 1995 Gray's anatomy 38th edn, Churchill Livingstone, London, with permission.*

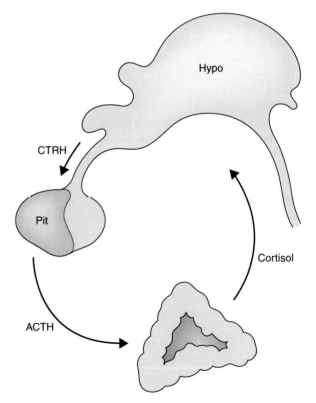

Fig. 7.7 • Corticotropin-releasing hormone (CTRH) is secreted by the hypothalamus (Hypo) into the capillary system, through which it reaches the anterior pituitary gland (Pit). In response, the pituitary releases adrenocorticotropic hormone (ACTH), which stimulates the adrenal gland to produce cortisol. Cortisol has a negative feedback effect on the hypothalamus.

the release of glucocorticoids and the reproductive steroids. This balance is maintained through daily circadian rhythms. When the locus ceruleus turns up the activity of the hypothalamus there is an increased production of CTRH, which shifts the adrenal gland from producing reproductive steroids to producing glucocorticoids. One of these glucocorticoids, cortisol, feeds back to turn down the activity in the pituitary and the hypothalamus.

Under stress, the body responds by producing and releasing cortisol. Cortisol stimulates the breakdown of glycogen and lipid stores into a ready energy supply. It enhances the effects of norepinephrine all over the body by potentiating the sympathetic nervous system – the flight or fight response. Cortisol blocks the production of prostaglandins. It suppresses the release of interleukins, interferons, tumor necrosis factor and other proinflammatory substances which would be used by the body for tissue repair. Increased levels of cortisol shift the body from a homeostatic state, where tissue breakdown and repair, energy storage and use, and cell death and regeneration, are balanced, to a state of readiness, where regeneration and repair are sacrificed. This state is called the general adaptive response. It is a physiological state which provides the individual with an efficient and effective means for short-term adaptation. Under normal conditions, a feedback mechanism is in place whereby the activity of the hypothalamus is downregulated under the influence of increased levels of cortisol. However, when the stimulus on the hypothalamus is constant or of sufficient magnitude, the feedback mechanism fails. Some authors have referred to this condition as a chronic hyperactivation state. While we have thus far limited our discussion to nociceptive input, the general adaptive response and its extreme, chronic hyperactivation of the hypothalamic–pituitary–adrenal (HPA) axis, can occur in the face of any physical, psychological or emotional stress of significant magnitude or duration.

EFFECTS OF CHRONIC HYPERACTIVITY OF THE HYPOTHALAMIC–PITUITARY– ADRENAL AXIS

There is much evidence that altered levels of CTRH can affect many aspects of homeostasis. As previously mentioned, McEwen & Stellar (1993) have coined the term allostatic load to describe a series of measurable physiological parameters which change in the presence of a chronic adaptive response. Although they have been followed primarily in adults, the mechanisms behind these changes are present in children.

Elevated levels of CTRH result in anorexia and, when sustained, may lead to anorexia nervosa (Gold et al 1986, Kaye et al 1987). In addition, prolonged activation of the HPA axis inhibits the production of growth hormone, somatomedin C and other factors necessary for normal growth. This is one of the mechanisms behind failure to thrive, a condition in which weight gain is not affected by caloric intake but by neuroendocrine factors. A severe form of failure to thrive, called psychosocial dwarfism, is due to severe emotional deprivation or harassment. The child will present with short stature and/ or delayed puberty, with or without signs of an affective disorder. These children have decreased levels of growth hormone, which is reversible if the child is removed from the negative environment (Albanese et al 1994). Intrauterine growth retardation is associated with activation of the HPA axis in developing fetuses (Nieto-Diaz et al 1996, Houang et al 1999).

During infection or stress, increased cortisol levels contribute to poor glucose control in diabetic patients by increasing gluconeogenesis and insulin resistance (Reaven 1988, Chrousos & Gold 1992). Chronic elevation of cortisol levels is associated with the development of diabetic neuropathy (Tsigos et al 1993). This highlights a very important aspect of osteopathic care. The development of diabetic neuropathy is a chronic process. Children with juvenile diabetes mellitus are at increased risk for this and other complications of diabetes later in life. Although there are no specific data concerning the role of musculoskeletal stress in any of the aforementioned conditions, the relationship between somatic primary afferent activity and activation of the HPA axis is well documented (Gold & Goodwin 1988a, b, Van Buskirk 1990, Gockel et al 1995, Vaccarino & Couret 1995). Osteopathic manipulation may provide a mechanism whereby one of the stimulants for HPA activity can be muted.

Increased activity of the HPA axis interferes with normal immune activity, and elevated CTRH has been linked to chronic immunosuppression (Gold & Goodwin 1988 a, b). Virtually every aspect of the immune response is affected by cortisol. This includes activity during times of acute response and diurnal activity. CTRH directly activates mast cells, which are involved with allergic reactions such as dermatitis, eczema and asthma. This may explain the empirical association between stress and atopic conditions.

There are several differences between the immune system of the newborn and young infant, and that of the adult. During early life, the immune system will be conditioned by experiences, and it will mature under the influence of hormones and neurotransmitters. Prior to birth, there is active transport of IgG across the placenta, so that the newborn's concentration equals that of the mother's. The level of IgG is directly proportional to the child's gestational age and birthweight. In addition, the fetus can synthesize IgA and IgM in response to intrauterine infection. Fetuses can also synthesize complement in the first trimester, although newborns have slightly diminished levels. Neutrophils demonstrate decreased chemotaxis, adherence, aggregation and deformability in the term newborn. This delays the neutrophilic response to infection. Respiratory distress, hypoglycemia, hyperbilirubinemia and sepsis will further diminish the neutrophilic response, as will elevated levels of CTRH. The macrophage population is decreased at birth, although monocytes are normal in the newborn and premature infant. Increased cortisol levels will indirectly inhibit macrophage production of antibody. Levels of interferon (IFN)-α and IFN-β are normal, but IFN-γ is diminished. Tumor necrosis factor-alpha (TNF-α) levels are normal, and interleukin-2 (IL-2) activity is higher than in adults. Increased cortisol has been shown to inhibit IL-2 activity and to adversely affect CD8 cell function (Norbiato et al 1994, Vago et al 1994, Corley 1995, Honour et al 1995, Nair et al 1995).

It is now known that although part of the stress response in individuals is genetically determined, environmental factors play a significant role. During infancy, childhood and adolescence, these systems are quite plastic, and early stressors may affect their thresholds for activation. For example, childhood sexual abuse is associated with altered activity in the HPA axis (De Bellis et al 1994), and signs of post-traumatic stress disorder (Lemieux & Coe 1995). As an adult, the sexually abused child is more likely to have chronic GI pain (Scarinci et al 1994), and melancholic depression (De Bellis et al 1994). CTRH inhibits gastric acid secretion and increases transit times while stimulating colon activity. It has been implicated in irritable bowel syndrome. Psychological health is influenced by the HPA axis. Elevated cortisol levels are found in individuals who are clinically depressed (Gold & Goodwin 1988a, b, McEwen 1987), and adult patients with chronic pain develop many of the criteria associated with clinical depression (Gold & Goodwin 1988a, b).

CONCLUSION

Many different types of stressors induce increased activity in the HPA axis and the release of CTRH. Under the influence of increased activity of primary nociceptive afferent neurons, the locus ceruleus is activated through the reticular formation.

In response, the hypothalamus: (1) stimulates activity in the sympathetic nervous system through direct projections; and (2) increases activity in the anterior pituitary, resulting in increased CTRH. In turn, CTRH orchestrates behavioral, neuroendocrine, autonomic and immunological responses to the stressful stimulus (De Bellis et al 1994). Under normal circumstances, there is a feedback mechanism in place which allows the individual to return to a functional baseline once the stress is removed. However, this mechanism can be irreversible when driven by a very large bolus of a single type of stimulus, by prolonged periods of low levels of stress, or by the summation effect of various stressors. This triggers a general adaptive response. The general adaptive response can be correlated with changes in physiological and psychological parameters. When prolonged, these changes lead to breakdown in the adaptive mechanisms of the neuroendocrine immune system. The contribution of somatic irritation to this process should not be underestimated. Research suggests that addressing the somatic component may favorably influence neuroendocrine immune function (Kiecolt-Glaser & Glaser 1991, Field et al 1996). This provides a great opportunity to the osteopathic physician, who can address musculoskeletal strains and stresses which may play a role in maintaining increased activity in the HPA axis. During childhood and adolescence, the nervous, endocrine and immune systems mature, developing patterns of response, and thresholds for activation. The influence of the nociceptive input in the maturation process should not be underestimated. When we see a child, we must expand our evaluation beyond the findings that are contributing to the child's current condition, and ask ourselves 'What are the long-term repercussions of our findings' and 'What is here that may influence the child's future health'. This is the essence of preventive care, and it is one of the cornerstones of osteopathic medicine. The application of osteopathic techniques with a goal of eliminating or dampening the primary nociceptor input should decrease the activity in the HPA axis, and facilitate the homeostatic mechanisms of the neuroendocrine immune system.

References

Albanese A, Hamill G, Jones J et al 1994 Reversibility of physiological growth hormone secretion in children with psychosocial dwarfism. Clin Endocrinol (Oxf) 40(5): 687–692.

Basbaum A I, Jessell T M 2000 The perception of pain. In: Kandel E R, Schwartz J H, Jessell T M (eds) Principles of neural science. McGraw-Hill, New York: 472–491.

Chrousos G P, Gold P W 1992 The concepts of stress and stress system disorders. Overview of physical and behavioral homeostasis. JAMA 267(9): 1244–1252.

Corley P A 1995 HIV and the cortisol connection: a feasible concept of the process of AIDS. Med Hypotheses 44(6): 483–489.

Craig A D, Bushnell M C, Zhang E T et al 1994 A thalamic nucleus specific for pain and temperature sensation. Nature 372: 770–773.

Craig A D, Reiman E M, Evans A et al 1996 Functional imaging of an illusion of pain. Nature 384: 258–260.

De Bellis M D, Chrousos G P, Dorn L D et al 1994 Hypothalamic–pituitary–adrenal axis dysregulation in sexually abused girls. J Clin Endocrinol Metab 78(2): 249–255.

Field T, Ironson G, Scafidi F et al 1996 Massage therapy reduces anxiety and enhances EEG pattern of alertness and math computations. Int J Neurosci 86: 197–205.

Gockel M, Lindholm H, Alaranta H et al 1995 Cardiovascular functional disorder and stress among patients having neck-shoulder symptoms. Ann Rheum Dis 54: 494–497.

Gold P, Goodwin F 1988a Clinical and biochemical manifestations of depression: Part II. N Engl J Med 319(7): 413–420.

Gold P, Goodwin F 1988b Clinical and biochemical manifestations of stress: Part I. N Engl J Med 319(6): 348–353.

Gold P W, Gwirtsman H, Avgerinos P C et al 1986 Abnormal hypothalamic–pituitary–adrenal function in anorexia nervosa. Pathophysiologic mechanisms in underweight and weight-corrected patients. N Engl J Med 314(21): 1335–1342.

Honour J W, Schneider M A, Miller R F 1995 Low adrenal androgens in men with HIV infection and the acquired immunodeficiency syndrome. Horm Res 44(1): 35–39.

Houang M, Morineau G, le Bouc Y et al 1999 The cortisol–cortisone shuttle in children born with intrauterine growth retardation. Pediatr Res 46(2): 189–193.

Karlamangla A S, Singer B H, McEwen B S et al 2002 Allostatic load as a predictor of functional decline. MacArthur studies of successful aging. J Clin Epidemiol 55: 696–710.

Kaye W H, Gwirtsman H E, George D T et al 1987 Elevated cerebrospinal fluid levels of immunoreactive corticotropin-releasing hormone in anorexia nervosa: relation to state of nutrition, adrenal function, and intensity of depression. J Clin Endocrinol Metab 64(2): 203–208.

Kiecolt-Glaser J K, Glaser R 1991 Stress and immune function in humans. In: Ader R, Felton D L, Cohen N (eds) Psychoneuroimmunology. Academic Press, San Diego, CA: 849–895.

Lemieux A M, Coe C L 1995 Abuse-related posttraumatic stress disorder: evidence for chronic neuroendocrine activation in women. Psychosom Med 57: 105–115.

McEwen B 1987 Glucocorticoid-biogenic amine interactions in relation to mood and behavior. Biochem Pharmacol 36: 1755–1763.

McEwen B S 1997 Hormones as regulators of brain development: life-long effects related to health and disease. Acta Paediatr Suppl 422: 41–44.

McEwen B S, Dhabar F 2002 Stress in adolescent females: relationship to autoimmune diseases. J Adolesc Health 30S: 30–60.

McEwen B S, Stellar E 1993 Stress and the individual. Arch Intern Med 153: 2093–2101.

Nair M P, Saravolatz L D, Schwartz S A 1995 Selective inhibitory effects of stress hormones on natural killer (NK) cell activity of lymphocytes from AIDS patients. Immunol Invest 24(5): 689–699.

Nieto-Diaz A, Villar J, Matorras-Weinig R et al 1996 Intrauterine growth retardation at term: association between anthropometric and endocrine parameters. Acta Obstet Gynaecol Scand 75(2): 127–131.

Norbiato G, Galli M, Righini V et al 1994 The syndrome of acquired glucocorticoid resistance in HIV infection. Baillières Clin Endocrinol Metab 8(4): 777–787.

Reaven G M 1988 Banting lecture 1988. Role of insulin resistance in human disease. Diabetes 37(12): 1595–1607.

Scarinci I C, McDonald-Haile J, Bradley L A et al 1994 Altered pain perception and psychosocial features among women with gastrointestinal disorders and history of abuse: a preliminary model [see comments]. Am J Med 97: 108–118.

Tsigos C, Young R J, White A 1993 Diabetic neuropathy is associated with increased activity of the hypothalamic–pituitary–adrenal axis. J Clin Endocrinol Metab 76(3): 554–558.

Vaccarino A L, Couret L C Jr 1995 Relationship between hypothalamic–pituitary–adrenal activity and blockade of tolerance to morphine analgesia by pain: a strain comparison. Pain 63(3): 385–389.

Vago T, Clerici M, Norbiato G 1994 Glucocorticoids and the immune system in AIDS. Baillières Clin Endocrinol Metab 8(4): 789–802.

Van Buskirk R L 1990 Nociceptive reflexes and the somatic dysfunction: a model. J Am Osteopath Assoc 90(9): 792–809.

Further reading

Buckingham J C, Loxey H D, Christian H C et al 1996 Activation of the HPA axis by immune insults: roles and interactions of cytokines, eicosanoids and glucocorticoids. Pharmacol Biochem Behav 54(1): 285–298.

Donnerer J 1992 Nociception and the neuroendocrine-immune system. In: Willard F H, Patterson M (eds) Nociception and the neuroendocrine-immune connection. American Academy of Osteopathy, IN: 260–273.

Esterling B 1992 Stress-associated modulation of cellular immunity. In: Willard F H, Patterson M (eds) Nociception and the neuroendocrine-immune connection. American Academy of Osteopathy, IN: 275–294.

Fischman H K, Pero R W, Kelly D D 1996 Psychogenic stress induces chromosomal and DNA damage. Int J Neurosci 84(1–4): 219–227.

Ganong W 1988 The stress response – a dynamic overview. Hosp Pract 23(6): 155–171.

Groenink L, Compaan J, Van Der Gugten J et al 1995 Stress-induced hyperthermia in mice – pharmacological and endocrinological aspects. Ann N Y Acad Sci 771: 252–256.

Häkkinen K, Pakarinen A 1995 Acute hormonal responses to heavy resistance exercise in men and women at different ages. Int J Sports Med 16(8): 507–513.

Herbert T B, Cohen S 1993 Stress and immunity in humans: a meta-analytic review. Psychosom Med 55: 364–379.

Host C R, Norton K I, Olds T S et al 1995 The effects of altered exercise distribution on lymphocyte subpopulations. Eur J Appl Physiol 72(1–2): 157–164.

Jemmont J B, Boryshenko M, Chapman R et al 1983 Academic stress, power motivation and decrease in secretion rate of salivary secretory immunoglobulin. Lancet I: 1400–1402.

Jevning R, Anand R, Biedebach M et al 1996 Effects on regional cerebral blood flow of transcendental meditation. Physiol Behav 59(3): 399–402.

Li H Y, Ericsson A, Sawchenko P E 1996 Distinct mechanisms underlie activation of hypothalamic neurosecretory neurons and their medullary catecholaminergic afferents in categorically different stress paradigms. Proc Natl Acad Sci U S A 93(6): 2359–2364.

Marsh J A, Scanes C G 1994 Neuroendocrine–immune interactions. Poultry Sci 73: 1049–1061.

Norbiato G, Bevilacqua M, Vago T et al 1992 Cortisol resistance in acquired immunodeficiency syndrome. J Clin Endocrinol Metab 74(3): 608–613.

Sabban E L, Hiremagalur B, Nankova B et al 1995 Molecular biology of stress-elicited induction of catecholamine biosynthetic enzymes. Ann N Y Acad Sci 771: 327–338.

Seeman T E, Singer B H, Rowe J W et al 1997 Price of adaptation – allosteric load and its health consequences. Arch Intern Med 157: 2259–2268.

Seidel A, Arolt V, Hunstiger M et al 1996 Increased CD56+ natural killer cells and related cytokines in major depression. Clin Immunol Immunopathol 78(1): 83–85.

Sternberg E M 1995 Neuroendocrine factors in susceptibility to inflammatory disease: focus on the hypothalamic–pituitary–adrenal axis. Horm Res 43: 159–161.

Sternberg E M, Chrousos G P, Wilder R L et al 1992 The stress response and the regulation of inflammatory disease. Ann Intern Med 117: 854–866.

Van Buskirk R L 1990 Nociceptive reflexes and the somatic dysfunction: a model. J Am Osteopath Assoc 90(9): 792–809.

Willard F H, Patterson M M 1992 Nociception and the neuroendocrine immune connection. International Symposium. American Academy of Osteopathy, Athens, OH.

Willard F H, Mokler D J, Morgane P J 1997 Neuroendocrine–immune system and homeostasis. In: Ward R C (ed) Foundations for osteopathic medicine. Williams & Wilkins, Baltimore: 107–135.

Chapter Eight

8

Labor, delivery and birth

CHAPTER CONTENTS

BIRTH PROCESS: TRANSITION FROM INTRAUTERINE TO EXTRAUTERINE LIFE

The fluid environment of the amniotic sac acts as a sensory deprivation tank. It provides protection from gravitational mechanics and allows the body to develop in a buffered environment where little or no sensory stimulation is present. Wave pressures are subdued as they pass through the fluid medium, so tactile stimulation is minimized. The amniotic fluid is at body temperature, which buffers temperature receptors from stimulation much like the sensation one gets when soaking in a very warm bath. Sound waves, which pass through the amniotic fluid, are mildly distorted but provide some auditory stimulus for the developing baby. (Myelination of the midbrain and auditory system is completed at approximately 22 weeks, but is probably somewhat sensitive to sensory input prior to that time.)

The chemical environment of intrauterine life differs from that of extrauterine life. The developing neonate is exposed to maternal hormones that are at higher levels than they would be in the baby. Maternal sympathetic stimulation affects vasomotor control of the placenta and fetus. Adrenergic effects in the lungs and gastrointestinal (GI) tract are also probable.

LABOR: 'THE PASSENGER ADAPTS TO THE PASSAGEWAY'

During labor, the head descends through the bony pelvis and its soft tissues. Engagement of the fetal head into the pelvis is most often in the left occiput transverse position; that is, the fetal occiput is on the left side of the mother's pelvis (Fig. 8.1). In this position, the sagittal suture lies

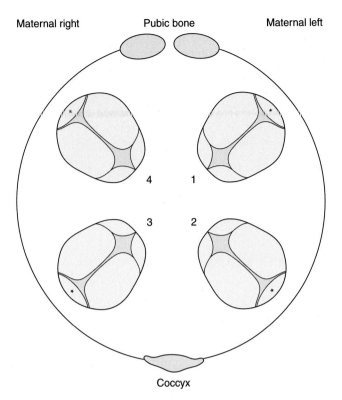

Maternal right   Pubic bone   Maternal left

Coccyx

Fig. 8.1 • Presentation of the fetal head is named according to the position of the fetal occiput in relation to the maternal pelvis. In this schematic diagram, the maternal pelvis is represented by the circle, with the pubic and coccyx bones labeled. There are four fetal heads present. The occiput in each is indicated by the asterisk. The fetal head marked (1) is in the left occiput anterior position. The occiput (*) lies on the maternal left, facing anteriorly, as compared with fetal head (2), where the occiput is also lying on the maternal left but faces posteriorly, towards the maternal coccyx. Note the right occiput posterior (3) and right occiput anterior (4) positions.

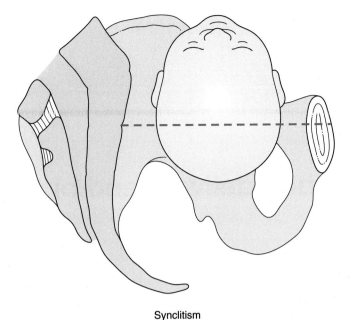

Synclitism

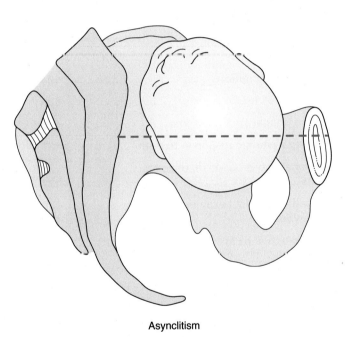

Asynclitism

Fig. 8.2 • Schematic representation of fetal head in synclitic and asynclitic positions.

along the transverse diameter of the pelvis; this is called synclitism. This occurs when the pelvis is roomy. When the sagittal suture lies in a position other than this, the head is in an asynclitic position. Asynclitism narrows the diameter of the head entering the pelvis because the head is tilted; this gives the baby an advantage. Asynclitism often occurs when the head is large. In fact posterior asynclitism is more common than synclitism. In most women the pregnant uterus is not perpendicular to the pelvic floor. As the head enters the pelvis the posterior parietal bone is more inferior than the anterior parietal bone. The biparietal diameter of the head is oblique to the plane of the pelvis. This is called posterior asynclitism. Anterior asynclitism occurs when the mother's abdominal muscles are weak and allow the uterus to tip anterior. Now the anterior parietal bone lies inferior to the posterior bone and enters the pelvis first (Fig. 8.2). Labor progresses as the increasing strength of uterine contractions pushes the presenting part of the fetus into the uterine fundus. In combination with chemical and hormonal changes this causes effacement and dilation of the cervix and stretching of the soft tissues of the pelvis.

During descent, the natural flexion of the neonate increases in response to resistance from the pelvic soft tissues. Flexion of the chin upon the chest shifts the presenting part, which is usually the head, from the left occiput transverse to the left occiput anterior (LOA) position. In the LOA position, most of the fetal engagement occurs in the right oblique diameter of the pelvis (Fig. 8.3). (The oblique while the occiput pivots upon the pubic symphysis. Once delivered, the head spontaneously returns to a neutral position with respect to the neck (restitution). As the baby's shoulders reach the pelvic floor, the anterior shoulder passes under the pubic symphysis and out of the vaginal canal. The posterior shoulder follows.

With each contraction of the uterus, vertical compressions are transferred through the neonatal body along a cephalocaudal axis. These forces are primarily absorbed in the cranial base and vertebral column. The occipitoatlantal articulation is the only true joint existing in the cranium at this time. Consequently, vertical forces are transmitted through the cranial bones and meet their first resistance at the craniocervical junction, which is typically locked into a flexed position. With the occiput flexed upon the atlas, rotational and side-bending forces are not easily accommodated at the occipitoatlantal joint. These torsional stresses must be absorbed by the condyles, cranial base and vault. The membranous quality of the intracranial architecture provides considerable accommodation. However, once the limits of accommodation are reached the visceroelastic properties of the tissues undergo deformation. This is probably the mechanism by which cranial base strains develop. William Sutherland DO developed a schematic representation of these strains as originating in the sphenobasilar synchondrosis (SBS). That area, articulating with C1, forms the only true functioning joint in the neonatal head and could thus create the fulcrum around which strains in the cranial tissues would occur. On gross visual inspection the child may have molding of the vault bones, asymmetry of the face, or a slight tilt to the head.

Depending on the vector of entry, vertical forces can also dissipate into the neonatal thorax and pelvis. Compressive forces are transferred from the periphery to the center of the body from the contracting uterus. The wider areas of the body, such as the pelvis, thorax, thoracic outlet, shoulders and head, are most vulnerable to these compressive forces.

As the neonatal body moves into and through the pelvis, rotational forces come into play. First, the head must turn towards its position of presentation from its position of lie. The compressive forces of the uterine contractions coax the presenting part of the fetus towards the pelvic opening. The fetal head comes up against the resistance of the geometry of the true pelvis. The resulting rotation, which is usually 45°, primarily occurs at the atlantoaxial joint, with some accommodation at the cervical–thoracic junction. Flexion at the thoracic inlet and the compressive forces on the rib cage will limit T1's ability to respond to this rotation, so forces may be dispersed into the clavicles. During delivery of the head through the perineum, the occiput acts as the fulcrum for the rotation of the cranium as it passes under the pubic symphysis. However, the actual torque is transmitted to the atlantoaxial joint. If this force cannot be accommodated at the atlantoaxial joint, it will have to be resolved at the occipital squama, which will affect the lateral masses, condyles and

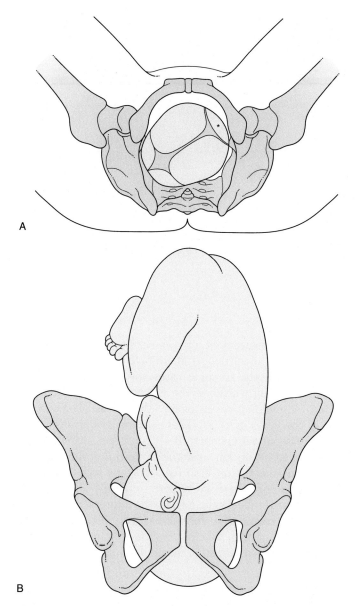

Fig. 8.3 • Schematic X-ray diagram (A) of maternal pelvis in the dorsal lithotomy position. The fetal head is in the LOA presentation. The occiput (*) is labeled. (B) The 45° rotation of the fetal head at the midpelvis position.

axis is named for the maternal posterior pole of origin.) At the midpelvis, the head rotates 45° to the right, turning the sagittal suture from a right oblique position to an anterior-posterior position. The shoulders remain in a left oblique position. This relationship persists until the head is delivered. One can immediately see the potential for tissue strain during prolonged deliveries.

In order for the head to deliver, extension must occur at the craniocervical junction and through the neck. Extension of the head occurs as a result of the continued pressure of the uterus pushing the neonate into the pelvic floor. The forehead, nose, mouth and chin are swept along the sacrum,

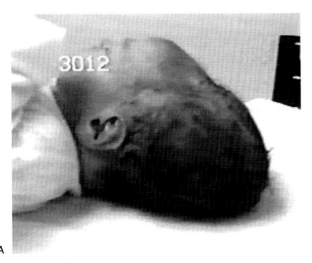 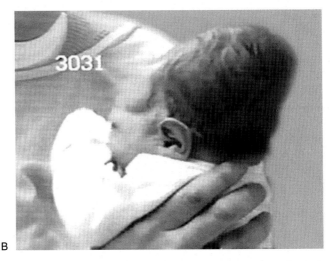

A   B

Fig. 8.4 • (A,B) Two photographs of a 6-hour-old newborn with extensive molding following prolonged labor and vaginal delivery. The baby was in a right occiput posterior (ROP) presentation.

occipitoatlantal joint. Torsional forces will stress all the vertebral junctions C1, C2, C3, C7–T1, T12–L1 and L5–S1.

MOLDING

Molding is the adaptation of the fetal cranium to the shape of the mother's pelvis and the path of exit. Molding occurs as the pliable bones of the fetal vault accommodate to the forces of labor. When molding is a normal adaptation of the head it is mild, there is no facial asymmetry, cephalohematoma, caput secundum or signs of bruising or abrasion, and involuntary cranial motion is balanced. Normal adaptive molding will resolve within hours after birth. Long protracted labors are often associated with significant molding of the neonatal skull (Fig. 8.4). In these cases there may be facial asymmetry, signs of bruising or abrasion, and most importantly cranial base mechanics are impaired. Molding that persists beyond the first or second day of life has one of two components: bone deformation with cranial base strain or bone deformation without cranial base strain. If no significant cranial base strain is present, then the deformation may have evolved over a period of time due to early engagement or uterine lie. If cranial base strain is present, then the molding may be due to uterine lie or early engagement, it may be secondary or compensatory to the cranial base strain, or it may be an adaptive pattern that is being maintained by the cranial base strain.

Molding can occur in the vault and base, and may produce connective tissue strains extending into the infant body. When the molding occurs as part of a normal adaptation to the vaginal canal, it and its associated strains will resolve spontaneously within a day or two after birth. Conversely when the molding is due to abnormal uterine

lie, prolonged engagement, or is associated with cranial base strain, it takes much longer to resolve and may not even resolve completely. In some cases the appearance of the deformation may worsen as the newborn grows. The same is true for molding occurring in other areas of the body, such as the limbs or chest. These strains have a soft tissue and an osseous component. Both must be addressed for correction to occur. For example in limb deformities such as metatarsus adductus, club feet and bow legs the tensile forces of the soft tissues contribute to the distorted growth pattern. The tensile forces need to be addressed as well as the articular relationship for normal growth to occur. This is the goal of casting, bracing, muscle training and manual therapies such as osteopathic manipulation.

ABNORMAL PRESENTATIONS

The most common abnormal position for the occiput is right occiput posterior (ROP) (Fig. 8.5). It produces a common pattern of adaptive molding in the vault. During descent, these newborns will typically rotate through 135° to the occiput anterior position. Usually, the shoulders follow the head through most of this turn, so that at extension the final angle is 45°. However, it may be greater. Labor is usually prolonged with occiput posterior presentations, because the rotation and flexion components are delayed. These infants usually present with slightly more torque in the junctional areas and, because of the prolonged duration of labor, the compression throughout the body is more pronounced.

In breech presentation (Fig. 8.6), the after-coming head may unseat the sacrum (A Wales, personal communication, 1996). In a true breech, the neonatal pelvis initiates passage through the birth canal. Rotational forces are much less than

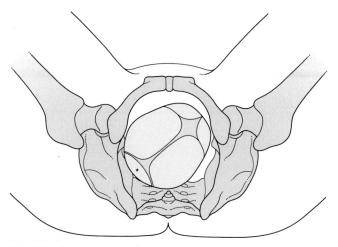

Fig. 8.5 • Schematic X-ray diagram of maternal pelvis in the dorsal lithotomy position. The fetal head is in the right occiput posterior (ROP) presentation. The occiput (*) is labeled.

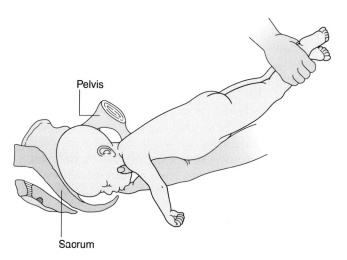

Fig. 8.6 • Schematic diagram of delivery of the infant head during breech presentation. The physician grasps the newborn's lower legs, while supporting the emerging head. The traction on the legs may induce strain in the pelvis and sacrum.

with cephalic presentation. However, vertical compressive forces are increased, especially in the neonatal pelvis. The ischial tuberosities are continuously meeting the resistance of the bony and soft tissue parts of the passageway, while vertical compressive forces are being transmitted through the cranium and spine directly to the sacrum, which is suspended between the innominates. The ischial tuberosities are forced medially, flaring the ilia, while the sacrum is forced inferiorly and into counternutation, which flattens the lumbar spine. Once the lower body is delivered, traction applied to the legs or pelvis may displace the innominates inferiorly. The sacrum takes a superior counternutated position in relation to the pelvis. This alters the mechanics at the sacroiliac joints, lumbosacral joint and thoracolumbar areas. Whether these changes resolve spontaneously with

newborn activity depends on the intensity and duration of the force which created them.

In brow presentation, the occiput is extended on the atlas and rotation at the atlantoaxial joint and the cervicothoracic junction are limited. The cranial base and vault receive much of the resulting stress. C3 is also vulnerable, because it is a functional transition point in the cervical spine. The upper thoracic area will flatten to accommodate forces transmitted through the thoracic inlet. This affects rib, diaphragm and clavicle function. The thoracolumbar area will compensate for the extended thorax, which also affects diaphragm motion. The stretch on the anterior and prevertebral tissues may be transmitted to the sternum, inducing a superior strain pattern.

In shoulder dystocia, the presentation is usually cephalic. Once the head is delivered, descent is arrested. Restitution of the head usually does not occur, and the head appears to recoil back into the pelvis. Normally, the shoulders enter the pelvis in an oblique lie, and then turn into the anterior–posterior position. If they enter the pelvis on the anterior–posterior axis, the superior shoulder will impact against the maternal symphysis. While in this position, the acute side-bent posture of the neck and prolonged compression of the chest impede venous return from the head. In severe cases anoxia may develop as well as hemorrhage and brain damage. Hemorrhage of the conjunctival vessels may be present. It is difficult to diagnose shoulder dystocia until after the head is delivered. Delivery may require gentle smooth traction without rotation or torsion of the head. If one or two attempts are unsuccessful, manual delivery of the anterior or posterior shoulder is attempted by placing the hand deeply into the pelvis. The clavicles are often compressed, with resultant tissue strain at the acromioclavicular and sternoclavicular joints. A greenstick fracture, or buckling of the clavicle, may also occur.

DELIVERY

As the head progresses down the vaginal canal, the bones of the cranial vault 'fold up' upon each other like the petals of a rosebud. After delivery, the normal processes of crying, respiration and suckling will resolve many of the stresses and strains absorbed by the tissues. Abnormal presentations and assisted deliveries involving forceps, manual traction or vacuum create strains, which are not easy for the body to resolve.

Low forceps deliveries provide a useful tool for the skilled practitioner. They are most often used to assist after prolonged pushing when the head continues to crown but does not emerge. By design, the forceps provide some compression to the neonatal head as the practitioner guides it out of the vagina. This may exacerbate or add to the tissue stress already experienced by the child which necessitated the forceps assistance to begin with. As a result these

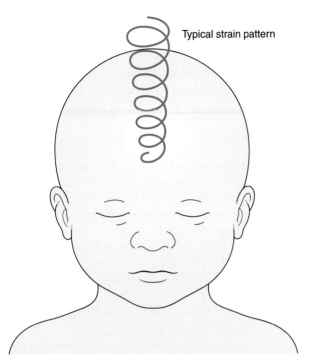

Fig. 8.7 • Schematic diagram depicting the typical cone-shaped, rotational strain seen at the site of vacuum placement. The depth of extension into deeper tissues appears to be dependent upon the duration and intensity of application of the device.

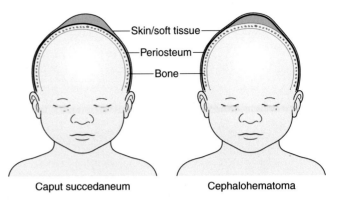

Fig. 8.8 • Schematic diagram comparing a caput succedaneum with a cephalohematoma.

newborns often have very complex cranial strain patterns involving SBS compression, and vertical or lateral shears with a compensatory torsion or side-bending rotation pattern. The SBS compression needs to be treated first. Once there is some motion present, the other patterns become easier to assess and treat.

The facial nerve is particularly vulnerable to forceps application. Unlike in the adult, where the mastoid process provides some lateral protection for the facial nerve, in the newborn the mastoid process has not yet developed. This leaves the stylomastoid foramen and facial nerve somewhat exposed. Newborns with facial palsy will present with facial asymmetry during crying (with deviation of the mouth away from the affected side) and/or difficulty latching onto the breast.

Vacuum extraction usually creates a membranous or soft tissue strain in the cranial mechanism. A cone-shaped rotational strain will be palpable, extending from the area of contact along the vector of traction (Fig. 8.7). Depending upon the force involved, the strain may be palpated into the thorax or pelvis. Compressive or shearing forces across the cranium may produce a cephalohematoma, a localized collection of blood between the periosteum of the skull and the calvarium.

Cephalohematomas do not cross sutures and usually resolve spontaneously, with the potential for calcification. They may be complicated by anemia, jaundice, infection,

leptomeningeal cyst and underlying fracture. Cephalohematomas occur in 1.5–2.5% of deliveries (Menkes & Sarant 2000). They may occur unilaterally or bilaterally. According to Menkes & Sarant (2000), linear skull fractures are seen in 5% of unilateral and 18% of bilateral cephalohematomas. Skull fractures generally do not require surgical treatment unless depressed (Menkes & Sarant 2000). Osteopathic treatment of the head should be avoided for the first 4 months. Fluid techniques directed to the vault from the sacrum or pelvis should be avoided through the first 6–8 weeks. However, fluid techniques can be directed at the cranial base and will help to alleviate strains contributing to vault distortion. Cephalohematomas are often absorbed within 8 or 9 months, although calcification does occur. Immediate complications include anemia and hyperbilirubinemia. Osteopathic treatments addressing respiratory mechanics, abdominal strains and visceral function are very important for maximizing the child's ability to handle the increased bilirubin load. Cephalohematomas need to be differentiated from caput succedaneum (Fig. 8.8), an area of scalp edema which extends beyond the suture line and usually resolves in a few days. Either of these conditions may occur in a protracted delivery; they are not necessarily associated with forceps or vacuums, although the incidence of cephalohematomas appears to have increased since the introduction of vacuum extraction.

Cesarean sections subject the neonate to a different set of conditions. If surgery is performed on a mother who has been laboring, the infant is rapidly taken from the high-pressure environment of the contracting uterus to a lower-pressure environment. The slow, gradual compressive and decompressive forces of the normal birthing process are replaced by a sudden change. This often creates a 'rebound' effect in the tissues, similar to the way in which a tissue contracts when it is suddenly stretched. This can most often be observed in the tissues of the head, neck and thorax, which feel more taut and often demonstrate clinical signs of facilitation.

The processes of labor and delivery affect systems other than the musculoskeletal system. The mechanical forces of labor impact on the fetal head, cerebral circulation, heart, umbilical cord and placenta. Valkeakari (1973) has reported echographic changes in the fetal brain as a result of normal cephalic delivery. Echography demonstrated midline shifts of the brain, which developed 3 h postbirth and resolved by 24 h. The direction of shift depended on the fetal lie and was thought to be induced by cerebral edema and was not necessarily associated with molding.

Both Schwartz et al (1969) and Mocsary et al (1970) have demonstrated that pressure on the fetal skull increases intracranial pressure. In humans, the fetal heart rate will remain stable up to pressures of 55 mmHg (Mocsary et al 1970). Pressures greater than 55 mmHg will result in rapid drops in heart rate. If cerebral perfusion decreases significantly, cerebral edema will result, further increasing the intracranial pressure. This may result in bradycardia. Uterine contractions also increase amniotic pressure, which may compromise umbilical vessels. Bradycardia may result from the decrease in oxygen delivery or through a baroreceptor reflex. Either condition may result in cerebral hypoxia and metabolic acidosis.

COMMON CRANIAL STRAIN PATTERNS

In the early part of the 20th century William Sutherland DO described a series of strain patterns in the cranial base that were found in both adults and children and which have since been found to be associated with various clinical syndromes (Frymann 1966, Upledger 1978, Heisey & Adams 1993, Degenhardt & Kuchera 1994, Mills et al 2002, Lassovetskaya 2003). Sutherland's cranial strain patterns may result from uterine lie, abnormal presentation, the forces of labor and delivery, or trauma to the head.

'These patterns are schematic representations that Dr Sutherland invented. He never meant them as an absolute' (A Wales, personal communication, 1994). By definition, the point of reference for these patterns (Fig. 8.9) is the sphenobasilar synchondrosis.

Torsions and side-bending rotations are considered 'physiological strains'. Torsions occur when the sphenoid and occiput rotate in opposite directions on an anterior–posterior axis, usually in response to a compression of the peripheral tissues in one quadrant. They are named by the superior greater wing of the sphenoid, as in 'greater wing high on the left'. Side-bending rotations occur when the occiput and sphenoid rotate in opposite directions on a vertical axis and in the same direction on the anterior–posterior axis. This usually results from excessive pressure on one side of the head. They are named by the side of the convexity, as in 'side-bending rotation convexity to the right'.

Vertical and lateral strains or shears are considered 'nonphysiological strains'. Vertical shears result when the sphenoid

moves into flexion while the occiput moves into extension (or vice versa). Blows to the head behind or in front of bregma may result in vertical strains. Compression of the condylar parts or facial compression, such as occurs in brow presentations, may also contribute to vertical strains. They are named by the position of the basisphenoid. Lateral strains create parallelogram-shaped heads. The sphenoid and occiput rotate in the same direction around a parallel vertical axis. Forceps placed diagonally may produce these strains. Like vertical strains, lateral strains are named by the position of the basisphenoid.

A more in-depth discussion of these strain patterns may be found in Magoun (1976) or Sutherland (1990).

ASSESSING SYSTEMIC RESPONSE TO BIRTH

The APGAR score (Table 8.1) reflects the stress experienced by the neonate during the birth process. It is assessed at 1 min and 5 min after birth. Five variables – heart rate, respiratory effort, muscle tone, reflex irritability and color – are given numerical values ranging from 0 to 2. An inverse relationship exists between the APGAR score and the degree of acidosis and hypoxia.

Hypoxia and acidosis may lead to brain cell injury or death. The threshold at which biochemical changes begin to occur in the central nervous system varies with individuals. During uncomplicated labor, ischemia and hypoxia are intermittent and moderate. Most infants seem to tolerate these episodes. However, if metabolic acidosis is prolonged or severe, the ability of the neonate to compensate is challenged. Episodes of sustained bradycardia indicate compromise. Fetal heart rate monitoring can provide a useful tool in assessing how well the infant is tolerating labor. Compression on the head may result in a decrease in fetal heart rate due to a vagal reflex. Late or prolonged decelerations suggest fetal stress, which may result from cumulative acidosis, hypoxia due to compromise of the umbilical vessels, or a myriad of other things. If the stress of labor and delivery has resulted in prolonged hypoxia or increased metabolic acidosis, it will be reflected in the APGAR score.

GESTATIONAL AGE IS BASED ON PHYSICAL FINDINGS (Fig. 8.10)

The gestational age and size are very important factors in evaluating the overall health of the newborn. The most reliable and accurate way to assess gestational age is by using the physical characteristics and neuromuscular behaviors of the infant. By definition, infants with gestational ages between 38 and 42 weeks are 'term infants'. Infants less than 38 weeks of gestational age are 'preterm', and those over 42

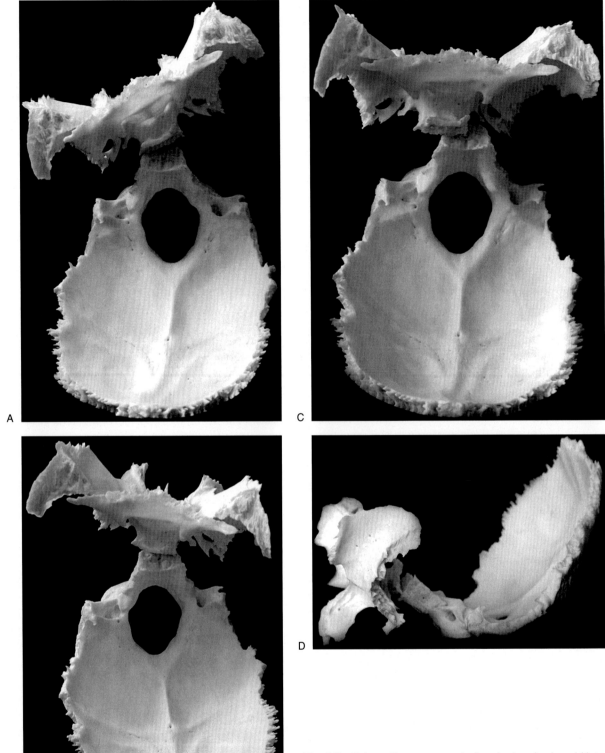

Fig. 8.9 • Schematic arrangement of occiput and sphenoid into the sphenobasilar synchondrosis (SBS) strains described by William Sutherland. (A) A right-side bending rotation pattern. (B) A right-torsion pattern. (C) A lateral strain. (D) A superior vertical strain.

Table 8.1 APGAR scoring chart to assess neonatal health

Variable/score	0	1	2
Heart rate	Absent	Less than 100 beats/min	More than 100 beats/min
Respiratory effort	Absent	Slow, irregular	Good, crying
Muscle tone	Limp	Some flexion extremity	Active motion
Reflex irritability	Absent	Grimace	Grimace, cough, sneeze
Color	Blue, pale	Acrocyanosis	Completely pink

weeks are 'post-term'. Infants within two standard deviations (plus or minus) from average for length, weight and head circumference are considered appropriate for gestational age (AGA). Those lower than two standard deviations from average are considered small for gestational age (SGA). Those greater than two standard deviations from average are considered large for gestational age (LGA). There are risk factors associated with both SGA and LGA infants.

Vernix is a thick white substance, with the consistency of soft cheese, that coats the baby's body. As gestation proceeds, the vernix disappears, so that by 40 weeks it is only present in the creases and folds of the skin. Lanugo is soft fine hair which covers the neonatal body. It first appears at approximately 20 weeks; by 33 weeks it has disappeared from the face, at 38 weeks it will only remain on the shoulders, and it should be completely gone by 42 weeks. True hair may first appear on the head at 20–21 weeks. Eyebrows and lashes appear at 24 weeks.

Neonatal skin is thin and translucent, with easily observed venous markings over the abdomen until 31 weeks. It then becomes smooth and pink, and the veins disappear over the next 8 weeks. It will become drier and starts to desquamate as gestation passes 42 weeks.

The ear is very soft and folds easily without recoil until 32 weeks, at which time it will slowly return to its original shape when folded. True recoil is not present until approximately 36 weeks. The ear is flat and shapeless until 34 weeks, and then gradually begins curling.

The areola of the breast is not prominent until 34 weeks. Early in gestation, the clitoris is larger than the labia, while in the male the testes are still in the inguinal canal and may not be easily palpated. In the hustle of the delivery room, this may lead to ambiguous gender assignment until closer examination. The testes will not enter the upper scrotum until approximately 36 weeks, and will descend further over the next several weeks. The labia majora is larger than the clitoris by 36 weeks and nearly covers it. By 40 weeks, it will cover the labia minor as well.

Neuromuscular reflexes and tone are also evaluated to determine gestational age. Posture should take on a more flexed position as gestation reaches 28 weeks. Prior to this, the infant is quite flaccid. This flexed posture begins in the lower extremities and progresses cephalad, so by 36 weeks the upper and lower extremities are flexed. By 38–40 weeks, the tone is very high and attempts by the examiner to straighten an arm or leg will be followed immediately by a recoil back to the initial posture. The leg and hip will resist heel-to-ear maneuvers. The popliteal angle will decrease from 150° at 28 weeks of gestation to 80° at 40 weeks of gestation, again because of the increased tone (Fig. 8.11). Dorsiflexion of the foot will increase with gestation, being most restricted prior to 32 weeks and least restricted in the term infant. The 'scarf sign' (Fig. 8.12), the ability to adduct the arm and shoulder across the chest, will become more limited as the child matures. Initially being unrestricted at 28 weeks, by 36 weeks the elbow may just pass the midline and at term only meet it. Active cervical muscle tone is also a good indicator of maturity in 32–40-week-gestation infants. Neck flexor and extensor control can be tested with the pull to sit and reverse to lie maneuvers.

The healthy newborn infant should be pink. Some mild acrocyanosis about the lips may be initially present but should resolve within a few minutes. Persistent acrocyanosis warrants cardiovascular work-up, as tissue perfusion and/or oxygenation may be compromised. This is especially true if acrocyanosis develops during crying or suckling. The infant cry should be vigorous. Soft, high-pitched or shrieking cries suggest a neurological problem. Hoarse cries are associated with hypothyroidism, and paralysis of the larynx. Trauma to the anterior tissues of the neck, such as may occur in a face or brow presentation, may also affect the sound of the cry.

In the first few hours, the infant will often assume a position similar to the one adapted while in the uterus. If the lie was particularly straining on the musculoskeletal tissues or if the position was held for a prolonged period of time, the child may continue to adopt this posture while sleeping, long after the post-birth period. Osteopathic treatment provided soon after birth alleviates most of this posturing.

OSTEOPATHIC PHYSICAL EXAMINATION OF THE TERM NEWBORN

There are six fontanels present in the newborn head. The anterior fontanel located at bregma should be soft, flat and less than 3.5 cm in diameter. The posterior fontanel at the parietal lambdoidal juncture should be quite small. Two other fontanels at asterion and pterion are also present but

	0	1	2	3	4	5
Skin	Gelatinous, red, transparent	Smooth, pink, visible veins	Superficial peeling and/or rash, few veins	Cracking, pale area, rare veins	Parchment, deep cracking, no vessels	Leathery, cracked, wrinkled
Lanugo	None	Abundant	Thinning	Bald areas	Mostly bald	
Plantar creases	No crease	Faint red marks	Anterior transverse crease only	Creases anterior two-thirds	Creases cover entire sole	
Breast	Barely perceptible	Flat areola, no bud	Stippled areola, 1–2 mm bud	Raised areola, 3–4 mm bud	Full areola, 5–10 mm bud	
Ear	Pinna flat, stays folded	Slightly curved pinna, soft, slow recoil	Well-curved pinna, soft but ready recoil	Formed and firm with instant recoil	Thick cartilage, ear stiff	
Genitals: male	Scrotum empty, no rugae		Testes descending, few rugae	Testes down, good rugae	Testes pendulous, deep rugae	
Genitals: female	Prominent clitoris and labia minora		Majora and minora equally prominent	Majora large, minora small	Clitoris and minora completely covered	

Maturity rating

Score	Weeks
5	26
10	28
15	30
20	32
25	34
30	36
35	38
40	40
45	42
50	44

Neuromuscular maturity

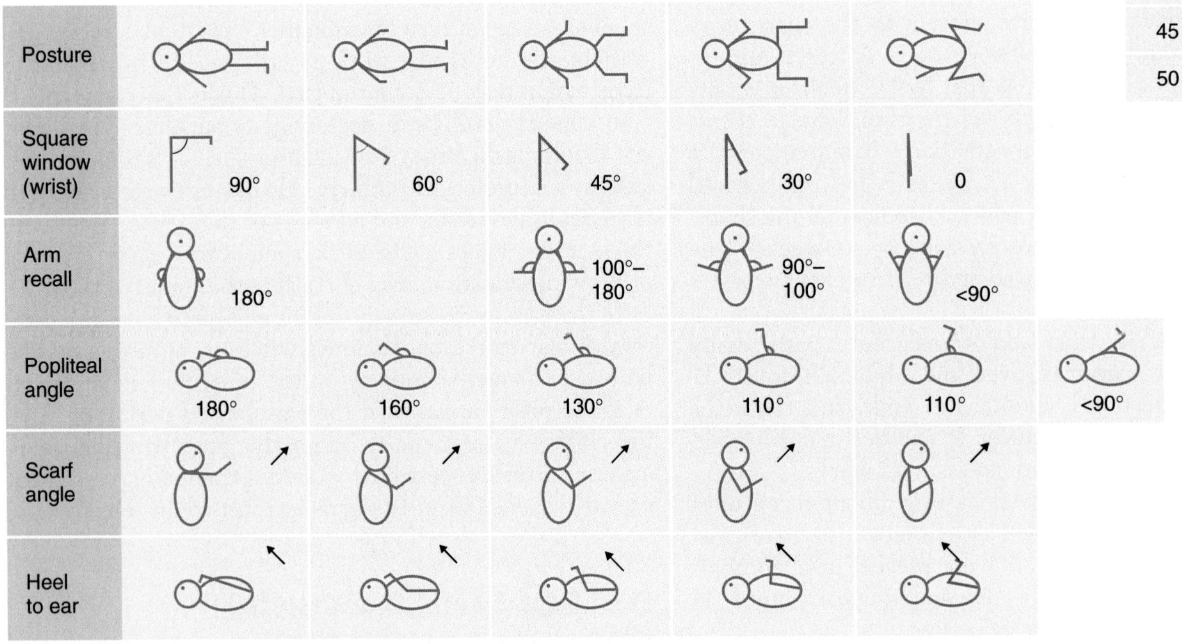

Fig. 8.10 • Chart for assessing gestational maturity. *With permission from Ballard et al 1979 A simplified score of assessment of fetal maturation of newly born infants. J Pediatr 95: 769.*

not palpable. The sutures should all be palpated for flexibility. Motion mechanics in the bones comprising the borders of the fontanels should be assessed. Overlapping sutures should be carefully evaluated to ensure that craniosynostosis has not occurred. The most common sites for overlap are the coronal and sagittal sutures, and these will often resolve spontaneously. Overlap at the lambdoidal suture is more difficult to resolve. This may be due to the current practice of

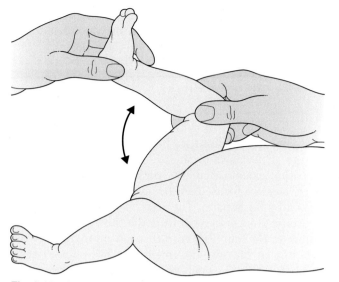

Fig. 8.11 • Assessment of popliteal angle. The hip is stabilized as the knee is extended.

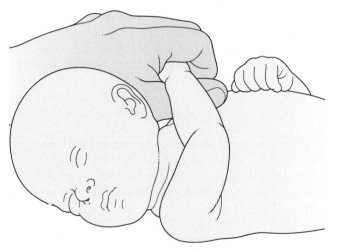

Fig. 8.12 • The arm is drawn across the chest to assess flexibility of the shoulder. This is the scarf sign.

keeping newborns and infants in the supine position during sleep. Increases in the occurrence of plagiocephaly may also be due to restricted positioning of newborns (Kane et al 1996, Peitsch et al 2002). Any asymmetry in cervical muscle tone will create a rotation of the neonate's head, so the child always lies on the same side of his head, producing a flattening on that side of the occiput. These problems are very difficult to treat osteopathically, because postural forces are creating them. Once the cervical muscle tension has been alleviated, the flattening will resolve as the child grows, provided that the child's sleeping position can be addressed. Encouraging parents to keep the child on his or her stomach, while awake and accompanied, will facilitate resolution of the plagiocephaly as well as contribute to development of

neck control and hand–eye coordination. A type of helmet made from lightweight material can be used in some cases to encourage correction of the vault. Often, the helmets are made of a Styrofoam material, although other lightweight materials can be used. When used appropriately helmets can support and facilitate the corrections occurring with osteopathic treatment.

Facial asymmetry may be due to uterine lie or labor and delivery. The presence of bruising or abrasion suggests the latter. Facial features should be observed during crying and suckling to detect paralysis or palsy, which present as asymmetry in muscle use. Forceps deliveries may rarely result in fracture of the zygoma, which may present with ecchymosis over the site, problems in sucking (secondary to pain), or a subtly asymmetric cry (reluctance to open the mouth wide). The eye on the affected side may be set slightly posterior and the globe may have a rounder shape. The zygoma should always be assessed osteopathically for strain or dysfunction at its articulations in any forceps delivery or face presentation.

Congenital ptosis of the eyelid may be present and unrelated to a neurological problem. Significant intraosseous strains of the sphenoid or between the sphenoid and frontal may be present which affect the origin of the levator palpebrae or the shape of the globe, resulting in a mild ptosis. Cranial nerve III innervates the superior levator palpebrae muscle. If irritated, it may result in a slight drooping of the eyelid when open. The oculomotor nerve travels through the subarachnoid space from the midbrain. It pierces the arachnoid and passes between the attached and free borders of the tentorium cerebelli just lateral to the posterior clinoid process. Continuing on, it pierces the dura and traverses the cavernous sinus. It divides into two rami which pass through the superior orbital fissure within the annular tendon. The superior rami will innervate the rectus superior and superior levator palpebrae. The oculomotor nerve may be affected by strains in the tentorium that alter the relationship between its two attachments, congestion within the cavernous sinus, or strains between the bones of the orbit which stress the annular tendon. Mild irritation may produce an ocular palsy, which is not easily tested in the newborn. A more noticeable finding would be the ptosis.

Inability to fully close the eye can occur with facial nerve injury or irritation. This irritation may be caused by direct injury or bruising of the peripheral nerve. More often, it occurs secondarily to compression of the nerve in the facial canal or at the point of exit. This compression may be due to venous congestion or adjacent connective tissue strain. The nerve travels through the facial canal with a dense venous plexus. The plexus drains in two directions: superiorly back into the petrosal sinus, and inferiorly into the external jugular plexus. Altered stresses and tensions in the muscles or connective tissues surrounding the venous plexus as it exits the foramen or drains into the jugular will lead to congestion in the vessels as they traverse the facial canal. Engorgement of this venous plexus may compress or irritate the facial nerve. One eye slightly opened in the newborn may be misinterpreted as ptosis.

The forces of labor and delivery may result in subconjunctival hemorrhage; severe forces may cause retinal hemorrhage or bleeding in the anterior chamber of the eye.

Nares should be evaluated for symmetry. Deviation of the septum may occur during labor, especially in the brow, face and occiput posterior presentations. Gently pushing the tip of the nose laterally should enlarge the ipsilateral nares if the septum is normal. The mouth should be examined for cleft palate by palpation. Cleft uvulas are often associated with cleft palate. The length of the frenulum also needs to be examined, as a short frenulum will interfere with normal suckling. The coordination and intensity of the suckling reflex can be assessed by placing a finger in the infant's mouth.

The neck should be evaluated for passive range of motion as well as more subtle tissue tensions and restrictions. Torticollis may result from a tight or shortened sternocleidomastoid muscle, although more commonly involvement of the scalene muscles results in a side-bending rotation position of the head which may not manifest immediately. Assessment of rib mechanics is essential in treating torticollis associated with scalene involvement. Muscle bruising may occur during labor. The subsequent scarring and fibrosis can create a torticollis. As the child grows, the torticollis may cause cranial deformation and postural development problems. Torticollis may also result from irritation to the accessory nerve as it exits the jugular foramen. Very often, plagiocephaly may be mistaken for torticollis until cervical range of motion is properly assessed. Passive motion testing of the torso and pelvis should be done to assess for fascial strains or posturing which my have resulted from uterine lie or delivery. The newborn is placed on her back with her face and head centered on her body. The newborn should maintain this position. Fascial strain will cause the baby to adopt a side-bent or tilted posture in less than a minute. The baby's position is straightened and the observation repeated. If the baby adopts the same distorted posture this suggests postural asymmetry (Phillippi et al 2006). Body on head rotation and passive side-bending of the pelvis and torso are then assessed for symmetry (see Carreiro: *Pediatric manual medicine*).

Integrity of all the joints should be assessed. Hip clicks or apparent laxity in the hip capsule may be due to congenital hip dysplasia, but more often is the result of biomechanical strain within the hip joint. The acetabulum is the place of convergence of the ischia, ilia and pubic bones. They are joined by cartilage at the center of the fossa. Stresses that alter the relationship between any of these bones will affect the origin and insertion relationships of the rotator cuff and articular capsule of the hip. This may present as altered range of motion or apparent laxity. However, ultrasound evaluation of the hip is usually normal in these patients. Rebalancing the relationships between the three bones and the associated tissues will often resolve the problem.

INITIAL FINDINGS AT BIRTH
(Carreiro 1993)

Initial palpatory findings at birth vary with the gestational age of the newborn and the mechanism of delivery. Osteopathic examination was performed on 1600 newborns. Evaluation focused on the involuntary mechanism as described by Sutherland. The response of the involuntary homeostatic process to birth from the time of delivery and severance of the umbilical cord through approximately the first 10 min of life was documented. These observations were made within the context of standard pediatric delivery room care. Some of the observations, especially those in compromised infants, may actually be the response of the involuntary mechanism to the medical treatment delivered. Approximately 80% of these infants were vaginal deliveries, the rest being cesarean births. Lack of definitive numbers is due to instances of inconsistent documentation, but is not thought to affect the data, which represent the most common patterns observed in the neonates corrected for age and birth mechanism.

All newborns were initially evaluated at birth, i.e. during the first 10 min after delivery. Each neonate was then placed on a schedule based on gestational age by Dubowitz assessment, history of prenatal complications, and abnormal palpatory, physical and medical findings. Exceptions to the devised schedule included four infants of 23 weeks' gestational age who were evaluated hourly due to their poor condition. One of these neonates was initially observed 20 min after birth, and then hourly for 24 h; he then went unobserved for 12 h. Hourly observation resumed for 12 h, then he was again unobserved for 12 h, during which time he died. Another infant of 23 weeks' gestational age was observed at birth and then hourly for 6 h and continuously for 30 min prior to death and 25 min after death. The third neonate was observed hourly for 24 h, then unobserved for 12 h, and then observed one or two times per day. A group of infants, who can be described as 'toxic', in that there was intrauterine exposure to infectious or chemical substances, were observed twice daily until discharge. Inclusion criteria for this group were based on specific palpatory findings that were confirmed by historical and laboratory data.

For infants greater than 26 weeks' gestational age, the first minute of life is a time of (re)organization. This process of (re)organization is observable by trained palpation. It occurs within the involuntary mechanism as well as between the involuntary and voluntary mechanisms. The primary respiratory mechanism, the motility of the central nervous system, the fluctuation of the cerebrospinal fluid, the mobility of the reciprocal tension membrane, and the articular mobility of the cranial bones and the sacrum between the ilia, become identifiable as distinct phenomena during the first moments of life in most viable newborns.

After the infant was delivered through the vaginal canal, the obstetrician handed the newborn to the observer. Occasionally, the umbilical vessels were still intact. On a palpatory level, the five phenomena of the involuntary mechanism were not differentiable. Qualitatively, the tissues were felt to be in extension, but the fluid was in a swelling phase. The cranial rhythmic impulse was not palpable. The tissues exhibited different phases of the involuntary mechanism, although no cyclical motion was present.

In infants, greater than 26 weeks' gestational age, there would then occur what can be described as a 'wind up', like the elastic band on a child's propeller toy. On a sensory level, this appears to occur within the meninges. It begins concurrently at bregma and the coccyx, and moves in a spiraling motion towards the center of the thorax in the area of the fourth thoracic segment on the right. Upon reaching this point, a fulcrum is created, a stillpoint, followed by a gradual expansion which spreads along the midline axis to the head and pelvis. It moves peripherally as well, but that is less impressive. The midline change is most obvious. When this expansion reaches bregma and the coccyx, a long flexion phase occurs. Then the five phenomena of the involuntary mechanism are distinctly observable. This is a purely palpatory experience, which occurred in less than a minute in most viable newborns.

Following this period of organization, and throughout the first 15–20 min of life, no identifiable strain patterns were discernible in viable newborns. The cranial base, vault, thorax, pelvis, extremities and reciprocal membrane functioned from physiological fulcrums. During these first minutes, no inertial fulcrums and no strains between or within the osseous or membranous structures were palpable in infants with spontaneous respirations, pulse rates greater than 100 beats/min, and good muscle tone. Quite often, however, there was a qualitative difference at the interface between the fluid and membranous structures within the cranium. This was associated with an increase in fluid potency at that area. Although accommodation of the cranial vault was often grossly apparent, within that geometrical context no strain was appreciated. The system functioned harmoniously within the geometry present. Re-examination of the newborns at 6 or more hours postbirth revealed strains in the sphenobasilar synchondrosis in 40%, while 70% had strains in the spine, sacrum, pelvis and/or vault.

Five term infants were diagnosed with trisomy 21 with associated physical appearance. During the time period following organization of the involuntary mechanism, no tissue strains were palpated. Most noticeably absent were the presphenoid/postsphenoid strain and the membranous torsion often seen in these patients. Similarly, a patient born with 'prune belly syndrome', congenital deficiency of the abdominal musculature, was observed to have no immediate tissue strain patterns. He later developed significant pelvic, lower back and diaphragmatic strain patterns with an inertial fulcrum in the posterior area of the right crura.

When the organizational period was prolonged, the five phenomena were noted to have decreased amplitude, low potency, and a sluggish tissue response. These findings were most often associated with anesthesia and complicated deliveries such as prolonged labor, premature rupture of membranes or assisted delivery. It is important to note that when the organizational process did not proceed completely, the infants were tachypneic and demonstrated retraction and grunting. Palpatory findings suggested a strain pattern in the area of the fourth thoracic segment. The fluctuation of the cerebrospinal fluid was in a relative expansion/inhalation phase, while the osseous and membranous components of the five phenomena were in an internal rotation/extension phase. Overall, the impression was one of exhalation, yet no cycling was present. Once recognized and balanced, the system would 'correct' and a long flexion phase, a longitudinal tide, would be sensed, followed by synchronistic cycles of flexion and extension of the five phenomena. In instances of no spontaneous respiration, a 'contradiction' in the phases between the sacrum and cranial base was readily apparent. (Sacrum in relative extension and cranial base in relative flexion.) Spontaneous respiration did not occur as long as the 'contradiction' remained. Often, manual stimulation such as rubbing or cardiac compression would resolve the contradiction. Once the thoracic fulcrum was established, the organizational period was prolonged. However, after it was completed and the five phenomena became distinct, there often remained a place of interference of strain at the tissue–fluid interface.

This organizational period was not observed in infants of less than 26 weeks' gestational age. Although cardiac activity was present and, occasionally, in the more mature infants, attempts at spontaneous respiration occurred, there was no appreciable organization of the involuntary mechanism. In neonates ranging in age from 19 to 23 weeks of gestation, the five phenomena could not be appreciated. Although there is something expressed other than cardiac and respiratory cycles, it cannot be described using the existing osteopathic terminology. During the period of 24 weeks of gestation to 26 weeks, a shift takes place, and gradually the phenomena become more easily discernible. The quality of their expression at this time actually lends itself to age assessment. It is difficult to describe the quality of the involuntary mechanism prior to 24 weeks of gestation. The palpatory quality of the tissue is very different from that of an older neonate. This may have something to do with the paucity of cellular components present in relation to intracellular space; perhaps the infrastructure cannot support itself against gravity. This is a purely subjective interpretation of the quality of the expression.

Included in the total population examined was a group of neonates that demonstrated a quality of the primary respiratory mechanism which differed from the rest. The patterns that were present were similar enough to be categorized into one of the previously mentioned age-based groups, but subtle differences allowed for subgrouping and comparison between groups. These subpopulations all presented with a subtle dissonance pattern that was not present in most newborns. This pattern became appreciable only after the five phenomena were distinguishable. The dissonance pattern had a high-frequency vibrational quality, which could be categorized further by its pitch. The dissonance existed in the fluid phenomena, extending into the fluid–potency interface. The prenatal histories of these children inevitably included intrauterine exposure to a 'toxin' such as an infectious agent, cocaine, marijuana, or heroin. Infants exposed to analgesic or anesthetic medications only during labor did not have a dissonance pattern. Subsequent experience suggests that these dissonance patterns are still appreciable in older infants and children.

In conclusion, five general observations of the involuntary mechanism in the neonate can be made:

- Immediately after birth in neonates greater than 26 weeks of gestational age, a fulcrum is established in the area of the fourth thoracic segment, after which there is a period of organization of the involuntary mechanism.
- The establishment of this fulcrum and the time over which the organization occurs has a relationship to the age of the patient, condition of the patient (APGAR score) and method of delivery.
- The five phenomena of the primary respiratory mechanism become distinguishable after this organizational process has been completed, yet strain patterns or inertial fulcrums are absent in most neonates for at least 6 h.
- The process was not observed in infants less than 24 weeks' gestational age.

- A high-frequency vibrational pattern was observed in infants with histories of intrauterine exposure to infectious agents, heroin, cocaine and marijuana.

In light of these observations, we must consider the possibility of the existence of a therapeutic window during which the neuromusculoskeletal system is adapting to the effects of the transition from a fluid environment to a gravitational field. We might term this 'proprioceptive priming'. The supple and resilient osseous structures literally float in a fluid matrix within membranous envelopes. The possibility that the neonatal body can resolve compressive and rotational forces rather than assimilate them into the structure needs to be considered. If this is the case, the role of the osteopath as a facilitator of the inherent homeostatic mechanism of the newborn becomes clear.

CONCLUSION

The mechanical structure and resiliency of the neonatal head and body are well suited for the process of labor and delivery, as many thousand years has proven. However, sometimes, natural processes are not as perfect as they could be and tissue deformation does occur. While the normal activities of breathing, crying and suckling aid the restitution of normal function, sometimes a little assistance is needed. Clinicians treating newborns with birth-related tissue strains would do well to remember that rarely are strains isolated to the apparent area of deformation. In most cases, other regions of the body have undergone some adaptation to the strain; limb deformations are usually associated with pelvic and torso strains and plagiocephaly with cervical and rib involvement. Rather than the traditional focused approach of casting, bracing and helmets, most infants will benefit from a comprehensive, whole-body osteopathic approach that addresses the obvious deformation and the not-so-obvious compensatory strains that contribute to it.

References

Carreiro J E 1993 Osteopathic evaluation of 1600 neonates. Paper presentation, Annual Convocation, American Academy of Osteopathy.

Degenhardt B F, Kuchera M L 1994 The prevalance of cranial dysfunction in children with a history of otitis media from kindergarten to third grade. J Am Osteopathic Assoc September: 10.

Frymann V M 1966 Relation of disturbances of craniosacral mechanism to symptomatology of the newborn. J Am Osteopathic Assoc 65: 1059–1075.

Heisey S R, Adams T 1993 Role of cranial bone mobility in cranial compliance. Neurosurgery 33: 869–877.

Kane A A, Mitchell L E, Craven K P et al 1996 Observations on a recent increase in plagiocephaly without synostosis. Pediatrics 97: 877–885.

Lassovetskaya L 2003 Osteopathic treatment of schoolchildren with delayed psychic development of cerebral-organic origin. J Osteopath Med (Australia) 6: 38.

Magoun H I S 1976 Osteopathy in the cranial field, 3rd edn. The Journal Printing Company, Kirksville, MI.

Menkes J H, Sarant H B 2000 Child neurology, 6th edn. Williams & Wilkins, Lippincott, Philadelphia.

Mills M V, Henley C E, Barnes L L et al 2002 Effect of osteopathic manipulative treatment (OMT) on recurrent acute otitis media in children [meeting abstract]. JAOA 102: 441.

Mocsary P, Gaal J, Komaromy B 1970 Relationship between fetal intracranial pressure and fetal heart rate during labor. Am J Obstet Gynecol 106: 407–411.

Peitsch W K, Keefer C H, LaBrie R A et al 2002 Incidence of cranial asymmetry in healthy newborns. Pediatrics 110: e72.

Phillippi H, Faldum H, Bauer K et al 2006 Patterns of postural asymmetry in infants: a standardized video-based analysis. Eur J Pediatr 165: 158–164.

Schwartz R L Strada-Saenz G, Althabe O 1969 Pressure exerted by uterine contractions on the head of the human fetus during labor. Scientific Publications No 185, Washington 115–126.

Sutherland W G 1990 Teachings in the science of osteopathy, 1st edn. Rudra Press, Portland, OR.

Upledger J E 1978 The relationship of craniosacral examination findings in grade school children with developmental problems. J Am Osteopathic Assoc 77: 760–776.

Valkeakari T 1973 Analysis of serial echoencephalograms in healthy newborn infants during the first week of life. Acta Pediatr Scand 242: 1–62.

Further reading

Amiel-Tison C, Stewart A 1994 The newborn infant: one brain for life. French National Institute of Health and Medicine, Paris.

Frymann V F 1998 Collected writings. American Academy of Osteopathy, IN.

Magoun H I S 1973 Idiopathic adolescent spinal scoliosis. The DO 13(6).

Magoun H I S 1976 Osteopathy in the cranial field, 3rd edn. The Journal Printing Company, Kirksville, MI.

Sutherland W G 1998 Contributions of thought, 2nd edn. Rudra Press, Portland, OR.

Volpe J J 1995 Neurology of the newborn, 3rd edn. W B Saunders, Philadelphia.

Chapter Nine

9

Posture, balance and movement

CHAPTER CONTENTS

OVERVIEW

If you close your eyes and extend your arms and try to touch your nose, it would be rare to actually miss it. The reason you can close your eyes and touch your nose is that in your brain you carry a map of your body and its relationship to space. When you close your eyes, information from the proprioceptive sensory receptors of your musculoskeletal system concerning the spatial relationships within your body at this moment is compared with the body map you created in your brain during development. Your brain compares the two maps to determine where your arm is in relationship to the rest of you and the muscular actions you will need to touch your finger to your nose. We have maps based on somatosensory, visual, auditory and vestibular information. The better coordinated the maps, the easier it is to maintain balance, execute movements and physically respond to our environment. If we look at disciplines such as yoga and the martial arts, one of the fundamental points of the discipline is to maintain a neutral balanced midline and orchestrate all movements around that midline. Using information from our visual, vestibular and musculoskeletal systems, which feeds into the spinal cord, brainstem and cortex, we are able to maintain our balance and move. At each of these levels of the nervous system there are maps. The information from these maps is interpreted and compared. When information from any of these systems is distorted, we can compensate for the distortion using information from one of the other systems. This implies some redundancy between the maps and the sensory systems which supply them. This redundancy can serve as a check and balance, fine-tuning the maps during development. A sensory system that is diseased or impaired may distort the organization of its own map and affect the development of other maps.

Posture is the ability of the body to control its position in space against the forces of the external world

(Shumway-Cook & Woollacott 2000). Posture is the product of an integrated orchestration between the sensory and motor systems of the body. Peripheral sensory systems provide an internal representation of the outside world. It is the function of the central nervous system to extract information from these internal maps and use it to guide the movements that make up our behavior. The neural networks in the central nervous system involved in mapping sensory experiences and integrating this information with the motor system constitute the postural control mechanism. This mechanism is capable of detecting the constantly changing external environment and adjusting our musculoskeletal system to respond to these demands. Normally, this mechanism, with its built-in redundant features, functions adequately throughout our life. However, diseases affecting sensory systems, central control systems, motor systems or structural elements of the body can lead to progressive failure of the postural mechanisms that will manifest as postural embarrassment. Nevertheless, numerous factors contributing to the demise of posture and balance can be addressed by the healthcare professional to improve the functional capacity of the patient.

SENSORY SYSTEMS AND THEIR ROLE AS POSTURE MODULATORS

Three sensory systems are involved in modulating the postural control mechanism: the visual system, the vestibular system and the somatic sensory system. The visual sensory system imparts information concerning the body's vertical orientation to the horizon as well as providing a mechanism for distance or depth perception. This information is mapped to the occipital portion of the cerebral cortex. Age-related changes in the visual system include alterations in visual acuity and depth perception. Visual acuity in the newborn is difficult to measure but has been reported to be 20/400 at birth. By 3 years it is between 20/30 and 20/20. Generally, there is little pupillary accommodation in newborns. Convergence is present and, under controlled conditions, infants between 8 and 10 weeks can track an object across approximately 180° (Olitsky & Nelson 2000). Both acuity and depth perception can affect postural stability, especially during movement-based activities. Depth perception involves taking a two-dimensional image and converting it into three dimensions (Wurtz & Kandel 2000). The ocular dominance columns of visual cortex segregate from each other at 4 months, and binocular depth perception emerges. Monocular depth perception relies more on experience than binocular depth perception and appears later.

Although visual acuity and depth perception are immature functions in young infants, movement and posture are visually triggered. For example, at 3 days of age, newborns will orient their eyes to a visual stimulus and track it as it moves, even though muscle synergies are too immature to support coordinated head movement (Shumway-Cook & Woollacott 2000). By 2 months of age, early signs of postural control can be recognized. An infant lying on her back will turn her head to look at something, and an infant lying on his stomach will begin to lift his head. These are visually triggered activities. Studies confirm that infants rely heavily on visual input in early postural control (Butterworth & Cicchetti 1978); however, vestibular and somatosensory inputs also have a role in maintaining balance (Woollacott et al 1987). By 2.5 months, visual fixation contributes to significant improvements in antigravity reflexes and the infant will respond to perturbations of balance with head control movements.

Visually activated muscle synergies precede those activated by the somatic sensory system. This suggests that the visual system maps to the motor system earlier than the proprioceptive system. Observations of the influence of visual cues on early posture and balance control confirm this hypothesis; infants under 1 year will sway in response to visual stimuli (Lee & Aronson 1974). Ten-month-old infants will make postural adjustments to optic flow while sitting. By 12 months, they will make postural adjustments while standing (Shumway-Cook & Woollacott 2000). In general, visual input appears to weigh more heavily than somatosensory cues when an individual is attempting a new task. Once the task becomes more automated, somatosensory input takes over (Lee & Aronson 1974) and visually triggered reflexes lessen.

The second system involved with posture is the vestibular system. The vestibular system supplies information regarding the direction of gravity and head motion in the sagittal, coronal and horizontal planes. Its information is mapped through the brainstem and onto the insular portion of the cerebral cortex. Each vestibular apparatus is located in the petrous portion of the temporal bone and is completely formed by 9.5 weeks of gestation (Fig. 9.1). The vestibular nuclei are functional by 21 weeks. Each vestibular apparatus is composed of three semicircular canals placed 90° from each other in superior, posterior and horizontal positions. The ampulla of each canal is lined with specialized hair cells, each of which is covered with many stereocilia and a single kinocilium that extend into the lumen of the canal. The canals are filled with endolymph. Movement of the head produces a relative movement of the endolymph located within the semicircular canals. The stereocilia of the hair cells are bent as they pass through the endolymph, like seaweed by a wave (Fig. 9.2). When the stereocilia are bent towards the kinocilium, the cell depolarizes. There is an increase in the release of neurotransmitter, and an increase in the rate of firing. When the stereocilia are bent away from the kinocilium, the cell hyperpolarizes and the release of neurotransmitter is decreased, as is the firing rate. The signal from the vestibular hair cells travels to the vestibular nuclear complex, four

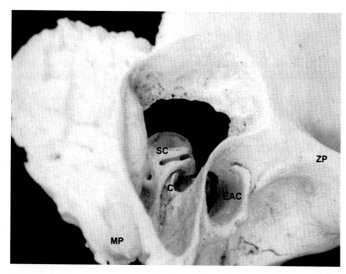

Fig. 9.1 • Adult temporal bone specimen. Parts of the squamous and mastoid have been drilled to reveal the vestibular–auditory apparatus. The semicircular canals (SC) can be seen through the drilled aperture. The cochlear (C) is located anterior–inferior and lateral. The remnant of the articular suture between the tympanic ring and petrous portion can be seen medial to the external auditory canal (EAC). MP, mastoid process; EAC, external auditory canal; ZP, zygomatic process. *Used with permission of the Willard & Carreiro Collection.*

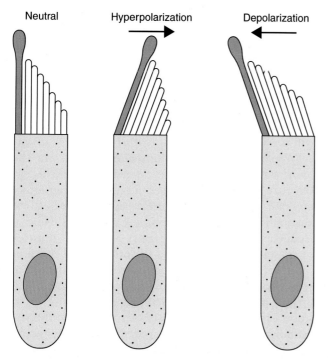

Fig. 9.2 • Schematic diagram of a hair cell. The kinocilium is depicted in black and the stereocilia in white. As the stereocilia bend towards the kinocilium, the cell depolarizes.

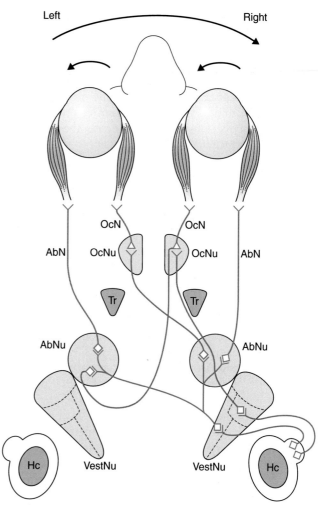

Fig. 9.3 • Schematic diagram of the vestibulo-ocular reflex when the head rotates to the right. The direction of head movement is indicated by the large arrow (pointing to the right). The direction of eye movement is depicted by the small arrows (pointed to the left). The connections shown on the right of each eye are inhibitory. The connections on the left are excitatory. OcN, oculomotor nerve; OcNu, oculomotor nucleus; AbN, abducens nerve; AbNu, abducens nucleus; Tr, trochlear nucleus; VestNu, vestibular nucleus; Hc, horizontal canal.

distinct nuclei with different architecture and functions. The lateral vestibular nucleus influences the extensors of the legs and flexors of the arms, and is involved with upright stance. This is termed the vestibulospinal reflex. The medial and superior nuclei mediate the vestibulo-ocular reflex. Signals from cells in these nuclei trigger the abducens and oculomotor nuclei, and the eyes are moved at an equal velocity but in an opposite direction to the movement of the head (Fig. 9.3). Fibers originating in the superior vestibular nucleus also terminate on motor neurons of the cervical musculature and influence neck position through the vestibulocollic reflex. The vestibulo-ocular reflex is intact at birth and, along with the vestibulocollic and vestibulospinal reflexes, will influence head and neck posture in the young infant. These three reflexes affect paraspinal muscle tone and can be used in specific muscle energy techniques for treatment of upper cervical somatic dysfunction (Goodridge & Kuchera 1997). Conversely, individuals with uncorrected visual acuity problems may develop increased tone in the upper cervical musculature, presumably through the same mechanism. As we pass through middle age, degeneration of the hair cells within the vestibular labyrinth organ affects the vestibular contribution to posture and balance.

The third system, the somatic sensory system, receives information from the skin, muscles and connective tissues of the body. This information is mapped onto the parietal portion of the cerebral cortex. Muscle afferent fibers are proprioceptive in function and relate information about change in spatial position. When these fibers are triggered by rapid tendon or muscle stretch, the resulting muscle contraction provides a quickly adaptive response to sudden positional change. Joint afferent fibers provide information regarding alterations in the relationship of joint surfaces. This includes changes in the orientation of the head to the neck and spine, and changes in the orientation of the limbs (appendicular skeleton) to the trunk (axial skeleton). Joint afferent fibers carry information about spatial relationships to the central nervous system. Many of these proprioceptors are located in the connective tissues of the cervical spine. The proprioceptive information from the cervical spine can actually override positional information from the eyes and vestibular system. Cutaneous afferent fibers carry information concerning pressure from the skin. Of particular importance to upright posture is information from the skin on the soles of the feet. Pressure on the plantar surface elicits a reflex movement of the foot towards the stimulus, and this increases tone in the extensor muscles of the limb and pelvis. In addition, neural signals concerning shearing forces on the skin of the plantar surface supply data on body motion to the central nervous system.

Alterations in the function of the somatosensory system may impede postural stability. For example, distortions in the proprioceptive information from diseased joints such as an arthritic knee (Barrett et al 1991) or spondylitic vertebrae will affect the individual's perception of position. Proprioceptive information can be altered by changes in joint mobility and gliding, increase in cervical lordosis and compression of vertebral disk spaces (Alexander et al 1992). This phenomena is not limited to joint proprioceptors. Diseases affecting cutaneous afferent fibers, such as diabetic neuropathy, will interfere with information about motion coming from the soles of the feet (Simoneau et al 1994). One study done by Woollacott et al (1998) suggests that children with spastic diplegia have altered postural strategies secondary to the altered biomechanical relationships rather than the neurological pathology (see Ch. 16). Although the effects of altered biomechanical relationships on posture have not been studied extensively, clinical experience suggests

a significant relationship between the two. In addition to the potential for altered proprioception, alterations in position sense require adaptations in movement strategies which are often difficult for the disabled or deconditioned patient, further compromising stability.

Posture is an expression of the integration of information from these three sensory systems: visual, vestibular and somatosensory. There appears to be a certain amount of redundancy between the systems, which allows for masking of deficits. However, when two systems are stressed, underlying dysfunctions are unmasked and balance is compromised.

MOTOR CONTRIBUTION TO POSTURE

The motor system consists of the neural connections from the cerebral cortex and brainstem to the spinal cord and from the spinal cord to the skeletal muscles. Through these connections, the brain can orchestrate the coordinated movement of both the axial muscles of the torso and the appendicular muscles of the limbs. To perform voluntary movement, the central nervous system, acting through the motor system, needs to accomplish three things: (1) make postural adjustments to the anticipated changing distribution of muscle mass; (2) execute accurately timed commands to agonist and antagonist muscles in the torso and limbs; and (3) integrate these commands into the pre-existing arrangement of the musculoskeletal tissues. The contraction and relaxation of agonist and antagonist muscle groups must be coordinated to effect smooth and precise movements. When posture is perturbed, the motor system must execute a rapid sequencing of muscular activation to maintain stability. This sequencing is often referred to as a postural strategy. Improper sequencing of agonist or antagonist muscle groups results in disjointed movement. This will present as increased sway during postural adjustments (Woollacott 1993) or clumsy movements. In the very young and the very old, onset latencies for muscle contractions may be altered. Increases in onset latencies affect the temporal sequencing of muscle response to postural perturbation (Woollacott & Shumway-Cook 1990). Normal adult sequencing patterns (strategies) of postural muscles are not present in newborns and infants. During development, these strategies are defined and refined through trial and error. Children with motor or sensory dysfunctions will develop postural strategies that vary from the norm.

Postural strategies coordinate sensory input from the visual, vestibular and somatosensory systems with motor activity. Therefore, postural control is dependent on the ability of the individual to interpret this sensory information and execute an appropriate motor response. An accurate motor response requires strength, flexibility and coordination, all of which (among other things) are influenced by muscle tone, joint range of motion and biomechanical relationships. Postural strategies can be divided into those that are engaged to maintain quiet balance, such as standing and sitting, and those engaged during active movement. Both require synchronized activity of muscle groups in response to sensory input and, to varying degrees, both are dependent on feedback and anticipatory control. Ghez (1991) uses the tasks of reaching for a cup and catching a ball to compare these two control mechanisms. In reaching for a cup, feedback control would compare visual and somatosensory information concerning the position of your arm in space with the location of the cup. Any necessary adjustments will be made on the basis of this information. Processing and responding to sensory information in a feedback loop is relatively slow; it takes almost as much time to process the information as to execute the movement. Feedback mechanisms are used to maintain or modulate slow movements or sequential acts. Actions requiring very rapid responses rely on feedforward control. Information is processed to anticipate the needed response. An example of feedforward control can be illustrated by reviewing the act of catching a ball. Visual information is used to assess the anticipated trajectory of the ball, its placement and the time until it reaches you. These visual cues will also be used to ready the musculoskeletal system by assuming an appropriate posture for impact (Ghez 1991). When a new task is being learned, feedback control will dominate the process. Once learned, feedforward control is involved with the initiation of the task, while feedback control is used to fine-tune the end movements (Ghez & Krakauer 2000).

Nashner (1976) found that muscle response to perturbations of stance generally occurred in a distal-to-proximal sequence. Two of the most common postural strategies used to correct for perturbation of stance are the ankle and hip strategies (Horak & Nashner 1986). The ankle strategy initiates in the muscles about the ankle and knee, resulting in small backward and forward sway. This strategy is usually employed when the support surface is stable and the perturbation relatively small. Hip strategies are initiated at the pelvis and hips with secondary response at the ankles. Large movements are generated at the pelvis and torso to adjust the position of the body mass. Hip strategies appear to be used when the support surface is narrow or unstable, or the perturbation large (Horak & Nashner 1986). Postural strategies are influenced by repeated experience (Nashner et al 1982). Unsuccessful components of the strategy are weeded out, and what remains is fine-tuned for efficiency and effectiveness. This is a form of learning.

Some postural strategies incorporate reflex movements such as the vestibulocollic and vestibulospinal reflexes. The vestibulocollic reflex engages when the head is rapidly moved forward without flexion of the neck. The posterior cervical muscles contract to raise the head. The vestibulospinal and

cervicospinal reflexes affect the upper limb musculature. Sudden forward movement of the head triggers contraction of arm extensors (Ghez 2000). Other reflexes such as the cervicocollic and cervicospinal are triggered through proprioceptors in the upper cervical vertebrae. The cervicocollic reflex causes cervical muscles to contract in response to sudden stretch. Cervicospinal reflexes are a bit more complex. Flexion of the neck results in flexion of the upper extremities, while tilting the head and the body forwards, as would happen in a fall, produces extension of the arms (Ghez 2000). Rotation of the neck will elicit extension of the ipsilateral arm and leg, and extension of the contralateral limbs. This maneuver is sometimes referred to as the asymmetric tonic neck reflex in newborns.

THE DEVELOPMENT OF POSTURE

Cognitive development in the early months revolves around coordination of simple action systems, which aid in establishing muscle synergies. The infant is beginning to develop movement strategies such as swiping and batting or turning the head. Learning is automated by repeated experiences. The mechanics of the extremities, thorax and neck are especially important during the early phase, because the infant is learning to use sensory feedback from the extremities in conjunction with visual input, to fine-tune action strategies. As the child actively engages muscle groups in coordinated patterns, new stresses are placed on the musculoskeletal system.

One of the earliest action systems to emerge involves head control. Initially, this is visually triggered. Between 32 and 34 weeks of gestation, newborns are able to orient their heads to a visual stimulus (Shumway-Cook & Woollacott 2000). By 2.5 months, improved coordinated muscle activity in the cervical area, in response to visual and vestibular interactions, allows for antigravity postural activity (Shumway-Cook & Woollacott 2000). This can be seen if one attempts to raise an infant by the arms from the supine position; during the newborn period the head will drop backwards, by 2.5 months the head travels in line with the back, and by 5–6 months the head will lead the shoulders (Fig. 9.4).

Sitting requires coordination between neck and trunk muscles to maintain the head in an upright position, along with improvements in lumbar and pelvic muscle control and relaxation in hip flexor muscles. Early sitting relies heavily on the visual system for postural cues. At 1–2 months of age, the infant will use visual cues to raise the head. By 3 months of age, there is improved control of the thoracic region but lumbar support is still lacking and the child relies on visual rather than proprioceptive cues for balance. In fact, young infants can maintain an unsupported, sitting position if their head is stabilized (Fig. 9.5). After 3 months, proprioceptive information from the hip and pelvis begins to dominate postural

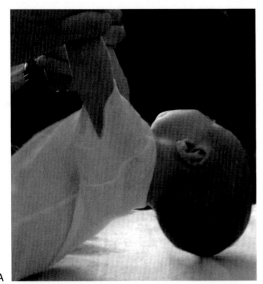
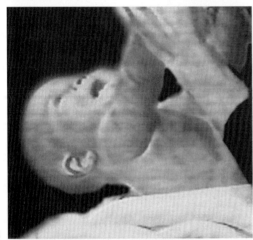
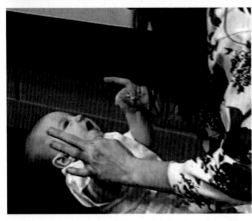

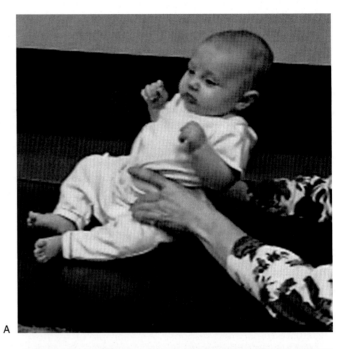
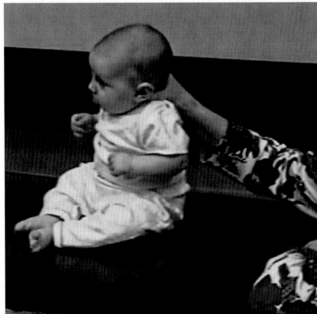

Fig. 9.5 • (A, B) A 2-month-old girl can maintain an upright unsupported seated posture if her head is stabilized. *Used with permission of the Willard & Carreiro Collection.*

Fig. 9.4 • (A–C) These three photographs compare the responses of the infants when we attempt to raise them from the supine position. The orientation of the ear to the shoulder alters as the child engages cervical muscles to raise the head. (A) A 10-day-old infant. The head falls back and there is no cervical muscle contraction or any resistance in the arms. (B) A 2-month-old infant. There is some cervical muscle contraction to lift the head. (C) A 4-month-old infant. Note the flexion of the elbows and the alignment of the ear and shoulder. *Used with permission of the Willard & Carreiro Collection.*

control. By 8 months, most children can sit successfully and are able to correct for sway with appropriate muscle activity in the trunk and neck (Shumway-Cook & Woollacott 2000). When balance is perturbed, they will use their extended arms to maintain stability (the protective equilibrium response). Somatic strain in the torso, hips or pelvis may interfere with independent sitting. Children with increased tone in the lower extremity muscles will have difficulty in extending the legs to stabilize the pelvis. Biomechanical strain in the pelvis, neck or torso may shift the child's center of gravity anterior to their base of support (the pelvis). This can occur in children with torticollis. Breech position can also place abnormal stresses on the pelvis and lumbar spine, resulting in delayed or awkward independent sitting (chart review and physician survey).

By 6 months, infants can raise their head and shoulders and most of their chest from a prone position. This is accomplished through head, neck and torso control, rather than lifting with their arms. The hip and leg flexors are more relaxed and the pelvis can lay flat on the ground. This is the position from which an infant will be able to initiate the commando crawl, wherein he uses his arms and torso to propel himself along the floor. In the early stages of this maneuver, an infant primarily relies on the sinusoidal motion of his body rather than leg activity. In recent years, since the advent of recommendations to avoid the prone position for sleeping infants, many overzealous parents have completely avoided placing infants on their stomachs. We have noticed that some of these children will substitute a rolling maneuver for the commando crawl, thereby using a form of torso coordination to propel themselves. In either case, as coordination of the lower extremity muscle groups develops, infants engage their legs in the activity. Once they can coordinate flexor and extensor activity in their legs, they need only to cultivate lumbar and pelvic control in order to raise their body and crawl on their hands and knees (creep) (Fig. 9.6). The ability to creep usually coincides with the ability to sit self-supported and the establishment of lumbar and pelvic control. Proprioceptive feedback is important in lumbopelvic mechanics. As previously mentioned, visual cues will strongly influence postural control in the first months of life; however, they will be quickly replaced by proprioceptive input.

If we review the progression of developmental stages, it would appear that mapping of the sensory systems begins in the neck and extends into the thorax, trunk, lumbar and pelvic areas. As these sensory maps become more firmly established, the child will rely more on somatosensory information and less on visual input. A child who cannot establish appropriate or effective somatosensory maps will use visual input to maintain balance. Anecdotally, most children with cerebral palsy will exhibit significant imbalance and unsteadiness if visual input is removed (clinical observation by the author and department staff). The development of postural control of the limbs involves an extension of sensory mapping to integrate limb movements (Ghez 1991). Up to 6 months, limb flexors show increased tone compared with extensors. This creates some restriction in range of motion kinetics. Sensory mapping requires many more degrees of freedom in movement to create an adequate representation of the limb's range of motion. Smooth, precise movements cannot be generated without appropriate sensory mapping. Prior to 6 months, infants fail

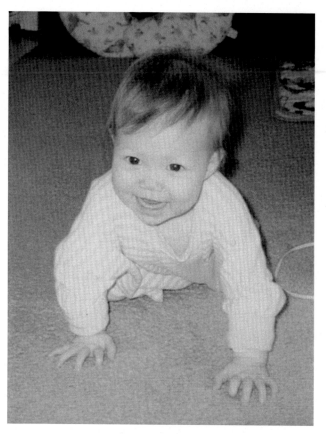

Fig. 9.6 • Creeping involves coordinated movement between the four extremities. *Used with permission of the Willard & Carreiro Collection.*

to stand; this is not due to muscle weakness, since lower extremity muscles have strength sufficient to support the child's weight (Roncesvalles & Jensen 1993). Rather, neural mechanisms controlling agonist and antagonist muscle coordination necessary for stance are not sufficiently developed. Electromyograms at 2–6 months demonstrate a lack of coordination between gastrocnemius, hamstrings, and tibialis anterior and quadriceps muscles when balance is threatened (Sveistrup & Woollacott 1993). By 7–9 months, there is improvement in ankle muscle control. This improvement will progress up the limb to include thigh and trunk muscles by 9–12 months (Shumway-Cook & Woollacott 1995: 158). Although practice on balance platforms will increase strength, it will not improve latency of activation, suggesting that the neural circuit must be mature in order to function (Sveistrup & Woollacott 1997).

The formation of the lumbar lordotic curve coincides with sitting upright and then becomes accentuated by standing. This helps children establish their center of gravity. Primitive tripod mechanics are often employed while the muscle activation sequences are being refined. During this time, children will rely on truncal sway to stabilize their posture. By 10 or 12 months, the child's balance is much improved, though postural strategies still involve torso and

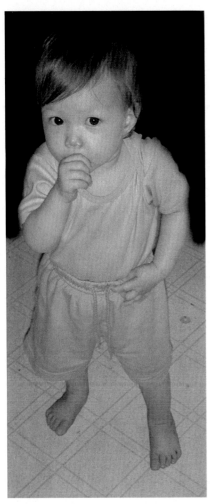

Fig. 9.7 • A 12-month-old child still uses visual input for postural stability during unsupported standing. *Used with permission of the Willard & Carreiro Collection.*

toe-off, swing phase, acceleration, midswing and deceleration are rudimentary at best. Early in gait development, a child will toe walk. This will continue until coordination of foot and ankle flexor and extensor muscles is established. (Children with lower extremity spasticity will continue to toe walk because of increased extensor tone.) Weight distribution in the foot should eventually occur in the following sequence: heel, rolling laterally onto the foot and then along the transverse arch (proximal to metatarsal heads), and then to longitudinal arch, freeing the heel for toe-off. While this sequence may not be mastered until the child is 5–6 years old, foot mechanics are being employed and refined. Functional relationships in the pelvis, hip, leg and ankle will influence the development of optimal foot mechanics. Eventually, through the coordinated effort of these areas, the child's balance strategies will move from the torso and pelvis into the foot and ankle. This occurs sometimes after 7 years of age (Shumway-Cook & Woollacott 2000).

Somatic strain in the cervical musculature may influence mechanics in the lumbar spine and lower extremities through the cervicospinal reflex. Alternatively, the development of a lumbar lordosis may influence the relationship and mechanics of the neck and craniocervical junction. Subtle cranial asymmetries and torticollis may be greatly exacerbated when the child begins to sit or stand. From an osteopathic perspective, the response of the lumbar spine and pelvis to the cranial base–cervical spine relationship may provide the foundation for later scoliosis (Magoun 1973).

MOVEMENT AND POSTURE

During voluntary movement, postural responses in the axial skeleton are triggered before the potentially destabilizing appendicular motion is performed. These movements in the axially and proximal limb muscles provide the base or platform for the movements of the distal extremities. As previously described, anticipatory or feedforward mechanisms predict disturbances in posture and produce preprogrammed responses that maintain stability. These responses can be modified by experience. An example of a feedforward mechanism would be postural adaptations preceding the execution of a voluntary limb movement such as picking up a gallon of milk. A shift in body mass occurs when the arm is extended and again as the milk is lifted. If the individual's center of gravity is not stabilized prior to each of these events, the person will lose his or her balance.

The large muscle groups of the limbs work in agonist and antagonist groupings (Fig. 9.8). Activation of an agonist group is coupled with an equal and balanced relaxation of its antagonist. This rapid process of adaptation and correction occurring between the muscle groups surrounding a joint produces smooth and coordinated movement. Temporal sequencing of muscle activation changes from birth through

pelvis. Protective mechanisms involving more controlled movement responses evolve. Posture and balance strategies improve in the trunk and arms, although leg and hip strategies are still quite immature. At this age, the child is still learning to use the integration of proprioceptive information from the spine, vestibular system, eyes and somatosensory system to maintain balance. While children of this age may pull themselves up to stand and accomplish supported standing, minor perturbations will easily disturb their stability. Even visual distraction can cause the 12–14-month-old child to lose balance (Fig. 9.7).

As ambulation becomes more coordinated and complex, the functional mechanics of the lower extremity are stressed. Evaluation of the innominate and femur relationship and the mechanics of the tibia and ankle are important during this period. Addressing tissue strains to maintain balanced biomechanical relationships should be emphasized. In the early stages of ambulation, normal adult gait mechanics such as stance phase, heel strike, foot flat, midstance,

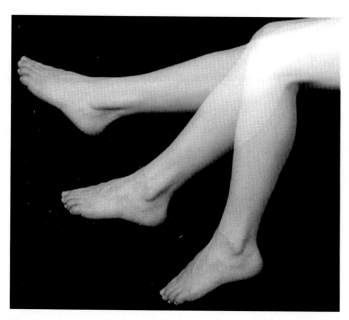

Fig. 9.8 • In this photograph of a leg extending, the quadriceps group is the agonist and the hamstring group the antagonist. *Used with permission of the Willard & Carreiro Collection.*

adulthood. This is due to maturation of latency times, motor unit organization and cortical processing. The process of myelination begins around gestation and continues through the first several years of life. Children have prolonged latency times because of incomplete myelination of the involved neural structures. In addition, the motor unit in the newborn and young child is less well organized than in the adult. Muscle fibers receive polyneural innervation; that is, the axons of two or more motor neurons synapse on the same fiber. The reverse is true in the adult, where the axons of a motor neuron will synapse on more than one muscle fiber, but each muscle fiber receives only one axon. In a mature motor unit, synchronized contraction of a group of muscle fibers is controlled by a single motor neuron, whereas in the newborn and infant, muscle contraction is often uncoordinated and random. Also interfering with the establishment of appropriate muscle coupling is the fact that the sarcoplasmic reticulum is immature and does not function optimally. This increases the contraction and relaxation times of muscle. Furthermore, neuromuscular junctional folds, postsynaptic membranes and some neurotransmitter receptors must undergo significant changes to reach the adult form which allows for coordination of muscle fiber contraction. In the young child, temporal sequencing is immature. It peaks between 10 and 20 years of age. After the age of 35, the ability to accurately coordinate muscle activity appears to decline. To be more precise, the latency periods for muscle activation increase with age, resulting in altered temporal sequencing. This may explain the larger, slower postural corrections often seen in older

people. Although some investigators have shown that when patients with subtle neurological pathology are excluded and direct muscular response through electromyography is assessed, there is no significant difference in response time in older adults (Woollacott et al 1986, Nardone et al 1995).

EARLY REFLEXES USE VESTIBULAR AND VISUAL INPUT TO INFLUENCE MUSCLE SYNERGIES

The ability to execute smooth, precise movements depends on synergistic muscle coordination – the functional coupling of muscle groups to act as a unit. These synergies are neural programs, which are activated by sensory stimuli. Often, parents erroneously think that their infant is too weak to successfully execute movements. The newborns have muscular strength sufficient to lift themselves; however, they lack the muscle coordination to accomplish the movement. All voluntary movement is the result of finely tuned sequenced patterns of muscle contraction. These patterns develop through trial and error, as inefficient and ineffective patterns are discarded and successful patterns are selected. Even relatively static movements such as sitting, standing or maintaining balance are the expression of muscle synergies that develop over time.

Generally, motor development proceeds from movements with low synergistic requirements to those with higher requirements. Simpler movement patterns are refined and integrated into more complex patterns. At birth, infants lack refined synergistic muscle control. Early reflexes such as the palmar grasp and Moro (startle) reflex represent segmental or vestibular reflexes, not voluntary movement patterns; however, the motions associated with the Moro may well be integrated into later protective responses. The Moro reflex is elicited by gently lifting the supine infant by the hands so that the head and neck are elevated. Then the child is allowed to gently fall back towards the supine position (Fig. 9.9) (please use a soft surface). This maneuver quickly changes the relationship of the head, neck and vestibular input. An infant will extend both arms rapidly and then flex them to his chest. There is usually a cry. This sequence of movements defines an intact Moro. Later in life, when that infant, now 33 years old, is walking along the street and trips, rapidly changing head, neck and vestibular input, his arms will reflexively extend, preventing him from breaking his nose on the pavement.

Other reflexes incorporate input from multiple sensory systems. As previously described, the asymmetrical tonic neck reflex develops at approximately 2 weeks and lasts until almost 6 months. It involves input from the vestibular system and proprioceptors of the neck, with coordination between arm and leg flexors and extensors (Fig. 9.10).

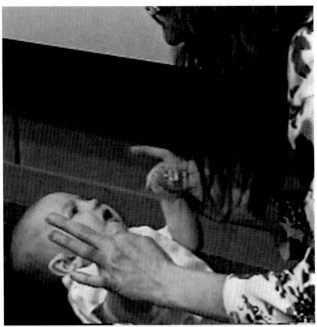

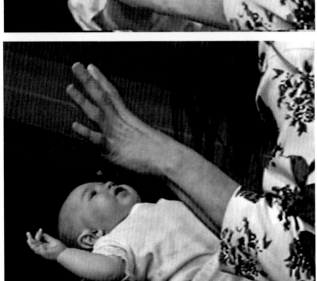

Fig. 9.9 • (A, B) The Moro or startle reflex. *Used with permission of the Willard & Carreiro Collection.*

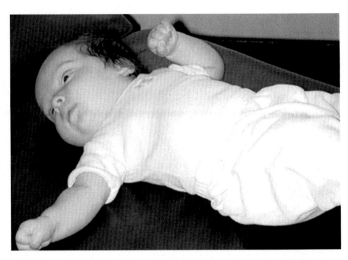

Fig. 9.10 • The asymmetric tonic neck reflex or fencer's pose; when the head is turned, the ipsilateral arm and leg extend and the contralateral limbs flex. It is usually fully present by 2 weeks and can remain intact until 6 months . *Used with permission of the Willard & Carreiro Collection.*

As the supine child's head is passively turned, the ipsilateral arm and leg extend while the contralateral limbs flex, similar to a fencer's position. The extended arm lies directly in the child's field of vision. Consequently, this reflex is often thought to be involved in hand–eye coordination.

NEUROBIOLOGICAL BASIS FOR EYE–HAND COORDINATION

In the adult, the intentional movement of a limb to a target involves three things: visual initiation of hand movement based on the target's position; ballistic arm movements towards the target which are dependent on the use of appropriate muscle synergies and sensory feedback; and anticipatory orientation of the hand's grasp to the target position, including closing the fingers as they approximate the target. Planning the trajectory of the movement occurs in the parietal cortex; the premotor cortex is involved in coordinating the intrajoint movements to accomplish the task (Levin 1996).

There are various theories on the development of eye–hand coordination, and a thorough analysis of each is beyond the scope of this chapter. However, a brief description of the most prominent theories will serve to set the background for the remainder of the chapter. Piaget emphasized the primacy of action over perception and of self-generated experience in development of coordination. His concepts of premotor development involved random movements where hand, eye and neck were not coordinated during the first 4 months of development. According to Piaget, it is only after this time that the first signs of coordination between perceptual systems become evident. Conversely, Gibson theorized that perception and action serve together to provide the individual with the capability to acquire experiences from the environment (Reed 1982). This assumes that perceptual and motor systems may have some degree of coordination early in development. Selection theory is a functionalist approach which claims that the anatomy of the brain is predetermined (hard-wired) and that the meaning of signals to the brain is fixed. Selectionists claim that the organism gains its ability to organize an unstructured world through variability in anatomy and function. An osteopathic perspective incorporates something from each of these schools of thought, while acknowledging the consistent yet adaptive nature of neural connections and the influence of motor system function on sensory processing.

During early life, movements progress from being visually triggered but guided by broad proprioceptive feedback (hitting the target) during the first weeks of life (von Hofsten & Fazel-Zandy 1984) to being guided by visual endpoint feedback between 4 and 5 months (von Hofsten & Fazel-Zandy 1984). At 12 weeks, undirected, flapping movements of an extended arm will hit a target. These movements are visually triggered but are guided by proprioceptive input; this is supported by the observation that using a glowing target as a trigger, these movements can be executed in the dark with the same accuracy as in the light (Clifton et al 1994). Frequent reversals of direction in hand trajectories during reaching movements begin to appear at 3.5–5 months, although they are not necessarily aimed at the target. These are probably visually directed. After 7 months, the infant begins to exhibit ballistic motion with visual endpoint guidance (Shumway-Cook & Woollacott 2000). During this period, modulation of motion-dependent torques with muscle torques develops. Visually guided movements of the extremities are emerging. The infant uses visual input to select muscle synergies. There is an increase in sequentially organized hand paths and a plateau in the number of hand reversals between 6 and 10 months. During this time, selective synergies develop in ballistic movements that use vision for endpoint guidance. Thus, visual input concerning accuracy is coordinated with proprioceptive input. Proprioception is used to fine tune. Although visualization is necessary to fix the target location, in the absence of vision, proprioceptive information can still guide the limb to the target (albeit somewhat clumsily). By 12 months, hand movements become smoother and are directed towards the midline of the toy. In early movements, children use muscle torques about the elbow and shoulder to generate excessive motion-dependent torques in the distal arm. By the end of the first year, they will use the muscle torques to control and counteract the motion-dependent torques and accomplish smoother movements.

Proprioception plays a major role in the guidance of limb movement. Consequently, the effect of limb trauma during birth, even when mild, is of concern to the osteopathic physician. Obviously, hand or shoulder presentations will place abnormal stresses on the infant's tissues which may affect biomechanical relationships and, subsequently, proprioceptive feedback from the affected extremity. More commonly, tissue strain will occur in the scalene, trapezius, upper ribs and shoulders when there is stretch placed on the neck as the shoulders and body are being delivered. This is especially true in larger babies. Upper extremity involvement may also be present when the child takes the first breath before the body and shoulders have been delivered. In this case, the rib and upper thoracic movement of attempted inhalation meets the resistance of the maternal vaginal tissues. These children often have significant respiratory complaints, so the shoulder involvement may be overlooked.

Adult grasp involves visually coding the object's size and orientation and converting this information into a motor pattern for orientation of the wrist, thumb and fingers. These size and orientation codes are processed in the parietal lobe and passed to the premotor cortex, where the patterns of movement are orchestrated (Ghez 1991). Information about size, shape and orientation is provided through visual and somatosensory input. The development of grasp involves several stages. The newborn's fingers will reflexively open when the arm is extended. This reflex is lost at 2 months, and the fingers now flex when the arm extends. Head and eye movements begin to be uncoupled after 2 months (Shumway-Cook & Woollacott 2000). This allows for greater flexibility and control. By 4–5 months, infants will begin to orient their hands towards the desired object (von Hofsten & Fazel-Zandy 1984); however, they do not appropriately size their open hand to the object until after the first year (Shumway-Cook & Woollacott 2000). By the age of 5 or 6 years, a child's ability to manipulate objects with the hands should be fairly well developed. Children without neurological problems who are observed to be awkward or clumsy in handling objects should be evaluated for mechanical stresses that may interfere with normal somatosensory input. Children with spasticity will develop mechanical stresses compensatory and secondary to abnormal muscle tone. These stresses may interfere with normal proprioceptive feedback, further alter muscle tone and impede optimum function. Addressing biomechanical stresses so that a child is able to express his or her fullest potential is very important. This does not mean that everything should be 'straightened out' or 'aligned' according to some textbook specifications. It does mean that the physician needs to assess the nature of the functional mechanics in the involved area and determine which characteristics are a manifestation of the child's brain injury and therefore the baseline from which he or she functions, which components have developed in compensation and may be necessary parts of altered movement strategies, and finally, which components have arisen in response to the compensation and are unnecessary.

SENSORIMOTOR INTEGRATION

The three sensory systems, used in posture and balance strategies, map to separate primary sensory areas of the cerebral cortex. Each primary area of the cortex communicates with the posterior parietal cortex where the sensory systems are integrated. These maps in the parietal cortex build a master plan of our body, its position in space and its spatial relationship to the external environment. These maps provide the necessary information for the motor cortex to control our movements.

The postural motor system can work very well using only two of the three sensory systems. This has been illustrated in studies where one or more sensory systems have been removed or altered. A study subject can mask the loss of one sensory system, but dysfunction of two sensory systems results in postural embarrassment. In practical terms we can use information from the functioning systems to mask a dysfunctional system. This is called compensation. So while there is redundancy between the sensory systems, the redundancy protects the individual. The plasticity of the nervous system allows us to compensate for degenerative changes in one system. However there is a limit beyond which failure of the postural motor system is expressed.

Abnormal posturing in newborns

Infantile postural asymmetry (IPA) is described as a condition of infancy involving changes to normal postural

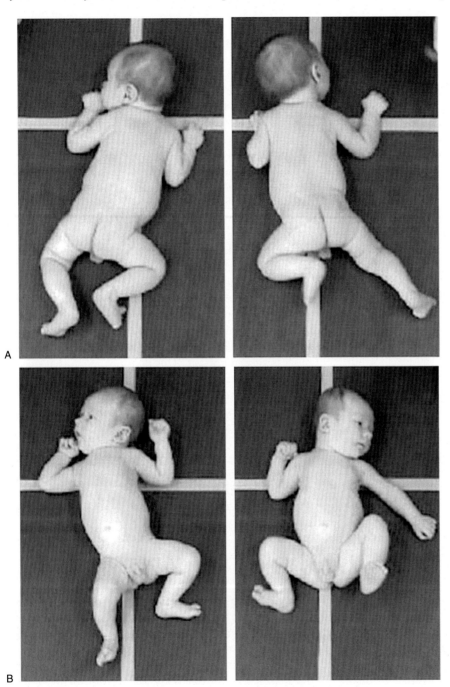

Fig. 9.11 • (A) Prone and (B) supine views of infant with fixed cervical side-bending. *Used with permission from Phillippi et al 2006 Patterns of postural asymmetry in infants: a standardized video-based analysis. Eur J Pediatr 165: 158–164.*

patterns and reflexes in the absence of organic disease such as cerebral infarction, neuromuscular disease, congenital malformation or tumor. The etiology and pathophysiology are unclear and described as idiopathic and postural or functional. There is some suggestion that early infantile asymmetry may be associated with plagiocephaly, temporo-mandibular joint dysfunction (St John 2002), progressive scoliosis (Canale et al 1982, Binder et al 1987), hip dislocation (Walsh & Morrissy 1998) and other structural asymmetries (Thompson 1980, Hamanishi & Tanaka 1994, Boere-Boonekamp & Van Der Linden-Kuiper 2001). Phillippi et al (2006) created a qualitative analysis scale of the asymmetry based on lateral flexion (truck convexity) and cervical range of motion during rotation. The presence of altered cervical rotation patterns and asymmetrical trunk convexity are the hallmarks present (Phillippi et al 2006), although other findings such as congenital plagiocephaly, hip dysplasia, foot malposition and/or torticollis may also be evident. Video analysis of infant response in the prone and supine positions was carried out (Fig. 9.11). Observers assessed the range of motion and appropriate coupling of cervical rotation and side-bending and the truncal response when the infant was stimulated to actively turn his head in one direction or the other (Table 9.1). Phillippi's video analysis (2006) showed that in infants younger than 4 months, active cervical rotation is associated with ipsilateral lateral flexion in the prone position, and contralateral side-bending in the supine position. Trunk convexity presented as asymmetric reactive movements in the trunk to the head orientation described above (Figs 9.12, 9.13). Phillippi categorized those children having predominantly asymmetric findings in truncal convexity as scoliosis type, while those children predominately having asymmetry in cervical rotation were categorized as torticollis type.

This simple tool for evaluating postural asymmetries has potential for use in the clinical setting for diagnosis, and perhaps more importantly, to assess the infant's response to treatment. The concept of IPA is very osteopathic in nature and accounts for the interrelatedness of body areas in many of the functional adaptations often seen in infants. In one small pilot study, infants with IPA who received osteopathic treatment had better outcomes than the control group (Phillippi et al 2006).

Table 9.1 Spinal convexity and rotation

Category	Description of spinal convexity
1	Equal convexity or no convexity
2	Convexity can be resolved to neutral and flexibility in other direction is present but slightly decreased
3	Convexity can be resolved to neutral and flexibility in opposite direction is present but obviously decreased
4	Convexity can only be resolved to neutral, resists movement to other direction
5	Convexity cannot be resolved to neutral, only a flattened curve
6	Convexity cannot be resolved
Category	**Description of active cervical spine rotation**
1	No restriction in motion
2	Slight decrease in active rotation in one direction, no preferential head position
3	Obvious decrease in active rotation to one side, but beyond midline. Able to overcome
4	Obvious decrease in rotation to one side, not beyond midline but may occasionally be overcome
5	Decrease in rotation to one side, not beyond midline and difficult to overcome

Adapted from Phillippi et al (2006).

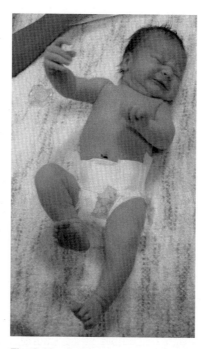

Fig. 9.12 • One-week-old boy with infantile postural asymmetry. Note cervical rotation to the left is coupled with torso side-bending to the right. Right rotation was restricted. *Used with permission of the Willard & Carreiro Collection.*

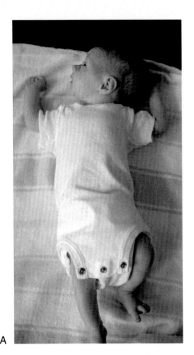
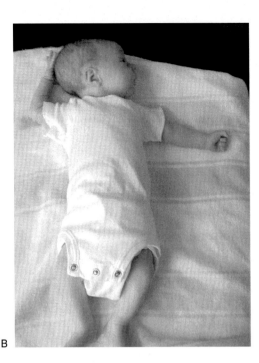

Fig. 9.13 • (A, B) Three-week-old girl with infantile postural asymmetry. *Used with permission of the Willard & Carreiro Collection.*

A

B

The center of gravity and posture

The relationship between the body's center of mass and the base of support must be maintained for postural stability. Shifts in mass distribution require changes in the position of the base of support. Feedback or compensatory mechanisms are evoked by sensory events following loss of balance. These are automatic postural adjustments influenced by vestibular information. These postural adjustments are reflexive and rapid, with relatively stereotyped spatial–temporal organization resulting in body sway. The spatial–temporal organization of these responses is referred to as a postural strategy. Strategies are scaled and refined through repetition. This represents a form of learning. Postural adjustments are typically initiated in structures closest to the base of support (Ghez 1991). Small movements at the ankles and knees will correct for perturbations in posture or balance. If the ankle or knee is unable to accomplish the necessary alteration in position, compensation must occur in the pelvis, hips or torso. This results in an exaggerated sway or torque as individuals attempt to correct and recover their balance. Elderly people tend to use their hips and trunks to stabilize their center of gravity, as opposed to younger people, who use their ankles. As the functional base of support declines there is an increase in sway while standing (King et al 1994). Elderly people also tend to make fewer but larger adjustments in muscle tension to combat sway, whereas young people make many, rapid, small adjustments in muscle tension (Panzer et al 1995). Children do not develop these mature strategies until the age of 7–10 years; prior to that time postural strategies are poorly organized.

A child's center of balance is higher (T12) than that of an adult (L5–S1). Consequently, the child requires more effort to maintain an erect stance and recover from perturbations. There is a rapid increase in postural responses during the first 4 years of life, and then a slight regression until adult-like reflexes are reached at approximately 7–10 years. Sensory systems play a vital role in these reflexes. Visual cues help to maintain posture in the 2–3-year-old. Removal or distortion of these cues results in shorter-latency postural reflexes. Vestibular input alone will not support postural reflexes in children under 7 years. However, as the postural system matures in the older child, posture and balance can be maintained through vestibular input. As would be expected, disturbances in vestibular function contribute to feedback dysfunction in the postural mechanism. Other factors adversely affecting the execution of appropriate postural strategies in children include visual abnormalities affecting depth perception, and joint restrictions, both physiological and iatrogenic. For example, when children with spasticity of the lower extremity are placed in orthotic devices which lock the ankle joint they will compensate for postural perturbations by using their hip and trunk strategies.

MECHANICAL ASPECTS OF POSTURE AND GAIT

When children begin walking, motor firing patterns in the hip stabilizers and muscles of the limbs are still immature.

This influences the phases of gait and the mechanics of the foot and ankle. During early walking, the swing phase is shortened to accommodate the instability of the standing limb by decreasing the time spent in single leg stance. As a result, stride length is shortened and cadence is increased. Young children also avoid cross-patterning movements between the upper and lower extremities, preferring to walk with the ipsilateral arm held stiff and slightly lateral. The wide-based gait and arm position reinforce stability. Foot mechanics in new walkers also differ. The plantar and dorsiflexors of the ankle lack mature firing patterns. This effects the eccentric contraction of the dorsiflexors as the foot moves from heel-strike to stance. Consequently most young walkers lack a true heel-strike phase, often

landing on the midfoot or preferring toe walking. The contribution of the toe-off phase is somewhat diminished as well. Most children initiate the stride from the hip and knee flexors rather than the foot. There is less knee flexion and ankle dorsiflexion during the swing phase, giving young walkers the appearance of a dropped foot. However, once the foot meets the ground, dorsiflexion actually increases and the knee is often kept in a slightly flexed position. The femur is externally rotated throughout the gait cycle. The external rotation in swing phase carries the pelvis laterally. As the pelvis rotates, the torso and arm are carried in the same direction. As previously described, this linear arrangement between the ipsilateral arm, torso, pelvis and leg is a stabilizing strategy (Fig. 9.14).

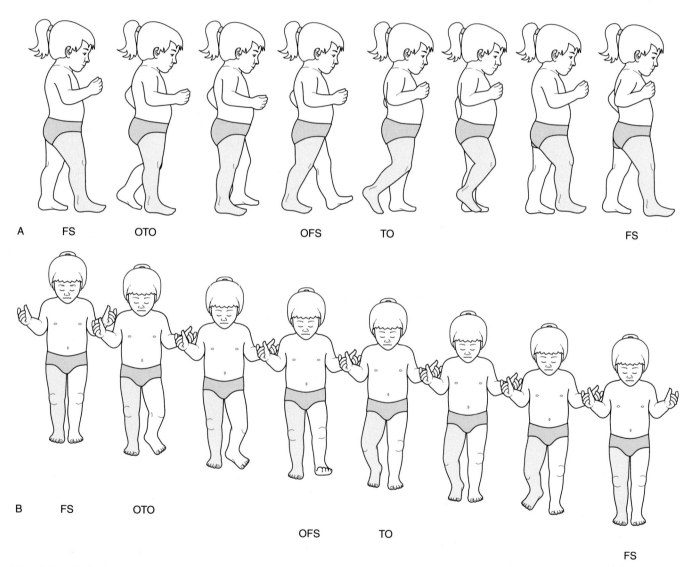

Fig. 9.14 • (A) Sagittal view of the gait of a 1-year-old girl. Tracings from individual move frames throughout one full gait cycle. The individual frames coincide with significant gait events. Gait cycle begins with right foot-strike (shaded) and ends with foot-strike of the same foot. (B) Frontal view. FS, foot strike; OTO, opposite toe-off; OFS, opposite foot-strike; TO, toe-off. *Reproduced with permission from Sutherland D H 1984 Gait disorders in childhood and adolescence. Lippincott, Williams & Wilkins, Baltimore.*

Maturing neurological processes affect coordination, stability and strength, all of which influence gait mechanics. Cross-patterning of the arms and legs emerges in most ambulating children by the second year of life (Burnett & Johnson 1971) and in all children by the fourth (Sutherland et al 1980). Children with upper extremity problems such as brachial plexus injuries or spasticity will often maintain the fixed arm position on the involved side while the uninvolved arm exhibits reciprocal swing. By 2 years of age the gastrocnemius and soleus muscles are better able to control the anterior momentum of the tibia as the foot contacts the ground. Deceleration of the tibia in concert with activation of the quadriceps produces knee extension as the leg moves

from stance to toe-off, although the propulsion of the toe-off phase is still rather insipid in the 2-year-old. By 2 years, maturing firing patterns in the muscles of the lower leg improve ankle control, resulting in better active dorsiflexion during the swing phase (Fig. 9.15). Since the ankle is now held in dorsiflexion as the foot meets the ground, a heel-strike pattern emerges. Improved coordination between the hip and pelvic stabilizers allows children to narrow their base of support, prolong the single leg stance phase and lengthen their stride. As the leg lengthens with growth, the stride will also lengthen. Children with leg length discrepancies may compensate with increased pelvic rotation and tilt during the swing phase of the short leg. Children with equal leg

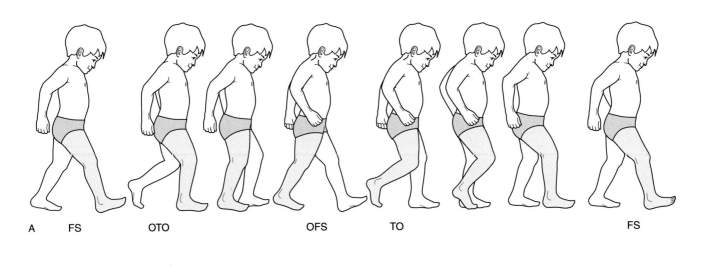

A   FS   OTO   OFS   TO   FS

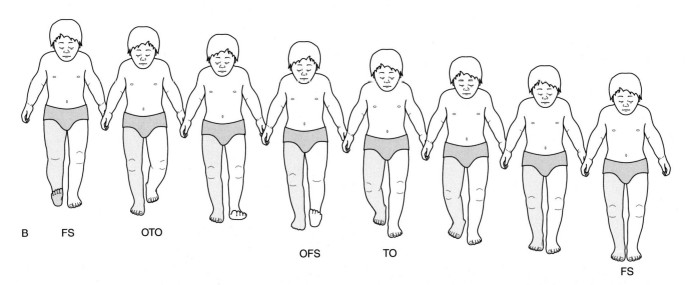

B   FS   OTO   OFS   TO   FS

Fig. 9.15 • (A) Normal gait pattern in a 2-year-old boy demonstrates the presence of heel-strike at the time of foot contact, reciprocal arm swing and increased step length. (B) Frontal view. FS, foot strike; OTO, opposite toe-off; OFS, opposite foot-strike; TO, toe-off. *Reproduced with permission from Sutherland D H 1984 Gait disorders in childhood and adolescence. Lippincott, Williams & Wilkins, Baltimore.*

lengths but variations in femoral and tibial height compensate with a combination of pelvic rotation and side-bending.

In adult walkers, there is a myofascial system of stabilization. It has been described by Vleeming and others (Gracovetsky 1985, Greenman 1990, Vleeming et al 1995a,b, Willard 1995) as extending from the foot through the lower limb via the peroneus longus, to the biceps femoris and ischial tuberosity, through the sacrotuberous ligament and the sacroiliac ligaments, crossing through the thoracolumbar fascias to the contralateral latissimus dorsi and the upper extremity. This system acts to absorb energy from one stride and release it into the next. This mechanism decreases the overall work of walking, posture and balance. Unfortunately this tensegrity mechanism is not well developed in young walkers, thus requiring a relative increase in energy expenditure when compared with an adult. Efficient and effective ambulation in children and adults relies on the orchestration of neurological and mechanical processes. Deficits or dysfunction in any of these components not only increase the workload of performing the task but also can severely compromise the child's functional ability to perform the task in a safe and reliable manner.

FACTORS WHICH ADVERSELY AFFECT THE POSTURAL MECHANISM

Ultimately, the failure of postural control mechanisms results in an increased incidence of falling. These individuals tend to sway more during quiet stance. They are unsteady when challenged by the environment, and have more difficulty in performing simultaneous motor tasks typically required in daily living. Body posture can be adversely influenced by diseases affecting the central nervous system, the peripheral nervous system, the eyes, the ears and the musculoskeletal system. The postural mechanism is also strongly influenced by the individual's body morphology, becoming adversely influenced as individuals gain weight above the appropriate value. There is some evidence that multiple factors can adversely affect the postural mechanism and that these factors are cumulative (Wolfson et al 1992). This cumulative effect is important to remember when evaluating children with handicaps. A child with very mild spasticity in the lower extremities may show significant signs of instability because of concomitant problems with visual acuity or depth perception. This can occur in association with corrective lens prescriptions that were too strong as well as those that were too weak. The influence of the visual system on posture cannot be emphasized enough.

Prescribing appropriate corrective lenses in the young child can be challenging. Close interprofessional cooperation between optometrists and osteopathic physicians can be very effective in corrective lens prescription.

The central nervous system contains the neural circuits that mediate sensorimotor integration and the postural control mechanism. Central processors are responsible for integrating sensory information about existing positional organization with postural requirements for voluntary movement. This integration has to play out against the backdrop of ever-changing spatial relationships. Impairment of central mechanisms will interfere with processing of sensory input and organization of motor output. The major diseases affecting the central nervous system involve ischemic, metabolic and degenerative processes. The most common factors affecting the central nervous system in children include cerebral insults such as cerebral palsy. Postural instability may result from ischemic insult to areas involved with proprioception, balance or motor coordination. Altered metabolism and absorption rates in the very young mean that pharmaceuticals causing minimal side effects in middle-aged people may produce clinically significant side effects in this population. Central nervous system degenerative disorders are rare in children but do occur. A good pediatric neurology text will give ample descriptions of these processes.

Sensory information, from skin, muscles and joints, is used to correct errors and adapt to changes in posture through feedback and feedforward mechanisms. Impaired function of the peripheral nerves carrying this sensory information will create deficits in feedforward control and consequently in the feedback control of posture. Demyelinating diseases may compromise function in the large, myelinated efferent nerves to muscles and can lead to demise of the postural control mechanism. Metabolic neuropathies such as those associated with nutritional deficits may alter sensory input. The function of afferent fibers is also influenced by compressive neuropathies.

The eyes provide a reference involving the horizontal plane of the earth. Loss or distortion of vision diminishes the transfer of this information to the postural control mechanism. Common factors affecting vision include degenerative diseases such as cataracts, errors of refraction (presbyopia), diseases of fluid imbalance (glaucoma) and restrictive diseases (strabismus).

The vestibular apparatus in the temporal bone uses a membrane-bound fluid system to detect the pull of gravity and movement of the head. Disease processes that alter this mechanism can produce dizziness, vertigo and postural embarrassment. The vestibular system is vulnerable to a loss of hair cells in the sensory organs as we age. Labyrinthitis, an acute and usually self-limiting disease of a viral nature, may cause severe vertigo and instability in patients. Similarly, Ménière's disease, a chronic disease thought to result from imbalances in endolymph production, will also result in postural instability.

The musculoskeletal system provides the vehicle through which the postural mechanism of the nervous system expresses itself. Defects in the musculoskeletal system result in compromise of posture as the system fails to respond to the appropriate neural commands. In addition, pain from musculoskeletal diseases can lead to restriction of motion of the limb, resulting in further compromise of posture. Postural control kinematics are the immediate response of the musculoskeletal system to motor signals. Muscle strength and the biomechanical relations of joints will affect an individual's ability to respond in an appropriate, efficient, effective and timely manner to perturbations in posture (Alexander et al 1992). In fact, assessment of stability during the performance of certain activities can be used to predict the risk of falling during related everyday activities (Topper et al 1993).

Factors affecting the musculoskeletal system in children include the muscular dystrophies, metabolic problems and developmental disorders of the muscle. More commonly, mechanical changes, degenerative and inflammatory diseases involving the joints and connective tissue structures, and structural changes such as scoliosis and unequal leg lengths, may affect posture. Scoliotic curves originating in the cervical and upper thoracic areas are often associated with cranial asymmetries, plagiocephaly or torticollis (Biedermann 1992). Thoracolumbar and lumbar scoliosis may be associated with leg length discrepancy. Sacral or pelvic unleveling results in abnormal muscle tensions and spinal curve compensation. This is especially true in growing children and adolescents. In the adult population, leg length discrepancies may present as pain in the back, neck or headache, and in some cases contribute to the development of arthritic changes in the vertebral column. Postural instability in children may contribute to various learning and behavior problems, including attention deficit disorder and pervasive developmental disorder. Many children who fall within these categories will demonstrate significant posture and balance dysfunctions when carefully tested. More often than not, the postural deficit is related to a biomechanical dysfunction, which can be addressed. Clinical evidence supports the use of various manipulative modalities to address joint imbalances and positional misalignments.

Deconditioning is a common factor in muscular weakness, restricted range of motion and altered movement strategies in patients of all ages. This can be addressed through reconditioning and postural alignment. Postural reconditioning exercise has been shown to be beneficial in improving balance and postural response. The program needs to be tailored to the patient's age and abilities. In infants, this may involve the parents placing the child's toys on one side of her body to encourage her to look or reach to that side. In older children, enthusiasm and interest have to be considered. It is easier to get children to participate in an activity that they enjoy. I often recommend swimming, tandem bike riding with a parent, early gymnastics, horseback riding or the martial arts. The benefits of dynamic and static postural training have been shown to persist for an average of 1.5 years in older patients. Province et al (1995) have shown that t'ai chi is beneficial in increasing postural stability in elderly patients. One study showed it to have greater long-term effects than physical therapy or weight training (Province et al 1995). Yoga and the Alexander technique are two other exercise programs that involve postural rebalancing. Large muscle group reconditioning has also been shown to improve postural adaptation and response to perturbed posture, especially in elderly patients, and should be considered in the adolescent or young adult. This can be accomplished through physical therapy (Hu & Woollacott 1994a, b) or weight lifting (McMurdo & Rennie 1994). The child's personality, abilities and interests need to be considered, to ensure that the child will engage in an activity at which he or she is most likely to be successful. Activities that can be employed to address the child's needs but avoid the boredom factor are especially desirable. I do not mean to imply that other therapeutic approaches should not be used. On the contrary, I see the aforementioned activities as supplementary and only to be used as a replacement where appropriate.

CONCLUSION

The postural system consists of three sensory systems and two motor systems integrated in the cerebral cortex to form the postural control mechanism. Defects in any of these components can lead to diminished postural function and increased instability, and eventually trauma from falling. Children have different postural strategies from adults. The maturation of appropriate postural mechanisms is influenced by the functional health of sensory and motor systems. Consequently, children with sensory or motor deficits continue to use immature mechanisms as they age. Regardless of age, individuals will alter postural strategies in response to pain or inflammation. The accumulation of defects in the components of the postural system accounts for a good deal of the postural embarrassment seen in patients. Facilitating optimum function of the components of the postural system will aid the child in meeting the demands of their environment and support the development of more appropriate strategies to use to meet their hidden potential.

References

Alexander N B, Shepard N, Gu M J et al 1992 Postural control in young and elderly adults when stance is perturbed: kinematics. J Gerontol 47: M79–M87.

Barrett D S, Cobb A G, Bentley G 1991 Joint proprioception in normal, osteoarthritic and replaced knees. J Bone Joint Surg [Br] 73: 53–56.

Biedermann H 1992 Kinematic imbalances due to suboccipital strain in newborns. J Manual Medicine 6: 151–156.

Binder H, Eng G D, Gaiser J F, Koch B 1987 Congenital muscular torticollis: results of conservative management with long-term follow-up in 85 cases. Arch Phys Med Rehabil 68: 222–225.

Boere-Boonekamp M M, Van Der Linden-Kuiper A T 2001 Positional preference: prevalence in infants and follow-up after two years. Pediatrics 107: 339–343.

Burnett C, Johnson E 1971 Development of gait in childhood II. Dev Med Child Neurol 13(2): 207–215.

Butterworth G, Cicchetti D 1978 Visual calibration of posture in normal and motor retarded Down's syndrome infants. Perception 7(5): 513–525.

Canale S T, Griffin D W, Hubbard C N 1982 Congenital muscular torticollis. A long-term follow-up. J Bone Joint Surg [Am] 64: 810–816.

Clifton R K, Rochat P, Robin D J et al 1994 Multimodal perception in the control of infant reaching. J Exp Psychol Hum Percept Perform 20(4): 876–886.

Ghez C 1991 The control of movement. In: Kandel E R, Schwartz J H, Jessell T M (eds) Principles of neural science. Elsevier, New York: 533–547.

Ghez C, Krakauer J 2000 The organization of movement. In: Kandel E R, Schwartz J H, Jessell T M (eds) Principles of neural science. Elsevier, New York: 653–673.

Goodridge J P, Kuchera W A 1997 Muscle energy techniques for specific areas. In: Ward R (ed.) Foundations of osteopathic medicine. Williams & Wilkins, Baltimore: 697–763.

Gracovetsky S 1985 An hypothesis for the role of the spine in human locomotion: a challenge to current thinking. J Biomed Eng 7: 205–216.

Greenman P E 1990 Clinical aspects of sacroiliac function in walking. J Manual Medicine 5: 125–130.

Hamanishi C, Tanaka S 1994 Turned head-adducted hip truncal curvature syndrome. Arch Dis Child 70: 515–519.

Horak F B, Nashner L M 1986 Central programming of postural movements: adaptation to altered support-surface configurations. J Neurophysiol 55(6): 1369–1381.

Hu M H, Woollacott M H 1994a Multisensory training standing balance in older adults: I. Postural stability and one-leg stance balance. J Gerontol 49: M52–M61.

Hu M H, Woollacott M H 1994b Multisensory training of standing balance in older adults: II. Kinematic and electromyographic postural responses. J Gerontol 49: M62–M71.

King M B, Judge J O, Wolfson L 1994 Functional base of support decreases with age. J Gerontol 49: M258–263.

Lee D N, Aronson E 1974 Visual proprioception and postural stability in infancy. Percept Psychophysiol 15: 529–532.

Levin M F 1996 Interjoint coordination during pointing movements is disrupted in spastic hemiparesis. Brain 119(1): 281–293.

McMurdo M E, Rennie L M 1994 Improvements in quadriceps strength with regular seated exercise in the institutionalized elderly. Arch Phys Med Rehabil 75: 600–603.

Magoun H I S 1973 Idiopathic adolescent spinal scoliosis. The D O 13(6).

Nardone A, Siliotto R, Grasso M et al 1995 Influence of aging on leg muscle reflex responses to stance perturbation. Arch Phys Med Rehabil 76: 158–165.

Nashner L M 1976 Adapting reflexes controlling human posture. Exp Brain Res 26: 59–72.

Nashner L M, Black F O, Wall C III 1982 Adaptation to altered support and visual conditions during stance: patients with vestibular deficits. J Neurosci 2(5): 536–544.

Olitsky S E, Nelson L B 2000 Growth and development of the eye. In: Behrman R E, Kliegman R M, Jenson H B (eds) Nelson textbook of pediatrics. W B Saunders, Philadelphia: 1895–1896.

Panzer V P, Bandinelli S, Hallett M 1995 Biomechanical assessment of quiet standing and changes associated with aging. Arch Phys Med Rehabil 76: 151–157.

Phillippi H, Faldum A, Jung T et al 2006 Patterns of postural asymmetry in infants: a standardized video-based analysis. Eur J Pediatr 165: 158–164.

Province M A, Hadley E C, Hornvrook M C et al 1995 The effects of exercise on falls in elderly patients: a preplanned meta-analysis of the FICSIT trials. JAMA 273: 1341–1347.

Reed E S 1982 An outline of a theory of action systems. J Mot Behav 14: 98–134.

Roncesvalles N, Jensen J 1993 The expression of weight bearing in infants between four and seven months of age. Sport Exerc Physiol 15: 568.

St John D, Mulliken J B, Kaban L B et al 2002 Anthropometric analysis of mandibular asymmetry in infants with deformational posterior plagiocephaly. J Oral Maxillofac Surg 60: 873–877.

Shumway-Cook A, Woollacott M H 1995 Motor control: theory and practical applications, 1st edn. Williams & Wilkins, Philadelphia.

Shumway-Cook A, Woollacott M H 2000 Motor control: theory and practical applications, 2nd edn. Lippincott, Williams & Wilkins, New York.

Simoneau G G, Ulbrecht J S, Derr J A et al 1994 Postural instability in patients with diabetic sensory neuropathy. Diabetes Care 17: 1411–1421.

Sutherland D, Olsen R, Cooper L et al 1980 The development of mature gait. J Bone Joint Surg [Am] 62: 354–363.

Sveistrup H, Woollacott M H 1993 Systems contributing to the emergence and maturation of stability in postnatal development. In: Savelsbergh G (ed.) The development of coordination in infancy. Elsevier, Amsterdam: 331.

Sveistrup H, Woollacott M H 1997 Practice modifies the developing automatic postural response. Exp Brain Res 114(1): 33–43.

Thompson S K 1980 Prognosis in infantile idiopathic scoliosis. J Bone Joint Surg [Am] 62-B: 151–154.

Topper A K, Maki B E, Holliday P J 1993 Are activity based assessments of balance and gait in the elderly population predictive of risk of falling and/or type of fall? J Am Geriatr Soc 41: 479–487.

Vleeming A, Pool-Goudzwaard A L, Stoeckart R et al 1995a The posterior layer of the thoracolumbar fascia: its function in load transfer from spine to legs. Spine: 753–758.

Vleeming A, Snijders C J, Stoeckart R et al 1995b A new light on low back pain: The selflocking mechanism of the sacroiliac joints and its implication for sitting, standing and walking. In: Vleeming A, Mooney V, Snijders C J et al (eds) The integrated function of the lumber spine and sacroiliac joints. European Conf Organ, Rotterdam: 149–168.

von Hofsten C, Fazel-Zandy S 1984 Development of visually guided hand orientation in reaching. J Exp Child Psychol 3: 378–388.

Walsh J J, Morrissy R T 1998 Torticollis and hip dislocation. J Pediatr Orthop 18: 219–221.

Willard F H 1995 The anatomy of the lumbosacral connection. Spine. State of the Art Reviews 9: 333–355.

Wolfson L, Whipple R, Derby C A et al 1992 A dynamic posturography study of balance in healthy elderly. Neurology 42: 2069–2075.

Woollacott M H 1993 Age related changes in posture and movement. J Gerontol 48: 56–60.

Woollacott M H, Shumway-Cook A 1990 Changes in posture control across the life span – a systems approach. Phys Ther 70: 799–807.

Woollacott M H, Shumway-Cook A, Nashner L 1986 Aging and posture control: changes in sensory organization and muscular coordination. J Aging Hum Dev 23: 97–114.

Woollacott M H, Debu B, Mowatt M 1987 Neuromuscular control of posture in the infant and child: is vision dominant? J Mot Behav 19: 167–186.

Woollacott M H, Burtner P, Jensen J et al 1998 Development of postural responses during standing in healthy children and children with spastic diplegia. Neurosci Biobehav Rev 22(4): 583–589.

Wurtz R H, Kandel E R 2000 Perception, motion depth and form. In: Kandel E R, Schwartz J H, Jessell T M (eds) Principles of neural science. McGraw-Hill, New York: S48–S69.

Further reading

Alexander N B 1994 Postural control in older adults. J Am Geriatr Soc 42: 93–108.

Angelaki D E, Hess B J M 1996 Adaptation of primate vestibuloocular reflex to altered peripheral vestibular inputs. 2. Spatiotemporal properties of the adapted slow-phase eye velocity. J Neurophysiol 76(5): 2954–2971.

Arendt R E, MacLean W E Jr, Halpern L F et al 1991 The influence of rotary vestibular stimulation upon motor development of nonhandicapped and Down syndrome infants. Res Dev Disabil 12: 333–348.

Arnold L E, Clark D L, Sachs L A et al 1985 Vestibular and visual rotational stimulation as treatment for attention deficit and hyperactivity. Am J Occup Ther 39(2): 84–91.

Balogun J A, Akindele K A, Nihinola J O et al 1994 Age-related changes in balance performance. Disabil Rehabil 16(2): 58–62.

Berg K O, Maki B E, Williams J I et al 1992 Clinical and laboratory measures of postural balance in an elderly population. Arch Phys Med Rehabil 73: 1073–1080.

Bertenthal B, von Hofsten C 1998 Eye, head and trunk control: the foundation for manual development. Neurosci Biobehav Rev 22(4): 515–520.

Black F O, Shupert C L, Horak F B et al 1988 Abnormal postural control associated with peripheral vestibular disorders. Prog Brain Res 76: 263–275.

Bundy A C, Fisher A G, Freeman M et al 1987 Concurrent validity of equilibrium tests in boys with learning disabilities with and without vestibular dysfunction. Am J Occup Ther 41(1): 28–34.

Butterworth G, Hicks L 1977 Visual proprioception and postural stability in infancy. A developmental study. Perception 6(3): 255–262.

Damiano D L, Abel M F 1996 Relation of gait analyses to gross motor function in cerebral palsy. Dev Med Child Neurol 38(5): 389–396.

De Negri M 1995 Hyperkinetic behaviour, attention deficit disorder, conduct disorder and instabilite psychomotrice: identity, analogies and misunderstandings. Commentary to Gordon's paper (Brain Development 1994, 15: 169–172) Brain Dev 17(2): 146–147.

Diener H C, Horak F B, Nashner L M 1988 Influence of stimulus parameters on human postural responses. J Neurophysiol 59(6): 1888–1905.

Forsstrom A, von Hofsten C 1982 Visually directed reaching of children with motor impairments. Dev Med Child Neurol 24(5): 653–661.

Freides D, Barbati J, Kampen-Horowitz L J et al 1980 Blind evaluation of body reflexes and motor skills in learning disability. J Autism Dev Disord 10(2): 159–171.

Freychat P, Belli A, Carret J P et al 1996 Relationship between rearfoot and forefoot orientation and ground reaction forces during running. Med Sci Sports Exerc 28(2): 225–232.

Gahery Y, Massion J 1985 Co-ordination between posture and movement. In: Evarts E V, Wise S, Bousfield D (eds) The motor system in neurobiology. Elsevier Biomedical Press, Amsterdam: 121–125.

Gimse R, Tjell C, Bjorgen I A et al 1996 Disturbed eye movements after whiplash due to injuries to the posture control system. J Clin Exp Neuropsychol 18(2): 178–186.

Goldberg M E, Hudspeth 2000 The vestibular system. In: Kandel E R, Schwartz J H, Jessell T M (eds) Principles of neural science. McGraw-Hill, New York: 801–816.

Greenman P E 1990 Clinical aspects of sacroiliac function in walking. Journal of Manual Medicine 5: 125–130.

Hansen P D, Woollacott M H, Debu B 1988 Postural responses to changing task conditions. Exp Brain Res 73(3): 627–636.

Harris N P 1981 Duration and quality of the prone extension position in four-, six-, and eight-year-old normal children. Am J Occup Ther 35(1): 26–30.

Hennessy M J, Dixon S D, Simon S R 1984 The development of gait: a study in African children ages one to five. Child Dev 55: 844–853.

Hills A P, Parker A W 1992 Locomotor characteristics of obese children. Child Care Health Dev 18: 29–34.

Horak F B, Diener H C, Nashner L M 1989 Influence of central set on human postural responses. J Neurophysiol 62(4): 841–853.

Horak F B, Nashner L M, Diener H C 1990 Postural strategies associated with somatosensory and vestibular loss. Exp Brain Res 82(1): 167–177.

Horak F B, Nutt J G, Nashner L M 1992 Postural inflexibility in parkinsonian subjects. J Neurol Sci 111(1): 46–58.

Janda V 1978 Muscles, central nervous motor regulation and back problems. In: Korr I M (ed.) The neurobiologic mechanisms in manipulative therapy. Plenum Press, New York: 27–41.

Jouen F 1984 Visual–vestibular interactions in infancy. Infant Behav Dev 7: 135–145.

Kandel E R 1991 Perception of motion depth and form. In: Kandel E R, Schwartz J H, Jessell T M (eds) Principles of neural science. Elsevier, New York.

Kandel E R, Schwartz J H, Jessell T M 2000 Principles of neural science, 4th edn. McGraw-Hill, Philadelphia.

Kantner R M, Clark D L, Allen L C et al 1976 Effects of vestibular stimulation on nystagmus response and motor performance in the developmentally delayed infant. Phys Ther 56: 414–421.

Katoh Y, Chao E Y S, Laughman R K et al 1983 Biomechanical analysis of foot function during gait and clinical applications. Clin Orthop Relat Res 177: 23–33.

Lesny I, Syrovatka A, Dourbravsky O 1975 Proceedings: Postural polymyography in children with minimal brain damage. Electroencephalogr Clin Neurophysiol 39(4): 440–441.

Lishman J R, Lee D N 1973 The autonomy of visual kinesthesis. Perception 2(3): 287–294.

McChesney J W, Sveistrup H, Woollacott M H 1996 Influence of auditory precuing on automatic postural responses. Exp Brain Res 108(2): 315–320.

McFarland D H, Lund J P, Gagner M 1994 Effects of posture on the coordination of respiration and swallowing. J Neurophysiol 12(5): 2431–2437.

Mills L 1919 The effects of faulty cranio-spinal form and alignment upon the eyes. Am J Ophthalmol 2: 493–499.

Mirka A, Owen Black F 1990 Clinical application of dynamic posturography for evaluation of sensory integration and vestibular dysfunction. Neurol Clin 8(2): 351–359.

Mitchell F L, Moran P S, Pruzzo N A 1979 An evaluation and treatment manual of osteopathic muscle energy procedures. Mitchell, Moran and Pruzzo, Valley Park, MO.

Nashner L M, Shupert C L, Horak F B 1988 Head–trunk movement coordination in the standing posture. Prog Brain Res 76: 243–251.

Nashner L M, Shupert C L, Horak F B et al 1989 Organization of posture controls:

an analysis of sensory and mechanical constraints. Prog Brain Res 80: 411–418.

Norre M E 1995 Head extension effect in static posturography. Ann Otol Rhinol Laryngol 104: 570–573.

Paige G D 1992 Senescence of human visual–vestibular interactions. 1. Vestibulo-ocular reflex and adaptive plasticity with aging. J Vestib Res 2: 133–151.

Petri J L, Anderson M E 1980 Eye and head movements in reading-disabled and normal children. Am J Occup Ther 34: 801–808.

Pyfer J L, Carlson B R 1972 Characteristic motor development of children with learning disabilities. Percept Mot Skills 35(1): 291–296.

Rider B A 1972 Relationship of postural reflexes to learning disabilities. Am J Occup Ther 26(5): 239–243.

Teixeira L F, Olney S J 1996 Relationship between alignment and kinematic and kinetic measures of the knee of osteoarthritic elderly subjects in level walking. Clin Biomech 11(3): 126–134.

Vleeming A, Pool-Goudzwaard A L, Stoeckart R et al 1995 The posterior layer of the thoracolumbar fascia: its function in load transfer from spine to legs. Spine 20: 753–758.

Weeks Z R 1979 Effects of the vestibular system on human development, Part I. Overview of functions and effects of stimulation. Am J Occup Ther 33: 376–381.

Weeks Z R 1979 Effects of the vestibular system on human development, Part II. Effects of vestibular stimulation on mentally retarded, emotionally disturbed, and learning-disabled individuals. Am J Occup Ther 33: 450–457.

Wells M R, Giantinoto S, D'Agate D et al 1999 Standard osteopathic manipulative treatment acutely improves gait performance in patients with Parkinson's disease [see comments]. J Am Osteopath Assoc 99(2): 92–98.

Westall C A 1986 Binocular vision: its influence on the development of visual and postural reflex eye movements. Ophthal Physiol Optics 6(2): 139–143.

Wheelwright E F, Minns R A, Elton R A et al 1993 Temporal and spatial parameters of gait in children. II: Pathological gait. Dev Med Child Neurol 35: 114–125.

Winter D A, Patia A E, Frank J S et al 1990 Biomechanical walking pattern changes in the fit and healthy elderly. Phys Ther 70(6): 340–347.

Wynne-Davies R 1975 Infantile idiopathic scoliosis. Causative factors, particularly in the first six months of life. J Bone Joint Surg [Br] 57(2): 138–141.

Zennou-Azogui Y, Xerri C, Leonard J et al 1996 Vestibular compensation: role of visual motion cues in the recovery of posturo-kinetic functions in the cat. Behav Brain Res 74(1–2): 65–77.

Chapter **Ten**

10

Movement, perception and cognitive development

CHAPTER CONTENTS

OVERVIEW OF THE PROCESS OF PERCEPTION

Our perception of the world in which we live is dependent on our senses. Each of our five senses, vision, hearing, taste, touch and smell, assist us in creating a map of the world we inhabit. We can think of our perception of the world as a map. Maps give us information about relationships. It may be the relationship between two cities, or between a mountain and a river, or between a chair and a table. Maps lay out a picture, which we use to navigate. Our perception of the world and the experiences we have are based upon and contribute to an inner map. The association cortex is a part of the brain which integrates information. It is involved in all learning: motor learning, visual learning, etc. The association cortex can be thought of as layers of information. Each layer of cells receives information from a different sensory system. As we develop and grow, the information carried by a sensory system is laid down like a map within that layer of cells. The different maps complement and enrich each other, creating a multisensory, multidimensional perception of our environment. We use this multisensory perception to interact effectively with the world. For example, if we are about to cross the street and we suddenly hear a loud car horn, we will quickly step back onto the pavement. Why? Because our auditory sense was stimulated by a sound frequency which somehow triggered an association with a large speeding vehicle, and for some reason this made us think of danger. Sensory experiences from our past – sound waves which were associated with a car, light waves which were associated with 1360 kg (3000 lb) of metal traveling very fast, perhaps even nociceptive stimulation from a past car accident – all converged to create an idea when we heard the car horn, resulting in a perception of danger.

Every minute of the day, in very subtle and very obvious ways, we use multisensory experiences from our past to interact effectively within the moment. These experiences converge to create a perception of what is happening and how to best respond. This is a form of learning. When the input from these sensory systems conflicts or a discrepancy exists between any of the sensory experiences, it may affect the individual's ability to interact with the environment.

Our perception of the world is plastic and it can change. Changes in perception occur in response to the type of stimulation experienced. This process continues throughout life, which is why a person can learn new skills, new concepts and completely new ways of thinking about things. Sensory stimulation concerning size, spatial relations, sounds, textures, taste, pain, comfort and a myriad of other experiences is collected and cataloged in the central nervous system. These records of experience can be thought of as 'maps' which can be compared and integrated. For example, information about size, color and shape, which allows us to recognize an object (the car), can be correlated with information about a physically painful experience (being hit by a car) to produce a very specific response. The neuromusculoskeletal system interacts in the process of creating our maps of the world. In fact, early in development, one of the most potent inputs into this process of mapping comes from the neuromusculoskeletal system. Problems that occur with sensory or motor control can have a large role in the person's ability to create maps and interact with their environment.

THE BIOLOGY OF LEARNING

The processes of proliferation, migration and aggregation of cells in the central nervous system begin very early in embryonic development and are completed prior to birth (see Ch. 1). Differentiation, synaptogenesis, remodeling and myelination begin later in the embryonic period and continue throughout life. These latter processes result in the formation, elimination and fine-tuning of intercellular connections. This is the physiological process of learning. All learning – emotional, physical, and cognitive – is accomplished by the formation, elimination and refinement of intercellular connections. The ability to pick up a cup of tea without spilling it, or lift a pen with the appropriate amount of tension so that it can still be moved across a piece of paper, are learned skills. Yet we do not have to think about these activities. They are spontaneous, almost unconscious movements which are based on incredibly complex processes. The ability to recognize the color blue, recall the word for a particular food, or add the numbers two and two, are also skills which for many people are spontaneous and almost unconscious. Yet these functions are also based upon incredibly complex processes. The ability to pick up a pen involves numerous chemical and electrical signals orchestrated in precise sequences and patterns which were learned and refined. The same is true for adding two plus two. Every time we learn something new,

we initiate the processes of differentiation, synaptogenesis and remodeling within the nervous system. A violinist is very sensitive to tone, vibration and pressure. Her receptor organs for tone, vibration and pressure will be highly developed. Cortical maps receiving input from hair cells, proprioceptors and touch receptors have a heightened sensitivity for receiving information about tone, vibration and pressure. A violinist will develop synaptic relationships from these sensory organs all the way to the cortex which enable her to precisely interpret tone, vibration and pressure. If we taught someone who did not play a musical instrument how to play the violin, that person's nervous system would use differentiation, synaptogenesis and remodeling to change the way in which tone, vibration and pressure are interpreted. If we took someone who played the violin and we prevented her from playing and listening for a period of time, she would lose some of her sensitivity to and ability to interpret tone, vibration and pressure; in other words, some of the intercellular organization which allowed her to play the violin would alter.

We are born with too many cells and too many intercellular connections in our nervous system. Through learning and development, we select out cells, and refine and define connections so that eventually we have many connections between fewer cells (Kandel et al 2000); this is called pruning. When we learn something new, such as standing, or jumping, or multiplying, instead of making a new cell, an existing cell will create new connections. Learning is a process of integration. The connections between interneurons in the spinal cord, the character of receptor sites present in the periphery and the interconnections developed in the cortex are all influenced by the type of stimulation experienced. A child who is taught a new skill will often learn the new task much more quickly than an adult. This becomes quite obvious on the ski slopes during school breaks. The adult will adapt previously learned skills to the new task. Unfortunately, familiar movement behaviors are often accompanied by familiar bad habits, which need to be corrected. The child, on the other hand, is learning a completely new skill and using the processes of differentiation, synaptogenesis and remodeling to perfect it. To some extent, the ease with which a person learns a new motor skill is influenced by his or her body type. A person who has long limbs will have long muscles. This person is working with long levers. A small movement proximally will create a large arc distally. A long lever requires greater precision than a short lever, so there is greater room for error. Consequently, children who are tall or long-limbed often seem ungainly or awkward until they 'grow' into their body.

A neural synapse can be thought of as a method of communication between cells. Many of the connections between cells are laid down before birth, creating a topographic map of the body. As the infant begins to move, interneurons are stimulated to plug into these circuits to refine the maps and the connections between them. The progression from random, spontaneous motions to planned intentional movements reflects the refinement of these connections. The accuracy and effectiveness of the infant's movements serve as a feedback control on the refinement of these maps and the connections between them, often resulting in alternative connections. As a result, people who do something well can do it in different ways that accommodate for different situations. If you drive to work every day, you learn that route very well, but you also know a few alternative routes. Those alternative routes are similar to different synaptic sequences which develop. In the same way if you do something frequently and you do it well, you have alternate means of doing it. Think about throwing a ball; you can throw overhand or underhand, you can throw soft balls and hard balls. Each of these activities requires a different series or sequence of connections, yet a professional pitcher will be able to successfully throw different-sized balls using different styles. Another example is tennis. Many people play tennis. They can hit the ball with a forehand stroke and a backhand stroke, overhand and underhand. I can only hit a tennis ball if it is on my right side (this is even after lessons!). My brother is quite good at tennis and has never been encumbered with such a limitation. When you can do something well, you are able to do that thing in many different ways. The same is true of more abstract skills such as doing mathematics or writing a sentence. If you are skilled at the task you can reach the same goal (determining the sum or constructing the sentence) through a variety of means. The ability to accommodate to different conditions is exactly why you are successful. You can create the same effect (hitting the tennis ball, adding the restaurant bill) by using various combinations of neuronal activities. In the former case, the activities are motor and in the latter they are cognitive, but in both cases you are dealing with a series of biochemical processes involving the internal maps of the parietal cortex. Children who have difficulties with motor or cognitive learning, and children who are handicapped, typically do not have a menu of options from which to choose. They may have one method, one strategy for accomplishing the goal. Any alteration in the conditions will disturb their ability to execute the skill effectively. Let us look at an obvious example.

Maura is a 9-year-old child with a mild spastic hemiparesis. Although initially delayed in developmental onset, she is now able to self-ambulate and perform virtually all self-care chores. When placed in a controlled environment such as the physician or therapist's office, Maura walks down the corridor with a slightly ataxic gait, but balance and stability are maintained. However, put this same child in a less pacific environment, i.e. the school yard or hallway, and her gait becomes quite unsteady, she falls to the side, flails her arms, trips, falls and despairs to her parents. Why? Maura has a very limited armamentarium of motor strategies. Under controlled conditions, when the stimulation around her is limited, she can execute these strategies effectively. However, when she is placed in an environment of spontaneous, random and varied stimuli, such as the unevenness of the ground, the movement of other people close by her, and the cheerful bellowing of her classmates, she is unable to adapt her motor strategies to accommodate and she loses her balance. Attempts can be made to remedy this unsteadiness by increasing postural stabilization through the use of rigid orthotic devices which lock the ankle, knee or hip to limit her sway. Unfortunately, these same orthotic devices interfere with the proprioceptive input she uses to aid her balance mechanisms. Furthermore, locking the ankle, knee or hip will impede the motor strategies she uses to maintain stability. This creates quite a dilemma for everyone trying to help.

Gross motor activities are not the only manifestation of limited options. Most cognitive processes are built upon the foundation of sensorimotor integration. Recognizing numbers and letters requires an understanding of shape and spatial relationships. Interpreting their meaning is an abstract process influenced by context and experience. In part, both logic and creativity evolve from conceptual frameworks which rely upon experiential knowledge. Children who have subtle difficulties with motor or sensory function often express cognitive learning disabilities because they cannot process information appropriately or easily. In effect they are limited in the variability of available strategies to process the information.

Internal maps

The nervous system is littered with maps – arrangements of cell bodies or axons which represent parts of our body, the external world and our emotional milieu. By far the majority of these maps are involved with sensory information, and mostly with somatosensory input. The axons of the dorsal root ganglia form a map of the body surface along the length of the spinal cord. Other maps exist in the brainstem, thalamus, cerebellum and cortex. Often, an area of the brain will have multiple maps, each receiving information from a specific sensory modality. For example, primary somatosensory cortex has many maps of the skin (Amaral 2000): one processes basic tactile information, another receives complex tactile input, and a third integrates tactile and proprioceptive signals to interpret the tactile recognition of objects (stereognosis). Though slightly different, each of these areas is primarily concerned with somatosensory information. They are considered unimodal association areas, because they focus on a single modality, touch (Amaral 2000). In turn, each of these unimodal areas will map information to adjacent cortical regions and so on and so on. Cortical areas which are integrating multiple types of information are called multimodal association areas. The multimodal association areas of the cortex are intimately connected to the hippocampus and play a significant role in creating a unified concept or perception, and representing it in memory (Amaral 2000). Multimodal sensory areas also project to multimodal motor areas that are involved with executing appropriate responses to the external world.

According to Saper et al (2000), 'multimodal association areas receive information from different higher order sensory areas and convey the information to higher order motor areas that organize planned action after appropriate processing ...'. Three areas of multimodal processing are of particular importance to perception and learning (Saper et al 2000). The posterior association cortex, composed of parietal, occipital and temporal lobes, is concerned with perception and language. This area is responsible for establishing a spatial map of the world around us. It integrates visual and somatosensory information, allowing us to maneuver around familiar spaces. The ability to get up in the middle of the night and go to the toilet without turning on any lights or causing any disasters is due to the posterior parietal cortex, as is the ability to pick up a pencil and move it across a piece of paper in a configuration which is a symbolic representation of a thought without tearing the paper or breaking the pencil. Through a somewhat more complex process, abstract ideas such as the ability to interpret 'same' versus 'equal' also involve the posterior parietal cortex.

The limbic area is involved with emotion and memory. The ability to convert short-term memory into long-term memory is mediated through this area. Emotional responses are weighted according to prior experience. Events which evoke memories of fear or joy are greeted with that same feeling. Events for which we have no preconceived emotional expectation are often met with nothing and a sense of 'having to process this'. Feeling 'nothing' is a very unfamiliar condition for most people of Western cultures, and many will refer to the person as 'being in a state of shock'.

Finally, the prefrontal cortex organizes movement and planning (Saper et al 2000). Phineas Gage is the classic example of an individual who had an injury to his frontal lobes, when a railroad spike pierced his skull. Although he survived the accident, his personality was irrevocably changed from that of a responsible, hard-working man to someone who was indecisive, unreliable, and prone to drinking. The prefrontal cortex is involved with decision making, weighing options and planning.

As can be seen, each of these areas is involved with multimodal processing – comparing and integrating information from primary sensory areas to construct a map, be it spatial, behavioral or emotional, which we use to respond to our world. Consequently, the association areas of the cortex are involved with all complex mental functions (Saper et al 2000). Damage to any of these areas of the cortex in an adult results in specific functional deficits. However, the situation is less clear when the damage occurs in the very young. Even in an adult, the brain is quite plastic and can demonstrate the ability to remodel so that function can be regained or alternative mechanisms can be expressed. The presence of many more cells, neurons and connections in the nervous system of the very young makes the potential for recovery that much greater. This is especially important to remember in young children with suspected cerebral injury from hypoxic or ischemic events. Even in the presence of magnetic resonance imaging (MRI) or computed tomography (CT) findings, the limitations of the child cannot be known completely. With appropriate stimulation and care, children may reach far beyond what the MRI scan predicts they can accomplish. Setting strict limitations is unfair to the child and the parents. Having said that, realistic and cautious guidance will help the parents and family set the tone for raising the child with appropriate stimuli, support systems and boundaries.

The complex workings of the many multimodal areas of the cortex are dependent on optimum function of the peripheral sensory system. If aberrant or distorted signals are carried to these association areas, then the maps, the process of integration and the appropriateness of the response will suffer. Consequently, anything interfering with the normal function of sensory receptors, their axons or interneurons in the spinal cord and brainstem may manifest in the child's ability to cognitively, emotionally or mechanically interact with his environment. Our perception of a stimulus will be influenced by the way in which it is integrated with everything we are experiencing at that moment. If we are using all of our attention to maintain our balance while sitting at our desk, we may not be able to attend to the teacher or the mathematics problem in our book. We may have to change our position every minute or two. If our internal map of the space around us is distorted, that may influence our ability to interpret letters on a page or a voice speaking across the room. Our response to and perception of a stimulus are affected by internal maps. And, as we have discussed, much of the information contained in these maps is derived from input coming from the musculoskeletal system in the form of proprioception, vibration, pressure, stretch, temperature, etc. In children with motor impairment, the information coming into the maps will be distorted, and consequently that child's perception of the stimulus and his or her response to it is affected.

NATURE VERSUS NURTURE

The nature–nurture question always arises when one begins to discuss learning and development. A child's tendency to excel in areas in which one or more parent excels is probably due to two major factors: genetics and exposure. An individual may be genetically predisposed to a certain response in a certain situation. Neurochemicals secreted under specific conditions may turn on a gene. When an individual possesses a specific skill, such as playing the violin, we need to look at the sensory and motor systems involved.

In this case, they would be vibratory, auditory, pressure sense and very fine motor control. The penchant for highly developed function of those systems may be present genetically, and when the child is placed in the proper stimulatory environment (his parents are both musicians), he is able to manifest the skill. This combination of genetic predisposition and environmental factors is also thought to be the mechanism behind many psychological and psychiatric disorders.

EARLY MOTOR AND SENSORY DEVELOPMENT ARE LINKED

The integration of the developing motor and sensory systems will influence perceptual and cognitive development (Bushnell & Boudreau 1993). Traditionally, sensory system development was considered as the key step in the ontogeny of motor behavior. Current research suggests that the development of motor behaviors is a permissive feature in the ontogeny of cortical sensory, cognitive and sensorimotor integration. Motor patterns emerge through dynamic and symbiotic interactions between the organism and its environment. Based on sensorimotor integration, the emergence of particular motor abilities may actually determine some aspects of perceptual and cognitive development. Motor control may serve as a control parameter in the development of the whole organism. The development of locomotion facilitates an expansion of perceptual development in the infant (Bushnell & Boudreau 1993). The development of self-generated locomotion in infants allows them to increase their perceptual and cognitive lives. The infant can start coding locations in terms of landmarks and not as an extension of self. Becoming mobile serves as a 'setting event', increasing the likelihood of other experiences.

Let us look at this from the beginning. The newborn infant plays a passive role in her environment. People, things and pets come into her field of awareness and leave again. The ability to interpret their significance will depend on her experiences with them. If every time the child is hungry her mother comes into view and nurses her, the infant will associate the scent of her mother with feeding, satiation and comfort. The parents hang a mobile over their child's crib, and eventually she notices it in her visual field. Weeks later, the flexor and extensor tone in her upper extremities begins to come into balance and she starts randomly moving her arms. Then one day the infant swipes her arm and hits the mobile. 'What was that?' She looks. 'It's that thing.' Proprioceptive information from the articular relationships at her shoulder, elbow, wrist and hand will provide a map of the position of her arm in space. This proprioceptive information comes together with visual information concerning the position of the mobile above her crib. Each time the child randomly hits the mobile, she confirms, corrects and compares the proprioceptive and visual input

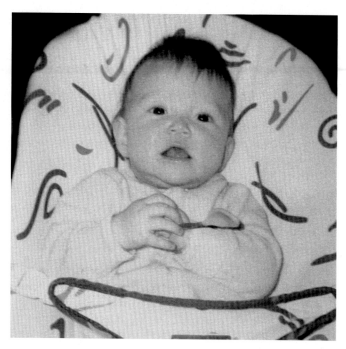

Fig. 10.1 • Hands meet, establishing the individual's midline.

which establishes the map of the spatial location of the mobile. Signals from her retina encoding information about size, shape, color and density are correlated and integrated with signals from her extremities regarding distance, density, shape and position. This is the beginning of understanding. The child's sense of space, distance and depth is initiated in the random swatting of the mobile. Eventually, she will be able to purposefully and accurately reach out and touch the mobile, but for now she will refine the necessary movement patterns through trial and error, using feedback from visual and somatosensory systems. What happens if one arm does not move as easily as the other? Suppose there was some damage to the motor system affecting an arm, or the child's clavicle was injured and the range of abduction was impaired. How does that affect the child's sense of her midline, or of distance or depth? A midline is not an esoteric idea. When, as infants, we bring our two hands together, we find the middle of our space, our physical midline (Fig. 10.1). Our arms extend equidistantly from that line, and information concerning joint position in space is bilaterally symmetrical. This construct helps us to establish our center of balance. It gives us a place that we can use to establish relationships between our self and something in our environment. What happens if our midline is shifted? How does that affect our ability to maintain balance? How does it affect our ability to learn?

In order to read, one must have a certain appreciation of the shape and the distance between letters and words. In order to write, a child needs a sense of the center of the page and boundary of the line to appropriately space letters and words. A child needs to be able to move the pencil smoothly across the paper with just enough pressure to make a lead marking but not tear the page. To read a book or write a sentence requires a certain amount of attention. The child needs to be able to maintain his or her balance in the chair without listing, tilting or becoming distracted. Each of these skills is influenced by vestibular, proprioceptive and visual interactions. From an osteopathic perspective, children who have difficulties in using their body are at risk of creating distorted spatial maps that may influence their effectiveness in a classroom environment.

VISUAL PERCEPTUAL DEVELOPMENT

When you touch someone you love, when you see something that is beautiful, or when you hear music which soothes, you are not touching with your hand, or seeing with your eyes, or hearing with your ears. You receive a stimulating signal of pressure, temperature, auditory frequency or light wave which results in an electrical impulse in your central nervous system and the secretion of chemicals. Your brain interprets the electrical stimulation and the chemicals which are secreted so that you feel you are touching someone you love, or you are seeing something red, or you are listening to Bach. If any of the connections from the peripheral receptor to the brain are disrupted, your ability to interpret the stimulation will be affected. We may all have different perceptions of blue; however, we have all learned to call it blue. Language is simply a symbolic representation of some chemistry happening in our brain.

For example, light focused on the retina through the cornea and lens is absorbed by the photoreceptors of the retina. These photoreceptors, the rods and cones, contain visual pigments which absorb the light, triggering a cascade of events which culminates in an alteration in the membrane potential of the photoreceptor cell (Tessier-Lavigne 2000). The photoreceptors transduce the absorbed light into electrical signals represented as a graded change in membrane potential, not as an action potential. This provides the photoreceptor with a certain amount of flexibility regarding the quality and quantity of the signal. An action potential can be seen as a binary signal: it is on or off. A cell capable of producing a graded change can generate a spectrum of signals. Interneurons such as bipolar, horizontal and amacrine cells transmit signals from the photoreceptors across lateral and vertical pathways to the ganglion cells of the optic nerve. The interneurons convey the signals to the ganglion cells in a spatiotemporal sequence related to the location of the signaling photoreceptor and the intensity of the stimulus. By this mechanism, the retinal signal is transformed into something that the cortex can use to interpret contrast and changing intensity (Tesser-Lavigne 2000). Obviously, focusing the light precisely on the retina

is of the utmost importance in this process. When the lens and cornea are unable to effectively focus light, the signals are affected and we perceive a blurred image. This is what happens in people with visual acuity problems.

The higher visual system is immature at birth and develops through appropriate stimulation and refinement. When higher centers receive disparate signals from the two retinas, the brain will suppress the aberrant input, leading to amblyopia. Amblyopia is cortical blindness. It can occur in children who have diplopia or significant differences in visual acuity between their eyes. Just like cells everywhere else in the nervous system, the cells of the visual cortex need to be stimulated to function. If stimulation does not occur, the connections and organization of the cells will be affected. In a child with esotrophia or exotrophia (an eye that deviates) to the extent that a double image is created, the brain will shut off the signal from the deviant eye. Cells in the visual cortex receiving signals from the photoreceptors of the deviant eye will be deprived of stimulation and will not develop. Although the eye, the retina and the nerves may be functional, the visual cortex cannot interpret the signal coming from that eye. This is referred to as cortical blindness. There is a window of opportunity during which amblyopia, or cortical blindness, can be reversed. Most texts place this between 3 and 5 years of age.

The cells of the visual cortex are organized into six horizontal rows based on function. They are then arranged into vertical columns called orientation columns, which respond to similar receptive fields (Wurtz & Kandel 2000). Dispersed between and within the orientation columns are blobs of cells which respond to color. Alternating with the orientation columns are ocular dominance columns which receive signals from a single eye and are responsible for binocular vision. Our brain takes the information from these columns, rows and blobs, and interprets it into a picture, which we recognize as shape, form, movement or color. Deciding what to call this interpretation, is a completely different process. First, we need to understand the signal as shape or form or movement or color; then we can name it.

Our ability to recognize a visual stimulus depends on associating shape, form, motion and color (Wurtz & Kandel 2000). Our sense of shape and form develop through our experiences with touch. The development of hand movements facilitates different stages of the ontogeny of touch perception (Bushnell & Boudreau 1993). For example, an infant seeing a block does not initially interpret it as such. Through holding it and playing with the block, the child gathers proprioceptive input from her joints and muscles and begins to form a map of the spatial relations within the object. This map can be integrated, compared and contrasted with the map formed from visual input. Have you ever noticed that you can reach for an object and your hand will conform to its shape and size? You do not even have to pay attention to the movement. Your arm does not overshoot the object, and you do not misjudge its size. This characteristic can be thought of as touch perception. The emergence of touch perception occurs during the first year of life. The perception of size arises at about 2 months, that of texture at 6 months, that of weight at 9 months, and that of shape configuration at 12–15 months (Shumway-Cook & Woollacott 1995). The inability to execute specific hand movements may serve as a barrier, adversely affecting perceptual and cognitive development. There are three phases of infant manual behavior: clutching (0–3 months), which is typical of the behavior used by adults to determine volume; rhythmical stereotypes (4–10 months), which is the behavior used by adults to assess hardness and texture; and complementary bimanual activity (>10 months), which requires the development of postural mechanisms and resembles movements used by adults to determine configurational shape.

At birth, the visual system is intact from the retina to the cortex. Visual acuity is estimated to be 20/400 at birth. By 3 years, it is between 20/30 and 20/20. In newborns, there is little or no accommodation; they maintain a fixed focus at approximately 20 cm (Harcourt 1974). Hyperopia is present at birth (5 diopters), reducing to 2.5 diopters at 3 years and 1 diopter by 8 years. Pupillary light reflex appears in the 29th to 31st week of gestation. Fixation and convergence reflexes are present at birth but are intermittent and poorly organized. By 6 weeks, the infant has conjugate vision but may still exhibit divergence. By 10 weeks, visual tracking is a smoother, controlled activity. Infants begin to recognize their mother's face at 4 months; prior to this, their visual acuity (contrast sensitivity) is too poor to resolve the details of the face. At 3.5 months, they will demonstrate visual expectations to regularity in slide show presentations (Harcourt 1974). Orientation selectivity is present at birth, and ocular dominance appears within the first few weeks. The ocular dominance columns of the visual cortex segregate from each other, and binocular depth perception develops at 4 months. In humans, susceptibility to visual acuity damage continues to exist until 6–8 years. During this time monocular vision or deprivation of visual stimulus will result in cortical blindness or amblyopia.

Motor development facilitates the ontogeny of depth perception in the visual system (Bushnell & Boudreau 1993). The development of depth perception is contingent on three cues: kinetic information, binocular information, and pictorial information. Movement of the head may be necessary for kinesthetic analysis of depth perception. There needs to be enough oculomotor control present for convergence, so that the infant may gain binocular information. Inconsistent vergence movements are first detected at 1 month, consistent movements are observed at 3 months, and saccadic eye movements will re-establish disrupted vergence at 6 months. Pictorial information is available from perceptualization of the image as well as prior knowledge.

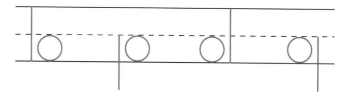

Fig. 10.2 • Reading requires an appreciation of shape and spatial relationships. The letters 'b', 'p', 'd' and 'q' are composed of a circle and a vertical line. The unique relationship between these geometrical figures gives each letter its identity. One cannot interpret the symbol 'b' until one can distinguish it from the symbol 'd', etc.

It first appears between 5 and 7 months. Manipulating the object in the infant's hand may be the motor skill required to promote prior knowledge of the object for use in pictorial cues for depth perception. Manipulative skills become prominent at 6 months.

Our ability to interpret shape and form from visual information is influenced by dexterity and manual development. Reading requires the accurate interpretation of the shapes of letters collected together to represent an idea such as 'dog'. The interpretation of 'd' is distinct from that of 'b' or 'p'. Each requires an appreciation of a circular and a linear component, and the relationship between the two (Fig. 10.2). Before a child can comprehend that a certain set of shapes (d–g–o) arranged in a particular pattern (d–o–g) represents an idea, he needs to recognize the individual shapes 'd', 'g', and 'o'. We understand the placement of the linear component by its orientation to the center of the circular component. We established our sense of center with the early random batting movements, and our sense of shape with object manipulation. Why does 'd' become 'b' or 'p' for some children? If the identification of the visual symbol 'd' is based upon a kinesthetic knowledge of shape and spatial relationships, then musculoskeletal impairment has the potential to influence a child's cognitive understanding of the different shapes 'd', 'b', and 'p'. Many children with learning disabilities will also have subtle balance and coordination impairments, which can be unmasked by stressing multiple sensory systems. Asking the seated, unsupported child with visual processing issues to 'look up over your head and close your eyes' will often result in the child falling backwards. Another test involves sitting the child at a table and giving him a task, such as drawing a house or adding numbers. Once the child is involved in the task, suddenly call his name or make a distracting sound. Often, the child will lose his balance in the chair. This is similar to an exaggerated startle response.

AUDITORY PERCEPTUAL DEVELOPMENT

Auditory perception is dependent on three things: the appropriate transduction of sound waves into electrical signals, filtering out of background noise, and the reconstruction of complex sound patterns into recognizable bytes. Small changes in air pressure move the tympanic membrane and its attached malleus, which shifts the stapes and incus. Movement of the incus against the oval window of the cochlea affects the fluid within the scala vestibuli and indirectly the scala tympani and scala media (Fig. 10.3). These changes affect the basilar membrane of the cochlea (Hudspeth 2000). Bony or connective tissue disruption within the external auditory canal or middle ear will impede this process and lead to conductive hearing loss. The basilar membrane is a small connective tissue structure, which varies in width and thickness along its 33 mm length. Because of this, various areas will be affected differently, based on the frequency, amplitude and intensity of the fluid wave (Hudspeth 2000). Depending on how the basilar membrane moves, the hair cells will be driven into excitatory, inhibitory or neutral positions. Therefore, through the action of the hair cell, the mechanical stimulus of the wave is transduced into an electrical signal. This signal is sent via the cochlea nerve to the cochlea nucleus and into the central auditory pathways to the cortex. Along this route, the signals are processed and analyzed (Hudspeth 2000). The process by which these electrical signals are translated into the symbolic context of language or vice versa involves many areas of the cortex, and is unclear and beyond the scope of this chapter. However, it is important to recognize that the processing of language involves many different areas of the cortex, including areas concerned with integrating visual or somatosensory information (Dronkers et al 2000). Consequently, abnormalities of language processing, such as dyslexia, may result from disturbances in the integration of visual or somatosensory information, or from distorted input.

At birth, the auditory system is functioning; however, the cerebral cortex has not reached a state of maturity sufficient to handle auditory sensory information for perception. Language is the symbol system for the exchange and storage of information. The development of language is dependent on: afferent neural input (hearing, vision), intact CNS function and neural output to functional vocal structures (Coplan & Gleason 1990). Normal hearing occurs in the range of 250–16000 Hz (cycles per second) or amplitude of 0–120 dB HL (decibels hearing level).

A review of the literature shows that between 4% and 20% of school-age children have hearing loss. Hearing loss may be unilateral or bilateral, and conductive or sensorineural. Conductive hearing loss results from dysfunction or interference in the transmission of sound to the cochlea, vestibule and semicircular canals. Air conduction is usually impaired. The most common causes include atresia of the canal, ossicular malformation, tympanic membrane abnormality, and blockage of the canal by a foreign body, cerumen impaction, and effusion in the middle ear. Conductive hearing loss affects all frequencies; however, bony conduction is usually preserved. Sensorineural hearing loss occurs when dysfunction or impairment of the cochlea hair cells or auditory nerve affects stimuli received through both air and bone conduction. Lower-frequency hearing may be less affected; however, one must remember that speech occurs in higher frequencies. Common causes of sensorineural hearing loss include hypoxia, intracranial hemorrhage, meningitis, hyperbilirubinemia, measles, mumps and, rarely, chicken pox.

Masking is the process by which the brain filters out background noise based on phase differences. Sound waves will reach the ears at slightly different times. This difference is used by the brain to screen out unwanted sound. Binaural hearing is required for masking. Children with unilateral deafness may have difficulties in isolating a sound

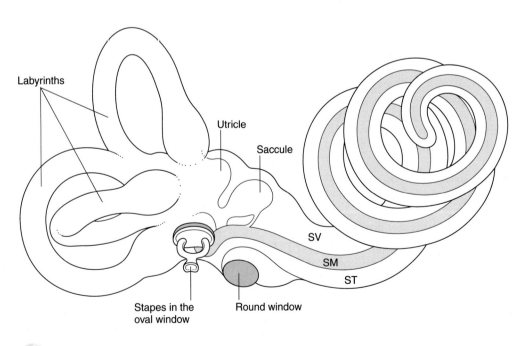

Fig. 10.3 • Schematic representation of the cochlea and labyrinths. SV, scala vestibuli; ST, scala tympani; SM, scala media. The shaded area represents the endolymph within the scala media.

Labyrinths

Utricle

Saccule

SV

SM

ST

Stapes in the oval window

Round window

such as the teacher's voice in a noisy environment like the first-grade classroom. This is especially true if the background noise occurs within the same frequencies as that to which the child is trying to attend. Partial hearing loss affects sibilants, which have high frequency and low amplitude, such as /s/, /sh/, /f/, /th/, while lower frequencies such as /r/, /m/, /v/ are unaffected. Children with a partial hearing loss may not be diagnosed until they enter school and exhibit an apparent learning disability.

Otitis media with effusion (OME) usually results in 10–50 dB hearing loss in acute cases; chronic otitis media results in 50–65 dB hearing loss, which includes most speech sounds. This hearing loss is usually temporary. However, during the first year of life, children with 130 days of OME will score one standard deviation lower on language skills than children with less than 30 days of OME.

Language disorders represent a dysfunction of cortical processes specifically involved with receptive and expressive function. A language disorder may be phonetic, such as deviant sound production, because the interpretation of sound is dysfunctional and children speak as it sounds to them. Another language disorder involves syntax, i.e. word order and grammar. The interpretation of word meaning and word relationships represents a disorder of semantics, while disorders of pragmatics affects the social appropriateness of language. Language disorders may involve one or more than one of these characteristics as an expressive or receptive function. Depending on the character of the disorder, sign language may be beneficial as a treatment and diagnostic modality. Often, language disorders are assumed to result from a problem with hearing. But, as we have seen, multiple sensory systems are involved with cognitive development. Think back to the example of the child who is unable to differentiate between the letters 'd', 'b', and 'p' because of a motor impairment. What will happen when that child is shown the letter 'd' and told the sound 'dah', then the letter 'b' and told the sound 'bah', and so on? How will the child discern the relationships between these letters and their sounds when he cannot consistently recognize the symbol for the sound?

Speech patterns are based on fluency, the rate and rhythm of the flow of speech. Very young children begin to mimic the speech patterns of their native language with early babbling. Fluency disorders (dysfluency) occur when there is impaired rate or rhythm of the flow of speech. Physiological dysfluency peaks between 2 and 4 years of age and then resolves. It is usually represented as phrase or whole-word repetition, such as 'can I–can I' or 'can–can'. A more abnormal form of dysfluency may also occur as part-word or initial-word sound; Wwwwwwwwwwhy? or wuh-wuh-wuh why? Alfred Tomatis reported that stuttering tends to be related to the length of the longest syllable of the spoken language. That is, the duration of the sound which the child stutters on is the same as the longest syllable.

Tomatis suggested that the child is somehow delayed in processing what he is hearing himself speak, and suggested 'abnormal cerebral representation of language and/or generalized abnormality of interhemispheric communication as the basis for stuttering' (Tomatis 1991). He reported that by using earphones to change the length of the stuttered sound, the child would revert to a smooth, uninterrupted speech pattern. Osteopaths have anecdotally found an association between mild head trauma and the development of stuttering (chart review and practitioner survey). The question of whether stuttering is a language dysfunction or a vocal dysfunction is an interesting one. Vocal disorders are not disorders of language or perception, but represent a dysfunction of the mechanical component of speech.

Receptive language skills precede expressive skills. Very early in life, children can demonstrate receptive language skills. This may manifest as looking for their bottle when a parent verbally indicates that it is time for feeding, or glancing at the family pet when its name is mentioned. Most children demonstrate the ability to point to an object before 10 months of age, although they often cannot name it until after the first year. Children will respond to the word 'no' before they can say it (often this ability is inexplicably lost between the ages of 2 and 18, but that is another story). The babbling speech of infants often contains the inflections found in the language to which they are exposed and probably represent the first attempts at mimicry. Tomatis (1991) reports that the babbling of infants also tends to fall within the frequency range of the home language. Children raised in multilingual homes are frequently slightly delayed in expressive language skills, although receptive skills are appropriate for age. As might be expected, once speech develops, these children seem to have a proficiency at learning new languages. In general, individuals appear to have greater fluency in languages that have frequency ranges which fall within the range of the native tongue.

Much of what is known about language was learned by studying people with language disorders secondary to cortical injury. Our understanding of the processes contributing to the formation, comprehension and expression of language is still vague. Localization of function is the phrase used to describe the condition by which any given area of the brain is involved with a specific process. For example, seeing a word, hearing a word, thinking of a word and speaking a word all involve different areas of the brain (Kandel et al 2000). Furthermore, the location of cognitive processes involved in each of these tasks is different from the sensory areas involved with language. For example, understanding the written word c–a–t does not occur in the visual cortex, but the visual cortex is needed to see the word. Language is a symbolic representation of a concept – a cat, a hug, to sleep. These are all concepts, and language is the means by which they are communicated. Whether spoken, written, drawn or signed, the message symbolizes an idea.

We can translate our ideas into any of these forms of language and we can interpret each of these forms into an idea. But each of these tasks occurs in a different area of the brain. Areas of association cortex in the frontal, parietal, temporal and occipital lobes of the dominant hemisphere are involved with language function (Dronkers et al 2000). The dominant hemisphere is the left in most people. The right or non-dominant hemisphere is concerned with the inflection, timing and rhythm of expressive language, which can be thought of as the emotional context.

THE VESTIBULAR SYSTEM AND COGNITIVE DEVELOPMENT

The vestibular apparatus is complete by 9.5 weeks of gestation, and the vestibular nuclei are functional by 21 weeks. The vestibular apparatus is composed of labyrinths, small delicate organs located in the petrous portion of the temporal bone and capable of sensing extremely small changes in position. They are of adult size and functional by the third trimester of pregnancy. From then on, any growth occurring in the child's body has to occur around these organs. As was discussed in previous chapters, this has a profound influence on growth and development. The vestibular labyrinth has five organs: a utricle, an ampulla and three semicircular canals oriented 90° from each other (Fig. 10.4). There is one labyrinth system in each temporal bone, and they act as mirror images of each other. The labyrinth system is lined by epithelial cells, which produce endolymph. Within each organ is a cluster of hair cells that can transduce physical movement into electrical signals (Goldberg & Hudspeth 2000). The hair cells are bathed by endolymph. As the head changes position, the hair cells are moved through the endolymph. Through a mechanism similar to that in the cochlea, the hair cells of the vestibular apparatus are stimulated and a signal is sent to the vestibular nuclei (Goldberg & Hudspeth 2000). The utricle and ampulla sense linear accelerations, while the semicircular canals, by virtue of their vertical, posterior and horizontal positions, sense rotational movements. Because the two vestibular organs are mirror images of each other, and when one is stimulated the other is inhibited, the brain can compare the signals to determine the direction of movement. A very simplified example can be used to illustrate this rather complex process; when you rotate your head to the right, the hair cells located in the right horizontal canal increase their rate of firing (Fig. 10.5). The hair cells in the left horizontal canal decrease the rate of firing. The signal from the right will be interpreted as right rotation of the head. If there is an abnormality in the system such that the signal from one side is decreased, then the brain will interpret that as an increased signal from the contralateral side and the person will experience a spinning sensation. Conditions which cause inflammation of the labyrinth or inner ear may produce similar symptoms (see Ch. 11). Early in life, our response to vestibular information is refined and integrated with information from other sensory systems to influence motor function and cognitive development.

An early reflex, the vestibulocephalicocular reflex, is involved with coordinating eye and head movement. When the head turns to the left, the eyes are moved at an equal velocity but in the opposite direction (see Ch. 9). By 6 months of gestation, myelination of the vestibular tracts is well underway. However, this and other vestibular-driven reflexes are inhibited until birth, preventing unnecessary

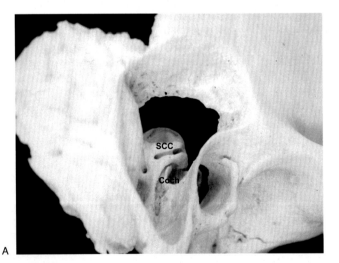
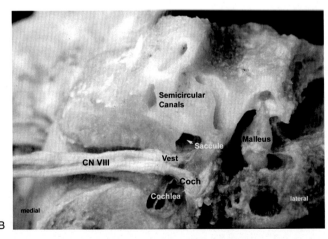

Fig. 10.4 • (A) Lateral view of a temporal bone with the squamous portion partially drilled to reveal the three semicircular canals (SCC) and the cochlea (Coch). (B) In this anterior view, the petrous portion of the temporal bone has been filed down to the level of the middle ear. The malleus can be seen; deep to it lie the incus and stapes. The saccule, cochlea and semicircular canals are clearly labeled. The vestibular (Vest) and cochlea (Coch) portions of cranial nerve VIII are also identified. *Used with permission of the Willard & Carreiro Collection.*

reflex movements in the womb. Nevertheless, movement behavior can be observed prior to birth. For example, while preterm infants lack signs of vestibular-related reflexes, they will change intrauterine position up to 20 times per hour in the first half of pregnancy. This frequency will halve during the latter half of pregnancy. In the term newborn, vestibular-ocular reflexes are intact, but lack somewhat in the fast saccade component. This may be related to the inadequate myelination of the involved cortical structures. The vestibular response is reduced in premature infants. They will also lack nystagmus but it will develop by 3–4 months post-birth.

Children between 5 and 10 years have a lower threshold of acceleration for eliciting nystagmus, as well as reduced latencies and increased amplitude of eye movements. Normal children will seek out vestibular and proprioceptive stimuli. Spontaneous vestibular stimulation will take the form of body-rocking, bouncing, swaying or head-shaking. This behavior usually develops at 6 months. Delays in onset are seen in children with Down's syndrome and cerebral palsy. Head-rocking, which begins between 6 and 8 months, can be associated with the rate of motor development. Delayed motor development has been associated with the absence of spontaneous vestibular stimulatory behaviors

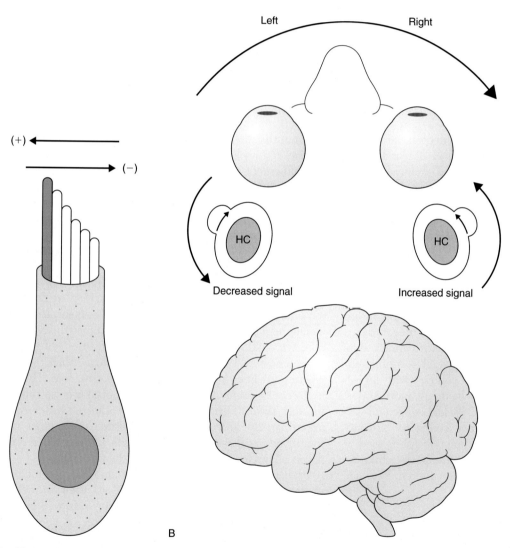

Fig. 10.5 • (A) Hair cells line the ampulla of the semicircular canals. Each hair cell has several rows of stereocilia and a single kinocilium (depicted in dark gray). When the stereocilia are bent towards the kinocilium, the cell depolarizes. When the stereocilia are bent away from the kinocilium, the cell hyperpolarizes. For the sake of convention, depolarization, the generation of a signal, is indicated by the (+) sign. The lack of signal hyperpolarization is indicated by the (−) sign. (B) The head is depicted rotating to the right. The small black arrow within each horizontal canal (HC) indicates the direction for depolarization of the hair cells. As the head rotates, the stereocilia are swept through the inert endolymph within the canals. The relative direction of movement of the stereocilia is depicted by the arrows at either side. Cells within the right horizontal canal will generate an increased signal. Signals are relayed to the brainstem, cerebellum and cortex.

due to damage to the labyrinth (Tsuzuku & Kaga 1992). Hyperactivity and emotional dysfunction have been associated with abnormal postrotatory nystagmus. Vestibular abnormalities have also been associated with learning disorders involving cognitive, perceptual and attention deficits. The somatosensory system, specifically the cervical musculature, can compensate and influence vestibular function. Poststroke patients or aged patients with vestibular dysfunction will rely upon sensory input from the cervical spine to maintain posture and balance. Conversely, the potential for abnormal sensory input secondary to biomechanical stresses to aggravate vestibular dysfunction must be considered. Anecdotally, we have found that children undergoing sensory integration therapy appear to show greater improvement when treated with osteopathic manipulation.

There is much evidence for the influence of the vestibular system on cognitive development in children (Weeks 1979). Appropriate vestibular stimulation appears to have a positive effect on motor system development; 'preambulatory normal human infants exposed to sessions of mild semicircular canal stimulation 2 days per week for 4 weeks demonstrated significant improvement in gross motor skills' (Clark et al 1977). Vestibular stimulation has been shown to decrease arousal in infants (Cordero et al 1986). Long-term vestibular therapy has been demonstrated to increase visual attentiveness in deprived, institutionalized infants. It has also been shown to increase motor development (reflexes and skills) (Clark et al 1977, 1988). Vestibular stimulation can be used to condition behaviors such as sucking. Sensory integration therapy, with emphasis on vestibular stimulation, may assist children with attention deficit, behavioral and cognitive disorders.

Vestibular abnormalities have been associated with early developmental delay and later learning disorders. For example, vestibular areflexia and delayed motor development are associated with instability while walking and speech delay. Caloric hyporeflexia has been associated with motor dysfunctions affecting reading and writing, and a subsequent loss of interest in school. In a group of children with speech delay, aphasia and dyslexia (without hearing abnormalities, mental retardation or brain lesion), 25% had congenital vestibular disturbances that could induce cerebellar dysfunction, delaying speech. Vestibular dysfunction (depressed or absent nystagmus) was frequent (63%) in aphasic children. In a study of 115 6–14-year-old dyslexic children, 97% had vestibular-cerebellar dysfunction.

OVERVIEW OF DEVELOPMENTAL MILESTONES

The primitive, clumsy, isolated reflexes of the newborn and young infant are the building blocks of later intelligence. The initiation and refinement of emotional and cognitive processes are influenced by motor and sensory learning. The integration of information from the motor and sensory systems influences the individual's perception of and ability to interact with the world. We can view development as an integrated event influenced by external and internal processes. The resulting behavior, or developmental milestone, represents the summation of many factors (Table 10.1).

At birth, flexor tone exceeds extensor tone. The flexed posture of the neonate is an expression of this phenomenon. As newborns develop, the flexor and extensor muscles will achieve a more balanced relationship, which will facilitate voluntary movements. Early reflexes, such as the Moro and asymmetric tonic neck reflex, rely on the activation of extensor muscles and relaxation of flexor tone. These early reflexes may provide the first example of agonist–antagonist muscle synergies. Early tactile and proprioceptive development, such as grasping and sucking, also involve the coordination of action systems. In the first 2–4 weeks of life, newborns begin to demonstrate primitive neck control, perhaps turning their head to a visual stimulus. The action systems responsible for cervical motion and head control begin to emerge, although head lag is still present. Over the next few months, these crude motions will evolve into smooth, precise and well-coordinated movement patterns through the refinement of action systems.

The ability to sit unsupported changes a child's relationship to her environment (Fig. 10.6). No longer in a passive posture, she can now initiate interactions with her surroundings. The ability to propel herself towards that which she desires makes the child master of all she surveys. This is a very important step in the development of the individual. Many developmentalists believe that the period from 8 to 36 months solidifies the potential capabilities of the individual. Up to this time, most development has been determined by neuronal myelination; now environmental stimulation assumes the dominant role. The child who is able to initiate her involvement with the environment will have a different experience than the child whose disabilities keep him in a more passive role. The ability to cruise closely follows loss of the plantar grasp reflex in the feet (Fig. 10.7). Fine motor control in the hands is also improving. By 12 months, most children can adduct their thumb independently of the other digits. Differentiated use of fingers allows for the development of the pincer grasp.

Prior to the development of early ambulation, children's perception of their world is limited to their immediate environment. The existence of something outside their field of awareness is quite limited. For example, if you show a 2-month-old a toy and then cover it with something, she will not attempt to find it. She will not look about for it, nor will she continue to stare at the cloth covering the toy, anticipating its return. There is no sense of object permanence. The cognitive processes which allow us to recognize that something continues to exist after it has been removed from our sensory environment has not yet developed in

Table 10.1 Milestones

Milestone	Age	Differential diagnosis
Moro grasp	NB	Brachial plexus palsy, clavicle fracture (UL), hypoxia (BL), hypoglycemia (BL), systemic problem
Rooting	NB	Facial palsy (UL), systemic condition (BL), i.e. hypoglycemia, hypoxia
ATNR	NB–5 months	Torticollis, extremity issue, IPA
Smiles, vocalizes	4–6 weeks	Visual and auditory systems (BL)
Pull to sit head lag	6–12 weeks	
Swiping batting	6–8 weeks	
Turns head to sound	12–16 weeks	Auditory (BL), torticollis (UL)
Lifts head prone	8 weeks	Torticollis, clavicle fracture
Rolling	5–6 months	
Stranger anxiety	6–8 months	
Sits	6–7 months	
Landau reaction	5–12 months	
Crawls	6–8 months	
Creeps	8–10 months	
Adduct thumb	8–10 months	
Protective reflexes	7 months++	
Pulls to stand	10–11 months	
Pincer grasp	12 months	
Stands unsupported	11–13 months	
Responds to 'no'	12 months	
Loses ability to respond to 'no'	24–30 months	
Walks	14–18 months	
Finds partially hidden toy	10–11 months	
Waves bye-bye	10–12 months	
Identifies pictures	14–20 months	
Geometric shapes	16–22 months	
2–4 word phrases	18–24 months	
Independence	24–30 months	
Stacks blocks	24 months	
Single limb stance	36 months	
Stairs sans support	36–48 months	
Copies shapes	36–48 months	

UL = unilateral; BL = bilateral; IPA = infantile postural asymmetry

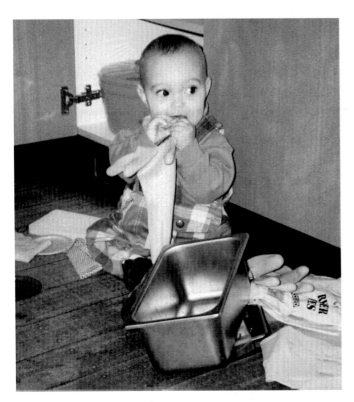

Fig. 10.6 • Unsupported sitting opens up new worlds of opportunity.

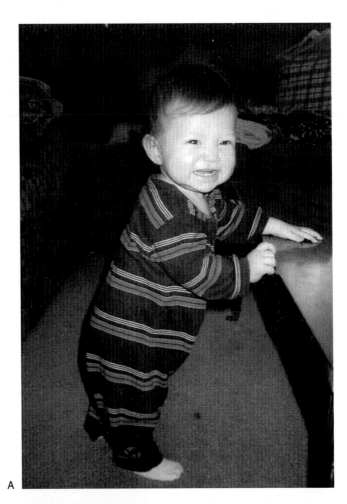

A

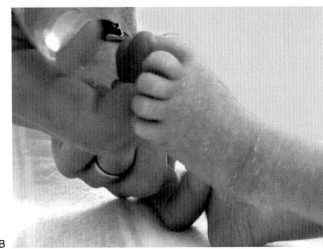

B

Fig. 10.7 • (A) Cruising. (B) The plantar grasp reflex.

young infants. Developmentalists believe that children's awareness of their environment enlarges with their ability to move through it. They learn that the existence of something is not contingent upon their being able to see it. Parents facilitate this learning through implementing hide-and-seek games, which introduce the concepts of object permanence. These games may lay the foundation for later understanding of the relationship between cause and effect.

Between 8 and 14 months, we begin to see early evidence of later cognitive skills. At 10 months, a child can easily find a partially hidden toy; by 12 months, children can find a completely hidden object, and usually enjoy the search as a game. The concept of object permanence first introduced with games of 'hide and seek' is now firmly established. Demonstrations of non-pretend or imitation play, such as using a comb or a pencil, are common within this age group. By 10 months, a child will use gestures appropriately. The first expression of this new-found skill usually occurs around 8 months, when children will shake their head for 'no'; by 14 months they can point to the object of rejection and shake their head.

Manual dexterity will initially manifest with tasks requiring isolated wrist mechanics, such as scribbling or the ability to turn a knob. During this time, coordinated mechanics within the components of the upper extremity and the integration of these mechanics with spinal movements become an important consideration for the osteopathic physician. As previously discussed, alterations or strains affecting any

of the components of the upper extremity will influence how the child uses the extremity and her perception of its use. Merzenich et al (1996) demonstrated that cortical representation of an extremity is altered in patients with musculoskeletal strains. This is presumably due to abnormal sensory input. It is easy to see the potential for biomechanical dysfunction to affect the development of cortical representation of the appendage. Prior to 18 months, children are ambidextrous and should not show hand preference. Those who demonstrate handedness prior to this age need to be evaluated for underlying pathology. Neurological and biomechanical etiologies affecting the extremity may manifest as a penchant to use the other extremity. Neurological processes which should be considered include an injury to the brachial plexus (wherein the child will generally use the hand but not the arm), the brain or the spinal cord. Biomechanical mechanisms can include undiagnosed fracture of the clavicle, thoracic outlet syndrome, shoulder dislocation, muscle spasm, rotator cuff strain, etc.

By 14 months, children can identify pictorial representations fairly easily. Their ideas of causality broaden, although often not enough to affect their increasing independence and 'boundary-testing' behavior. At some time between 18 and 24 months, the child will become comfortable with using 2–4-word phrases in speech, although grammar and syntax may not be appropriate. Speech development can vary considerably if a child has older siblings or parents who 'interpret' for them. Identity formation, the concept of 'self', begins to appear between 18 and 24 months. By 18 months, the child has established early identity formation, the idea of self, although the concept of 'I' is still overshadowed by second-person perspectives; that is, children will often call themselves by name – 'Pick up David' – or use the second person to address themselves – 'Pick up me'. By 24 months, most children can recognize and sort by color and shape. The seeds of this appreciation of geometry began in early touch perception and primitive hand movements.

By 3 years, most children's awareness of their body has reached sufficient levels to allow for successful toilet training. Younger children often lack consistent awareness of their bodily sensations and/or the ability to accurately interpret them. Posture and balance are fairly stable by 3 years, allowing the child to move on to more daring endeavors, such as hopping, kicking and jumping. By this age, most children can maintain their balance with forward and backward movement, although motions may still be rather jerky. Fine motor skills improve rapidly between 3 and 4 years, such that by the age of 4 most children can recognizably copy squares, circles and most letters. Language advances to five- and six-word sentences, and grammar improves during the fourth year also. Stuttering is not uncommon at this age, and should resolve by the age of 5 if purely developmental.

A 3–4-year-old child cannot always distinguish between reality and fantasy. Fears of monsters and wild animals may be present, especially when encouraged by older siblings who find the child's response entertaining. Three- to four-year-old children will begin to show some ability to negotiate solutions to problems, and while they are more independent, they are (thankfully) more cooperative than they were at 2. Slowly, a sense of time and abstract thought will evolve, although it is still immature and reasoning is concrete.

Creativity is primarily expressed through play in the toddler and young child. At some time between 24 and 36 months, a child will begin to participate in pretend play, using unrelated objects to represent the intended article. Often the child will announce his intention: 'This box is my car'. This represents an expansion of his understanding of symbolic capabilities and the concrete expression of intention. He has a plan. Slowly, the child will incorporate more abstract ideas into play, drawing from experiences and observations. Between the ages of 4 and 5 children may tell their first stories to interested audiences. During this same time, a child's sense of humor for the absurd will often appear. By the fifth year, a child can skip and throw accurately. Minimal assistance is needed for dressing, but facewashing and tooth-brushing often require supervision, due to the reluctance factor. A 5-year-old can copy triangles and print letters. If he is asked to draw a person, there is usually a head, body and simple extremities. Abstract thought is maturing, and the child will use future tense in her speech, as well as devising plans and schemes. The maturation of abstract thought facilitates verbal language skills. This step cements the foundation for communication and cognitive learning which was first laid down by the primitive sensory and motor systems of the newborn.

CONCLUSION

The somatosensory system is intricately linked to the development of perception and cognition throughout life. The foundation for the way we interpret and interact with our world rests upon the maps we develop early in life. The musculoskeletal system plays a major role in creating and refining those maps. While some literature explores the impact of gross musculoskeletal conditions (spasticity, hypotonia, etc.) on cognitive function, there is scant research delving into the influence of more subtle dysfunctions or the summative effect of dysfunctions in the early formative period. The osteopathic philosophy recognizes the contribution that biomechanical dysfunction may have on structural and physiological processes. Those of us caring for the very young must consider the potential effects that somatic dysfunction may have on developing maps and neural relationships. Does cranial base compression play a role in the development of attention deficit disorder? What about depression? Can torticollis or cervical strain in the newborn affect spatial perception? There are many questions to be answered and possibilities to be considered. From the osteopathic perspective, the relationship between structure and function is obvious, and the potential for dysfunction to have a negative impact on growth and development warrants osteopathic intervention. This is the epitome of preventive care. Do no harm.

References

Amaral D G 2000 The functional organization of perception and movement. In: Kandel E R, Schwartz J H, Jessell T M (eds) Principles of neuroscience. McGraw-Hill, New York.

Bushnell E W, Boudreau J P 1993 Motor development and the mind: the potential role of motor abilities as a determinant of aspects of perceptual development. Child Dev 64: 1005–1021.

Clark D L, Kreutzberg J R, Chee F K 1977 Vestibular stimulation influence on motor development in infants. Science 196(4295): 1228–1229.

Clark S A, Allard T, Jenkins W M et al 1988 Receptive fields in the body-surface map in adult cortex defined by temporally correlated inputs. Nature 332(31): 444–445.

Coplan J, Gleason J R 1990 Quantifying language development from birth to 3 years using the Early Language Milestone Scale. Pediatrics 86(6): 963–971.

Cordero L, Clark D L, Schott L 1986 Effects of vestibular stimulation on sleep states in premature infants. Am J Perinatol 3: 319–324.

Dronkers N F, Pinker S Damasio A 2000 Language and aphasias. In: Kandel E R, Schwartz J H, Jessell T M (eds) Principles of neuroscience. McGraw-Hill, New York.

Goldberg M E, Hudspeth A J 2000 The vestibular system. In: Kandel E R, Schwartz J H, Jessell T M (eds) Principles of neural science. McGraw-Hill, New York.

Harcourt B 1974 Strabismus affecting children with multiple handicaps. Br J Ophthalmol 58: 272–280.

Hudspeth A J 2000 Hearing. In: Kandel E R, Schwartz J H, Jessell T M (eds) Principles of neuroscience. McGraw-Hill, New York.

Kandel E R, Schwartz J H, Jessell T M 2000 Principles of neural science, 4th edn. McGraw-Hill, Philadelphia.

Merzenich M, Wright B, Jenkins W et al 1996 Cortical plasticity underlying perceptual, motor, and cognitive skill development: implications for neurorehabilitation. Cold Spring Harb Symp Quant Biol 61: 1–8.

Saper C B, Iverson S, Frackowiak R 2000 Integration of sensory and motor function. In: Kandel E R, Schwartz J H, Jessell T M (eds) Principles of neuroscience. McGraw-Hill, New York.

Shumway-Cook A, Woollacott M H 1995 Upper extremity manipulation skills: changes across a life span. Motor control: theory and practical applications. Williams & Wilkins, Baltimore 12: 377–397.

Tessier-Lavigne M 2000 Phototransduction and information processing in the retina. In: Kandel E R, Schwartz J H, Jessell T M (eds) Principles of neural science. McGraw-Hill, New York: 400–420.

Tomatis A A 1991 The conscious ear. Station Hill Press, Barrytown, New York.

Tsuzuku T, Kaga K 1992 Delayed motor function and results of vestibular function tests in children with inner ear anomalies. Int J Pediatr Otorhinolaryngol 23: 261–268.

Weeks Z R 1979 Effects of the vestibular system on human development, part 2: effects of vestibular stimulation on mentally retarded, emotionally disturbed, and learning-disabled individuals. Am J Occup Ther 33: 450–457.

Wurtz R H, Kandel E R 2000 Perception, motion depth and form. In: Kandel E R, Schwartz J H, Jessell T M (eds) Principles of neural science. McGraw-Hill, New York.

Further reading

Arnold L E, Clark D L, Sachs L A et al 1985 Vestibular and visual rotational stimulation as treatment for attention deficit and hyperactivity. Am J Occup Ther 39(2): 84–91.

Byl N, Wilson F, Merzenich M et al 1996 Sensory dysfunction associated with repetitive strain injuries of tendinitis and focal hand dystonia: a comparative study. J Orthop Sports Phys Ther 23(4): 234–244.

Gazzaniga M S 1993 The cognitive neurosciences, 1st edn. The MIT Press, Cambridge, Massachusetts.

Ghez C 1991 The control of movement. In: Kandel E R, Schwartz J H, Jessell T M (eds) Principles of neural science. Elsevier, New York: 533–547.

Ghez C, Krakauer J 2000 The organization of movement. In: Kandel E R, Schwartz J H, Jessell T M (eds) Principles of neural science. McGraw-Hill, New York.

Harcourt B 1970 Hereditary nystagmus in early childhood. J Med Genet 7: 253–256.

Harcourt B 1971 Functional and organic visual defects: the differentiation in schoolchildren. Proc R Soc Med 64: 619–621.

Harcourt B 1973 The association of visual and other handicaps in childhood. Proc R Soc Med 66: 612–616.

Harcourt B 1975 The education of visually handicapped children in Great Britain. Child Care Health Dev 1: 359–361.

Harcourt B 1975 Clinical ophthalmic assessment in visually handicapped children. Child Care Health Dev 1: 315–324.

Harcourt B 1976 Squint. BMJ i: 703–705.

Kantner R M, Clark D L, Allen L C et al 1976 Effects of vestibular stimulation on nystagmus response and motor performance in the developmentally delayed infant. Phys Ther 56: 414–421.

Kantner R M, Kantner B, Clark D L 1982 Vestibular stimulation effect on language development in mentally retarded children. Am J Occup Ther 36: 36–41.

O'Brien C, Clark D 1994 Ocular biometry in pre-term infants without retinopathy of prematurity. Eye 8: 662–665.

Savelsbergh G, von Hofsten C, Jonsson B 1997 The coupling of head, reach and grasp movement in nine months old infant prehension. Scand J Psychol 38(4): 325–333.

Sveistrup H, Woollacott M H 1993 Systems contributing to the emergence and maturation of stability in postnatal development. In: Savelsbergh G (ed) The development of coordination in infancy. Elsevier, Amsterdam: 331.

Tallal P, Merzenich M, Miller S et al 1998 Language learning impairment: integrating research and remediation. Scand J Psychol 39: 197–199.

Tsuzuku T, Kaga K 1991 The relation between motor function development and vestibular function tests in four children with inner ear anomaly. Acta Otolaryngol Suppl 481: 443–446.

Woolley S M, Rubin A M, Kantner R M et al 1993 Differentiation of balance deficits through examination of selected components of static stabilometry. J Otolaryngol 22(5): 368–375.

Chapter Eleven

Otolaryngology

CHAPTER CONTENTS

OTITIS MEDIA

Chronic otitis media and recurrent acute otitis media with effusion are two of the most frequent illnesses of early childhood. Countless office visits, antibiotics and sleepless nights owe their existence to this culprit. By the age of 7, most children have experienced at least one episode of otitis media, and approximately a third have had recurrent episodes of acute otitis (Bluestone & Klein 1995). There is some suggestion that speech, language and learning disabilities may be related to recurrent or chronic otitis media with effusion. Generally speaking, 40% of children presenting with acute otitis media with effusion will continue to have effusion 1 month after the acute infection has cleared. Of the initial group, 20% will continue to have effusion after 2 months and 10% after 3 months (Bluestone & Klein 1995). Furthermore, a strong correlation has been drawn between the existence of persistent effusion and recurrent acute infection. A list of the possible etiologies of middle ear effusion and its chronicity is certainly extensive; however, a common denominator among many of them is the presence of eustachian tube dysfunction. The eustachian tube plays an important role in the health of the middle ear, and its dysfunction has been implicated in the development of many diseases of the middle ear. From an osteopathic perspective, the anatomy of the cranial base and its related tissues may influence eustachian tube function. Furthermore, empirical data suggest that osteopathic treatment of these tissues affects eustachian tube function. Consequently, for the purposes of this chapter, we will primarily focus on the role of eustachian tube dysfunction in otitis media with effusion.

Diagnosis

Otitis media is an inflammation of the middle ear (Fig. 11.1), and may occur with or without effusion. Otitis media with

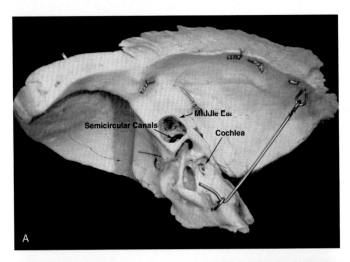

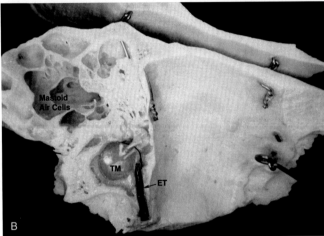

Fig. 11.1 • (A) Disarticulated temporal bone viewed from above. The petrous portion has been preferentially drilled over the semicircular canals, middle ear and cochlea. The superior petrosal sinus is illustrated by the shaded area, as is the sigmoid sinus.
(B) View into the petrous portion of the same specimen, revealing the contents of the middle ear. The incus, malleus, tympanic membrane (TM), eustachian tube (ET) and mastoid air cells are labeled. *Used with permission of the Willard & Carreiro collection.*

and effusion, an acute onset of signs and symptoms, the presence of middle ear effusion, and signs and symptoms of middle ear inflammation (American Academy of Pediatrics and American Academy of Family Physicians 2004). One of the following signs of middle ear effusion must be present: bulging tympanic membrane, limited or absent movement of the tympanic membrane, air–fluid level behind the tympanic membrane or otorrhea. Middle ear inflammation presents as injected vessels, or erythema. The acute symptoms may or may not be preceded by a prodrome of upper respiratory symptoms. In addition it has become clearer that acute otitis media is a somewhat different disease in children under 2 years than in older children. Acute otitis media is often the result of viral infection rather than bacterial infection, although bacterial overgrowth may occur. Until recently, most children with acute otitis media were given antibiotics; however, recent studies have demonstrated that this is unnecessary in the majority of older children, and the current recommendation in the USA and much of Europe is to delay initiation of antimicrobial therapy unless specific criteria are met.

Chronic otitis media with effusion occurs when middle ear effusion persists for more than 3 months. Systemic signs are often absent, and there may or may not be recurrent acute infections. Chronic otitis media with effusion is often asymptomatic, although the child may be seen playing with or digging at his or her ears. Otitis media with effusion is not necessarily associated with an infection. In fact, erythema and injection of the tympanic membrane is usually absent. Bulging or retraction may be present in some children, and air–fluid levels and/or bubbles may be visualized behind the tympanic membrane. In some cases, the tympanic membrane is opaque, due to thickening or swelling from the persistent irritation. Otitis media with effusion may be acute, subacute or chronic in presentation; however, it differs from acute otitis media in that there are no systemic signs or symptoms.

Etiology

For a complete discussion, see one of the excellent texts cited at the end of this chapter.

Otitis media with effusion is a relatively common disease, occurring in up to 20% of infants and young children. It is typically seen in children between the ages of 6 months and 6 years, with a significant decline in occurrence after the sixth year. During the first 3 years of life, the incidence tends to increase. After the eighth year of life, it is rare. It is also known that 40% of all children presenting with acute otitis media will have middle ear effusions which will last 4 weeks, and 10% of those initially presenting will have effusions lasting for 3 months (Bluestone & Klein 1995). We need to ask ourselves why. The etiology and pathophysiology of otitis media are multifactorial. Immature or impaired immune responses, allergy, passive smoking, exposure to

effusion refers to the presence of fluid within the middle ear. The effusion may be thin and serous, thick, viscous and mucoid, or purulent. The character of the fluid provides the clinician with clues concerning its etiology and chronicity. Thick viscous fluid is usually present with chronic processes. Purulent fluid suggests an acute bacterial infection. Thin, relatively clear fluid is more common in early viral processes. Otitis media with effusion will present differently, depending on whether it is acute or chronic. Systemic signs such as fever, malaise, appetite changes, ear pain or other signs of illness accompany acute infections. In fact, under current standards of medical practice, the diagnosis of acute otitis media requires that there is a rapid onset of symptoms accompanied by signs of middle ear inflammation infected children, presence of concurrent infection and eustachian tube dysfunction have all been implicated as contributing factors in the development of this disease. Regardless of the inciting event, the role played by the anatomy of the pediatric eustachian tube, temporal bone and musculoskeletal components of the pharynx in the etiology of chronic otitis media and recurrent acute otitis media with effusion cannot be underestimated.

Eustachian tube physiology

The eustachian tube has several functions which are important to the middle ear: first, it acts to equilibrate middle ear pressure with atmospheric pressure, which aids in sound transmission; second, it prevents reflux of secretions and bacteria found in the nasopharynx into the middle ear space; and last, it drains fluids produced in the middle ear. Each of these activities is dependent upon a patent, functioning eustachian tube. At rest, the eustachian tube is collapsed. In the adult, pressures in the middle ear and the atmosphere are maintained at an equilibrium through the periodic opening and closing of the eustachian tube which occur with swallowing and other activities. In children, middle ear pressures are slightly negative (Bluestone & Klein 1996), and most children, even those without middle ear disease, have difficulty in maintaining appropriate pressure. The ability to maintain appropriate pressure appears to be related to the stiffness of the eustachian tube. The fact that the tube is relatively pliable in children is thought to be responsible for the increased incidence of middle ear disease in this age group (Bylander 1980, Bylander & Tjernstrom 1983). Deficits in eustachian tube function impede normal drainage to the nasopharynx (Takahashi et al 1989) and create a negative pressure within the middle ear as compared with atmospheric pressure. The resulting negative pressure may promote insufflation, aspiration or reflux of nasopharyngeal secretions into the middle ear.

Eustachian tube dysfunction can be divided into the following categories: abnormal patency, extrinsic obstruction and intrinsic obstruction. Abnormal patency is generally thought to be secondary to a flexible tube, which is more common in the child than in the adult. Intrinsic obstruction arises when the lumen narrows because of hypertrophy or swelling of the wall. This may result from inflammation or congenital processes. Extrinsic obstruction is commonly thought to result from the adenoids or tumor. However, from an osteopathic perspective, adjacent musculoskeletal tissues may also have a role in extrinsic obstruction of the tube.

Eustachian tube dysfunction is associated with recurrent infection. Overgrowth of adenoidal tissue is frequently implicated as the culprit; however, current research suggests that it may not be the size of the adenoidal tissue but perhaps the bacterial reservoir in the tissue which contributes

to reinfection (Gates et al 1988). Adenoidectomy reduces the incidence of acute infection, but the presence of middle ear effusion is not affected by adenoidectomy (Gates et al 1988). Other treatment approaches include myringotomy and tympanostomy tubes. Tympanostomy tubes can be inserted to improve ventilation and drainage of the middle ear (Handler 1994, Berman 1995), but do nothing to prevent reflux or insufflation (Bluestone & Klein 1996). Short-term success rates are reported, but follow-ups at 6, 12 and 18 months suggest recurrence of otitis media with effusion, necessitating re-treatment (Philippe et al 1991, Berg & Stool 1994, Handler 1994). The presence of middle ear effusion undoubtedly increases the risk for recurrent infection as well as hearing and speech difficulties. Drainage of the eustachian tube becomes a prophylactic measure in the control of acute otitis media.

Functional anatomy

At birth, the temporal bone is in three parts: the squamous portion, the petrous portion and the tympanic ring. These three parts are joined by cartilage. The eustachian tube travels from the middle ear through the petrous portion of the temporal bone, across the articulation between the sphenoid and petrous tip, through the pharyngeal musculature, to open in the lateral wall of the nasopharynx. The diameter of the tube is narrowest at the junction of the osseous and cartilaginous parts. This junction occurs just as the tube leaves the temporal bone and traverses under the petrosphenoid articulation (Fig. 11.2). Within the pharynx, the eustachian tube closely approximates the tensor veli palatini and levator veli palatini muscles as well as the salpingopharyngeus muscle (Bluestone & Klein 1995, Standring 2004).

The mucosa of the eustachian tube and middle ear is an extension of the respiratory mucosa of the nasopharynx, and likewise is ciliated columnar epithelium with secretory glands which progresses to a cuboidal mucosa deep in the middle ear. This tissue lines the eustachian tube, mastoid air cells, middle ear and ossicles. Mucous secretions provide nourishment and help to trap antigens and other unwanted materials. The nasopharynx and middle ear are related via the mucosal-associated lymphoid tissue present in both, so irritants or antigens triggering increased mucus secretion in the nasopharynx will result in increased production in the middle ear; that is, if your nose is congested, your ears are congested. Under optimal conditions, this excess mucus would be drained through the eustachian tube. However, when tube function is compromised or drainage obstructed, the fluid will accumulate in the middle ear, leading to otitis with effusion. Although the effusion is initially a serous-type fluid, the prolonged retention will alter its character. Accumulation of inflammatory mediators and cellular waste products will change the pH in the middle ear, affecting secretory activity. Chronic effusions typically become more

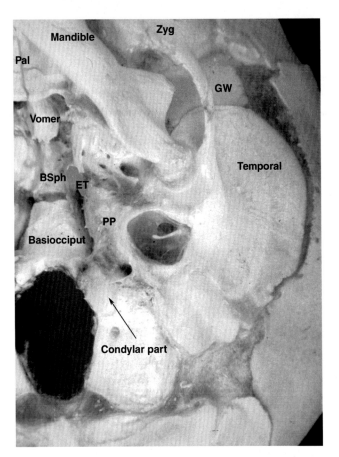

Fig. 11.2 • Inferior view of a newborn skull. Note the location of the eustachian tube (ET) between the petrous portion (PP) of the temporal bone and basisphenoid (BSph). The palate (Pal), greater wing (GW) and zygoma (Zyg) are labeled. *Used with permission of the Willard & Carreiro collection.*

viscous over time, and findings on visual examination of the tympanic membrane will change. A serous effusion will give a gray or amber color to the tympanic membrane. Light reflex is absent, because light from the otoscope is absorbed by the fluid rather than reflected.

The eustachian tube is surrounded by three intraoral muscles, which have varying attachments to the tubal cartilage. The salpingopharyngeus muscle arises from the inferior cartilage of the eustachian tube at its distal end and blends with the palatopharyngeus muscle inferiorly. This muscle may have a role in eustachian tube function, although this is unclear. The lateral bundle of the tensor veli palatini muscle has some posterior inferior fibers that originate from the tubal cartilage. In fetal specimens, the majority of this muscle bundle attaches to the posterior one-third to one-half of the membranous wall of the eustachian tube, which becomes the cartilaginous portion in the adult (Proctor 1967, Rood & Doyle 1978, Standring 2004). The medial bundle of the tensor veli palatini muscle (the dilator tubae) lies immediately adjacent to the lateral membranous wall of

the eustachian tube. When contracted, this muscle pulls the lateral wall inferolaterally and opens the lumen of the tube (Proctor 1967, Rood 1973, Rood & Doyle 1978, Standring 2004). Honjo and Okazaki have demonstrated that contraction and relaxation of the tensor palatini produces a pumping function of the eustachian tube, which expels fluid into the nasopharynx (Honjo et al 1980a, b, 1981a, b).

We tend to think of the muscles of the palate as small and relatively inconsequential because of their relative size in the adult. However, in the infant, these muscles are relatively large when compared with the eustachian tube (Fig. 11.3). Abnormal tensions may affect tube function in two ways. Muscle flaccidity or a mechanical arrangement that distorts muscle biomechanics may impede opening. However, increased tone may result in one of two problems, depending on the compliance of the tubal cartilage. Spasm or shortening of the tensor veli palatini will open the tube, resulting in a patulous tube. This will occur in adults, because the tubal cartilage of the medial wall resists the pull of the muscle while the lateral wall is pulled away. Unlike in the adult, the eustachian tube of the infant is quite pliable, and rather than opening in response to muscle activity, the entire tube will be pulled by the contracting muscle and distort (Bluestone & Klein 1996). Consequently, shortening of the same muscle in the infant is likely to obstruct the tube by distorting its shape.

A fourth muscle, and one which is often neglected in discussions of the eustachian tube, is the medial pterygoid. This relatively large muscle lies in close proximity to the tube and may have fibrous attachments to the lateral wall in some individuals (Willard FH & Carreiro JC, unpublished observation 1993, Standring 2004). During contraction of the medial pterygoid, the increased bulk of muscle will compress the eustachian tube (Ross 1971, Bluestone & Klein 1996). It seems perfectly reasonable that increased pterygoid bulk secondary to biomechanical factors would also act to compress the tube. Furthermore, in those individuals in whom there are attachments between the pterygoid muscle and eustachian tube, increased tone in the muscle might act to distort the pliable tube. Pterygoid spasm can be ascertained in older children and adults by observing mandibular movements during opening and closing of the mouth. If there is asymmetrical tone in the pterygoid muscles, the mandible will deviate towards the muscle as it engages. The pterygoid can also be palpated intraorally to compare tension.

Postnatal changes

At birth, the eustachian tube is orientated more horizontally than in the adult. Throughout the first few years of life, there are changes in the orientation of the basicranium and the temporal bone composite (Bosma 1986). These changes were discussed in Chapter 3, but will be briefly reviewed here. In the infant, the basicranium has a fairly oblique

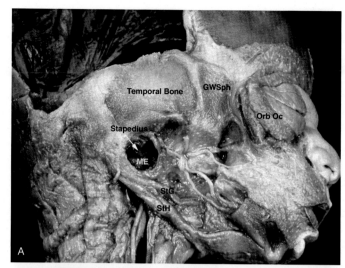

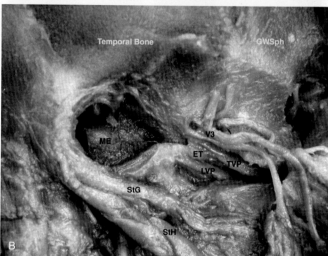

Fig. 11.3 • (A) Lateral view of neonatal dissection. The mandible and zygoma bones have been cut and the muscles of mastication removed. The tympanic membrane has collapsed, revealing the middle ear (ME) and malleus. The styloglossus (StG) and stylohyoid (StH), orbicularis oculi (Orb Oc), mandibular branch of the trigeminal (V3) and greater wing of the sphenoid (GWSph) are labeled. (B) Close-up of area indicated by the arrow in (A). The lateral aspect of the temporal bone has been drilled away to reveal the eustachian tube (ET) surrounded by the tensor veli palatini (TVP) and levator veli palatini (LVP) muscles. Note the relative size of the muscles as compared to the eustachian tube. The middle ear (ME), styloglossus (StG), stylohyoid (StH), greater wing of the sphenoid (GWSph), and ophthalmic branch of the trigeminal nerve (V3) are labeled. *Used with permission of the Willard & Carreiro Collection.*

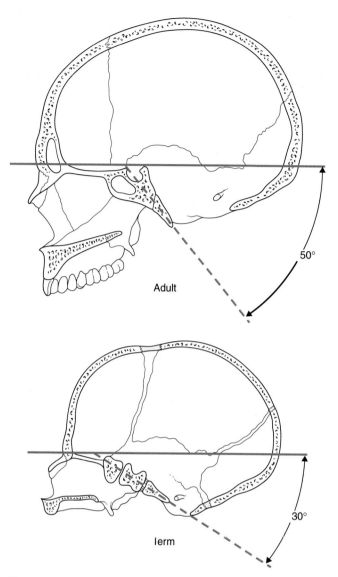

Fig. 11.4 • A comparison of the orientation of the newborn and adult cranial base as measured in relation to the axial plane passing through the glabella and inion. *Used with permission of the Willard & Carreiro Collection.*

orientation, whereas in the adult it is more flexed (Fig. 11.4). Vertical orientation and enlargement of the pharynx, as well as longitudinal growth of the mandible, are correlated with postnatal developments in the temporal bone. Appositional growth within the petrous portion of the temporal bone results in a lateral displacement of the temporomandibular fossa and superior displacement of the tympanic cavity

(Fig. 11.5) (Bosma 1986). The external auditory meatus shifts from the horizontal to the sagittal plane (Fig. 11.6). Within the basiocciput, growth at the spheno-occipital synchondrosis is greater that at the basisphenoid margin, thereby extending the basiocciput posteriorly (Bosma 1986). In effect, this growth pattern produces a flexion in the cranial base and a lateral–superior rotation of the temporal bones, which shifts the orientation of the eustachian tubes from a horizontal to a slightly anterior declined plane (Bosma 1986, Bluestone & Klein 1995, Standring 2004).

As the eustachian tube passes from the middle ear to empty in the posterior wall of the pharynx, it is surrounded by the muscles, fascias and other soft tissue structures of the pharynx and cranial base. Many of these tissues are

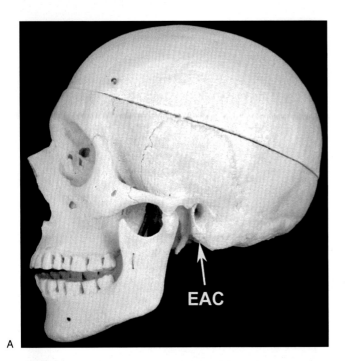

A

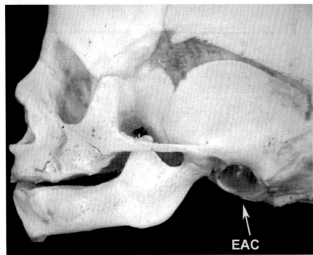

B

Fig. 11.5 • Comparison between orientation of adult (A) and infant (B) external auditory canal (EAC). *Used with permission of the Willard & Carreiro Collection.*

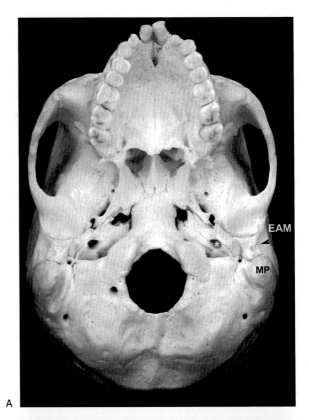

A

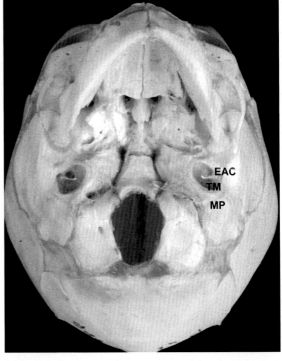

B

attached to the cartilaginous portion of the tube and can exert an influence on it. The eustachian tube is at its narrowest where it crosses beneath the articulation between the petrous portion of the temporal bone and the sphenoid. It is enveloped in a connective tissue hammock that is suspended from this junction. In the newborn and infant, the petrosphenoid junction is cartilaginous and vulnerable to mechanical stress. Tissue strains transferred from the cartilaginous structures into the fascial tissues of this area may influence eustachian tube function. An association between middle ear infections and cranial strain patterns has been reported (Degenhardt & Kuchera 1994, Mills et al 2002, 2003).

Fig. 11.6 • Views of the inferior aspect of the cranium in adult (A) and infant (B) specimens. The external auditory canal/meatus (EAC/M) is placed more inferiorly in the infant than in the adult. Note the positions of the mastoid processes (MP) in the adult and mastoid portion (MP) in the infant. The foramen for the carotid artery is indicated with an asterix in the adult specimen but is less obvious in the infant. TM, tympanic membrane. *Used with permission of the Willard & Carreiro Collection.*

Epidemiological data demonstrate a significant decline in chronic serous otitis media after the age of 6 years (Bluestone & Klein 1995). This correlates closely with maturation of the eustachian tube position. A hypothesis of the pathogenesis of chronic serous otitis media must include discussion of the postnatal developmental changes and functional anatomy of the area which potentially affect eustachian tube drainage. During early life, horizontal placement of the eustachian tube may affect drainage. Furthermore, muscle tension in the tensor veli palatini, dilator tubae, medial pterygoid and salpingopharyngeus, tissue edema and abnormalities of the surrounding or tissue structures may compromise the diameter of the eustachian tube at the isthmus as well as affect patency. Addressing soft tissue function with gentle osteopathic manipulative medicine may decrease tissue edema and muscle tension, thereby facilitating normal eustachian tube function. Changes in tympanograms and acoustic reflectometry in children with chronic serous otitis media can be seen following osteopathic treatment and suggest a causative relationship (Fig. 11.7). Acoustic reflectometry (AR) is an easy-to-use method of measuring middle ear pressure and predicting middle ear effusion. The AR has been shown to be a reliable and valid alternative to tympanograms for predicting middle ear effusion (Block et al 1998).

A pilot study

Patients ranging in age from 18 months to 5 years were referred to the practice with a diagnosis of chronic otitis media with effusion. A few of the children were self-referred, but the majority were referred by an otolaryngologist or pediatrician. Each child was treated with osteopathic manipulative medicine, specifically balanced ligamentous and balanced membranous tension techniques. Each patient received a complete osteopathic examination and treatment. There is no single specific treatment for chronic serous otitis media; rather, a total body screening examination was performed, with application of osteopathic techniques to those anatomical areas most closely related to proper function of the middle ear and eustachian tube. No dietary restrictions were imposed. Antibiotics were administered if the patient's clinical picture suggested acute bacterial infection. No antihistamines were used, but in four cases the child was prescribed a decongestant/mucolytic. Clinical response was determined by visual inspection of the tympanic membrane with and without pneumatic otoscopy, time to first recurrence of acute infection, time to first recurrence of effusion, and duration of effusion when it recurred.

Twelve of the children involved in the study had complete resolution of the effusion by the fourth treatment visit. The time frame for this ranged from 4 weeks to 6 weeks. The children in this group remained free of acute otitis media symptoms during this period. Antibiotics were

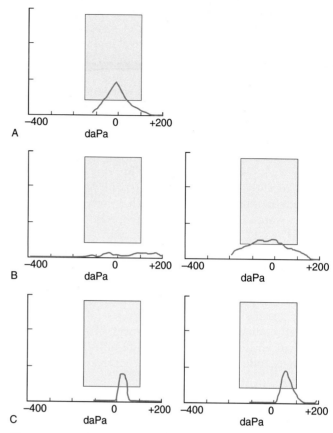

Fig. 11.7 • Comparison of tympanograms in a 13-month-old baby boy with a 9-month history of chronic serous otitis media with recurrent infection. (A) A normal reflex in an age-matched control provided for reference. (B) A reflex measured prior to osteopathic manipulative treatment. (C) A reflex immediately following osteopathic manipulative treatment; (C) was performed 20 min after (B).

not used, although, if indicated, decongestants were used during upper respiratory tract infections. Four children entered the treatment program on prophylactic antibiotics. These children remained on the antibiotics until the medication was discontinued by the referring/prescribing physician. This generally occurred once the effusion had cleared, generally within 4–6 weeks of initiating osteopathic manipulative treatment.

Once the effusion had cleared, these 16 children had no recurrence of acute otitis media as of the 18 months after initial clearing. However, more than half of them were seen for follow-up treatment during that 18-month period. Follow-up occurred either at the request of the referring physician for recurrence of effusion without infection, because of parental concern or at the discretion of the treating osteopath. No child was seen more than eight times during the 18-month period. Of the 18 children involved in the study, two showed no improvement in clinical presentation, including no appreciable change in the findings of the osteopathic examination after manipulative treatment. This indicated poor response or lack of response to osteopathic manipulative medicine. These children were referred back to the otolaryngologist for surgical management. Although this study dealt with a very small population, it was a useful preliminary tool in the investigation of alternative approaches to chronic otitis media with effusion. While a control group was not created specifically for the study, much data already exist concerning treatment outcomes for this population (Gates et al 1988, Goldie et al 1993, Handler 1994, Bluestone & Klein 1995).

More recently Mills et al (2003) published data on a pilot study in which 57 children with recurrent acute otitis media were randomized to an osteopathic manipulative treatment (OMT) or a standard treatment group. Patients in the OMT group had fewer reoccurrences, fewer surgical procedures, an increased frequency of improved tympanograms, and less antibiotic use than those in the standard treatment group (Mills et al 2003). However, in order to properly discuss the suggested efficacy of osteopathic manipulative medicine in the treatment of chronic otitis media with effusion or recurrent acute otitis media, larger prospective studies are needed.

CHRONIC SINUSITIS

Chronic sinusitis may be due to allergic inflammation or persistent infection. In young children, it will present as cough, stuffiness or congestion with or without nasal discharge. In addition, headaches, facial pain and mild facial edema may be present in adolescents (Kenna 2000). The cough is often worse at night or when the child is supine due to pharyngeal irritation from the postnasal drip. There may be morning nausea or loss of appetite. The child may complain of toothache if the maxillary sinuses are involved, or pain behind the eye if there is frontal, sphenoid or ethmoid involvement. The latter two may also present as headache over the top of the head or behind the eyes. The mechanism for this pain referral is discussed in Chapter 16.

On physical examination, there may be tenderness over the involved sinus. The pharynx may be erythematous with signs of postnasal drainage. Lymphoid hyperplasia may be visible as a cobblestone appearance of the posterior pharyngeal wall. This effect is produced by lymphadenopathy of the deep pharyngeal nodes draining the sphenoid and ethmoid sinuses. Transillumination of the maxillary and frontal sinuses can be helpful but is often difficult to interpret. Visualization of the nasal passages usually reveals swelling of the nasal turbinates, an erythematous mucosa which may be injected. Thin, stringy mucus suggests allergy, whereas more purulent discharge implies chronic infection. Having said that, chronic allergic rhinorrhea may appear thickened in the child having long-term treatment with antihistamines

or if the child is slightly dehydrated. Evaluation by X-ray, computed tomography (CT) scan or magnetic resonance imaging (MRI) may be required in complicated or recalcitrant cases. In cases of unresponsive or chronic infection with complications, aspiration of the sinus may be necessary to obtain definitive identification of the microbe.

Functional anatomy

Like the middle ear, the sinuses are part of the respiratory tract and are lined with pseudostratified columnar epithelium with cilia. Secretory cells are dispersed throughout. The secretory cells produce a mucous layer which coats the epithelium. The mucous layer has two parts. A superficial viscous gel layer traps particulate matter and other unwanted substances such as bacteria. Beneath it is a thinner sol layer, through which the cilia protrude. The cilia move through the sol layer, gently moving the particulate matter of the gel layer towards the ostium.

Mucus and debris exit the sinus at the ostia. This mechanism of clearance acts to protect the deeper respiratory tract from exposure to potentially harmful material, and the spaces created by the sinuses are involved with sound generation and transmission of speech. Obstruction of the ostia, paralysis or impaired function of the cilia or alterations in the quality of the mucous secretions will impede this mechanism and lead to sinusitis.

Rudimentary sinuses are present at birth and develop slowly over the next 12–14 years. However, in most people the sinuses continue to enlarge throughout life (Annon et al 1996, Standring 2004). The sinus ostia are quite small throughout life and lined with respiratory mucosa. The ostia may be obstructed due to mechanical obstruction from polyps, congenital anomalies, deviated septum, foreign body or traumatic injury. More commonly, obstruction is due to mucosal swelling. In fact, inflammation of the mucosa secondary to viral infection or allergic response is considered the most common cause of ostial obstruction (Wald 1996). Most often, there is partial obstruction which leads to delayed removal of secretions and inadequate aeration. When complete obstruction occurs, there is an initial increase in intraspinal pressure, which is followed by the development of negative pressure. When the ostium reopens, usually as a result of sniffling, sneezing or blowing one's nose, secretions can be insufflated from the nose back into the sinus. This is the most common mechanism for bacterial colonization of the sinus.

The ostium of the maxillary sinus is located on the superior medial wall (Fig. 11.8). Ciliary action is required to move secretions towards it. According to Sutherland's model of facial bone mechanics, movement of the zygoma on the maxilla acts to create a pumping mechanism in the sinus which facilitates the movement of fluids towards the ostium (Magoun 1976, Sutherland 1990). The ethmoid

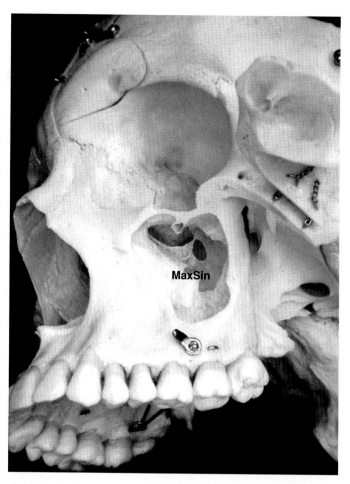

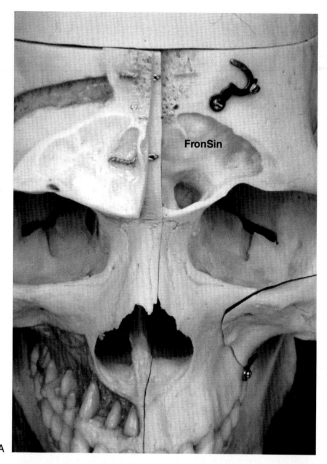

A

Fig. 11.8 • Adult skull revealing maxillary sinus (MaxSin); the lateral wall of the maxilla has been drilled away. The maxillary ostium has been artificially enlarged. *Used with permission of the Willard & Carreiro Collection.*

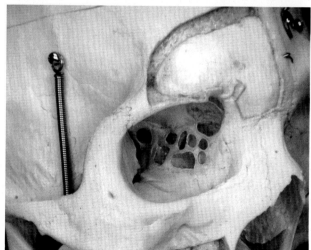

B

Fig. 11.9 • (A) Frontal sinus (FronSin) in an adult skull. (B) Ethmoid air cells viewed through medial wall of the orbit. *Used with permission of the Willard & Carreiro Collection.*

and frontal sinuses both drain into the nose through the nasofrontal duct (Fig. 11.9). Secretions enter the duct through scattered ostia in the inferior walls of the sinuses. Fenestrations in the walls of the ethmoid air cells may also allow passage of some secretions. The ostia of the sphenoid sinuses are located on the anterior–inferior walls of the sinuses. Although placement of the ostia in these latter sinuses suggests a potential for gravitational facilitation of mucous drainage it should be remembered that the mucous layer is a viscous gel which is moved by the cilia. Having said that, there is still some controversy regarding the effect of the supine position on mucous drainage (Bluestone & Klein 1996).

Mucociliary transport system

The mucociliary transport system provides the means for drainage of secretory products and particulate matter out of the sinuses. It is dependent on proper ciliary function and mucus viscosity. The cilia beat in a fixed direction but not in unison, and have been shown to clear substances from the nasal mucosa in 10–20 min (Cressman & Naclerio 1996). As the cilia pass through the gel layer, they elongate and straighten to move particulate matter towards the ostia. Then the cilia bend and pass through the thinner sol layer to return to the starting position. This coordinated motion is dependent on normal function of the cilia and normal consistency of the mucus. Ciliary motion can be impeded by congenital or acquired diseases of cilia motility. Viruses tend to affect the cilia as well. There is a decrease in ciliated cells after exposure to viral substances. Alterations in mucus viscosity will also impair mucociliary clearance. Thickening of mucous secretions occurs with chronic inflammation, cystic fibrosis, and some viral and other infections. Anticholinergic medications will increase mucus viscosity and delay mucociliary clearance. Likewise, antihistamines will thicken mucus and paralyze cilia. Conversely, guaifenesin is thought to decrease viscosity and facilitate clearance (Cressman & Naclerio 1996).

The mucociliary transport system of the upper respiratory tract receives parasympathetic and sympathetic innervation. The parasympathetic fibers synapse in the sphenopalatine ganglion and then traverse via the vidian nerve to the glands and vasculature of the mucosa. Parasympathetic stimulation causes increased secretion and vasodilation. Sympathetic innervations arise in the hypothalamus, and then travel to the superior cervical ganglion, where they synapse. Fibers then travel with the carotid arteries to join the parasympathetic fibers in the vidian nerve. Sympathetic stimulation causes vasoconstriction. Other neurotransmitters are also involved with upper respiratory mucosal function. They are part of the non-adrenergic–non-cholinergic system. Many of these have been discussed in Chapters 5 and 6, and are mediators of inflammation. Vasoactive intestinal polypeptide, substance P and calcitonin gene-related peptide are a few examples which seem to have a role in chronic sinusitis. Though the mechanism is unclear, the common presence of these proinflammatory substances may explain the clinical observation that chronic sinus congestion appears to be associated with gastroesophageal reflux.

Osteopathic evaluation

Facial mechanics are typically restricted in children with chronic sinusitis. The tissues of the pterygopalatine area are edematous and tender. The space between the pterygoid muscles and the connective tissues of the fossa is often quite narrow on one or both sides. In a cooperative child, use of the maxillary spread technique and zygoma techniques described by Sutherland (1990) and Magoun (1976) will go far towards resolving these strains. Compression at the ethmoid notch is usually present, especially in children with a history of congestion as infants. It is not unusual to find an intraosseous strain of the sphenoid between the lesser wings and the body. In the younger child, this may be perceived deep in the anterior cranial area, due to the position of the ethmoid. Restriction of base mechanics and

venous sinus system is usually present. Although it may be difficult to determine the primary dysfunction, normalizing base mechanics prior to addressing the other findings often proves successful. Vault restriction is often secondary to the findings in the cranial base. Dysfunction in the suboccipital muscles may be due to facilitation from pain referred from the sphenoid or ethmoid sinuses, via the trigeminal–cervical reflex (see Ch. 16).

Of special interest to the osteopathic practitioner is the role of sinusitis and upper respiratory tract congestion in triggering an asthmatic event. Sinusitis or congestion usually worsen the asthmatic symptoms and can interfere with bronchodilator treatment (Wald 1995). Undiagnosed chronic sinusitis may present as recalcitrant asthma (Kercsmar 1998). In these children, osteopathic treatment needs to focus on facial mechanics and factors that may be contributing to the sinusitis or upper airway congestion, in addition to dysfunction in other areas involved with respiratory activity.

Treatment

Chronic sinusitis due to recalcitrant infection should be treated with appropriate antimicrobials, and prophylaxis may be necessary. Mechanical obstruction should be dealt with appropriately, usually through surgical intervention. In viral or allergic exposures, as with the others, osteopathic treatment to resolve the associated mechanical dysfunction may help to facilitate mucociliary clearance of the sinuses and promote overall health. In addition to the traditional osteopathic description of the role of bony and tissue mechanics in sinus drainage and aeration, tissue edema, as noted by tissue texture changes and motion restriction, may have a role in persistent sinusitis through the non-adrenergic–non-cholinergic system previously described.

PERSISTENT NASAL CONGESTION IN THE NEWBORN

Newborns are obligate nose breathers for the first 2 or 3 months of life. Obstruction of the airways can result in cyanosis and even apnea. Consequently, nasal congestion in the newborn can be a real worry for parents. Typically, the child is noted to be congested very soon after birth. Although nasal drainage is usually scarce, parents can often use a manual suction bulb to aspirate thickened mucus from the nares several times throughout the day. The baby is typically described as snuffling and snorting during feeding. Cough is not present in the very young infant, because the reflex has not developed. Persistent nasal congestion does increase the risk of apnea and sudden infant death syndrome. There may or may not be a history of occiput posterior position, facial bruising with delivery, or abnormal trauma. Frequently, the mother will report that labor progressed slowly and then suddenly accelerated. This can occur when the baby is in an asynclitic position, which slows the progress of labor. If the baby can turn or shift, passage through the pelvis will accelerate. Nevertheless, the earlier forces of labor have entered the neonatal head and neck while in an abnormal position, and the tissues may not have been able to easily accommodate for this.

Physical examination is normal, except for mucus in the nasal passages and occasionally the mucosa being erythematous. Congenital abnormality, including deviated nasal septum, must be ruled out. In the majority of cases of chronic neonatal congestion, no causative etiology can be found and the congestion is explained away by the infant's undersized nasal passages. Theoretically, the sinuses are too small to be involved.

Osteopathic examination usually reveals compression at the frontoethmoid–sphenoidal junction, or the ethmoid notch. One must remember that this is an extremely small space in the newborn. Compression of the base may be present in some infants who are more than a few days old. However, in very young neonates and premature infants, the compressive strain may not be appreciable yet. Empirically, vertical strain patterns at the sphenobasilar synchondrosis and intraosseous strains in the sphenoid between the lesser wings and the body also appear to be associated with chronic congestion.

References

American Academy of Pediatrics and American Academy of Family Physicians 2004 Subcommittee on management of acute otitis media clinical practice guideline. Diagnosis and management of acute otitis media. Pediatrics 113(5): 1451–1465.

Annon J B, Rontal M, Zinreich S J 1996 Embryology and anatomy of the paranasal sinuses. In: Bluestone C D, Sylvan S E, Kenna M A (eds) Pediatric otolaryngology. W B Saunders, Philadelphia: 319–335.

Berg A O, Stool S E 1994 Managing otitis media with effusion in young children. Am Fam Physician 50(5): 1003–1010.

Berman S 1995 Otitis media in children. N Engl J Med 332(23): 1560–1565.

Block S L, Mandel E, McLinn S et al 1998 Spectral gradient acoustic reflectometry for the detection of middle ear effusion by pediatricians and parents. Pediatr Infect Dis J 98 17(6): S560–564.

Bluestone C D, Klein J O 1995 Otitis media in infants and children. W B Saunders, Philadelphia: 5–16, 39–54.

Bluestone C D, Klein J O 1996 Otitis media, atelectasis and eustachian tube dysfunction. In: Bluestone C D, Sylvan S E, Kenna M A (eds) Pediatric otolaryngology. W B Saunders, Philadelphia: 388–583.

Bosma J F 1986 Anatomy of the infant head, 1st edn. Johns Hopkins University Press, Baltimore.

Bylander A 1980 Comparison of eustachian tube function in children and adults with normal ears. Ann Otol Rhinol Laryngol 89: 20.

Bylander A, Tjernstrom O 1983 Changes in eustachian tube function with age in children with normal ears: a longitudinal study. Acta Otolaryngol Stockh 96(467).

Cressman W C, Naclerio R M 1996 Nasal physiology. In: Bluestone C D, Sylvan S E, Kenna M A (eds) Pediatric otolaryngology. W B Saunders, Philadelphia: 738–744.

Degenhardt B F, Kuchera M L 1994 The prevalence of cranial dysfunction in children with a history of otitis media from kindergarten to third grade. J Am Osteopath Assoc 94: 754.

Gates G A, Avery C A, Prihoda T J 1988 Effect of adenoidectomy upon children with chronic otitis media with effusion. Laryngoscope 98: 58–63.

Goldie P, Jung T K T, Hellstrom S 1993 Arachidonic acid metabolites in experimental otitis media and effects of anti-inflammatory drugs. Ann Otol Rhinol Laryngol 102: 954–960.

Handler S D 1994 Current indications for tympanostomy tubes. Am J Otolaryngol 15(2): 103–108.

Honjo I, Okazaki N, Ushiro K et al 1980a Cineradiographic analysis of eustachian tube function. Experimental study. Ann Otol Rhinol Laryngol 89(3 Pt 1): 276–278.

Honjo I, Okazaki N, Kumazawa T 1980b Opening mechanism of the eustachian tube. A clinical and experimental study. Ann Otol Rhinol Laryngol Suppl 89(3 Pt 2): 25–27.

Honjo I, Ushiro K, Okazaki N et al 1981a Evaluation of Eustachian tube function by contrast roentgenography. Arch Otolaryngol 107(6): 350–352.

Honjo I, Okazaki T, Ushiro K et al 1981b Experimental study of the pumping function of the eustachian tube. Acta Otolaryngol 91: 85–89.

Kenna M A 2000 Upper respiratory tract. In: Behrman R E, Kliegman R M, Arvin H B (eds) Nelson's textbook of pediatrics. W B Saunders, Philadelphia: 1258–1259.

Kercsmar C 1998 Asthma. In: Chernick V, Boat T (eds) Kendig's disorders of the respiratory tract in children. W B Saunders, Philadelphia.

Magoun H I S 1976 Osteopathy in the cranial field, 3rd edn. The Journal Printing Company, Kirksville, Missouri.

Mills M V, Henley C E, Barnes L L et al 2002 Effect of osteopathic manipulative treatment (OMT) on recurrent acute otitis media in children [meeting abstract]. JAOA 102: 441.

Mills M, Henley C, Barnes L et al 2003 The use of osteopathic manipulative treatment as adjuvant therapy in children with recurrent acute otitis media. Arch Pediatr Adolesc Med 157: 861–866.

Philippe A M, Bernard T N, Stenstrom R J et al 1991 Randomized, controlled trial comparing longterm sulfonamide therapy to ventilation tubes for otitis media with effusion. Pediatrics 88(2): 215–222.

Proctor B 1967 Embryology and anatomy of the eustachian tube. Acta Otolaryngol 86: 51–62.

Rood S R 1973 Morphology of the muscle tensor veli palatini in a five month old human fetus. Am J Anat 38: 191.

Rood S R, Doyle L W 1978 Morphology of tensor veli palatini, tensor tympani, and dilator tubae muscles. Ann Otol 87: 202–210.

Ross M 1971 Functional anatomy of the tensor palatini – its relevance in cleft palate surgery. Arch Otolaryngol 93: 1.

Standring S (ed.) 2004 Gray's anatomy, 39th edn. Churchill Livingstone, New York.

Sutherland W G 1990 Teachings in the science of osteopathy, 1st edn. Rudra Press, Portland.

Takahashi H, Hayashi M, Sato H et al 1989 Primary deficits in eustachian tube function in patients with otitis media with effusion. Arch Otolaryngol Head Neck Surg 115: 581–584.

Wald E R 1995 Chronic sinusitis in children. J Pediatr 127: 339–347.

Wald E R 1996 Rhinitis and acute and chronic sinusitis. In: Bluestone C D, Sylvan S E, Kenna M A (eds) Pediatric otolaryngology. W B Saunders, Philadelphia: 843–859.

Further reading

Bluestone C D, Klein J O (eds) 1995 Otitis media in infants and children. W B Saunders, Philadelphia.

Bluestone C D, Klein J O 1996 Otitis media, atelectasis and eustachian tube dysfunction. In: Bluestone C D, Sylvan S E, Kenna M A (eds) Pediatric otolaryngology. W B Saunders, Philadelphia: 388–583.

McMyn J K 1940 The anatomy of the salpingopharyngeus muscle. J Laryngol Otol 1–22.

Magoun H I S 1951 Osteopathy in the cranial field, 1st edn. The Journal Printing Company, Kirsville, Missouri.

Mills M, Henley C, Barnes L et al 2003 The use of osteopathic manipulative treatment as adjuvant therapy in children with recurrent acute otitis media. Arch Pediatr Adolesc Med 157: 861–866.

Parsons D S, Wald E R 1996 Otitis media and sinusitis: similar diseases. Otolaryngol Clin North Am 29(1): 11–25.

Weinberg B, Bosma J F 1970 Similarities between glossopharyngeal breathing and injection methods of air intake for esophageal speech. J Speech Hear Disord 35(1): 25–32.

Ophthalmology

INTRODUCTION

When you touch someone you love, when you see something that is beautiful or when you hear music which soothes, you are not touching with your hand, or seeing with your eyes or hearing with your ears. A signal of pressure, temperature, auditory frequency or light wave results in an electrical impulse in your central nervous system and the secretion of chemicals. Your brain interprets the electrical stimulation and the chemicals that are secreted. As a result, you feel someone you love, or you see something red or you hear Bach. If any of the connections from the peripheral receptors to the brain are disrupted, your ability to receive the stimulation will be affected. Our interpretation of the signal is based on other information, including prior experience and language. We may all have different perceptions of blue; however, we have all learned to call it blue. Language is simply a symbolic representation of some chemistry happening in our brain. For example, the sensory receptors in the retina of the visual system are stimulated by the frequency of light waves. They fire onto primary visual cortex located in the occipital lobe. The nerve cells arrange themselves in vertically oriented columns, which respond to a certain frequency of light. They then arrange themselves in horizontal rows based on the intensity of the stimuli. Our brain takes these areas and interprets them to form a picture that we recognize as shape or form or color. The process by which we interpret visual input is influenced by many factors and is discussed in the chapter on perception. The mechanism by which this input reaches the nervous system (the retina) involves the structures of the bony orbit, its muscular and connective tissue components and the globe.

DEVELOPMENTAL ANATOMY

The orbit and its contents develop from various embryonic tissues (Bosma 1986). The retina is an extension of the forebrain, the lens is ectoderm and the sclera is mesoderm. The extraocular muscles, their fascias and the circulatory system also derive from mesoderm. The orbital skeleton is composed of bones, which develop in membrane. Early in development, the globe is oriented laterally and the optic nerve lies in the frontal plane. As the face develops, the eyes are turned medially and anteriorly so at birth they are facing forwards. The optic nerve changes its position following the movement of the globe, eventually coming to lie in an oblique plane. The bony orbit will also alter its position and shape, although this process continues after birth.

At birth, the eyes are disproportionately large for the size of the face. The globe and orbit are quite round and shallow in the infant and toddler. In the adult, the orbital opening takes on a quadrangular shape, due in part to the elongation of the frontal processes of the zygoma and maxillary bones (Fig. 12.1). During the first year of life, an increase in facial and orbital width occurs through growth at the midpalatal sutures that affects the maxillae at the intranasal sutures, and increases the depth and width of the orbit, and growth at the metopic and frontal sutures, which affects the length of the supraorbital rim (Standring 2004). It is interesting to note that initial postnatal growth occurs along the midline of the face.

Inferior wall of the orbit: zygomae and maxillae

The infraorbital margin and floor of the orbit consist of the zygomatic rim laterally and the maxillary rim medially. In the newborn and infant, the zygoma is rather flat, lacking the characteristic prominence seen in most adults, which develops in response to forces from the zygomaticus minor and major, and the masseter muscles. The intraorbital articulatory surfaces of the zygomae are primarily cartilaginous in the infant and young toddler. However, unlike the other walls of the orbit, the inferior wall is complete and relatively stable. Intraosseous strains in the zygoma are rare unless there has been molding consequent to an abnormal uterine lie. From an osteopathic viewpoint, the articulation of the zygoma with the frontal appears to be rather stable when compared with other areas of the orbit, probably because the articulation is better defined and less vulnerable to membranous influences, whereas the medial wall of the orbit is primarily membranous with an often discontinuous surface and ill-defined osseous borders. As is the case with most bones of the orbital cavity, growth of the zygoma occurs at the periphery with deposition of bone on the facial surface (Standring 2004). The characteristic sailboat shape of the zygomae is achieved through expansion of

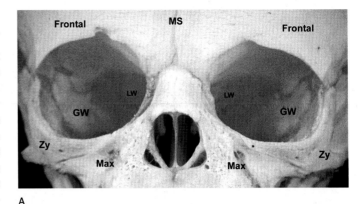

Fig. 12.1 • Comparison of the infant (A) and adult (B) orbital rims. MS, metopic suture; LW, lesser wing of the sphenoid; Zy, zygoma; Max, maxilla; GW, greater wing of the sphenoid. *Used with permission of the Willard & Carreiro Collection.*

the body, and lengthening of the maxillary and frontal processes. When comparing an infant and adult zygomae, most of the growth appears to occur at the sites of articulation with the maxilla, frontal and sphenoid, and relatively less at the temporal process.

At birth the maxilla is short and broad, the transverse and anteroposterior diameters being greater than the vertical. The plate of the maxilla forming the floor of the orbit is mature bone, and, although thin, it is completely formed and stable. The body of the maxilla contains no air sinuses, and the bulk of it houses the alveolar arch and the tooth sockets. In fact, there is very little bone between the tooth sockets and the orbital floor. The primitive maxillary sinus is only a groove on the nasal surface, perhaps twice the size of the nasolacrimal groove. The alveolar process and sinus will greatly increase in size, resulting in the pyramidal-shaped bone familiar in adults (Fig. 12.2). Growth of the alveolar process lengthens the medial rim of the orbit and enlarges and encloses the canal for the nasolacrimal duct.

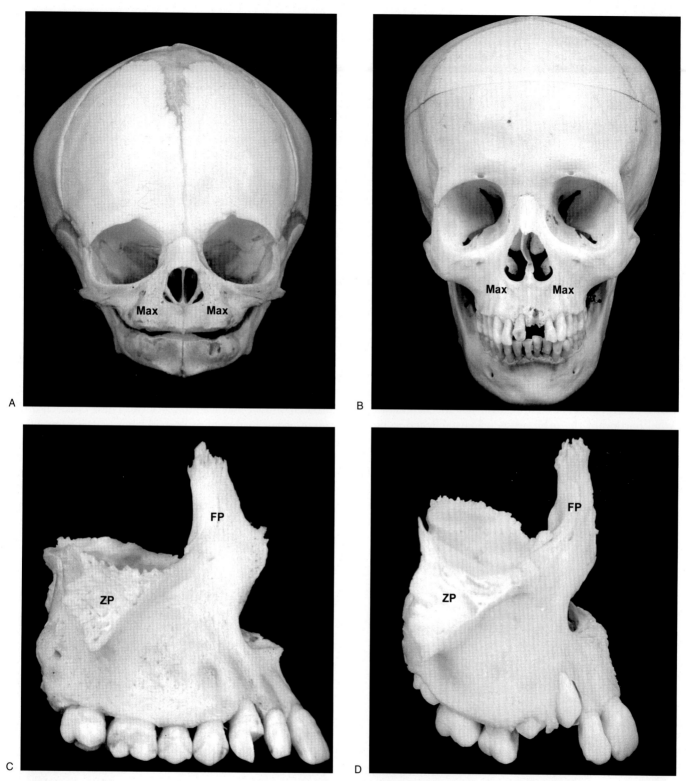

Fig. 12.2 • Anterior views of the infant (A) and adult (B) skulls. The disarticulated maxilla from an adult (C) and an older child (D) are also shown. The frontal process (FP) and zygomatic process (ZP) are labeled in each. Note the comparative sizes of the alveolar arch and frontal process in the different specimens. These changes occur through most of early life and account for the change in midface appearance during life. *Used with permission of the Willard & Carreiro Collection.*

Medial wall of the orbit: lacrimal, ethmoid, palatine, sphenoid

Ethmoid

The anterior portion of the medial wall of the orbit forms the partition between the apparatus of the eye, which is almost mature in size, and the nasal chamber, the size of which will increase fourfold to sixfold by adulthood. This area of the orbit undergoes significant change after birth. The lacrimal and ethmoid bones that are predominantly involved in these changes are formed in membrane and they are still cartilaginous at birth. The ethmoid accounts for much of the lateral margins of the nose and undergoes tremendous remodeling as the nasal passages widen and the conchae develop. The medial wall of the orbit may be fenestrated and incomplete (Fig. 12.3). The conchae may erode through the orbital plate of the ethmoid to become adjacent to the facial bones, which had once articulated with the ethmoid (Bosma 1986). Ethmoid and frontal air cells may also erode through this area. Because the medial wall is often incomplete and less stable, great caution should be used when addressing this area with manual techniques. Its cartilaginous and incomplete nature lends itself to strains that may be torsional or compressive. The mechanics of the medial portion of the orbit are poorly established at birth and remain so in the young child. By 7 years of age, growth of the upper nasal cavity is almost complete, providing some stability to the area, although the face continues to grow into adulthood.

It is important to remember that the cribriform plate of the ethmoid is shorter in newborns and infants. This means that the crista galli lies on the same plane as the lesser wings of the sphenoid. Consequently, the ethmoid notch area is relatively more compressed than in the adult, and the anteroposterior length of the medial wall of the orbit is less.

Lacrimal

The lacrimal bone is a small delicate structure which articulates anteriorly with the frontal process of the maxilla, posteriorly with the orbital plate of the ethmoid, superiorly with the frontal bone and inferiorly with the orbital surface of the maxilla. The lacrimal bone is influenced posteriorly and superiorly by the cranial base and anteriorly by the face. Consequently, the lacrimal bone can become a place where conflicting stresses are resolved. The most common problem involving this area is dacryostenosis, a blocked lacrimal duct. This usually presents quite soon after birth, as thickened discharge in the area of the lacrimal punctum. Under normal conditions tears secreted by the lacrimal gland pass through the conjunctival sac, aided by blinking, to the lacrimal canaliculi and into the lacrimal sac. From here the fluid is eliminated through the nasolacrimal duct. *Gray's anatomy* (Standring 2004) describes the process as being facilitated by contractions of the orbicularis oculi, which has a small attachment to the lacrimal bone. These contractions occur with blinking movements. Restriction at the site of the canaliculi or duct may lead to blockage. These children often present with a history of prolonged labor or cranial molding. Forces exerted upon the cranial vault may be transmitted through the frontal or ethmoid bones and absorbed at the junction between lacrimal, maxilla and ethmoid. It must also be remembered that in the newborn this area is incompletely formed and extremely thin, which makes it vulnerable to membranous-type strains. The osseous canal of the lacrimal duct (Fig. 12.4) is formed by the maxilla, lacrimal bone

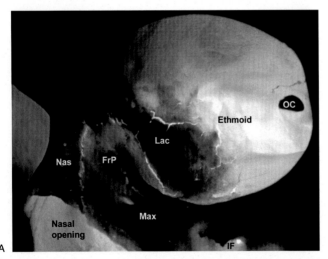
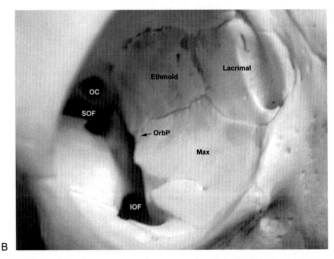

Fig. 12.3 • Transilluminated left infant orbit (A) is presented for comparison with a right adult orbit (B). Note the thinness of the medial wall in the infant, and fenestration in the adult. OC, optic canal; Lac, lacrimal; FrP, frontal process of the maxilla; Nas, nasion; Max, maxilla; IF, infraorbital foramen; OrbP, orbital process of the palatine; SOF, superior orbital fissure; IOF, inferior orbital fissure. *Used with permission of the Willard & Carreiro Collection.*

and inferior nasal concha. Because the maxilla is primarily influenced by the sphenoid via the palatine bones, forces imparted onto the sphenoid may affect the facial mechanism and the relationship between the lacrimal and maxilla. Facial presentations are also common in children with dacryostenosis, for obvious reasons. If the frontal process of the maxilla

is driven posteriorly or the lacrimal anteriorly, the duct will be narrowed. More often, the strain seems to be posterior, coming from the ethmoid into the lacrimal, probably because face presentations are rare. Intraosseous strains between the supraocciput and intraparietal occiput may be conveyed through the falx and/or tentorium to the developing crista galli of the ethmoid and into the lacrimal.

Sphenoid

Postnatal development of the sphenoid was discussed in Chapter 3. Here we will only review changes as they relate to the eye.

The sphenoid comprises the posterior aspect of the inferior and lateral walls of the orbit. The zygoma and maxilla form the anterior aspect. The lateral wall is shorter than the medial wall, which tends to direct the newborn's eyes laterally. With growth of the lateral bones and elongation of the frontal processes of the maxilla, the eyes will set more medially. According to Magoun (1976), non-union of the presphenoid and postsphenoid will produce a slant to the eyes. This can be seen in children with Down's syndrome. The superior and inferior fissures are relatively larger in the newborn than in the adult (Fig. 12.5). In the infant, the superior orbital fissure is more elongated and narrow than in the adult, where it assumes a triangular shape. Its borders consist of the body of the sphenoid medially, the lesser wing superiorly and laterally, and the greater wing inferiorly

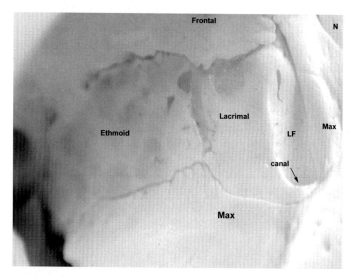

Fig. 12.4 • Lacrimal fossa (LF) and canal in an adult specimen. It is almost imperceptible in the infant specimen (see Fig. 10.3 A). Max, maxilla; N, nasion. *Used with permission of the Willard & Carreiro Collection.*

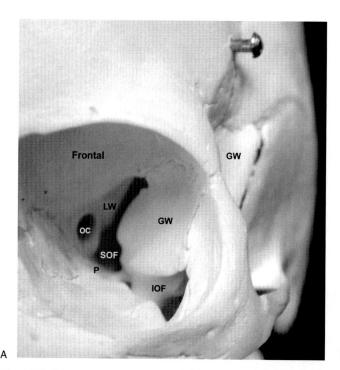

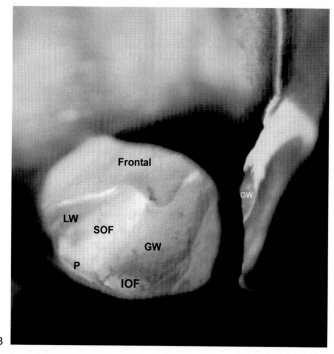

Fig. 12.5 • View of the orbit in the adult (A) and the infant (B). The shape and orientation of the superior orbital fissure (SOF) and inferior orbital fissure (IOF) can be compared. LW, lesser wing; GW, greater wing; OC, optic canal; P, palatine bone. *Used with permission of the Willard & Carreiro Collection.*

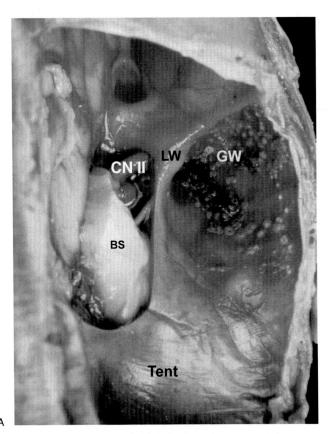
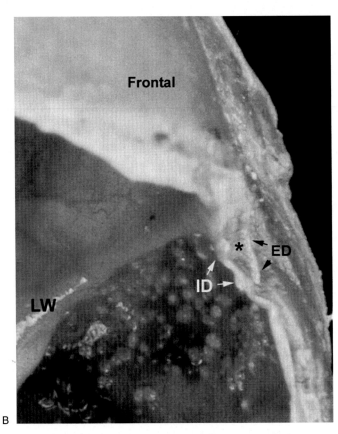

A

B

Fig. 12.6 • (A) Photograph of a newborn specimen. The camera is positioned posterior and to the right of the head. The right hemisphere of cortex has been removed to expose the tentorium (Tent) and the cut brainstem (BS). The greater wing (GW) and lesser wing (LW) of the sphenoid are labeled. The optic nerve (CNII) is also labeled. (B) is a close-up of the cut coronal suture. The external dural layer (ED) and internal dural (ID) layer are indicated by the arrows. Between them lies a space (*), which will eventually be lost as the cranium matures. The continuity between the lesser wing and coronal suture in the newborn is evident. *Used with permission of the Willard & Carreiro Collection.*

and laterally. These three parts of the sphenoid are not fused at birth and exist as separate structures joined by very thin cartilage. At birth, the lesser wing is embedded in the remnant of the anterior dural girdle. A cross-section of this area clearly shows the lesser wing as a cartilaginous structure, out of which extends a thickened connective tissue band, which sweeps coronally over the anterior vault (Fig. 12.6). The greater wing, which is also immature, is embedded in the periosteum of the anterior cranial fossa, and lies on the same plane as the crista galli and anterior clinoid processes. The periosteum of these structures can also be seen to extend from this remnant of the anterior dural girdle. Intraosseous strains within the sphenoid may result from forces acting on the cranial base which transmit through the basisphenoid or from forces acting upon the vault which are transmitted through the membranous cranium, i.e. the anterior dural girdle, into the paired structures of the sphenoid. In addition, these same forces may be distributed into the ethmoid or the basisphenoid. Intraosseous strains generated through the cranial base tend to involve the sphenoid body and lesser wing component on

the greater wings, and are often associated with compression within the basisphenoid. Intraosseous strains generated through the vault tend to involve the greater wing on the body–lesser-wing unit and tend to be unilateral. Often there is a torsional strain passing into the ipsilateral pterygoid and primitive palatine. Intraosseous strains of the sphenoid will alter the shape of the superior orbital fissure. The superior and inferior ophthalmic veins, frontal, lacrimal, nasociliary and cranial nerves II, III and VI, may be affected. The latter four nerves travel through the common tendon of the extraocular muscles, which extends from the optic canal across the inferior aspect of the superior orbital fissure (Fig. 12.7). Alterations in the relationship of the parts of the sphenoid may also indirectly affect the rectus muscles of the eye, which have their origin in the common tendon.

The optic canal is a small foramen bounded on each side by a cartilaginous bridge connecting the lesser wing to the sphenoid body. The optic nerve and ophthalmic artery pass through this space surrounded by a connective tissue netting. Intraosseous strains involving the lesser wing and body may affect these structures. All vessels and nerves are

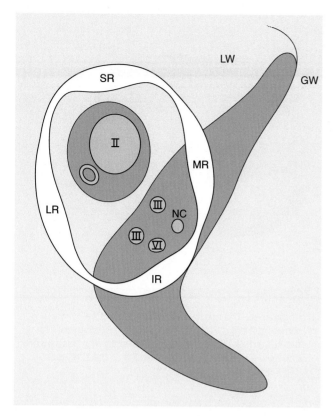

Fig. 12.7 • Schematic diagram of the common tendon and its attachments. LW, lesser wing; GW, greater wing; SR, superior rectus muscle; MR, medial rectus muscle; IR, inferior rectus muscle; LR, lateral rectus muscle.

supplied by tiny arteries, veins and nerves that travel with them. Slight compressive forces on these miniscule structures may impede their function, leading to changes in the action potentials and depolarization properties of the nerves they supply. In addition to all the aforementioned structures, intraosseous strains may alter the shape of the orbit, influencing the mechanical efficiency of the oblique muscles or the levator palpebrae.

Palatine

The palatine extends a very small, but quite important, process into the floor of the orbit. According to Sutherland (1990) and Magoun (1976), this process is involved with maintaining a balanced tension in the maxillary nerve throughout the flexion and extension cycles of the cranium. The action of the orbital process maintains the tension of the maxillary nerve. At term, the orbital and sphenoidal processes are made of cancellous bone. The grooves for the maxillary and greater palatine nerves are smooth and well formed. While the palatine will undergo extensive postnatal remodeling, the area associated with the maxillary groove is relatively stable. However, it may be affected by changes

happening elsewhere. Most of these will involve the components related to the naso-oral pharynx.

At birth, the horizontal plates are mere veneers, described by Bosma (1986) as 'vanes', which the *Oxford dictionary* (Brown 1993) defines as a projection to be acted upon by air or liquid. The transverse surface, which attaches to the maxilla, has no serration or digitation and overlaps the maxilla. The pyramidal process extends slightly laterally to meet the lateral pterygoid plates of the sphenoid. At birth, the dimensions of the horizontal and perpendicular plates are almost equal, whereas in adults the length of the perpendicular plate is twice the width of the horizontal plate (Standring 2004). This accounts for much of the difference between the neonatal and adult oropharynx. Other changes involve the invasion of maxillary and ethmoid sinuses into the orbital partition. The anteromedial aspect of the orbital process communicates with the sphenoidal sinus in the adult. This sinus is not formed in the infant, so this is an aspect of the orbital process which will undergo remodeling.

The palatines form a functional partition between the mouth and pharynx, and between the face and cranial base. The former partition is muscular and functional in nature and is described in detail in Chapters 11 and 14. The latter is osseous and mechanical in nature, and is well described by Magoun (1976).

Frontal

The entirety of the superior wall of the orbit consists of the frontal bones, which extend slightly along the lateral margin to articulate with the zygomae. At birth, the frontals are paired structures joined at the metopic suture (Fig. 12.8). During postnatal development, the frontal bones must accommodate changes occurring in the adjacent structures. Development of the frontal lobes and enlargement of the vault influence the frontal bones through the falx cerebri, culminating in the formation of a metopic ridge and usually fusion of the suture. The roof of the orbit is thin and may be incomplete, while the superior orbital ridge is quite thickened and well developed. Postnatally, the articulatory surfaces adjacent to the lacrimal bone mature sooner than those adjacent to the sphenoid and parietal bones. Initially, these sutural areas are smooth, with ill-defined boundaries. The bone itself differentiates into two layers of cortical bone with a layer of cancellous bone sandwiched between. The primitive sinuses appear during the first year of life. They will invade the bone, sometimes erupting through the wall into the orbital space. Vertical growth of the frontal at its maxillary and zygomatic processes contributes to changes in the shape of the orbit. The relation of the frontal articulation with the cribriform plate will also alter in response to changes in the nasal chambers and this will affect the medial aspect of the orbit.

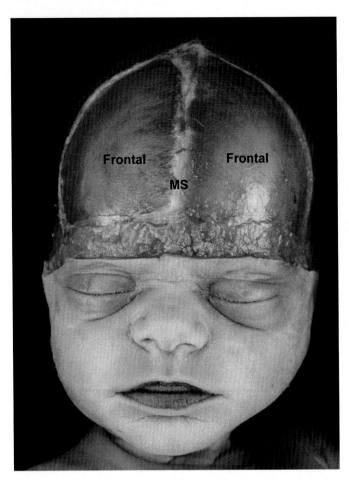

Fig. 12.8 • The metopic suture (MS) in a newborn specimen. *Used with permission of the Willard & Carreiro Collection.*

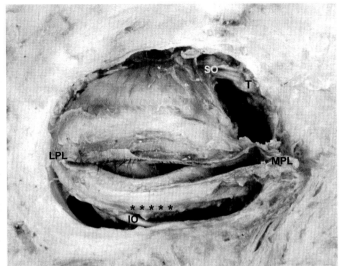

Fig. 12.9 • An anterior view of the dissected ocular ligaments of an adult specimen. The inferior oblique (IO) and superior oblique (SO) muscles can be seen. The medial palpebral ligament (MPL) and lateral palpebral ligament (LPL) are also evident. T = trochlea. The check ligaments lie deep to the palpebral ligaments. The suspensory ligament is marked (*****). *Used with permission of the Willard & Carreiro Collection.*

The lacrimal gland is immature at birth. It is suspended from the lateral aspect of the orbital roof in the lacrimal fossa of the zygomatic process of the frontal bone.

Fascia

The contents of the orbit are protected and supported by the surrounding fat and fascia. Although continuous, the fascial sheaths are given various names, depending on location, attachment and who discovered them. A sheath of fascia covers the optic nerve and extends forwards with it to the back of the eye. Here it spreads out, becoming the fascia of the posterior aspect of the globe. Wherever it reaches an extraocular muscle, it turns onto the muscle, becoming the muscle sheath. Posteriorly, where the recti muscles attach to the common tendon, this same fascia merges into the tendon. Where the oblique muscles attach to the bony orbit, their fascial sheaths merge with the periosteum. The orbital fascia forms the periosteum of the orbit, but it is only loosely attached to the bones (Standring 2004). This space provides one of the potential routes for

the spread of infection from the face and periorbital area into the cranium. The fascial sheath of the superior rectus muscle blends with that of the superior palpebral muscle. The fascial sheaths of the lateral and medial rectus thicken as they approach the bone and firmly attach to the zygoma and maxilla as the medial and lateral check ligaments. Slung between the check ligaments and beneath the eye is a thickened fascial hammock called the suspensory ligament of the eye (Fig. 12.9). The interrelatedness of the fascial arrangements of the eyes creates a support system for eye movement, limiting and guiding motion to some extent. This can be seen in nerve palsies, where the eye will drift back to a neutral position when the unaffected antagonist muscle relaxes. The influence of these fascial structures on the eye may be important in understanding astigmatism, refractive errors in the lens created by the shape of the lens and presbyopia (the loss of the ability of the lens to accommodate).

MUSCLES OF THE EYE

There are six extraocular muscles (EOMs), four of which are oriented towards cardinal directions and called recti, and two which are oblique (Fig. 12.10). The four recti muscles have a common origin in the fibrous common annular tendon. The common tendon surrounds the optic canal and crosses the superior orbital fissure to attach to the greater wing of the sphenoid. It will be influenced by the mechanics of the lesser wing, greater wing and body of the sphenoid. The four recti muscles arise from this tendon, although

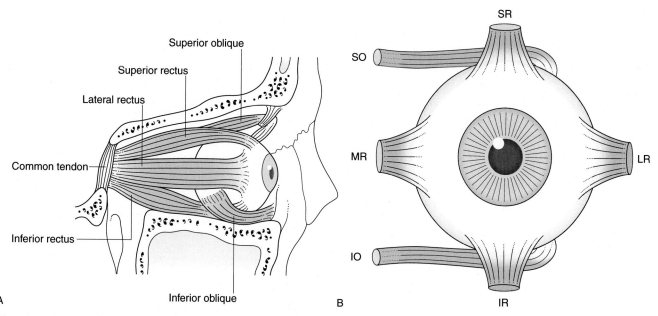

Fig. 12.10 • Schematic diagrams depicting the extraocular muscles from a lateral (A) and cut anterior (B) view. SO, superior oblique; IO, inferior oblique; MR, medial rectus; LR, lateral rectus; SR, superior rectus; IR, inferior rectus. In the lateral view (A), the muscles are depicted attached to the common tendon.

the lateral rectus also has a head that originates from the greater wing of the sphenoid lateral to the common tendon (Standring 2004). An analysis of the actual mechanics of the EOMs of the eye can be quite complicated. However, a general understanding of their function and effect on eye position is needed to interpret clinical and palpatory findings. The position of the eye is named by the position of the pupil. The medial and lateral recti adduct (medial) and abduct (lateral) the eye across the horizontal plane of the visual field. These four muscles (two on each eyeball) act through a complicated neurological sequence to produce conjugate vision; coordinated movement of both eyes along the horizontal plane, convergence; movement of both eyes towards the midline, or divergence; and movement of both eyes away from the midline. The superior and inferior rectus muscles move the eyeball on the vertical axis and they each influence the horizontal plane, so that the resultant motion is superior medial for the superior rectus and inferior lateral for the inferior rectus. The oblique muscles also influence motion on the vertical and horizontal planes. The isolated effect of the inferior oblique muscles is to move the eye up and out, while that of the superior oblique is to position the pupil down and in. In concert with the superior and inferior recti, the oblique muscles can elevate and depress the eyes along the midline.

The two oblique muscles attach directly to the bony orbit. The superior oblique originates from the body of the sphenoid, above and medial to the optic canal. The muscle travels forwards, passing through the trochlea, a fibrous ring

attached to the frontal bone. Thus the superior oblique is affected by the mechanics of the sphenoid and the frontal bones. The trochlear nerve innervates the superior oblique. Increased tone or contraction of the superior oblique turns the eye downwards and medially. The inferior oblique lies along the inferior orbital surface. It has its origin on the maxilla just lateral to the nasolacrimal groove. The muscle weaves posterior and laterally first between the inferior rectus and the orbital floor and then between the lateral rectus and the globe, before inserting on the eye. Along with the superior, inferior and medial recti, the inferior oblique is supplied by the oculomotor nerve. Contraction of the inferior oblique turns the eye upwards and laterally. In the presence of oculomotor nerve injury, the forces of the superior oblique and lateral rectus would be unopposed and the eye would deviate downwards and outwards.

Osseous strains of the orbit or strains affecting the connective tissue structures surrounding the eye may influence the biomechanical efficiency of the EOMs. Most strabismus is responsive to surgical correction of the positioning of the EOMs, suggesting a mechanical rather than neurological cause.

At birth, the attachments of the EOMs on the globe are essentially in their adult position. However, the myriad of changes occurring to the bony structures to which they attach will alter the relationship of the globe and the EOMs to the orbit. The trochlear of the superior oblique will be displaced anteriorly as the orbital plate of the frontal grows. The attachment of the inferior oblique will move anteriorly with expansion of the maxilla. The origin of the oblique muscles is closer to the coronal plane in the infant than in the adult (Bosma 1986).

The superior levator palpebrae muscle, which elevates the eyelid, has voluntary and autonomic functions. It has its origin on the lesser wing of the sphenoid and inserts into the distal margin of the lid. Except for blinking, the levator palpebrae must maintain contraction for many hours. Most ptosis in newborns and infants is mild, covering less than one-quarter of the visible surface of the eyeball. It generally does not obscure the visual field. When it does, amblyopia may develop. Mild ptosis may be seen in children with intraosseous strains involving the lesser wing of the sphenoid that affect the biomechanical efficiency of the muscle. This is more likely to be the etiology if the ptosis is intermittent or associated with fatigue. Constant ptosis, which covers one-half to three-quarters of the height of the eye, can be related to injury of the oculomotor nerve and is rare.

INNERVATION OF THE STRUCTURES OF THE EYE

The optic nerve carries information from the ganglionic cells in the retina; it and the retina are an extension of the brain. They are covered with oligodendrocytes, not Schwann cells. The optic nerve passes back through the optic canal to enter the intracranial space. The two nerves join at the optic chiasm, which is positioned just superior to the sella turcica, the center of the five-pointed star. Within the orbital space, the nerve is slightly longer than the distance from the optic foramen to the eye. This gives it a rather sinuous appearance. The optic nerve is enveloped in the layers of the cranial meninges: pia, arachnoid and dura. This is a potential route of access for the invasion of bacteria from the eye into the brain, though normally the eye is aseptic. There is an arterial plexus in the pial sheath of the nerve, which, along with some intraneural arteries, provides necessary nutrients to the nerve and retina. According to *Gray's anatomy* (Standring 2004), the pia sends a process into the substance of the nerve. Because of these connections, meningeal irritation may present with severe eye pain and photophobia.

The oculomotor nerve supplies all the muscles concerned with the eye, except the lateral rectus and superior oblique. It carries proprioceptive fibers from the trigeminal ganglion, as well as motor and autonomic fibers from cranial nuclei along a convoluted path towards the globe. The nerve exits the ventral side of the midbrain and travels through the subarachnoid space covered by a pial sheath. It passes between the superior cerebellar and posterior cerebral arteries, which in older individuals may expand and take on a tortuous appearance, compressing the nerve. (This is rare in children.) The nerve travels through the interpenduncular

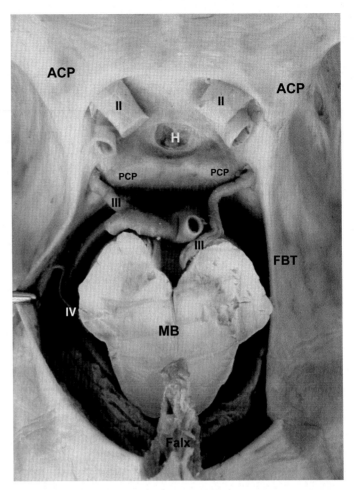

Fig. 12.11 • View into the cranium. The cortex has been removed to reveal the midbrain (MB). The cut edge of the falx cerebri (Falx) can be seen. The anterior clinoid processes (ACPs) are labeled, as is the free border of the tentorium (FBT). The oculomotor nerve (III) can be seen passing between the free and attached borders of the tentorium, just posterior to the posterior clinoid processes (PCPs). Forceps are lifting the edge of the tentorium to expose the trochlear nerve (IV) as it pierces the inner dura. The cut hypophysis (H) lies in the sella turcica. The optic nerve (II) lies over the ophthalmic artery. *Used with permission of the Willard & Carreiro Collection.*

cistern with the posterior communicating artery, and then pierces the arachnoid and passes between the free and attached borders of the tentorium (Fig. 12.11). Here it penetrates through the inner layer of dura near the posterior clinoid process and migrates between the inner and outer dura to enter the cavernous sinus. Within the cavernous sinus, the oculomotor nerve receives sympathetic fibers from the internal carotid plexus. It then enters the orbit, dividing into a superior and inferior ramus. The superior ramus travels laterally, sending branches to the rectus superior and levator palpebrae muscles. The inferior ramus supplies the medial and inferior recti and the inferior oblique muscles. The branch to the inferior oblique also sends fibers to the

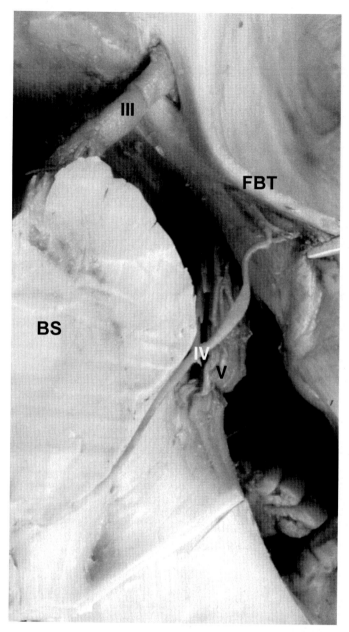

Fig. 12.12 • A close-up view of the trochlear nerve (IV) piercing the free border of the tentorium (FBT). The trigeminal (V) and oculomotor (III) nerves can be seen. *Used with permission of the Willard & Carreiro Collection.*

ciliary ganglion. Obviously, the oculomotor nerve is in a vulnerable position for compression and irritation throughout its long, dangerous traverse. Areas of particular importance are where it crosses the borders of the tentorium and where it pierces the inner dura. Both of these areas would be susceptible to osseous and membranous strains. Again, we need to remember that irritation or compression of the tiny nervi vasorum of the nerve will impede delivery of oxygen and nutrients to the nerve, adversely affecting conduction. The nerve need not be greatly compressed for its function to be compromised.

The trochlear nerve innervates the superior oblique muscle and also has an interesting path. Within the brainstem, the tracts decussate and exit the dorsal side of the brainstem. The nerve moves anteriorly by wrapping around the cerebral peduncle and passing between the superior cerebellar and posterior cerebral arteries with the oculomotor nerve. It then pierces the inner dura just inferior to the free border of the tentorium (Fig 12.12). Traveling through the cavernous sinus, the nerve is accompanied by the oculomotor and ophthalmic division of the trigeminal. Crossing the oculomotor, it enters the orbit through the superior orbital fissure, above the common tendon. Within the sinus, the trochlear nerve receives fibers from the trigeminal. True trochlear paralysis presents with an inability to look down and out; the child will compensate by extending the head and neck and side-bending away from the side of involvement.

The lateral rectus muscle receives its supply from the abducens nerve, which exits the ventral portion of the brainstem. It pierces the inner dura and ascends over the apex of the petrous portion of the temporal bone beneath the petrosphenoid ligament. It passes through the cavernous sinus and enters the orbit via the common tendon. This nerve is at greatest mechanical risk in two areas: as it crests the petrous portion, where abnormal position of the temporal may place stretch on the nerve or the ligament may compress it, and passing through the annular ligament, where the mechanics of the orbit may affect the shape of the ligament or the position of the surrounding muscles and fascia. Complete paralysis of the lateral rectus results in an esotropia, and the eye will deviate medially.

INHERENT MOTION OF THE EYE AND ORBIT

The orbit is pyramidal in shape. Magoun (1976) implies that the bony apex is at the optic foramen; however, visual inspection and measurement of adult and infant skulls suggest that it is at the inferior medial portion of the supraorbital fissure (Fig. 12.13). During the flexion phase, the anterior–posterior (AP) length of the orbit decreases, while the superomedial–inferolateral diameter increases. Simply put, the orbit gets broader and flatter. The physiological motion of the globe is somewhat different. Being an extension of the brain, the eyeball will express motion patterns similar to those described by Sutherland for the central nervous system. During the flexion phase, the globes will converge towards lamina terminalis, decreasing its AP diameter and increasing its transverse. The fulcrum of globe motion is the optic nerve. During the extension phase of cranial base motion, the globe moves away from the lamina terminalis, the AP diameter increases, and the transverse decreases. Consequently, when

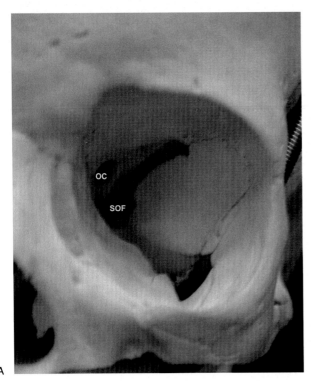 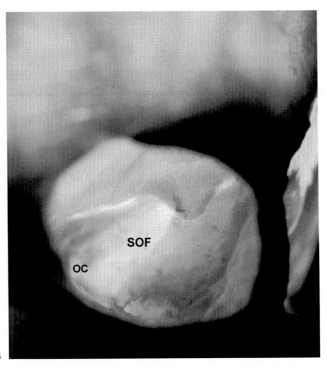

A   B

Fig. 12.13 • Views of the left orbit in an adult (A) and transilluminated in an infant (B), demonstrating the bony apex. OC, optic canal; SOF, superior orbital fissure. *Used with permission of the Willard & Carreiro Collection.*

evaluating the intrinsic motions of the structures in this area, the observer needs to be aware that the fulcrum of motion is different for the eye and its bony house. Placing the pads of your fingers along the orbital rim, you would observe that the orchestrated movements of the involved bones seem to orient almost directly posterior to the center of the external orbital surface, whereas the inherent motion of the globe is superior and medial to that point. This is important to remember in cases of astigmatism, where the shape of the lens is distorted. One can compare the functional position of the globe with that of the orbit to determine if the problem lies within the relationship of the eyeball to its origin or is an indirect result of bony strains. Comparing the orientation of the globe to that of the orbit will also provide useful information when evaluating myopia and hyperopia.

VISUAL ACUITY

Rays of light entering the eye are refracted by the cornea and lens and focused onto the retina. The refractive properties of the lens bend rays of light towards a focal point. Near-sightedness and far-sightedness result when the axial length of the eye is either too short (hyperopia) or too long (myopia) for the refracting power of the lens. The focal point of the rays of light is either behind or in front of the

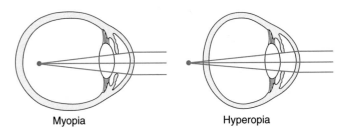

Myopia   Hyperopia

Fig. 12.14 • Schematic diagram depicting the focal point of light in myopia and hyperopia.

retina (Fig. 12.14). Consequently, the light is dissipated and the image is blurred. The focal point will also be affected by distortions in the lens that create differences in refractive power between meridians. This is called astigmatism.

Hyperopia may result when the mechanics of the orbit or central nervous system as described by Sutherland (1990) restrict free movement into the exhalation phase. Conversely, myopia may result when movement towards the inhalation phase is restricted. If the problem is due to a refractive error in the lens, the eye itself may strain into the appropriate phase to accommodate the focal point (Fig. 12.15). Corrective lenses aim to adjust the refractive power of the ocular lens and shift the focal point onto the retina. Glasses that are too strong or too weak will create

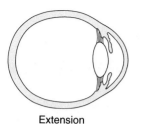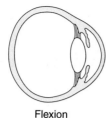

Extension Flexion

Fig. 12.15 • Schematic diagram depicting the relative shapes of the globe during the extension and flexion phases described by Sutherland (1990). The extent of the distortion is obviously exaggerated.

strains in the inherent motility of the eye as it attempts to compensate for the position of the focal point. This may lead to all sorts of complaints, including, but not limited to, headaches, hyperactivity, postural strains, depression and fatigue. Osteopathic findings suggesting paradoxical motion between the eyes and central nervous system or strains within the globe itself may be due to the aforementioned mechanisms and warrant further investigation. Training in this aspect of osteopathy is available and should be pursued. The ability to prescribe corrective lenses using this information will ensure that the entire mechanism benefits from the therapeutic process.

STRABISMUS

If we look at the ontogeny of eye movements, there is some evidence that eye movements in the first few months are affected by the rapidly changing anatomy of the globe (Bushnell & Boudreau 1993). As previously stated, the globe and orbit are quite round and shallow. The relationships between the EOMs and their origins and insertions are slightly different from those found in an older child or adult. The position of each EOM determines the mechanical effect it will have on the globe. The EOMs maintain a dynamic, tonic relationship with each other, which translates into positional stability and smooth movement of the globe. The relationship between the origin and insertion of each muscle will influence its effectiveness in balancing the forces exerted by the other EOMs. Distortions in the geometry of the bony orbit may arise from biomechanical strains. For example, if a child has a tissue strain which alters the relationship between the body of the sphenoid and the frontal bone, the relationship between the origin and insertion of the superior oblique muscle will also be affected. If the origin and insertion are abnormally close, then over time the muscle may develop a shorter resting length, and be more resistant to lengthening, and may actually have a harder time contracting against the forces of the opposing muscles (Frank–Starling principle). If the origin and insertion are further apart than usual, then the resting length

is longer, and the muscle will have to use more metabolic energy to contract against the forces of opposing muscles. In either scenario, the efficiency of muscle work is altered, resulting in fatigue and an eye that drifts away from the target. In point of fact, most cases of strabismus occur due to restrictive rather than neurological factors. This accounts for the high success rate of corrective surgery, whereby the relationship between the EOMs is corrected such that the biomechanical effectiveness of the muscle is enhanced.

Strabismus is misalignment of the visual axes. It may be comitant, where the angle of misalignment remains constant regardless of the direction of gaze, or non-comitant, when the amount of misalignment varies with the direction of gaze. Non-comitant strabismus is associated with muscular paralysis and may indicate neurological or orbital injury. Comitant strabismus is usually due to mechanical factors. Strabismus can also be classified into phorias, which are misalignments of the visual fields that can be elicited by the cover-uncover test. Phorias are usually controlled by the normal fusion mechanism. Mild heterophoria, the tendency of one eye to deviate when not focusing, is normal, especially in children. However, heterophoria, which presents with binocular tracking, may represent an orbital asymmetry, which may be treated osteopathically. Trophis are misalignments which usually result from abnormal muscle function, either biomechanical or neurological. These are more significant and more likely to create problems for the child.

Strabismus will present differently at different ages. In the very young infant, it may go completely undetected. Prior to 4 weeks, there is a lack of coordination between the EOMs, and infants of this age may appear cross-eyed. As the infant grows and the visual system matures, accommodation, tracking and convergence are somewhat easier to evaluate, although prior to 2 years of age the experience of the examiner is the determining factor in the success of the examination. However, there are certain clues which, when present, suggest the need for a thorough ophthalmological evaluation. Any infant developing a torticollis, wryneck or abnormal head position that appears to resolve during sleep and worsens during wakeful periods deserves an ophthalmological examination (Hertle & Zhu 2000). An infant or child with strabismus may compensate by altering the position of her head (Fig. 12.16). In the presence of esotropia or exotropia, this may manifest as a cocked position of the head. During sleep, the visual stimulus for the head position is removed and the head and neck move towards neutral. In muscular torticollis, a child will maintain the head and neck position even in sleep, and will often awaken or become fussy if forced to lie with his head in the opposite position. Although there is centrally driven torticollis that improves during sleep, this is rare in children and is suspected to be the consequence of infarctive events. While there appears to be a familial component to strabismus (Abrahamsson et al 1990, Aurell & Norrsell 1990), clues in the child's history

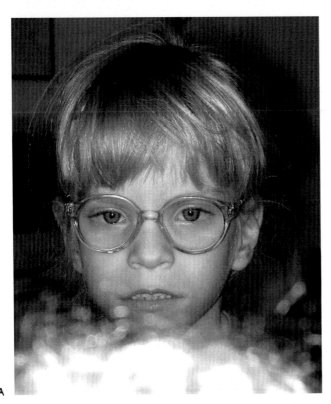

A

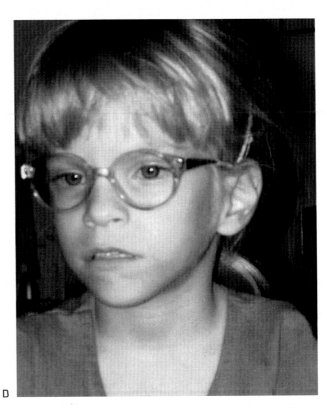

D

Fig. 12.16 • (A, B) In these two photographs, the child was asked to look at a small doll that the examiner held directly in front of her. After approximately 90 s, the child began to turn her head to maintain her focus. This is an example of postural adaptation to a strabismus. The child has esotropia in the right eye. *Used with permission of the Willard & Carreiro Collection.*

may suggest a mechanical etiology. Face presentations, deliveries where forceps were placed near the greater wings of the sphenoid or on the face, excessive molding, gross asymmetries in the shape or position of the orbits, and facial malformations or asymmetries may affect the structure of the bony orbit, and influence the position of the EOMs and compromise their mechanical effectiveness.

AMBLYOPIA

Amblyopia is cortical blindness. It occurs in approximately 2% of children and it is preventable. It needs to be recognized and addressed prior to 5 years of age. Amblyopia is unilateral defective vision, uncorrectable by lenses. It may occur when two eyes are misaligned, as in strabismus. In this case, the visual information from one eye is suppressed. Fifty percent of children with amblyopia have strabismus. Significantly different refractive errors between the two eyes may also be a cause, as well as occlusion of the visual axis. Risk factors for amblyopia include less than 32 weeks of gestation, family history, worsening astigmatism, strabismus and significant refractive errors between the eyes (Sjöstrand & Abrahamsson 1990, Levartovsky et al 1995,

Eibschitz-Tsimhoni et al 2000). Photoscreen photography can be used to screen low-risk children; others should be referred to an ophthalmologist.

Amblyopia can occur in children when there is aberrant or contradictory information coming from a retina. The brain will selectively inhibit development of the cortical cells receiving the aberrant input. Just like cells everywhere else in the nervous system, the cells of the occipital lobe need to be stimulated to function. If the cells are not stimulated, the connections and organization of the cells will be affected. This may occur if a child has a strabismus severe enough that a double image is created. The brain will shut off the signal from the deviant eye. Cells in the occipital cortex receiving signals from this eye will be deprived of stimulation and will not develop. Although the globe, the retina and the nerve pathways may be functional, the occipital lobe cannot interpret the signal they carry. Amblyopia may also occur when the visual acuity in one eye is significantly less than in the other. If undetected, the brain will selectively inhibit the input from the affected eye. There is a critical window of opportunity during which the process of amblyopia can be reversed; many investigators place this time period between 5 and 10 years, although definitive studies are scarce. If the problem is addressed during this time, then the child has a fairly good chance of developing normal function in the involved cortical cells.

Amblyopia is generally treated with occlusion therapy or lenses. Recent studies suggest that visual acuity improves in strabismic amblyopia in the first 6 months of therapy and plateaus thereafter (Cleary 2000). Successful outcome (visual acuity of 20/40) is reduced in the presence of fixed strabismus and worsening astigmatism (Beardsell et al 1999).

VISION AND POSTURE

Our eyes are involved with balance. They give us information about our relationship to the horizon. Basically, your brain wants you to see the horizon as level. Along with plagiocephaly and torticollis, strabismus may be a risk factor for scoliosis. In each of these conditions, the orientation of the visual axis to the horizon is disrupted. In response to the deviated position of the head, reflexes presumably mediated through the oculovestibular system create changes in the resting length of paraspinal muscles, leading to abnormal joint position and changes in posture. In other words, the brain will twist the spine to keep the eyes level. Children with significantly different refractive errors between their eyes, or amblyopia, may also be at risk for developing scoliosis.

The vestibular system influences the eyes through the vestibulocephalic reflex. While studies have not investigated the precise mechanism for the effect of visual stimulus upon the vestibular system, we all know from experience that discrepancies between the two often result in nausea and/or dizziness. This can also be a problem in individuals in whom the postural mechanisms are compromised, specifically children with motor problems, spinal deformity, or congenital problems of the head or neck. As was previously discussed, proprioceptive input from mechanoreceptors in the neck and low back provide much of the information used to establish and maintain posture. When visual problems arise in these children, the ability to maintain balance and postural integrity may be compromised. These children frequently show decompensation of postural strategies (see Ch. 9). Changes in the postural mechanics of the head and neck are frequently the most noticeable. If corrective lens prescription is inappropriate, many of these children will develop complaints of headache, dizziness or vague gastrointestinal symptoms. When at-risk children present with the aforementioned complaints and the etiology is unclear, look to the visual system.

BEHAVIORAL OPTOMETRY AND VISION

Although the globes, extraocular muscles, associated cranial nerves and vessels of the eye are almost mature at term gestation, the ability to organize and interpret impulses passing from the retina is still immature. This process occurs in visual cortex and different parts of the cortical hemispheres and takes longer to mature. Vision, the ability to recognize and derive meaning from visual stimuli, is influenced by the development of other sensory systems, movement, posture and experience. It is part of the greater process of perception. Having said that, we can turn it around and 'look' at vision as a tool for effecting changes in perception and the way we interact with the world.

Behavioral or functional optometry is a branch of optometry which places great emphasis upon the role of vision in the development and expression of who the patient is, and how he or she processes the world. Collaboration with someone trained in behavioral or functional optometry can be most rewarding to patient and practitioners.

OCULAR EVALUATION

A general examination of the eyes in even the youngest child must include an evaluation of pupillary reactions to rule out optic nerve damage, lens displacement, and cataracts. The presence of conjugate gaze and accommodation can be ascertained by enticing the child with a bright toy which generates a sound. For very young babies, a black and white object is easiest. Holding the object 30 cm from a child and moving it across his field of vision best assesses tracking. I often draft one of the parents into the game, and nonchalantly try to assess the eyes while the father entertains the child. The position of the reflected corneal light should be symmetrically placed in each eye (Fig. 12.17). Any asymmetry

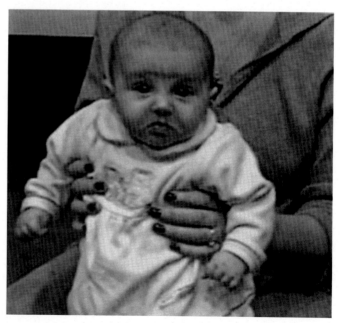

Fig. 12.17 • The light reflected from this infant's corneas is symmetrical. *Used with permission of the Willard & Carreiro Collection.*

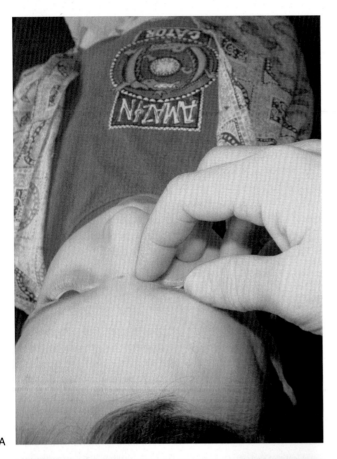

A

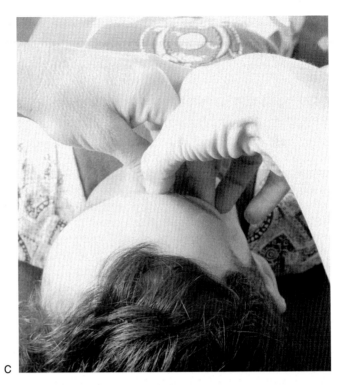

C

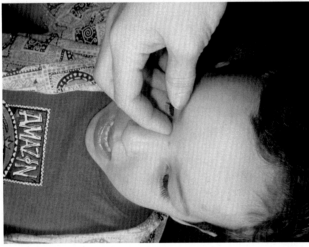

B

Fig. 12.18 • Hand placement for evaluation and treatment of the orbit and eye. The first hand is placed so that the distal pads rest upon the bones of the orbital rim: maxilla, frontal, zygoma, lacrimal/nasal. Two views are shown (A, B). The thumb and index (and if possible middle) finger of the second hand (C) are slipped under the first hand to gently rest upon the globe. In this manner, the globe and orbit can be assessed simultaneously. *Used with permission of the Willard & Carreiro Collection.*

needs further investigation, as it may be due to strabismus. The cover test can be used with children who can maintain focus, usually between 8 and 10 months. In children under 1 year, retinal evaluation is very tricky unless you are quite skilled, and it is best to refer the child if needed. As a result, the entire examination can be performed in a naturally lit room or one with soft lighting. This in itself makes the evaluation easier, as the child is less agitated.

The shape of the bony orbit should be ascertained through both visual and palpatory inspection. Special attention should be paid to those areas associated with either the origin or insertion of a muscle. Although most cases of strabismus are restrictive, the relationships between the bones of the cranial base may give clues towards undesirable influences upon cranial nerves IV, V and VI. The relationship of the petrosphenoid ligament and abducens nerve may be inferred by findings in the sphenoid and temporal areas. The examiner should have a high index of suspicion for interosseous strains affecting bones of the orbit or middle cranial fossa in any child with suspected heterophoria.

The maxilla and palatine are sometimes forgotten when evaluating the orbit; however, these bones and the adjacent structures may also have a role in strabismus. The globe will accommodate to the shape of its bony house. This may create strains in the inherent mechanics of the globe or in the tissues residing between it and the orbit. The ability of the eye and orbit to integrate can be ascertained by comparing the mechanics inherent in each of these structures and the adaptations taking place. The examiner places the pads of the thumb and fingers of the ipsilateral hand on the rim of the bony orbit. The pads of the thumb and middle finger of the contralateral hand are slipped beneath the first hand and gently placed upon the closed eye (Fig. 12.18). This hand position allows the examiner to observe the mechanics of the globe and orbit simultaneously.

Osteopathic treatment will be much more effective if the fulcrum of any apparent strain can be precisely localized to the appropriate tissue of origin – bone, membrane, etc. In infants under 8 months, the strain is almost exclusively membranous in origin, with osseous compensation. After 8 months, the osseous component is generally more significant in the strain pattern. This probably occurs because the bony mechanics, which are directed and guided by the membranous mechanics, become more fixed as the child grows. The osseous fulcrum has a more rigid nature than that of the membrane and is often more apparent. Nevertheless, the osseous findings are a result of compensation to the membranous strain, with the latter being primary.

Strains originating in the globe or central nervous system phenomena (as described by Sutherland (1990)) are also possible but rare. These children usually have other congenital findings, most often including retinopathy. Primary fluid strains influencing eye mechanics are usually associated with pathogen or chemical exposure during gestation and, again, other congenital findings are present. Rarely, a fluid strain in the orbit or globe may be associated with vacuum extraction, but the pattern is localized and quite distinct, with force vectors oriented towards the site of the vacuum placement.

CONCLUSION

Integral to a thorough osteopathic evaluation of the eyes and orbits is the knowledge that these structural relationships are changing. With growth and development, new forces are placed upon the musculoskeletal structures, sometimes altering the existing relationships. A strain, especially an interosseous one, may go undetected during an initial evaluation, only to be exacerbated when the next growth spurt or developmental milestone is reached. A comprehensive understanding of the orbit and visual development affords the practitioner the information needed to anticipate changes and their potential effects.

References

Abrahamsson M, Fabian G, Andersson A K et al 1990 A longitudinal study of a population based sample of astigmatic children – I. Refraction and amblyopia. Acta Ophthalmol (Copenhagen) 68(4): 428–434.

Aurell E, Norrsell K 1990 A longitudinal study of children with a family history of strabismus: factors determining the incidence of strabismus. Br J Ophthalmol 74(10): 589–594.

Beardsell R, Clarke S, Hill M 1999 Outcome of occlusion treatment for amblyopia. J Pediatr Ophthalmol Strabismus 36(1): 19–24.

Bosma J F 1986 Anatomy of the infant head, 1st edn. Johns Hopkins University Press, Baltimore.

Brown L (ed.) 1993 The new shorter Oxford English dictionary, Vol. 2. Oxford University Press, Oxford: 3544.

Bushnell E W, Boudreau J P 1993 Motor development and the mind: the potential role of motor abilities as a determinant of aspects of perceptual development. Child Dev 64: 1005–1021.

Cleary M 2000 Efficacy of occlusion for strabismic amblyopia: can an optimal duration be identified? Br J Ophthalmol 84(6): 572–578.

Eibschitz-Tsimhoni M, Friedman T, Naor J et al 2000 Early screening for amblyogenic risk factors lowers the prevalence and severity of amblyopia. J Am Assoc Pediatr Ophthalmol Strabismus 4(4): 194–199.

Hertle R W, Zhu X 2000 Oculographic and clinical characterization of thirty-seven children with anomalous head postures, nystagmus, and strabismus: the basis of a clinical algorithm. J Am Assoc Pediatr Ophthalmol Strabismus 4(1): 25–32.

Levartovsky S, Oliver M, Gottesman N et al 1995 Factors affecting long term results of successfully treated amblyopia: initial visual acuity and type of amblyopia. Br J Ophthalmol 79(3): 225–228.

Magoun H I S 1976 Osteopathy in the cranial field, 3rd edn. The Journal Printing Company, Kirksville, Missouri.

Sjöstrand J, Abrahamsson M 1990 Risk factors in amblyopia. Eye 4(Pt 6): 787–793.

Standring S (ed.) 2004 Gray's anatomy, 39th edn. Churchill Livingstone, New York.

Sutherland W G 1990 Teachings in the science of osteopathy, 1st edn. Rudra Press, Portland, Oregon.

Further reading

Abrahamsson M, Fabian G, Sjöstrand J
1990 A longitudinal study of a population
based sample of astigmatic children – II.
The changeability of anisometropia. Acta
Ophthalmol (Copenhagen) 68(4): 435–440.

Bosma J F 1975 Introduction to the
symposium. In: Bosma J F, Showacre J
(eds) Development of upper respiratory
anatomy and function. National Institutes
of Health, Bethesda: 5–49.

Bosma J F 1986 Anatomy of the infant head,
1st edn. Johns Hopkins University Press,
Baltimore.

Bosma J F, Showacre J (eds) 1975 Symposium
on development of upper respiratory
anatomy and function: implications for
sudden infant death syndrome. National
Institutes of Health, Bethesda.

Levartovsky S, Oliver M, Gottesman N et al
1998 Long-term effect of hypermetropic
anisometropia on the visual acuity of
treated amblyopic eyes. Br J Ophthalmol
82(1): 55–58.

Magoun H I S 1951 Osteopathy in the
cranial field, 1st edn. The Journal Printing
Company, Kirksville, Missouri.

Magoun H I S 1973 Idiopathic adolescent
spinal scoliosis. DO 13(6).

Chapter **Thirteen**

13

Pulmonology

CHAPTER CONTENTS

INTRODUCTION

The respiratory system is an engine of gas exchange. Its primary function is to replace waste products that are dissolved in the blood with oxygen. This occurs through a process of diffusion that is influenced by the partial pressure of oxygen, the permeability of the alveoli–capillary barrier and the time available for equilibration. Decreased oxygen saturation or availability, thickening or obstruction of the alveolar wall or increased respiratory rates and decreased functional residual capacity (FRC) adversely interfere with this function. The result is increased carbon dioxide and hydrogen ion concentrations, and decreased oxygen levels in the blood. In the extreme case, this results in respiratory failure. Diseases of the respiratory system may interfere with ventilation, perfusion and/or gas exchange across the alveoli wall. The impediment of any of these tasks will increase the work of breathing. The work of breathing can be thought of as the ability of the child to generate gas volumes against the elastic and resistive forces of the lung. Under normal conditions, the work of breathing in very young infants and children is complicated by the compliancy of the chest wall, the immaturity of neuronal mechanisms, and the heightened tone of the pulmonary vasculature. Therefore, the ability of the young child to compensate for increased workload during times of stress is compromised.

When discussing problems of the respiratory system, we need to remember the factors present in the child which have a bearing on the clinical picture. First, children have more elastic recoil in the lung parenchyma and the distal airways are more compliant. This translates into an increased vulnerability for collapse and atelectasis. Second, the bronchial smooth muscle is thicker and more reactive, with a tendency for bronchospasm when irritated. Third, the musculoskeletal structures involved with breathing are mechanically and neurologically less effective. Finally, the infant lung has more secretory glands, so that when inflammation does occur, mucus production increases to a greater extent than in the adult (O'Brodovich & Haddad 2001).

Diseases of the middle and lower respiratory system can be classified into two broad categories: restrictive diseases that affect the elastic properties of the lung and obstructive diseases that affect gas exchange (Haddad & Mellins 1984). Restrictive disease occurs when the ability of the lung to attain appropriate air volume is impeded; that is, the elastic recoil of the lung increases. This may result from increases in the surface tension of the alveoli, decreases in the compliancy of lung parenchyma or filling of the alveolar spaces. Examples of this would be respiratory distress of the newborn, interstitial edema or pneumonitis, infectious processes and congenital problems affecting the chest wall or thorax. Obstructive disease occurs when the ability of the lung to exchange gas is impeded, either through turbulent flow or increased resistance to exhalation. The common denominator in obstructive lung disease is narrowed airways and increased work of breathing. In general, children with obstructive and restrictive disease present differently. According to Haddad and Perez Fontain (1996), children with restrictive disease tend to compensate by increasing the rate and decreasing the depth of breathing. There is often an expiratory grunt present. Children with obstructive disease will compensate by taking slower and deeper breaths with a prolonged exhalation phase with recruitment of accessory muscles. An inspiratory stridor, wheeze or rales may be present.

Because children need to expend considerably more work to meet respiratory demands, careful evaluation of the acute patient's condition is warranted so that appropriate intervention may occur. In the remainder of this chapter, we will discuss acute and chronic respiratory conditions which may present for osteopathic evaluation and management. Pathophysiology, clinical presentation and appropriate treatment will be reviewed in the context of the child's ability to compensate and the body's tendency towards self-healing.

NEONATAL RESPIRATORY DISTRESS SYNDROME

Neonatal respiratory distress syndrome (NRDS) or hyaline membrane disease (HMD) is a direct result of immaturity of the newborn lung. Contributing factors include anatomical immaturity of the lung, increased compliance of the chest wall and inefficiency of the premature pulmonary lymphatics, coupled with decreased surfactant function or production. Approximately 30% of all neonatal deaths result from complications of HMD. Risk factors include prematurity, low birthweight, maternal diabetes, asphyxia, cesarean section delivery, cold stress and multiple gestation pregnancies (Verloove-Vanhorick et al 1986, Cotran 1989, Kliegman 1996, Montan & Arul-Kumeran 2006). Surfactant deficiency

results in high surface tensions in the alveolar spaces. The infant is unable to develop a sufficient functional residual capacity and the affected alveoli tend to collapse. Blood is shunted away from the involved area, which then becomes ischemic. The resulting inflammation causes capillary leakage and deposition of fibrin and protein into the alveolar spaces, with the formation of a hyaline membrane, which obstructs gas exchange (Maitra & Kumar 2005).

Signs of surfactant deficiency present almost immediately after birth, with grunting, nasal flaring, sternal and intercostal retractions, and tachypnea. Administration of surfactant can improve mortality but does not appear to decrease bronchopulmonary dysplasia (Kliegman 2007). Bronchopulmonary dysplasia is marked by thickening of the alveolar walls accompanied by peribronchial and interstitial fibrosis (Cotran 1989), which adversely affect gas exchange and ventilation. In the neonatal intensive care unit (NICU), therapeutic measures include mechanical ventilation, exogenous surfactant, and appropriate measures to maintain pH and blood pressure. Mechanical ventilation of infants with NRDS frequently includes the addition of positive end-expiratory pressures (PEEPs), which increase residual volume and improve oxygen saturation. In the neonate with NRDS, the chance of developing bronchopulmonary dysplasia increases with mechanical ventilation and the use of PEEP. This presents quite a dilemma for the treating physician, who needs to maintain oxygen levels in the baby without contributing to alveolar damage.

The potential role for osteopathic manipulative treatment of these children has only been explored empirically. Osteopathic treatment directed at improving lymphatic drainage from the lung may help to decrease the elastic recoil of the interstitial tissue and decrease surface tension in the alveolar space, both of which decrease the need for PEEP. PEEP has been shown to decrease venous return to the heart, which affects cardiac output and leads to mild hypoxia, and pulmonary vasoconstriction. Tissue strains in the abdomen and pelvis which could potentially decrease venous return to the caval system need to be addressed so that they will not contribute to the overall effect of PEEP. The relative static posturing required for both ventilation and nasal continuous positive airway pressure (CPAP) places constant compression on the compliant neonatal torso. Mechanical dysfunctions at the costovertebral and costochondral junctions are common, and in many cases rib deformity can develop. Osteopathic treatment may alleviate biomechanical dysfunction in these areas and aid in decreasing the mechanical work of breathing. Neonates on mechanical ventilation provide some unique challenges to osteopathic treatment, and only after the infant is stabilized should osteopathic manipulative techniques be considered. The following may complicate the beneficial effects of osteopathic treatment, and special care needs to be taken to avoid adverse consequences: the presence of persistent hypotension in the child increases the risk of intraventricular bleed, techniques in the head and neck should be avoided, as well as fluid fluctuation techniques; endotracheal tube placement may be disturbed, with movement of the head or neck resulting in obstruction or trauma; and finally, catheterization of the umbilical artery increases the child's risk for embolism, and, while rare, vascular trauma, visceral techniques should be avoided and abdominal and anterior pelvic techniques should only be used with great caution in experienced hands.

BRONCHOPULMONARY DYSPLASIA

Bronchopulmonary dysplasia (BPD) is the most common form of chronic lung disease in infants. The clinical presentation consists of radiographic abnormalities, oxygen dependence and respiratory symptoms (Hazinski 1998). Pathological changes include thickened alveolar walls, interstitial fibrosis and narrowing of the airways (Cotran 1989). Emphysematous changes may occur in distal airways, while the walls of pulmonary arterioles thicken, leading to right ventricular hyperplasia (Hazinski 1998). Long-term problems include increased incidence of respiratory infection, reactive airway disease, cardiac involvement, and aspiration with or without gastroesophageal reflux (Hazinski 1998).

BPD usually results from lung injury sustained due to the mechanical ventilation. The oxygen and mechanical ventilation adversely affect alveolar and vascular development in the lung parenchyma. While in the past it was common in most infants receiving PEEP, the use of antenatal steroids has fortunately reduced the incidence and mostly confined development of the condition to low weight premature infants of less than 28 weeks' gestational age (Northway et al 1976, Smith et al 2005, Van Marter 2005). BPD manifests as decreased oxygen saturation levels on room air. It has four stages: acute lung injury, exudative bronchiolitis, proliferative bronchiolitis, and obliterative fibroproliferative bronchiolitis. Treatment includes nutritional support, hydration, oxygen supplementation, and pharmacotherapeutics. The age at which the infant can wean from oxygen supplementation correlates with the prognosis for recovery. The long-term prognosis is dependent on the ability of the lung to grow and the alveoli to undergo normal septation and development.

In the majority of infants with BPD, the condition improves, although many are left with chronic reactivity and bronchial asthma (Bader et al 1987, Gibson et al 1988). Many infants experience generalized developmental delay, including growth, during the first 24–36 months, but catch up as the disease process abates (Meisels et al 1986). During the chronic phase of BPD there is fibrosis of the alveolar septa. There is also mucous gland hypertrophy and squamous metaplasia (Hazinski 1998). Smooth muscle hypertrophy around pulmonary arteries and bronchioles is present. These infants have a tendency towards right ventricular hypertrophy. Once stabilized, a child with BPD may be discharged on oxygen, and, when appropriate, diuretic and/or bronchodilator therapy. Corticosteroid therapy is also prescribed in some cases, although its use is more controversial (Hazinski 1998). Most children have persistent radiographic changes and recurrent symptoms into early childhood. These children face an increased workload of breathing. Common problems include growth delay, transient psychomotor retardation, and complications from medication use. Less common but more devastating long-term risks include developing pulmonary hypertension, cardiac hypertrophy and right-sided failure, emphysema, respiratory distress and necrotizing bronchiolitis (Kliegman 2007).

The goal of osteopathic treatment in these children is to minimize the work of breathing so that minimal medication is needed, decrease cardiac afterload so that right-sided work is not increased, and maximize ventilation–perfusion match and gas exchange. Factors that may adversely affect pulmonary bronchial smooth muscle tone and pulmonary vascular tone include vagal irritation and somatic findings that may influence autonomic tone, such as spinal facilitation in the thoracic area. Techniques which normalize biomechanical relationships in the torso may promote respiratory muscle efficiency. Specific attention should be paid to the mechanics of the ribs and their associated vertebrae, the sternum, pelvis, diaphragm, quadratus lumborum, and the scalene muscles and their cervical attachments. The mechanics of the nasopharynx and their role in maintaining patency of the upper airway also need to be considered. This includes the cranial–cervical junction and cranial base because of the role this area has in oropharyngeal function. Fascial restrictions may have a role in tissue congestion. Nociceptive stimulation may generate segmental restrictions in paraspinal muscles and may facilitate autonomic drive to smooth muscle of the airways and vasculature. Cell bodies for sympathetic fibers innervating pulmonary smooth muscle are located in the lower cervical and upper thoracic cord. Paraspinal muscle spasm in the lower cervical and upper thoracic areas would contribute to spinal facilitation in these levels. Fluid mechanics within the pulmonary lymphatics should also be monitored. Finally, optimal neuroendocrine immune function can be supported by decreasing any somatically induced nociceptive input. Environmental exposures which might exacerbate bronchial muscle reactivity need to be eliminated; these may include smoke (wood and tobacco), pets, certain foods and any other substance to which the child may be sensitive.

TRANSIENT TACHYPNEA OF THE NEWBORN

Transient tachypnea of the newborn (TTN) occurs when the removal of intrapulmonary fluid from the neonatal lung is delayed. Under normal conditions, the alveolar fluid would be removed by the pulmonary lymphatics in the hours after birth. When removal is delayed, the child presents with tachypnea, mild retractions and cyanosis (Avery et al 1966, Adams et al 1971). TTN is a benign, self-limiting condition. In the healthy term newborn, fetal lung fluid triggers the J receptors, which increase respiratory rate. As the fluid is absorbed, the rate decreases. The condition usually resolves within 48 h after birth, but in severe cases may continue for 3 or more days. There is a higher incidence of TTN in children delivered by cesarean section, presumably because the thoracic compression occurring during vaginal delivery facilitates movement of pulmonary fluids (Milner et al 1978, Lee et al 1999). Alterations in intrathoracic pressures facilitates lymphatic drainage from the thorax. The majority of children with TTN who have been examined osteopathically (chart review of newborns examined in the newborn nursery at the Waterville Osteopathic Hospital, 1988–1993) present with restriction of normal newborn respiratory mechanics, usually involving the thoracolumbar and pelvic areas, particularly the quadratus lumborum muscles. Dysfunction in the mechanics of the scalene muscles is also frequently found. While there are no published data on the efficacy of osteopathic treatment in this condition, anecdotal data suggest that osteopathic evaluation and treatment focused on improving fluid mechanics in these children will almost always result in a fairly rapid resolution of the tachypnea.

APNEA

Apnea is defined as a pause in respiration, its clinical significance being determined by its length. Most normal infants and children experience pauses, sighs and irregular respiration during rapid eye movement (REM) sleep which are asymptomatic (Alvarez et al 1993, Kirkpatrick & Mueller 1998). Premature infants often exhibit period breathing, which is characterized by a 3–10 s pause followed by 15 s of breathing. Then the cycle is repeated. Its etiology is unknown and assumed to be related to immaturity of brainstem function. It, too, is considered benign (Kirkpatrick & Mueller 1998). True apnea or clinical apnea is accompanied by cyanosis, bradycardia and signs of respiratory distress (O'Brodovich & Haddad 2001). Apnea may be due to central, peripheral or mixed processes (Marchal et al 1987).

Apnea occurring during sleep may be due to upper airway obstruction (UAO). When this occurs in older children, there is usually an associated anatomical abnormality. Children with UAO may present with disturbed sleep habits, snoring, failure to thrive and developmental delay. Older children with undiagnosed UAO frequently do poorly in school, and some have enuresis (O'Brodovich & Haddad 2001). The most common factor in UAO is tonsillar adenopathy (Potsic et al 1986, Laurikainen et al 1992). Studies have shown that tonsillectomy is the most appropriate and effective choice of treatment

in most children (Guilleminault et al 1981, Brouillette et al 1982). However, when conditions warrant surgery being delayed or avoided, there are other, albeit somewhat less effective, options. Tonsillar adenopathy may develop secondary to allergen exposure. This can occur in toddlers and young children who are still breastfeeding. If weaning has occurred, then other food sensitivities should be investigated. The time frame for reduction of allergic tonsillar adenopathy will vary and may be insufficient to alleviate the obstruction; nevertheless, it should be considered when surgery is not an option. Other effective strategies for UAO include CPAP administered through a nasal cannula. CPAP has been shown to be effective in the long-term treatment of UAO (Schmidt-Nowara 1984, Guilleminault 1987), although it often interferes with sleep, and children frequently pull the apparatus off. When UAO is associated with obesity, weight loss improves the clinical picture. In the presence of congenital abnormalities, surgical intervention is warranted.

Apnea may also be associated with spitting up. In this case, gastroesophageal reflux into the esophagus stimulates vagal activity, resulting in bradycardia and constriction of the airways. This presentation is more common in premature infants but may also occur in infants. Symptomatic treatment includes placing the child in an upright position during and after feeding, and while sleeping; if severe, medication may be used to increase gastrointestinal transit time and/or increase lower esophageal sphincter tone. From an osteopathic viewpoint, the child should be evaluated and treated for tissue strains which may interfere with the functional relationship between the diaphragm and the lower esophageal sphincter, the mechanics of which are described in Chapters 6 and 14. The child's breathing mechanics, particularly abdominal use, need to be assessed. Increased intra-abdominal pressures act to displace the lower esophageal sphincter cephalad, compromising the effect of the diaphragm. Factors which may influence peristalsis and transit times within the gastrointestinal tract also need to be addressed. Within the osteopathic concept, these would include fluid mechanics and autonomic tone, both sympathetic and vagal. Functional assessment of the cranial base and upper cervical and thoracic areas is of particular importance. Paraspinal muscle spasm reflecting viscerosomatic reflex should be assessed and treated appropriately, with the goal of decreasing afferent drive into the associated spinal segments. The focus of osteopathic treatment is to address factors influencing the reflux and vagal response, which should help to decrease the frequency and intensity of the apneic episodes.

SUDDEN INFANT DEATH SYNDROME

Sudden infant death syndrome (SIDS) is one of the leading causes of infant mortality in the industrialized countries. By definition, SIDS is a diagnosis of exclusion. All other causes of sudden death must be ruled out by autopsy, clinical history and examination of the scene of death (Zylke 1989). There are many theories surrounding the mechanism for SIDS, most of which propose that the infants experience recurrent hypoxic events prior to the final incident. With this in mind, the presence of any apneic event (apparent life-threatening event (ALTE)) warrants close follow-up. Autopsy findings on SIDS victims suggest a role for UAO. Other evidence suggests immature sensitivity to increased carbon dioxide levels (Kinney & Filiano 1988). Factors contributing to the risk for SIDS include low birthweight, prematurity, lying in the prone position, maternal smoking and illicit drug use. Of these, the factor most intriguing to the osteopath is the infant's sleeping position.

During diaphragmatic contraction, the oropharyngeal muscles contract to maintain the patency of the upper airway against the negative pressures generated in the thorax. In the prone position, the head and cervical spine are flexed. In the flexed position, the walls of the pharyngeal tube approximate. This increases the forces and workload of the oropharyngeal muscles during inhalation. As previously discussed, the muscle composition and innervation patterns in the infant lend themselves to discordant muscle firing, prolonged recovery time and fatigue (Haddad & Perez Fontain 1996). The combination of the increased workload and tendency to fatigue add up to catastrophe. However, the question remains as to why this combination fails to produce apnea in all children. Placing children in the supine position to sleep has significantly reduced the incidence of SIDS worldwide (Willinger et al 1994), but it has not eliminated it, even in children without other risk factors. What is interesting from an osteopathic viewpoint is the relationship of the cranial base to the upper airway. The oropharyngeal muscles are suspended from the temporal, sphenoid and basiocciput bones. These are the attachments from which the muscles will leverage themselves to open the airway. Since we know that flexion of the head or neck alters the biomechanical efficiency of the muscles, we need to consider how the mechanics of the cranial base might also influence these structures. It seems logical that tissue strains which disrupt the relationships of the components of the cranial base will alter the mechanical efficiency of the oropharyngeal muscles.

In the infant, the pharynx is short when compared with the length of the cervical spine, and because of the position of the sphenoid and occiput, the upper part of the pharynx adjacent to the basilar portion of the occiput (Bosma 1975), whereas in the adult it drops vertically just behind the sphenoid sinus. This occurs due to the developmental flexion of the basisphenoid–basiocciput area discussed in Chapter 3. The muscle mass of the pharynx in the infant is proportionately larger than in the adult, and the mouth, nasopharynx and oropharynx are smaller. Because the mouth is so short on the vertical dimension, the uvula and epiglottis meet (Bosma 1975). The hyoid and epiglottis are on the same horizontal plane. In the infant, maintenance of the laryngeal portion of the airway is accomplished through coordination of the hyoid, tongue and mandibular musculature (Bosma 1975). This is necessary because the mandible offers little stability due to the fact that the temporal fossa is undeveloped. Consequently, the position of the oral space is maintained through muscular and not osseous structures. The mandible is stabilized through lateral pterygoid, temporalis and masseter muscles. The hyoid is held in place through the submental muscles and its attachment to the temporal bone (stylohyoid). Finally, the tongue is suspended from the hyoid, mandible and styloid process through muscular attachments (Bosma 1975). According to Bosma (1975), the spatial relations in the cervical spine and cranium 'constitute the gross background for the more discriminating positioning … of the airway which is accomplished by the actions of the tongue, hyoid and mandibular muscles'.

Osteopathic findings (results were gathered via general survey and chart review) in infants who have experienced apneic events usually include compression in the cranial base with restriction of normal mechanics at the craniocervical junction, positional strains of the hyoid which are usually associated with abnormal temporal bone mechanics, and decreased mobility of the upper cervical complex frequently associated with occipital falx involvement with or without an intraosseous strain of the occiput. These and any other areas which may affect respiratory function should be evaluated and treated in all infants, whether or not apnea has occurred.

MECONIUM ASPIRATION

Meconium is a waste product of the fetal gut. It is usually passed by term infants in the first 24 hours after birth; however, in up to 20% of deliveries, the meconium is passed in utero and the amniotic fluid is meconium stained. Meconium passage in utero may be a normal event in some term deliveries, but often it is indicative of fetal distress (Kirkpatrick & Mueller 1998). Approximately 5% of infants born with meconium staining will experience aspiration (Kliegman 2007). Aspiration may occur prior to delivery when continued hypoxia causes the fetus to gasp, aspirating the stained amniotic fluid. More often, it happens with the first breath. Meconium in the pharynx is drawn into the lungs with the first inhalation. Suctioning of the infant's nose, mouth and posterior pharynx prior to arousal is a standard preventive measure done in the delivery room. In the past it was thought that infants born with thick meconium staining or with evidence of fetal distress benefited from deep suctioning of the trachea (Kirkpatrick & Mueller 1998). However, the 2007 recommendations for cardiopulmonary resuscitation in neonates advise against deep suctioning and vigorous stimulation (Sung & Hsieh 2007).

Aspirated meconium will obstruct alveoli and small airways, resulting in atelectasis and air trapping. Within several hours, tachypnea, retraction, grunting and cyanosis may develop. If severe, the air trapping may lead to localized hyperinflation and pneumothorax (Kirkpatrick & Mueller 1998). Infants with meconium aspiration syndrome often require mechanical ventilation. PEEP may be necessary but increases the risk of pneumothorax (Kliegman 2007). Meconium promotes bacterial growth, so these children are also at risk for pneumonia. Clinical outcome is worse for premature infants or infants born with low APGAR scores (Kliegman 2007). Long-term complications of severe meconium aspiration syndrome may last 5–10 years, and include wheeze, cough and hyperinflation (Kliegman 1996). Osteopathic manipulative care of the child with a history of severe meconium aspiration syndrome should include a focus on pulmonary lymphatic function, the neuroendocrine immune system and eliminating any somatic findings which may contribute to airway hyperactivity, which would increase hyperinflation.

ASTHMA

Asthma is a chronic inflammatory disease of the respiratory system resulting in non-specific hyperactivity of the tracheobronchial tree (Kercsmar 1998, American Academy of Allergy, Asthma and Immunology 2002, National Asthma Education and Prevention Program 2002, Husain & Kumar 2005). It is an obstructive disease process marked by exacerbation and remission of bronchospasm. Bronchial narrowing usually presents as dyspnea, expiratory wheeze or cough. Asthma often begins in childhood and is due to a combination of environmental and genetic factors. Frequently an environmental exposure triggers the initial reaction. Young children may be predisposed to inflammatory responses to common respiratory antigens because of their immature immune system. Inflammation and abnormal tissue repair results in airway hyperresponsiveness and decreased air flow, both of which affect lung growth. The asthmatic lung undergoes mucosal edema, bronchospasm and mucus plugging. This narrows the airway and increases resistance to airflow. Sufficient expiratory pressures to overcome these factors cannot be generated, and the exhalation phase is prolonged and the lung becomes hyperinflated. The increased intra-alveolar pressure decreases blood flow to the affected area, and when combined with hypoxia-driven vasoconstriction, alters the ventilation–perfusion match. Chronic hyperinflation may affect the developing thoracic cage, resulting in a 'barrel chest', pectus excavatum and/or pseudorickets (Gillam et al 1970). Inflammatory changes are the hallmark of asthma (Vogel 1997). Infiltration of eosinophils, CD4+ cells and mast cells and the release of proinflammatory substances are thought to initiate the asthmatic event (Boushey et al 2000). Chronic asthma produces smooth muscle hypertrophy, alterations in secretory cells, subepithelial fibrosis, and increases in the size and number of blood vessels (Boushey et al 2000). This airway remodeling is thought to occur in response to successive episodes of acute inflammatory exacerbation or chronic inflammation (Boushey et al 2000).

Many studies support an association between reactive inflammatory conditions and asthma (Kercsmar 1998, Husain & Kumar 2005). For example, elevated serum IgE is commonly present in patients with asthma as well as in those with atopy and allergic rhinitis. Whether or not this represents a generalized hyperreactivity of the respiratory immune system that is genetically linked is unclear. The association between gastroesophageal reflux and asthma is well documented in clinical and basic science literature (Shimizu et al 1996). The mechanism is thought to be a vagally mediated reflex, although whether gastroesophageal reflux acts as a trigger for asthma or as part of the initiating pathology is unclear. Even less well understood is the relationship between the gastrointestinal-associated lymphoid tissue (GALT) and the bronchus-associated lymphoid tissue (BALT) and its potential to stimulate hyperreactivity of the airways. Sinusitis and upper respiratory tract congestion also have a role in triggering an asthmatic event. Sinusitis or congestion will also worsen asthmatic symptoms and can interfere with bronchodilator treatment (Wald 1995). Undiagnosed chronic sinusitis may present as recalcitrant asthma (Kercsmar 1998). In these children, osteopathic treatment needs to focus on facial mechanics and factors which may be contributing to the sinusitis or upper airway congestion. There are many other triggers for acute asthmatic attacks. A partial list includes allergens that stimulate IgE, bronchial irritants including pollution, infectious processes, exercise, cold weather, and endocrine factors. It is important to limit the child's exposure to environmental allergens that may exacerbate the asthma.

Osteopathic care of the child with asthma is an ongoing process directed at maintaining function and balance in the non-acute child and assisting the body's innate ability to heal during times of exacerbation. Fitzgerald and Stiles (1984) reported a 14% reduction in hospital length of stay when osteopathic manipulative treatment was added to the management of adult patients with asthma. In addition, Howell and Allen (1974) demonstrated that osteopathic manipulative treatment of adult patients with chronic obstructive pulmonary disease improved oxygen saturation, total lung capacity and residual volume. A more recent study investigating the efficacy of chiropractic treatment of specific thoracic vertebrae in children with asthma provides an interesting perspective. While there was no statistical difference between the children receiving chiropractic treatment and the control group, it must be noted that the control group received 'sham' treatment composed of techniques which were quite similar to osteopathic soft tissue techniques (Balon et al 1998).

It is important to remember that asthma is an obstructive lung disease. Thus the child has the greatest difficulty in generating adequate expiratory forces, rather than inspiratory forces. Furthermore, because these children usually experience hyperinflation of the lungs, techniques aimed at increasing inhalation mechanics should be avoided, i.e. techniques which use sudden rapid inhalation forces to establish tissue fulcrums. The primary and accessory muscles of exhalation and their attachments should be evaluated and treated. Optimum function of pulmonary lymphatics is important to maintain fluid balance. Musculoskeletal findings that may affect vagal tone through neural and/or mechanical mechanisms also need to be addressed. This would include the mechanics of the cranial base and cranial–cervical junction. In addition to the above, osteopathic evaluation and treatment of children with concurrent gastroesophageal reflux and asthma should include factors influencing lower esophageal sphincter tone, muscle spasm reflecting facilitated spinal segment, and findings affecting gut transit times.

CYSTIC FIBROSIS

Cystic fibrosis is a genetic disorder of exocrine gland function. Although it affects multiple systems, chronic lung disease is the hallmark and principal cause of morbidity (MacLusky & Levison 1998, Boucher et al 2000). Cystic fibrosis is described in almost every race, although there is a somewhat higher prevalence in those with European ancestry (MacLusky & Levison 1998). Numerous mutations of a gene responsible for encoding the cystic fibrosis transmembrane regulator (CFTR) are responsible for the syndrome and its variations (Boucher et al 2000). Dysfunction of the CFTR leads to elevated levels of inorganic ions being secreted from serous glands. This results in increased viscosity of mucus and eventual loss of glandular function (MacLusky & Levison 1998). The most common presentation of patients with cystic fibrosis is recurrent lung infection. Other presentations include chronic airway obstruction, pancreatic insufficiency, gastrointestinal manifestations, chronic sinusitis, nasal polyps, biliary cirrhosis and failure to thrive (Rosenstein & Cutting 1998, Boucher et al 2000). The median survival for patients in the USA is approximately 30 years (Fiel 1993).

The CFTR is involved in regulation of cellular chloride channels and some other ion channels. Failure to secrete chloride into the respiratory lumen reduces sodium content in the lumen fluid. This leads to decreased water content, dehydration and thickened secretions. The viscous mucus accumulates in the organ passages, obstructing airways and promoting infection (Cotran 1989). Within the pancreas, dysfunction of the CFTR causes decreased secretion of bicarbonate ion. Generally speaking, the CFTR decreases epithelial membrane permeability to anions, resulting in obstruction and dilation of secretory ducts and flattening of epithelium. Infiltration of fibrous tissue and fat into the affected areas is common in the pancreas. In the lung, there is hypertrophy of submucosal glands, bronchiectasis, and, less often, emphysematous changes (Boucher et al 2000).

The degree of CFTR activity determines the patient's clinical picture and ultimately, their outcome. Children with approximately 10% residual activity of the CFTR gene are more likely to have respiratory disease, idiopathic chronic pancreatitis and, if male, absence of the vas deferens. Children with 5% residual activity have greater chance of developing respiratory disease without pancreatic involvement, while children with 1% activity levels are more likely to develop pancreatic insufficiency in addition to the respiratory disease.

Recurrent infection resulting from failure to clear mucus appropriately is the primary pathophysiology in the lungs (Boucher et al 2000). The most common initial clinical presentation is cough, which is worse at night and on awakening. The cough progresses to become productive, and then paroxysmal with gagging and emesis (Boucher et al 2000). Hyperinflation of the lungs is common, as is chronic sinusitis and airway hyperactivity due to mucus plugging. Diagnosis is usually made before the teenage years. The life expectancy for children with cystic fibrosis is less than 30 years (MacLusky et al 1985). Osteopathic treatment can be used to support the body's attempts to compensate for and respond to the sequelae of the dysfunctional CFTR. Often, children with cystic fibrosis also have tissue strain affecting facial and respiratory mechanics. When present, these findings need to be properly addressed. Restricted facial mechanics may impede sinus drainage. Other areas to be examined include somatic findings which may influence the neuroendocrine immune system, pulmonary lymphatic function, and respiratory mechanics which emphasize exhalation activity. As with other diseases with an obstructive component, it is prudent to avoid using techniques which may exacerbate hyperinflation.

CONCLUSION

Breathing mechanics differ in the newborn, toddler, child and teenager. Consequently, one must know what to expect in the child's age group. Whereas profound abdominal exertion would be normal in the 2-year-old, it would be of concern in a 12-year-old. It goes without saying that any child presenting with respiratory disease needs to have pulmonary and cardiovascular status stabilized before osteopathic treatment is initiated. When examining the child with respiratory disease, be it acute or chronic, several common areas need to be addressed. In addition to respiratory rate, rhythm, effort and efficacy, the actual mechanics of breathing should be systematically evaluated. This includes not only the diaphragm and thoracic cage, but all the musculoskeletal tissues influencing the work of respiration. Breathing can be considered a total body activity, and recognizing this can be especially significant in compromised individuals.

References

Adams F H, Yanagisawa M, Kuzela D et al 1971 The disappearance of fetal lung fluid following birth. J Pediatr 78(5): 837–843.

Alvarez J E, Bodani J, Fajardo C A et al 1993 Sighs and their relationship to apnea in the newborn infant. Biol Neonate 63(3): 139–146.

American Academy of Allergy, Asthma and Immunology 2002 Pediatric asthma: promoting best practice. American Academy of Allergy, Asthma and Immunology, Milwaukee, WI, www.aaai.org.

Avery M E, Gatewood O B, Brumley G 1966 Transient tachypnea of newborn. Possible delayed resorption of fluid at birth. Am J Dis Child 111(4): 380–385.

Bader D, Ramos A D, Lew C D et al 1987 Childhood sequelae of infant lung disease: exercise and pulmonary function abnormalities after bronchopulmonary dysplasia. J Pediatr 110(5): 693–699.

Balon J, Aker P D, Crowther E R et al 1998 A comparison of active and simulated chiropractic manipulation as adjunctive treatment for childhood asthma. N Engl J Med 339(15): 1013–1020.

Bosma J F 1975 Introduction to the symposium. In: Bosma J F, Showacre J (eds) Development of upper respiratory anatomy and function. National Institutes of Health, Bethesda, MD: 5–49.

Boucher R C, Knowles M R, Yankaskas J R 2000 Cystic fibrosis. In: Murray J, Nadel J A (eds) Textbook of respiratory medicine. W B Saunders, Philadelphia.

Boushey H A, Corry D B, Fahy J V 2000 Asthma. In: Murray J, Nadel J A (eds) Textbook of respiratory medicine. W B Saunders, Philadelphia.

Brouillette R T, Fernbach S K, Hunt C E 1982 Obstructive sleep apnea in infants and children. J Pediatr 100: 31.

Fiel S B 1993 Clinical management of pulmonary disease in cystic fibrosis. Lancet 341(8852): 1070–1074.

Fitzgerald M, Stiles E 1984 Osteopathic hospital's solution to DRGs may be OMT. DO 97–101.

Gibson R L, Jackson J C, Twiggs G A et al 1988 Bronchopulmonary dysplasia. Survival after prolonged mechanical ventilation. Am J Dis Child 142(7): 721–725.

Gillam G L, McNicol K N, Williams H E 1970 Chest deformity, residual airways obstruction and hyperinflation, and growth in children with asthma – II. Significance of chronic chest deformity. Arch Dis Child 45(244): 789–799.

Guilleminault C 1987 Obstructive sleep apnea syndrome and its treatment in children: areas of agreement and controversy. Pediatr Pulmonol 3(6): 429–436.

Guilleminault C, Korobkin R, Winkle R 1981 A review of 50 children with obstructive sleep apnea syndrome. Lung 159(5): 275–287.

Haddad G G, Mellins R B 1984 Hypoxia and respiratory control in early life. Annu Rev Physiol 46: 629.

Haddad G G, Perez Fontain J J 1996 Development of the respiratory system. In: Behrman R E, Kliegman R M, Arvin H B (eds) Nelson's textbook of pediatrics. W B Saunders, Philadelphia.

Hazinski 1998 Bronchopulmonary dysplasia. In: Chernick V, Boat T (eds) Kendig's disorders of the respiratory tract in children. W B Saunders, Philadelphia: 364–389.

Howell R K, Allen T W 1974 The influence of osteopathic manipulative therapy in the management of patients with chronic lung disease. J Am Osteopath Assoc 75: 757–760.

Husain A, Kumar V 2005 The lung. In: Kumar V, Abbas A, Fausto N (eds) Robbins and Cotran pathologic basis of disease. Elsevier Saunders, Philadelphia: 711–772.

Kercsmar C 1998 Asthma. In: Chernick V, Boat T (eds) Kendig's disorders of the respiratory tract in children. W B Saunders, Philadelphia: 688–731.

Kinney H C, Filiano J J 1988 Brainstem research in sudden infant death syndrome. Pediatrician 15(4): 240–250.

Kirkpatrick B V, Mueller D G 1998 Respiratory disorders in the newborn. In: Chernick V, Boat T (eds) Kendig's disorders of the respiratory tract in children. W B Saunders, Philadelphia.

Kliegman R 2007 Perinatal and Neonatal Medicine. In: Kliegman R, Behrman R E, Jenson H B et al (eds) Nelson's textbook of pediatrics. Saunders Elsevier, Philadelphia: 93–109.

Laurikainen E, Aitasalo K, Erkinjuntti M et al 1992 Sleep apnea syndrome in children – secondary to adenotosillar hypertrophy? Acta Otolaryngol Suppl 492: 38–41.

Lee S, Hassan A, Ingram D et al 1999 Effects of different modes of delivery on lung volumes of newborn infants. Pediatr Pulmonol 27(5): 318–321.

MacLusky I, Levison H 1998 Cystic fibrosis. In: Chernick V, Boat T (eds) Kendig's disorders of the respiratory tract in children. W B Saunders, Philadelphia.

MacLusky I, McLaughlin F J, Levison H 1985 Cystic fibrosis: part II. Curr Prob Pediatr 15(7): 1–39.

Maitra A, Kumar V 2005 Diseases of infancy and childhood. In: Kumar V, Abbas A, Fausto N (eds) Robbins and Cotran pathophysiologic basis of disease. Elsevier Saunders, Philadelphia: 469–508.

Marchal F, Bairam A, Vert P 1987 Neonatal apnea and apneic syndromes. Clin Perinatol 14(3): 509–529.

Meisels S J, Plunkett J W, Roloff D W et al 1986 Growth and development of preterm infants with respiratory distress syndrome and bronchopulmonary dysplasia. Pediatrics 77(3): 345–352.

Milner A D, Saunders R A, Hopkin I E 1978 Effects of delivery by caesarean section on lung mechanics and lung volume in the human neonate. Arch Dis Child 53(7): 545–548.

Montan S, Arul-Kumeran S 2006 Neonatal respiratory distress syndrome. Lancet 367: 1878–1879.

National Asthma Education and Prevention Program 2002 NAEPP guidelines for the diagnosis and management of asthma – update on selected topics. Washington, DC: NIH pub no 02–5075.

Northway W H, Rosan R C, Porter D Y 1976 Pulmonary disease following respiratory therapy of hyaline-membrane disease. Bronchopulmonary dysplasia. N Engl J Med 276: 357–368.

O'Brodovich H M, Haddad G G 2001 The functional basis of respiratory pathology and disease. In: Chernick V, Boat T (eds) Kendig's disorders of the respiratory tract in children. W B Saunders, Philadelphia: 27–74.

Potsic W P, Pasquariello P S, Baranak C C et al 1986 Relief of upper airway obstruction by adenotonsillectomy. Otolaryngol Head Neck Surg 94(4): 476–480.

Rosenstein B J, Cutting G R 1998 The diagnosis of cystic fibrosis: a concensus statement. J Pediatrics 132: 589–592.

Schmidt-Nowara W W 1984 Continuous positive airway pressure for long-term treatment of sleep apnea. Am J Dis Child 138(1): 82–84.

Shimizu T, Mochizuki H, Tokuyama K et al 1996 Relationship between the acid-induced cough response and airway responsiveness and obstruction in children with asthma. Thorax 51(3): 284–287.

Smith V C, Zupanoc J A F, McCormick M C et al 2005 Trends in severe bronchopulmonary dysplasia rates between 1994–2002. J Pediatr 146: 469–473.

Sung D S, Hsieh K S 2007 The key changes in pediatric and neonatal cardiopulmonary resuscitation. Acta Paediatr Taiwan 48: 52–56.

Van Marter L J 2005 Strategies for preventing bronchopulmonary dysplasia. Curr Opin Pediatr 17: 174–180.

Verloove-Vanhorick S P, Verwey R A, Brand R 1986 Neonatal mortality risk in relation to gestational age and birth weight. Lancet 1: 55–57.

Vogel G 1997 New clues to asthma therapies. Science 276: 1643–1645.

Wald E R 1995 Chronic sinusitis in children. J Pediatr 127(3): 339–347.

Willinger M 1995 SIDS prevention. Pediatr Annu 24(7): 358–364.

Willinger M, Hoffman H J, Hartford R B 1994 Infant sleep position and risk of sudden infant death syndrome: report of meeting held January 13th and 14th. Pediatrics 93: 814–819.

Zylke J W 1989 Sudden infant death syndrome: resurgent research offers hope. JAMA 262(12): 1565–1566.

Further reading

Adams F H, Latta H, el Salawy A et al 1969 The expanded lung of the term fetus. J Pediatr 75(1): 59–66.

Avery M E, Gatewood O B, Brumley G 1966 Transient tachypnea of the newborn. Am J Dis Child 11: 380.

Bosma J F, Showacre J (eds) 1975 Symposium on development of upper respiratory anatomy and function: implications for sudden infant death syndrome. National Institutes of Health, Bethesda, MD.

Chernick V, Boat T (eds) 1998 Kendig's disorders of the respiratory tract in children. W B Saunders, Philadelphia.

Chessare J B, Hunt C E, Bourguignon C et al 1995 A community-based survey of infant sleep position. Pediatrics 96(5 Pt 1): 893–896.

Donner M W, Bosma J F, Robertson D L 1985 Anatomy and physiology of the pharynx. Gastrointest Radiol 10(3): 196–212.

Guilleminault C, Stoohs R 1990 Obstructive sleep apnea syndrome in children. Pediatrician 17(1): 46–51.

Guilleminault C, Stoohs R 1990 Chronic snoring and obstructive sleep apnea syndrome in children. Lung 168(suppl): 912–919.

Guilleminault C, Pelayo R, Leger D et al 1996 Recognition of sleep-disordered breathing in children. Pediatrics 98(5): 871–882.

Haddad G G, Perez Fontain J J 1996 Congenital abnormalities. In: Behrman R E, Kliegman R M, Arvin H B (eds) Nelson's textbook of pediatrics. W B Saunders, Philadelphia.

Haddad G G, Perez Fontain J J 1996 Regulation of respiration. In: Behrman R E, Kliegman R M, Arvin H B (eds) Nelson's textbook of pediatrics. W B Saunders, Philadelphia.

Hageman J R, Adams M A, Gardner T H 1984 Persistent pulmonary hypertension of the newborn. Trends in incidence, diagnosis, and management. Am J Dis Child 138(6): 592–595.

Hageman J R, Adams M A, Gardner T H 1985 Pulmonary complications of hyperventilation therapy for persistent pulmonary hypertension. Crit Care Med 13(12): 1013–1014.

Haouzi P, Marchal F, Huszczuk A 1995 Muscle perfusion and control of breathing: is there a neural link? Adv Exp Med Biol 393: 363–368.

Hondras M A, Linde K, Jones A P 2000 Manual therapy for asthma. Cochrane Database Syst Rev(2): CD001002.

McNicol K N, Williams H E, Gillam G L 1970 Chest deformity, residual airways obstruction and hyperinflation, and growth in children with asthma – I. Prevalence findings from an epidemiological study. Arch Dis Child 45(244): 783–788.

Meisels S J, Plunkett J W, Pasick P L et al 1987 Effects of severity and chronicity of respiratory illness on the cognitive development of preterm infants. J Pediatr Psychol 12(1): 117–132.

Murray J, Nadel J A 2000 Textbook of respiratory medicine. W B Saunders, Philadelphia.

Nicolai T, Von Mutius E 1996 Risk of asthma in children with a history of croup. Acta Paediatr 85(11): 1295–1299.

Plunkett J W, Meisels S J, Stiefel G S et al 1986 Patterns of attachment among preterm infants of varying biological risk. J Am Acad Child Psychiatry 25(6): 794–800.

Schmidt-Nowara W W 1988 Body position does not affect apnea frequency. Sleep 11(4): 402.

Schmidt-Nowara W W 1990 Cardiovascular consequences of sleep apnea. Prog Clin Biol Res 345: 377–385.

Schmidt-Nowara W W, Appel D 1983 Periodic breathing and sleep apnea. Am Rev Respir Dis 127(4): 524–525.

Schwartz J, Weiss S T 1995 Relationship of skin test reactivity to decrements in pulmonary function in children with asthma or frequent wheezing. Am J Respir Crit Care Med 152(6 Pt 1): 2176–2180.

Stiles E 1981 Manipulative management of chronic lung disease. J Am Osteopath Assoc 9(8): 300–304.

Wald E R 1996 Diagnosis and management of sinusitis in children. Adv Pediatr Infect Dis 12: 1–20.

Weese-Mayer D E, Hunt C E, Brouillette R T et al 1992 Diaphragm pacing in infants and children. J Pediatr 120(1): 1–8.

Chapter Fourteen

Gastroenterology

CHAPTER CONTENTS

SUCKLING

The function of the gastrointestinal tract starts in the mouth, where the tongue, teeth and salivary glands begin the process of digestion. In the newborn, sucking is an essential component of this process. Sucking can be divided into two categories: nutritive and non-nutritive sucking. Non-nutritive sucking is a pattern of oral activity which can first be observed as spontaneous mouthing movements at 18 weeks of gestation (Boyle 1992). These movements are precursors to nutritive sucking. Non-nutritive sucking does not generate enough pressure to effectively draw milk into the mouth. It may occur spontaneously or reflexively, as occurs with a pacifier. Premature infants born before 32 weeks of gestation lack the ability to produce a coordinated and effective suck, but display non-nutritive sucking movements. Consequently, infants born before 32 weeks of gestation often cannot nurse effectively and usually need to be tube-fed. Those born between 32 and 36 weeks also have an immature sucking pattern, but it is somewhat more effective (Boyle 1992, Milla 1996). A mature nutritive sucking pattern usually evolves within 1–2 weeks after birth in the former group and in less than a week in the latter. There is some evidence that in premature infants nutritive sucking behavior can be stimulated by non-nutritive sucking (Bernbaum et al 1983). Non-nutritive sucking may also stimulate weight gain and decrease the length of hospital stay in premature infants (Measel & Anderson 1979, Field et al 1982, Bernbaum et al 1983).

Nutritive sucking behavior is mechanically different from what an adult would do to suck fluid through a straw. The nutritive suck of the infant involves coordinated movement of the tongue, hyoid, mandible and lower lip, which brings the tongue vigorously against the palate at a very rapid rate. A mature nutritive sucking pattern consists of a burst of activity with 10–30 sucks at a rate of two per second.

Interspersed within the burst would be one to four swallows (Boyle 1992). This pattern of activity depends on coordination between the many muscles of the tongue, pharynx and submental triangle. The body of the infant tongue must fully approximate the palate and then rapidly move away to generate the negative force needed to draw milk into the oropharynx. One can think of the tongue as a piston within the cylinder of the mouth (Boyle 1992). In order for this to be accomplished smoothly and effectively, the root of the tongue needs to be stabilized from below as the body moves back and forth against the palate (Fig. 14.1). Stabilization of the root is achieved through the coordinated actions of the hyoid bone, mandible and their associated muscles.

The tongue is a complex muscular structure consisting of intrinsic and extrinsic muscles. The intrinsic muscles are concerned with changing the shape of the tongue, which allows for fine manipulation of the food bolus and articulation of speech. In the newborn and infant, the extrinsic muscles are involved with the coordinated activity of sucking. Unlike the intrinsic muscles, the extrinsic muscles have a bony attachment to the mandible, temporal bone and/or hyoid (Fig. 14.2). They can use these attachments to stabilize their position and coordinate actions between the tongue and these structures (Bosma 1986, Standring 2004). The quality and character of movements resulting from contraction of the genioglossus, hyoglossus and geniohyoid muscles will be influenced by the biomechanics of the mandible and hyoid, and indirectly by those of the upper extremities and thorax. The hyoid is suspended from the temporal bones by the stylohyoid ligament, and the stylohyoideus and digastric muscles (Fig. 14.3). In the

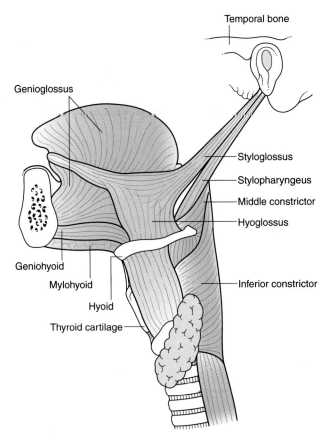

Fig. 14.2 • Parasagittal view of the oral pharyngeal muscles and their relationship to the temporal, mandible and hyoid bone. Note how the entire oropharyngeal system is virtually suspended from the cranial base, with the hyoid and mandible acting as anterior buttresses.

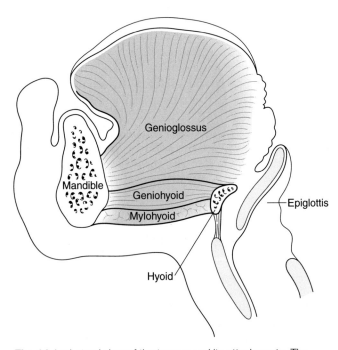

Fig. 14.1 • Lateral view of the tongue and its attachments. The genioglossus, geniohyoid and mylohyoid are labeled.

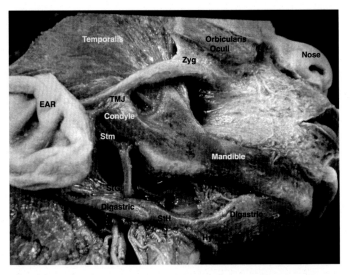

Fig. 14.3 • Right facial dissection in a term specimen. The camera is positioned slightly posterior and lateral. The ear and nose are marked for orientation. The inframandibular muscles are labeled as follows: StH, stylohyoid; digastric; StG, styloglossus. The hyoid bone (Hy) and stylomandibular ligament (Stm) are also visible. *Used with permission of the Willard & Carreiro Collection.*

adult, the hyoid lies in the anterior cervical tissues below the mandible. In newborns and infants, the hyoid lies within the arch of the mandible, level with the submental muscles which lie in a transverse plane (Bosma 1986). The hyoid is also influenced by the superficial muscles of the throat, which lie inferior to it (Fig. 14.4). Finally, the shoulders and clavicles, through the omohyoid and sternohyoid muscles, can affect the hyoid (Fig. 14.5). Biomechanical strains affecting any of these structures may interrupt effective sucking.

For example, asymmetry in the position of the clavicles or the scapula due to birth-related trauma may affect tone in the omohyoid or sternohyoid muscles. This could result in lateral and inferior displacement of the hyoid bone, thus compromising the biomechanical efficiency of the extrinsic muscles attached to the hyoid. The end result would be that the tongue would move asymmetrically in the oral cavity. Rather than neatly approximating the palate and pulling away, the infant exhibits a discordant sucking pattern. A similar problem, albeit a more symmetrical pattern, can be seen when the child has a short frenulum.

Effective sucking can also be compromised neurologically. True palsy of the vagus nerve or glossopharyngeal nerve will affect suck and swallow. Hypoglossal nerve or nucleus damage, which is uncommon in newborns, results in paresis of the ipsilateral muscles. It presents immediately after birth with a markedly discordant sucking pattern due to the asymmetrical tongue movement. The tongue will deviate towards the damaged side. Magoun (1976) describes irritation of the hypoglossal nerve at the level of the hypoglossal foramen resulting in weakened or poor sucking activity. Likewise, irritation of the glossopharyngeal, vagus or spinal accessory nerves as they pass through the jugular foramen may also compromise suck or swallow. These nerves or, more likely, their microscopic vascular supply may be compromised by abnormal strains and tensions in the soft tissues or cartilaginous components of the cranial base. This could result in altered conduction and depolarization characteristics. In Chapter 3, the neonatal skull is described as largely cartilaginous, especially at bony articulations. The hypoglossal nerve exits the skull through the hypoglossal foramen

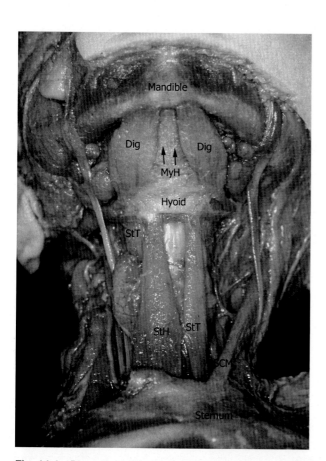

Fig. 14.4 • Dissection of the neonatal anterior cervical structures. The camera is positioned to look up from the chest towards the submandibular area. The mandible, sternum and hyoid bones are clearly labeled: Dig, digastric; MyH, mylohyoid; StT, sternothyroid; StH, sternohyoid; SCM, sternocleidomastoid. *Used with permission of the Willard & Carreiro Collection.*

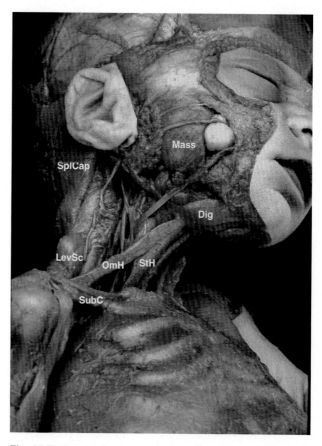

Fig. 14.5 • Lateral view of superficial infant dissection depicting omohyoid (OmH), subclavius (SubC), levator scapulae (LevSc), splenius capitis (SplCap), masseter (Mass), digastric (Dig) and sternohyoid (StH). *Used with permission of the Willard & Carreiro Collection.*

located on the inferior surface of the skull. In the adult, this is a well-defined bony canal which begins on the medial surface of the foramen magnum deep to the occipital condyle and terminates on the external surface (Fig. 14.6). In the newborn and infant, this area is cartilaginous. The condyle is in two parts, so the size and shape of the lumen of the canal may be compromised by distortions between the two parts. Many connective tissue and muscular structures attach near this area. During labor and delivery there is tremendous flexion and rotation of the cranial–cervical junction and cervical spine. If the child's head is in an asynclitic position during the birth process, these suboccipital and cranial tissues may be strained and inflamed (see Ch. 8). Because of the close proximity of these tissues, congestion and muscle spasm in this area have the potential to affect the hypoglossal nerve by creating vascular congestion or mild hypoxia.

The jugular foramen carries the jugular vein, and cranial nerves IX, X, and XII. In the newborn infant, the foramen is a poorly defined space located within the cartilaginous junction of the occiput and temporal bones (Fig. 14.7). The glossopharyngeal nerve passes along the wall of the foramen, creating a notch in the bone as it does so. On the external surface, the deep postural muscles of the head and neck, and the pharyngeal column, have their attachments close to the foramen. Abnormal tissue tensions or strains in the

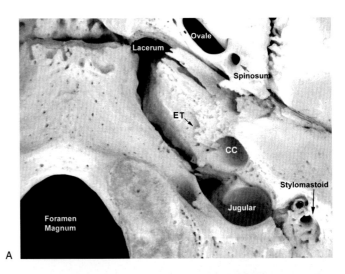

A

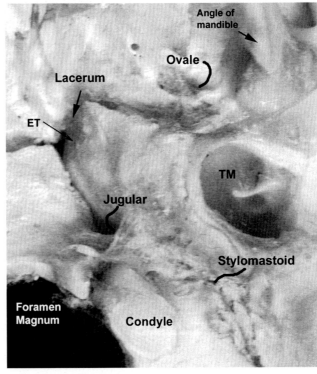

B

Fig. 14.6 • Disarticulated occipital bone from an adolescent specimen. The internal surface is presented. The basiocciput (BaO), hypoglossal canal (HypC), grooves for the superior saggital (SupS), transverse (Trn), and confluence of sinuses (CS) are labeled, as is the attachment of the cerebellar falx (CF). *Used with permission of the Willard & Carreiro Collection.*

Fig. 14.7 • Comparison close-up views of the inferior surface of an adult (A) and infant (B) cranium. The walls of the jugular foramen are formed by the occiput and temporal bones. The eustachian tube (ET), tympanic membrane (TM) and carotid canal (CC) are labeled. *Used with permission of the Willard & Carreiro Collection.*

connective tissue, muscles or cartilaginous components may irritate the delicate structures passing through the foramen.

The infant's sucking pattern can easily be assessed during the physical examination by gently placing the distal phalanx of the smallest finger into the infant's mouth. A firm, coordinated suck is readily evident. Both sides of the tongue should approximate the infant's palate simultaneously. Movement between the mandible, tongue and palate should be smooth and coordinated. The hyoid can be palpated within the arch of the mandible. It should be seated in the midline, and move synchronistically with the mandible as the tongue moves against the palate. If the hyoid deviates laterally, there may be involvement of the digastric or omohyoid muscle on the ipsilateral side. If one cornus is positioned slightly inferior to the other, the sternohyoid muscle and clavicle should be evaluated on the inferior side, and the stylohyoid muscle, temporal bone and cranial base mechanics on the superior side. In general, strains at the cranial–cervical junction do not appear to directly affect hyoid mechanics, although there may be irritation to the hypoglossal nerve from the resultant tissue strain. Osteopathic treatment should be initiated to normalize tissue relationships. Studies suggest that osteopathic manipulation improves sucking effectiveness in infants with sucking dysfunction (Fraval 1998).

When there is an abnormal or ineffective suck pattern, the infant should be evaluated osteopathically, and consultation with a lactation specialist should be initiated. Often, maternal postures, nipple characteristics and poor technique can play a role in sucking problems. Recommendations to keep the child nursing on one breast for the entire feed should be considered to afford maximum opportunity for the infant to obtain high-fat breast milk (Woodward et al 1989). Studies suggest that the 'hind breast milk' has a higher fat content than the 'fore breast milk' (Jensen et al 1978, Woodward et al 1989, Boersma et al 1991).

SWALLOWING

Although the fetus is able to swallow amniotic fluid, coordination of oral, pharyngeal and esophageal phases of swallowing is lacking until 34 weeks of gestation. In normal children and adults, the initial phase of swallowing, the oropharyngeal phase, is voluntary; however, in the term and premature newborn, swallowing, like sucking, is a reflexive movement influenced by neurological development. As previously mentioned, studies have shown that reinforcement of non-nutritive sucking in premature infants is associated with accelerated development of mature suck and improved intestinal transit time (Bernbaum et al 1983).

The mechanics of swallowing involve three phases: an oral phase, a pharyngolaryngeal phase, and an esophageal phase (Boyle 1992, Reynolds 1995, Guyton 1996, Milla 1996). The oral phase involves the tongue manipulating the bolus of milk or food towards the back of the oropharynx. When the bolus enters the posterior area of the oropharynx, receptors in the tonsillar pillars and pharynx trigger a cascade of events involving the trigeminal, glossopharyngeal, vagus and hypoglossal nerves. This initiates the second phase of swallowing. The soft palate elevates against the hard palate, effectively closing the nasopharynx. Simultaneously, the styloglossus and hyoglossus muscles pull the tongue posteriorly as the epiglottis folds over the larynx and the vocal cords are pulled together. As the larynx is pulled superiorly towards the epiglottis, the proximal portion of the esophagus is pulled forwards. Then the middle and inferior constrictor muscles propel the bolus inferiorly as the upper esophageal sphincter relaxes. This phase of swallowing lasts less than 2 s, and although respiration is halted during that time, it generally goes unnoticed. The third phase of swallowing is called the esophageal phase and involves a propagation of the peristaltic wave initiated in the pharynx by the constrictor muscles, which propel the food bolus along. This primary peristaltic wave generally lasts 8–10 s, by which time the bolus of food has reached the terminal end of the esophagus. In the event that the food does not pass with the primary wave, secondary waves triggered by esophageal distention will facilitate further movement. There is a concurrent relaxation of the stomach and duodenum in response to the primary peristaltic wave. Thus the food bolus is easily manipulated into the awaiting gastrum.

In the fetus, swallowing appears towards the end of the first trimester. However, it is still uncoordinated at birth, even in the term infant. Refinement of the phases of swallowing evolves over several days following birth, although the rate and velocity of the pharyngolaryngeal phase surpass those of an adult. In the newborn and infant, the mechanics of swallowing are modulated through local sensory mechanisms to a much greater extent than in the adult (Stevenson & Allaire 1991, Milla 1996). Esophageal motility disorders may present in children with severe neurological impairment from cerebral palsy motor neuron disease, muscle disease, congenital malformations and metabolic diseases. Difficulties in swallowing are termed dysphagia and usually involve a problem with motility, whereas painful swallowing is called odynophagia. Odynophagia may present in toddlers and small children due to foreign bodies, infection, inflammation or mass-occupying lesions.

GASTROESOPHAGEAL REFLUX

Gastroesophageal reflux (GER) is a condition in which acidic secretions and gastric contents flow backwards from the stomach into the esophagus. Although some reflux occurs in almost everyone, it is usually asymptomatic, sporadic and clinically irrelevant. However, when reflux is chronic or severe, the protective mechanisms in place to prevent tissue injury may be overwhelmed, resulting in breakdown and inflammation of the esophageal mucosa. Reflux is particularly prevalent in infants and young children, due in part to conditions of immaturity in the gastrointestinal tract.

In newborns, GER most often presents as spitting up or vomiting, which may occur after or between feedings. Eighty-five percent of infants with GER will present with excessive vomiting in the first week of life (Herbst 2000). In toddlers and children, GER may also present as chest pain, chronic cough, recurrent pneumonia, wheezing or anorexia. Although GER appears to be prevalent in asthmatic patients and patients with aspiration pneumonia, the actual role which GER may play in respiratory diseases such as asthma, infant apnea and sudden infant death syndrome (SIDS) is unclear (Allen 1984, Kahn et al 1992, Herbst 2000). The probable mechanism for bronchial irritation or inflammation with GER is through a vagovagal reflex or the mucosal-associated lymphoid system.

The most common complication of GER is inflammation of the esophageal mucosa, which may lead to esophagitis (Fig. 14.8). A severe condition called Barrett's esophagus is a dysplasia of the gastroesophageal junction secondary to chronic irritation. Both esophagitis and Barrett's dysplasia are dependent on the extent, duration and chronicity of the reflux. Mechanisms of limiting mucosal exposure to the acidity, such as saliva production and esophageal clearance, may be able to neutralize small amounts of chronic reflux. Other complications in children with long-term GER include esophageal strictures and cancer.

Natural barriers to GER

Under normal conditions, pressures in the stomach exceed those in the esophagus, increasing the likelihood of backflow of gastric contents into the esophageal lumen. The lumen of the esophagus is lined with a stratified squamous epithelium lacking the protective adaptations present in the gastric mucosa. The highly acidic nature of refluxed gastric contents make them especially damaging to the epithelium. There are three inherent mechanisms in place to protect the esophagus from this acid trauma (Altschuler 1992, Ogorek 1995). The first is the existence of a high-pressure zone at the gastroesophageal junction to prevent reflux of gastric contents into the esophageal lumen. The second is esophageal peristalsis, which can clear the esophagus by moving the refluxed secretions back into the stomach. The third is the increased production of saliva in response to lowered esophageal pH. The saliva acts as a buffer, neutralizing the acidity of gastric backflow. The increased production triggered by esophageal acidity may explain the phenomenon of water brash seen with GER (Ogorek 1995).

The high-pressure zone (HPZ) of the lower esophagus is probably the most potent antireflux mechanism present.

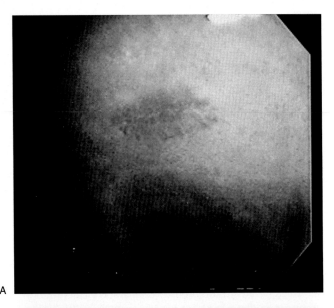

A

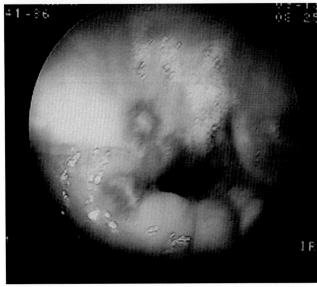

B

Fig. 14.8 • Endoscopic photographs of the gastroesophageal junction. (A) An area of inflammation; note the erythematous mark on the mucosa. (B) Esophagitis; note the blanched areas surrounded by an erythematous ring. The blanched areas represent severe mucosal inflammation and localized tissue disruption. *Used with permission of the Willard & Carreiro Collection.*

In the adult, the high-pressure zone stretches over an area of 3–4 cm. It occupies a somewhat smaller area in the newborn. In the adult, resting pressures in this area measure between 15 mmHg and 35 mmHg above gastric pressure (Welch & Gray 1982, Pelot 1995). In the premature and term newborn, pressures at the HPZ are generally lower, with the lowest pressures in the most premature patients. As might be expected, pressures in the HPZ increase as the infant matures (Boix-Ochoa & Canals 1976, Euler & Ament 1977, Kenigsberg et al 1981, Milla 1996). Nevertheless, neonates are capable of generating effective pressures in the HPZ regardless of gestational age. This is probably due to the anatomical relationships at the esophageal hiatus and the contribution of the diaphragmatic crura.

The lower esophageal HPZ is created through the concerted efforts of the lower esophageal sphincter (LES), the crura of the diaphragm and the phrenoesophageal ligament. This zone must have sphincter-like qualities which allow it to relax during swallowing and contract while at rest; this is accomplished through the presence of a functional sphincter. Although the presence of a distinct anatomical muscular sphincter at the distal esophagus is controversial, the existence of a functional sphincter is beyond doubt (Altschuler 1992, Ogorek 1995, Milla 1996). Altschuler (1992) describes the LES as an area of intrinsic smooth muscle with distinctive mechanical and electrical characteristics, unique responses to hormones and drugs, and a specialized innervation pattern. The area of the LES as defined by manometer extends over 2–3 cm (Ogorek 1995). Under the influence of vasoactive intestinal polypeptide, nitrous oxide, cholecystokinin, esophageal peristalsis or distention of the esophagus, resting LES pressure decreases. Various other substances, such as reproductive hormones, prostaglandins and fat, also cause relaxation of LES tone (Altschuler 1992, Ogorek 1995, Reynolds 1995). Vagal stimulation seems to be involved in both inhibition and excitation of smooth muscle activity of the LES (Ogorek 1995). Although one might assume that resting LES pressures would be decreased in newborns and infants, studies measuring lower esophageal pressures in infants have reported decreased and normal levels, and one study even showed elevated pressures (Euler & Ament 1977, Herbst et al 1979, Arasu et al 1980). However, it is difficult to accurately measure LES pressures in infants, because the manometer exerts a certain amount of stretch on the small, narrow esophagus. This may account for the discrepancies reported.

The LES is aided in generating the HPZ through the assistance of the crura of the diaphragm and the phrenoesophageal ligament. These two components may be of especial significance in the newborn and infant, in whom organization of the neural and chemical systems responsible for modulating LES tone may still be immature. The crura of the diaphragm form a sling around the lower esophagus as it passes through the esophageal aperture (Fig. 14.9). Oscillations in pressure at the HPZ correlate with respiratory cycles (Welch & Gray 1982, Altschuler 1985, Boyle et al 1985, Mittal & McCallum 1988). During inspiration, contraction of the diaphragmatic crura around the lower esophagus augments LES pressures. During swallowing, pressure in the LES decreases and there is a concurrent decrease in the magnitude of contraction of the crura (Altschuler 1992). Studies performed in humans and mammals with functional esophageal characteristics similar to those in humans have shown that electrical activity in the crura

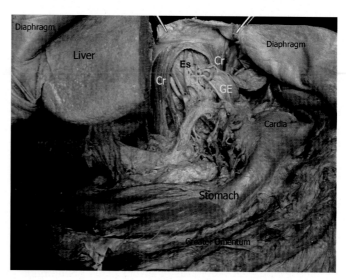

Fig. 14.9 • An overview for orientation. The greater omentum has been removed, the liver has been bisected, and the diaphragm trimmed back to reveal the esophageal hiatus. The two crura of the diaphragm (Cr) can be seen forming the walls of the opening, with the esophagus (Es) passing through. The gastroesophageal junction (GE) is seen distal to the hiatus. The cardiac portion of the stomach is clearly indicated.

of the diaphragm is selectively inhibited during activities requiring relaxation of the HPZ, while activity in the costal portion remains unchanged (Titchen 1979, Harding & Titchen 1981, Altschuler et al 1985). The body and crura of the diaphragm can function independently. This needs to be kept in mind when evaluating diaphragm mechanics. Normal thoracic cage and respiratory function may not be affected by crural dysfunction. Tissue relationships in the thoracolumbar area may provide better clues of crural mechanics than evaluation of the anterior or lateral thoracoabdominal region.

The third contribution to the HPZ is generally thought to come from the phrenoesophageal ligament. Fascia from the inferior surface of the diaphragm combines with transversalis fascia to form a cone around the terminal esophagus, the fibers of which then blend into the submucosa (Standring 2004). The phrenoesophageal ligament creates the angle of His, the junction between the intrathoracic and intra-abdominal esophagus. When the ligament has a more caudal insertion into the esophagus, there is shortening of the intra-abdominal section of the esophagus, which may be related to reflux (Ogorek 1995). The incidence of this anomaly is unclear. From a mechanical perspective, the relationship at the diaphragmatic aperture differs in the infant and adult. The angle of His is less acute in the newborn because of the relative flattening of the diaphragm.

The contributions of the diaphragmatic crura and phrenoesophageal ligament to the HPZ are thought to be more significant in infants and young children than in adults. Once the neural and myogenic control systems mature, tone in the LES becomes the primary protection against GER.

Pathophysiology of GER

The three most common findings associated with GER have been described based on observations and measurements of lower esophageal pH, pressure in the HPZ, esophageal motility and swallowing (Altschuler 1992). The findings include transient elevation of intra-abdominal pressure, spontaneous reflux, and transient relaxation of the LES. Of the three, the last is most commonly involved (Dodds 1982).

Transient relaxation of the lower esophageal HPZ occurs when resting tone in the HPZ falls below that of the stomach and esophageal peristalsis is absent. This phenomenon is present in children and adults and is the most commonly accepted mechanism for GER. Studies have shown that during transient relaxation there is a sudden decrease in pressure at the HPZ associated with a decrease in both respiratory-induced oscillations and end-expiratory pressures. Transient relaxations may last almost 30 s, but reflux only occurs during the few seconds while pressure is at zero and there are no respiratory-induced oscillations. The mechanism for transient relaxations of the HPZ is unclear (Mittal & McCallum 1988). It has been suggested that they may be a result of subthreshold levels of activity in the esophagus which are too low to stimulate full deglutition but nevertheless trigger HPZ relaxation (Paterson et al 1986, Mittal et al 1996).

The second common phenomenon observed in symptomatic GER is transient elevation in intra-abdominal pressure. In patients without GER, transient increases in intra-abdominal pressure trigger a vagally mediated contraction of the smooth muscle at the LES proportional to the increase in gastric pressure. At the same time, crural activity is inhibited by the elevations in intra-abdominal pressure. This suggests that, under normal conditions, the mature LES is capable of accommodating increased abdominal pressure. In order for increased intra-abdominal pressure to result in reflux, the pressure at the LES must be diminished to begin with. Gastric distention does not change resting LES pressure; it does, however, increase the incidence of transient relaxation of the sphincter (Ogorek 1995). Transient increases in intra-abdominal pressure may result from delayed gastric emptying. In adults, there is an association of retention of gastric contents with reflux. In general, the intensity and duration of reflux are inversely correlated with the transit time through the stomach. Infants have delayed gastric emptying when compared with adults, and there is some evidence that in premature infants gastric emptying is delayed even further (Gupta & Brans 1978). In infants, gastric distention can trigger relaxation of the LES (Holloway et al 1985), and result

in reflux. Although the method of feeding does not appear to influence gastric emptying in newborns, the composition of the feed does (Boyle 1992). For example, breast milk is emptied from the stomach more quickly than cow's milk formula (Cavell 1979, 1981), which may have a role in the anecdotal increase in the incidence of GER in formula-fed babies.

When one or more of the three components of the HPZ is compromised, resting pressure may be abnormally low and delayed gastric emptying time and increased pressures may overcome the sphincter without triggering transient relaxation. This may account for GER of the newborn, which resolves as the gastrointestinal system and diaphragm function mature. Hypotonic LES may account for GER in a small number of patients. This is usually associated with neurological impairment, connective tissue disease, surgery at the gastroesophageal junction and esophagitis (Dodds et al 1981, Williams 1989).

Diagnosis of GER

Conventional diagnosis of GER is made through history and normal findings on physical examination. The astute clinician trained in palpatory diagnosis might confirm the diagnosis by the presence of viscerosomatic reflexes between the levels of T5 and T7 (Beal & Dvorak 1984, Beal 1985). More invasive testing includes an esophageal pH probe, which will register changes in pH due to refluxed gastric contents in the distal esophagus. Another test frequently employed is the barium swallow X-ray. While the sensitivity of barium swallow is good, the specificity is low, due to the incidence of false negatives. Plain radiographs and computed tomography (CT) scans may show evidence of hiatal hernia but, because they are not dynamic studies, functional capacity of the LES cannot be evaluated. Gastroesophageal endoscopic evaluation will provide information concerning inflammatory changes at the gastroesophageal junction, and concomitant tissue biopsy can be done.

From an osteopathic perspective, GER in children is often associated with one or more of the following: diaphragmatic restrictions, strains at the thoracolumbar junction, altered respiratory mechanics in the thorax, strains at the craniocervical junction, and cranial findings suggesting vagal irritation (surveyed results from osteopathic clinicians) (Magoun 1976). Concurrent with these findings are the presence of the aforementioned viscerosomatic reflexes.

If we compare what is known about the pathogenesis of GER with the more common osteopathic findings, we can see a logical relationship between the two. The HPZ at the gastroesophageal junction is maintained through the combined efforts of the LES, the diaphragmatic crura and the phrenoesophageal ligament. Tone in the LES is modulated by the vagus, which also influences gastric emptying time and acid secretion. Somatic strains at the craniocervical junction or cranial base have the potential to irritate one or both of the vagus nerves, either through compression of the vasa nervorum by adjacent tissue structures and subsequent changes in conductive activity, or via irritation of the nervi nervosa, which results in local inflammatory changes that may affect nerve function. Furthermore, vagal dysfunction will affect peristalsis, secretory activity and emptying time in the stomach. As previously described, the crura of the diaphragm are capable of acting independently of the costal portion. The role of the phrenic nerve in this process is not well described. However, one must consider the potential influence of somatic strains in the midcervical area, C3–C5, and the resulting increase in spinal cord activity and/or altered sensory input at those levels, upon phrenic nerve function. Although these neural mechanisms are understood in general terms, specific responses at particular levels are not well described.

The effectiveness of the crural contribution to the HPZ is determined by the mechanical efficacy of the crural muscles, and the positional relationship between their origin and insertion. Biomechanical strains at the thoracolumbar junction will involve the areas of attachment of the crural muscles, potentially compromising their ability to contract effectively around the esophageal hiatus. Altered respiratory mechanics may be a result of biomechanical strain in any part of the thoracic cage, the diaphragm or the crura. Each of these may affect competency of the HPZ. Restricted diaphragm motion, regardless of its etiology, will affect the relationship of the phrenoesophageal ligament to the esophagus, and possibly the acuity of the angle of His. This may compromise the ability of both to contribute to the HPZ. Furthermore, if diaphragmatic mechanics are altered, functional isolation of the crura from costal portions may be undermined.

Differential diagnosis of GER

The newborn infant with GER typically presents with excessive spitting up, which may or may not be associated with feeding. The differential diagnosis for this presentation would include pyloric stenosis, duodenal stenosis or atresia, and tracheoesophageal fistula. Pyloric stenosis may present with projectile vomiting, depending on the extent of the stenosis and size of the feeds. On physical examination, a firm palpable mass is usually present in the right upper quadrant at the site of the pyloric sphincter. It may be pea-sized or larger. Weight gain is often poor with pyloric stenosis, whereas GER usually does not affect weight gain.

In cases of duodenal atresia or stenosis, spitting up is delayed after feeding. The vomitus is usually curdled or partially digested. Weight loss or poor weight gain is the norm. On physical examination there may be no abnormal findings. Barium swallow or plain film radiograph can be diagnostic in each of these cases.

Treatment of the infant and child with GER

All osteopathic findings should be considered with special attention to viscerosomatic reflexes, which could potentially mediate continued symptoms through neurological mechanisms. In the premature and newborn infant, balanced ligamentous and balanced membranous techniques are very useful. Fluid techniques may be directed at the findings in the cranium. Dietary sensitivities should be elucidated and addressed to ensure optimum gastrointestinal function. The child should have small and frequent feeds with the head elevated, and it should remain so after eating. Studies done with a pH probe have shown that elevating the infant's head in the prone position reduces the incidence of reflux as compared with positioning in an infant seat (Orenstein & Whitington 1983). If the baby is receiving formula, adding a thickener such as rice cereal may be helpful, in that crying and vomiting decrease, and sleeping increases, although reflux is unchanged. It should be kept in mind that a complication of thickened formula can be increased respiratory symptoms (Orenstein et al 1987, 1992). If breastfeeding, the mother may need to try an elimination diet to deduce what substances may be aggravating the clinical picture. Cow's milk antigens do cross into breast milk.

H_2 blockers and antacids are often used for the treatment of severe GER in infants. These reduce the acidity of the refluxed gastric secretion and may prevent esophagitis. Cisapride, a prokinetic agent that increases LES pressure and rate of gastric emptying, has been shown to be effective in treating GER. It works through the enteric nervous system by stimulating the release of acetylcholine from neurons in the myenteric plexus, so there are few central side effects.

COLIC

Colic is a symptom complex in infants consisting of crying or irritability which does not respond to soothing, signs of gastric discomfort including gastric distention, pulling legs to belly and excessive gas, and facial expressions indicating discomfort. Studies investigating maternal behaviors and ability to discern these phenomena have shown that there is no relationship between these signs and care-giving practices (Barr 1990, Barr et al 1991), and that mothers can consistently distinguish colic behaviors from 'normal' behaviors (Forsyth 1989, Sifter & Braungart 1992). The duration and quality of the infant's crying is a hallmark of colic. Traditionally, the duration of symptoms should be 3 h/day for 3 days/week for 3 weeks (Wessel et al 1954). Even if the duration does not meet these criteria, the quality of the cry may be indicative of colic (Barr et al 1992, Alvarez & St James-Roberts 1996). In most infants, signs of colic begin some time in the first month of life, peak at 2 months, and, even if untreated, resolve by 4 or 5 months of age (Wessel et al 1954, Illingworth 1955). Infantile colic has been associated with maternal prenatal and postnatal smoking (Canivet et al 2008), prenatal maternal anxiety (Canivet et al 2005), sensitivity to cow's milk protein (Leung & Lemay 2004), dyscoordinate sucking patterns and gastroesophageal reflux (Miller-Loncar et al 2004). Interestingly, in a 4-year follow-up study Canivet et al (2000) reported that children who had colic in infancy demonstrated more negative emotions (especially during meals) and stomach ache than controls. Colic is a diagnosis of exclusion, so other etiologies for the presentation must be ruled out through history and physical examination.

A model for the pathophysiology of colic

Theories concerning the etiology and pathophysiology of colic are broad and varied, ranging from food sensitivities to gut and nervous system immaturity to poor care-giving techniques. From an osteopathic perspective, each of these has some merit, and in fact the clinical presentation of colic may represent different pathologies manifesting with a similar symptom/sign complex, the way in which many different pathological processes manifest as headache. Furthermore, there is no clear-cut pathology or treatment for colic, with equivocal responses to diet change. Perhaps there are different causes of colic, with some children having gastrointestinal-related symptoms, others experiencing a state of hyperactive/irritability, and an additional group having some combination of the two. From an osteopathic perspective, this makes the most sense.

Colic typically appears early in life sometime around the first month. This is a time when both the nervous and gastrointestinal systems are immature. This may play out in several ways. Older children and adults have the ability to screen out and prioritize sensory information. The reader sitting in her chair, engrossed in this discussion, is not necessarily aware of the pressure of her ischial tuberosities on the chair, or the weight of the book in her hands, or the sensation of her socks on her feet. The reader has the ability to ignore the input from those various sensory receptors even though they may be firing. The ability to ignore, or prioritize sensory input is something that develops with maturation of the nervous system. We are not born with it; it is learned. A newborn does not possess this capability and is consequently bombarded with sensory stimuli. Any component of the nervous system receiving continuous or excessive stimuli can become sensitized. And what was once non-noxious may soon become noxious. The nociceptive system functions with scant myelination when mature, while other systems are heavily myelinated. The gating reflex at the level of the spinal cord is dependent on the speed of conduction of large-calibre (heavily myelinated) fibers to 'gate' the signals from the slower C fibers. With

this lacking, C-fiber activity may have the potential to go 'unchecked', rendering it more capable of signaling higher areas. The ability of the nociceptive system to respond to a stimulus may be more akin to a mature system while the ability of other systems is not.

Most of the body maps used to localize sensory input are absent or poorly formed at birth. The ability to localize noxious and non-noxious stimuli is compromised. When newborns are exposed to continuous stimulus, be it noxious or non-noxious, they are probably not able to localize the stimulus. With constant stimuli coming in from tactile, pressure, visual, auditory, temperature, and proprioceptive receptors, as well as stretch and chemoreceptors in the gut, areas of brainstem and cortex become awash with activity, creating a sensory barrage. Newborns with their poorly defined sensory maps and immature gating mechanisms are left with little ability to differentiate the myriad of signals they are receiving, and may instead interpret the heightened activity as noxious.

The gastrointestinal and nervous systems share many components throughout life. The enteric nervous system of the gut influences and is influenced by processes occurring in the nervous, respiratory, endocrine, dermatological and immunological systems. In the newborn these systems are not well differentiated and often exhibit reactions to processes occurring in another system. One example of this is the relationship between sleep cycle and digestion. The immaturity of both of these systems lends itself to a confluence of influences: heightened activity or responses occurring simultaneously in multiple systems and having a summative effect on multiple systems.

An osteopathic perspective on colic

Children presenting with colic fall into three groups based on osteopathic evaluation (chart review): somatic dysfunction findings suggesting persistent nociceptive or painful stimuli; findings suggesting functional gastrointestinal disturbance; and findings suggesting some combination of the two. This hypothesis is based on the observation that the somatic dysfunction present in the baby with colic is similar to findings in older patients who are able to communicate their complaint. It is probable that the somatic dysfunction produces a similar symptom in the infant, who has limited means of communication.

From an osteopathic perspective, findings suggesting functional gastrointestinal disturbance include strains in the thorax, abdomen or pelvis which could be equated with irritable bowel, constipation or dietary sensitivity. Commonly, there is also dysfunction at the cranial base which is often interpreted as vagal irritation, via the vasa nervosum or nervi nervosum, but may also represent a source of trigeminal irritation. As previously discussed, gut motility and function are immature. Increased transit times and immature hormone and enzyme function may promote the production of intestinal gases. Function of the colon is not well developed at birth, which may affect gas absorption. Poor mucosal barrier function may lead to antigen exposure and subsequent inflammatory response in the gut wall, affecting peristalsis, digestion and absorption.

In traditional osteopathic teaching, colic has been described as resulting from vagal nerve irritation associated with tissue strain patterns in the cranial base, petrobasilar and occipitomastoid areas. Interestingly, the classic symptoms of colic usually arise sometime between the second and fourth weeks of life in the term infant. This period of time coincides with initial development of voluntary control of the posterior cervical muscles. Infants of this age will begin to lift their heads if placed prone. These are the very muscles which attach to the areas of the cranium commonly found to have mechanical strain in infants with colic. One hypothesis might be that the engagement of the posterior cervical muscles exacerbates minor tissue strains in this area.

There is a second group of infants with colic often described by osteopathic clinicians based on palpatory observation and atypical presentation (survey, meeting reports). This group demonstrates a high level of irritability in the primary respiratory mechanism, which, using Sutherland's model, can be described as being localized to the palpatory phenomena of the potency-fluid interface or the central nervous system (CNS). Coincidently, the medical literature also recognizes a subgroup of infants with colic whose symptom complex suggests immaturity or irritability of the CNS. The nervous system of the newborn infant is still immature at birth, and the ability to screen out stimuli is poor, as is organization of the sleeping and waking states. In the normal child and adult the conscious awareness of stimuli only occurs when the stimulus attains the necessary threshold to be mapped to cortical areas and reach the association cortex. Prior to that the stimulus may still be received by receptors, and mapped to the spinal cord and brainstem, but it is in essence 'ignored' by our awareness. This hierarchical response to stimulus is not present at birth. In fact, as discussed in Chapter 10, the process of appropriately mapping and interpreting stimulus develops over the first few years of life. Consequently, whereas while reading this book you may not be aware of your gut peristalsis, the static contraction of your erector spinae muscles or the dryness in the room, the nervous system of a very young infant is aware of all these things and more. Furthermore, if you actively choose to bring these things to your conscious attention, you will soon find that they can be rather irritating. Now imagine you have just spent 9 months in a sensory deprivation tank, you have been pushed through a tight canal, and you are lying in clothes and a nappy in a dry heated room with some banging in the background. You see my point.

The last subgroup of infants with colic also has an atypical presentation that is not necessarily related to feeding. Parents often report that symptoms began immediately,

rather than in the second or third week. Osteopathic evaluation of these children often reveals somatic dysfunction in the upper cervical, cranial–cervical or cranial base areas. Tissue palpation usually elicits signs of irritability from the newborn. Similar somatic strains in an older child or adult would typically be associated with cephalgia and trigeminal irritation. Primary afferent nerves carrying nociceptive information are functional in the newborn. However, how the immature brain interprets the signal is unclear. Nevertheless, nociceptive stimulus is known to increase activity in the hypothalamic–pituitary–adrenal axis. In the adult, this can generate a state of hyperarousal, with anxiety and irritability. Modulation of many of the neurotransmitters and hormones involved in this mechanism is immature in the newborn and may not be able to compensate for nociceptive input. Furthermore, as already mentioned, sleep and waking states are poorly organized. The potential for a non-gastroenterological etiology such as muscle spasm or cephalgia needs to be taken into account. For example, a 'colicky' infant demonstrating aversion to loud sounds and bright lights, and 'gastrointestinal symptoms', may be exhibiting the photophobia, hyperacusis and nausea of headache. The reported association of colic in infancy and migraine cephalgia in later life would support this notion.

Many of the aforementioned factors mature by 4 or 5 months, which coincides with the time at which untreated colic usually resolves. Nevertheless, osteopathic treatment of associated findings may help the infant compensate until these systems mature, and give the parents a much-needed break (Hayden & Mullinger 2006).

CONSTIPATION

Constipation is a frequent concern for parents of infants and toddlers, and accounts for one-quarter of visits to pediatric gastroenterologists (Taitz et al 1986). Yet the clinical syndrome of constipation is not well defined or understood. The term constipation may be used to describe a condition of prolonged time between bowel movements or abnormally hard stools. In either case, parents report perceived discomfort in their child and anxiety in themselves. There is a relationship between constipation in childhood and irritable bowel syndrome in adult life, although inconsistencies between the two exist (Davidson & Waserman 1966, Fielding 1977, Murphy & Clayden 1996). Clinical presentation of abdominal distention, hard stools, abdominal pain and abnormal frequency are similar between the two groups. However, childhood constipation appears to be evenly distributed between girls and boys, while irritable bowel syndrome is more prevalent in females. This may reflect hormonal influence, but that is unclear. Fortunately, serious clinical sequelae of constipation in childhood, such as enterocolitis, are rare and usually related to massive retention.

The presence of encopresis or fecal soiling may complicate the clinical picture in children with constipation. The term encopresis is generally used to describe the socially unacceptable passage of a bowel movement; examples would include passing normal stool into clothing or into the bed. Fecal soiling refers to involuntary passage of stool which is usually quite loose and frequent. Fecal soiling is usually caused by overflow due to chronic constipation, but may occur acutely in infectious gastroenteritis with diarrhea. Encopresis may be associated with improper toilet training, developmental delay, psychological trauma or disturbance and neurological abnormalities.

Normal stool frequency for adult and preschool children in Western societies falls within the rather broad range of three bowel movements daily to three weekly (Connell et al 1965, Drossman et al 1982, Weaver & Stevens 1988). Bowel movements in term infants of less than 5 months occur between one and seven times per day, although fewer movements are still considered normal. In fact, delays of 10 days or more have been reported in healthy breast-fed babies (Murphy & Clayden 1996). During the first 2 months of life, bowel movement frequency is greater in breastfed infants than in those being bottle-fed; however, this appears to even out once solids are introduced (Weaver & Stevens 1988). As would be expected, stool frequency, size and consistency vary with diet in adults and the same would be anticipated in children (Burkitt et al 1980, Kelsay et al 1981, Walker & Walker 1985, Davies et al 1986).

Differential diagnosis of chronic constipation

Constipation may occur as a result of organ disease, which can usually be ruled out through history and physical examination. Intestinal obstruction will present with acute onset of the constipation and signs of paralytic ileus: guarding and rigidity, abdominal distention, absent bowel sounds, and, if severe, rebound pain. Plain abdominal X-rays will usually rule out obstruction when physical examination is equivocal. Pseudo-obstruction occurs in cases of dysmotility, and may be secondary to a systemic disease process. Signs and symptoms of obstruction may be present without the existence of an obstructing lesion.

Hirschsprung's disease is congenital aganglionosis in Meissner's and Auerbach's plexuses which presents with chronic constipation. The extent of involvement of the colon varies, although typically it is restricted to the rectum and anal sphincter. When involvement is extensive, clinical symptoms present soon after birth and are severe, including vomiting of fecal matter. In the majority of cases, the child has partial obstruction and presents later with chronic constipation and abdominal distention. On physical examination, stool is absent from the rectum. The abdomen is usually distended, and stool is palpable through the abdominal wall proximal to the area of involvement. In Hirschsprung's disease, the affected area is tonically contracted due to the absent influence of the enteric nervous system. Progressive and chronic retention of fecal matter leads to distention of the colonic wall and megacolon or megarectum. Other congenital abnormalities of innervation in the colon may present with chronic constipation but are rare, and physical findings and presentation are similar to those for Hirschsprung's disease.

Chronic constipation is also associated with congenital spinal cord lesions such as tethering of the cord and myelomeningocele, and acquired lesions from trauma, tumor and infection. Spina bifida occulta can be associated with underlying cord abnormalities which lead to chronic constipation.

Finally, anatomical anomalies of the colon and anus such as stenosis or stricture must be considered but can generally be ruled out on physical examination.

Precipitating factors in functional constipation

Neural components of mesenteric and submucosal plexus in the distal colon are immature at birth and remain so throughout the first 2 years of life. They appear to mature completely by 5 years (Murphy & Clayden 1996). In general, gut motility is not fully functional at birth and, as previously discussed, does not take on adult characteristics until some time later. Furthermore, transit time is significantly delayed in children with constipation, with most prolonged clearance times occurring in the distal colon or rectum (Arhan et al 1981, 1983).

The anatomy of the pelvic area has a role in maintaining competency of the anal sphincter. The sigmoid colon becomes the rectum at the level of the third sacral segment, and runs along the anterior surface of the sacrum and coccyx. Just beyond the coccyx, the rectum turns posteroinferiorly and narrows as it passes through the pelvic diaphragm, becoming the anal canal as it does so. The angle formed at this juncture is important in maintaining fecal continence. The puborectus muscle forms a sling around the anus, supporting it from the pubic ramus. Under normal conditions, this sling can contract and draw the rectum anteriorly to close the lumen; this action contributes to competency of the external sphincter. The internal and external sphincters lie in the perineal portion of the pelvic diaphragm. The internal sphincter is under autonomic control, and the external under voluntary. The external sphincter has deep and superficial portions, both of which are extensions of the perineal body of the pelvic diaphragm. Fibers from the puborectus muscle merge into the external sphincter, as do fibers from the anococcygeal ligament (Standring 2004). The external sphincter receives its innervation from the lower sacral segments. In children with chronic constipation, the anal canal is positioned more obliquely, which is thought to affect function of the external sphincter such that delays in fecal elimination are due to the altered relationships at this junction. Placement of the anal canal may be abnormally forward, creating a palpable shelf distal to the orifice, or quite subtle, without gross anatomical change, but nevertheless affecting sphincter function (Kerremans et al 1974, Hendren 1978, Leape & Ramenofsky 1978, Kiely et al 1979, Reisner et al 1984). Alterations in the relationship between the pelvic bones and the sacrum will affect the pelvic diaphragm and its muscular components. Increasing the obliquity of the angle at the anorectal junction has been shown to alter electromyographic and manometric characteristics of sphincter mechanics (Kerremans et al 1974). Soft tissue strains also have the potential to alter function of the sphincter by the same mechanisms. From an osteopathic viewpoint, tissue stresses and dysfunction in the sacral and pelvic area are common findings in children with chronic constipation. Resolution of these strains appears to be related to improvement in symptoms. Other common findings include altered mechanics in the lower thoracic and upper lumbar areas which may be related to viscerosomatic reflexes and/or autonomic modulation of lower gut motility.

HYPERBILIRUBINEMIA/NEONATAL JAUNDICE

Jaundice is a yellow discoloration of the sclera and skin which occurs in the presence of elevated levels of serum bilirubin. Bilirubin, a yellow-green pigment, is one of the major byproducts of the breakdown of the hemoglobin in red blood cells. Hemoglobin is catabolized in two steps, resulting in bilirubin. Bilirubin is then transported to the liver via albumin, where it is conjugated with one or two glucuronide groups to form bilirubin monoglucuronide or diglucuronide, i.e. conjugated bilirubin. Unconjugated bilirubin is lipophilic and can cross cell membranes but is not easily excreted. The addition of the glucuronide molecule makes bilirubin water soluble, so it can enter into the bile and be excreted in the fecal matter. Bilirubin levels are traditionally measured by blood or urine sampling. Two methods exist for serum measurements, each with its own terminology. The older, diazo method measures direct (conjugated), indirect (unconjugated) and total bilirubin, but does not differentiate conjugated bilirubin bound to albumin, delta-bilirubin. A second method, the Ektachem method, accounts for all three types of bilirubin and the total. Normal values between the two methods of serum testing vary, as do values for the same method in different laboratories. But, in general, hyperbilirubinemia can be defined as total serum levels of bilirubin greater than

34.2 μmol/l (2 mg/dl) in the diazo method and greater than 22.2 μmol/l (1.3 mg/dl) in the Ektachem method.

Jaundice can result from elevated levels of conjugated or unconjugated bilirubin. Discoloration is usually first seen in the sclera of the eye when total serum bilirubin levels exceed 34.2–51.3 μmol/l (2–3 mg/dl). Using the diazo scale in the newborn, icterus of the face can be seen at total bilirubin levels of 102.6 μmol/l (6 mg/dl), torso involvement presents at levels exceeding 136.8 μmol/l (8 mg/dl), and the palms and soles become discolored when bilirubin reaches 342 μmol/l (20 mg/dl). Hyperbilirubinemia may result from increased production of bilirubin, decreased conjugation of bilirubin, or decreased elimination of conjugated bilirubin. Increased production will occur in the presence of hemolytic diseases such as hemolytic disease of the newborn. Decreased conjugation may result from obstruction of the biliary system, insufficient albumin levels or binding sites, or dysfunction or inadequacies of the conjugation system. Elimination is affected by the frequency of stool passage and the presence of intestinal flora.

Physiological jaundice

In utero, the conjugation system for bilirubin is dormant. Unconjugated bilirubin can pass through the placenta and enter maternal excretion systems. After 20 weeks of gestation, some bilirubin will pass into the stool, where it can be reabsorbed and transferred back to the liver – enterohepatic recirculation. After birth, it takes several days for the conjugation system in the smooth endoplasmic reticulum to activate. During that time, many newborns experience physiological jaundice. This probably results from a combination of factors: immaturity of the conjugation system, reabsorption of bilirubin via enterohepatic circulation because of delay in passage of stools, caloric intake of substances which may alter albumin-binding sites and/or levels of albumin, and absence of intestinal flora which enzymatically alter conjugated bilirubin, preventing reabsorption (Cashore 1992, Rosenthal 1992, Keating 1996). Physiological jaundice appears early in life and resolves spontaneously within a few days. Total bilirubin levels, which peak by the third day, generally do not exceed 205.2 μmol/l (12 mg/dl), and there is no elevation in conjugated bilirubin.

Breast milk jaundice

Jaundice occurs in approximately 13% of breastfed newborns and is characterized by an elevation in unconjugated bilirubin (Gourley 1992). Breastfed infants are three times more likely to experience moderate jaundice and six times more likely to experience severe jaundice than their formula-fed counterparts (Kivlahan & James 1984, Osborn et al 1984, Maisels & Gifford 1986, Schneider 1986). Breast milk jaundice may present in one of two ways. The first is most probably due to inadequate intake of milk, and appears during the first several days of life, as a result of a rise in unconjugated bilirubin levels. This usually resolves with increased milk intake. The second type of breast milk jaundice is also a result of unconjugated bilirubin levels but presents during the second week of life (Keating 1996). The mechanism for this is unclear, but it resolves spontaneously with increased feedings and sunlight. If bilirubin levels remain high, phototherapy may be instituted.

Differential diagnosis

The differential diagnosis of hyperbilirubinemia must include abnormalities and diseases of the liver, biliary system and hematopoietic system. Generally speaking, these can be differentiated from physiological and breast milk jaundice by the bilirubin fraction and clinical presentation.

Elevations in unconjugated bilirubin can result from overload of the hepatic conjugating system due to red blood cell hemolysis. This may occur secondary to cephalohematoma or other concealed hemorrhage. Pallor, signs of anemia and hepatosplenomegaly may be present. The most dangerous and dramatic condition is hemolytic disease due to Rh incompatibility. Jaundice appears soon after birth and unconjugated bilirubin levels climb very quickly. Complications include congestive heart failure, hypoxia, encephalopathy and kernicterus. This is a medical emergency. Although improved diagnostic and therapeutic precautions have almost eliminated hydrops fetalis in most of the Western world, it can still be seen in patients emigrating from underdeveloped areas. Other conditions, albeit less worrisome, which are associated with perinatal jaundice include pyloric stenosis and Gilbert's syndrome. Moderate elevations in unconjugated bilirubin may be present with pyloric stenosis. Accompanying signs include excessive spitting up, weight loss, and palpatory changes in the right upper quadrant. The jaundice is transient and resolves once the stenosis is remedied. A second consideration in unconjugated hyperbilirubinemia is Gilbert's syndrome, a benign familial condition consisting of intermittent asymptomatic mild jaundice concurrent with mild infection or stress. The mechanism for Gilbert's syndrome is unclear. Diagnosis is based on history and physical examination, so the diagnosis is usually not made until the child is older.

Hyperbilirubinemia involving the conjugated fraction of bilirubin occurs with conditions affecting the liver and biliary systems, such as infection or congenital abnormality. Biliary atresia is the most common hepatic disorder in newborns. Jaundice appears in the first week of life due to elevations in conjugated bilirubin. Other signs of hepatic disease may not appear for several months. Cholestasis from bile plugs or other ductal obstruction also needs to be considered with increased conjugated bilirubin. Ischemic injury to the hepatocytes may result from heart disease, or fetal

distress. In the infant and older child, hepatitis will present with jaundice with an elevated conjugated fraction. Other conditions associated with jaundice include hypothyroidism, liver enzyme deficiencies, and congenital infarction.

Complications of hyperbilirubinemia

The most serious complication of hyperbilirubinemia is the toxicity of unconjugated bilirubin to the brain. Unconjugated bilirubin can cross the blood–brain barrier because of its lipophilic nature. Furthermore, unconjugated bilirubin appears to have a natural affinity for proteins in the cell membrane and synaptosomes. It is hypothesized that the bilirubin is taken up at the synapse and carried through retrograde transport to the cell body (Cashore 1992). Under normal conditions, unconjugated bilirubin is bound to albumin, which cannot cross into the brain. However, when levels of unconjugated bilirubin exceed the binding capacity of serum albumin, or if the blood–brain barrier is damaged, free bilirubin may cross into the CNS. Bilirubin appears to impair water and ion transport across cell membranes, as well as enzyme activities in the cell. Nerve conduction, transmission and cell membrane potential are affected (Cashore 1992).

Bilirubin encephalopathy occurs when bilirubin deposits in the brain. It usually presents 2–5 days after birth, but may present later in premature and low-birthweight infants. The infant appears ill. There is loss of muscle tone, and newborn reflexes, and a weak, high-pitched cry. A weak suck and poor feeding are present, and inability to maintain basal temperatures can occur. As the condition progresses, spasticity, opisthotonos and seizures may develop. If the child survives, the neurological syndrome of kernicterus is usually present, with choreoathetosis, involuntary muscle spasm, seizures, dysarthric speech, extrapyramidal signs, severe cognitive delay and hearing loss. Partial syndrome may occur in less severe cases with extrapyramidal signs, hypotonia, and ataxia. A very mild form involves incoordination and minimal brain dysfunction.

Treatment of jaundice

The risk of kernicterus is directly related to the level of unconjugated bilirubin and indirectly proportional to the gestational age and weight of the infant. Consequently, bilirubin levels in low-weight and premature infants are monitored much more closely than in full-term infants. Standard therapy for hyperbilirubinemia consists of exposure to blue light. Unconjugated bilirubin absorbs blue light photons, which excite the bilirubin molecule. One of three things can happen: the bilirubin molecule can release heat, emit a photon, or undergo photochemical conversion. Photochemical conversion produces one of three products, all of which can be excreted through either the urine or the gut (Ennever 1992). Generally speaking, in the uncomplicated full-term neonate phototherapy for hyperbilirubinemia should be implemented immediately if jaundice appears before the first 24 h of life. During the first 2–5 days of life, bilirubin levels reaching or exceeding 256.5 μmol/l (15 mg/dl) warrant phototherapy. In very low-birthweight infants, therapy is instituted earlier, with levels of 171–205.2 μmol/l (10–12 mg/dl) requiring treatment. When bilirubin levels are unresponsive to phototherapy, or exceed 342–427.5 μmol/l (20–25 mg/dl), or signs of encephalopathy develop, exchange transfusion may be necessary to prevent long-term sequelae.

References

Allen C 1984 Gastroesophageal reflux and chronic respiratory disease. Am Rev Respir Dis 129: 645–647.

Altschuler S M, Boyle J T, Nixon T E et al 1985 Simultaneous reflux inhibition of the lower esophageal sphincter and crural diaphragm in cats. Am J Physiol 249: G586–591.

Altschuler S M 1992 Pathophysiology of gastroesophageal reflux. In: Polin R, Fox W (eds) Fetal and neonatal physiology. W B Saunders, Philadelphia: 1033–1039.

Alvarez M, St James-Roberts I 1996 Infant fussing and crying patterns in the first year in an urban community in Denmark. Acta Paediatr 85(4): 463–466.

Arasu T S, Wyllie R, Fitzgerald J F et al 1980 Gastroesophageal reflux in infants and children: comparative accuracy of diagnostic methods. J Pediatr 96(5): 798–803.

Arhan P, Devroede G, Jehannin B et al 1981 Segmental colonic transit time. Dis Colon Rectum 24(8): 625–629.

Arhan P, Devroede G, Jehannin B et al 1983 Idiopathic disorders of fecal continence in children. Pediatrics 71(5): 774–779.

Barr R G 1990 The normal crying curve: what do we really know? Dev Med Child Neurol 32(4): 356–362.

Barr R G, Konner M, Bakeman R et al 1991 Crying in Kung San infants: a test of the cultural specificity hypothesis. Dev Med Child Neurol 33(7): 601–610.

Barr R G, Rotman A, Yaremko J et al 1992 The crying of infants with colic: a controlled empirical description. Pediatrics 90(1 Pt 1): 14–21.

Beal M C 1985 Viscerosomatic reflexes: a review. J Am Osteopath Assoc 85(12): 786–801.

Beal M C, Dvorak J 1984 Palpatory examination of the spine: a comparison of the results of two methods and their relationship to visceral disease. Manual Medicine 1: 25–32.

Bernbaum J C, Pereira G R, Watkins J B et al 1983 Non-nutritive sucking during gavage feeding enhances growth and maturation in premature infants. Pediatrics 71: 41–45.

Boersma E R, Offringa P J, Muskiet F A et al 1991 Vitamin E, lipid fractions, and fatty acid composition of colostrum, transitional milk, and mature milk: an international comparative study. Am J Clin Nutr 53(5): 1197–1204.

Boix-Ochoa J, Canals J 1976 Maturation of the lower esophagus. J Pediatr Surg 11: 749–856.

Bosma J F 1986 Anatomy of the infant head, 1st edn. Johns Hopkins University Press, Baltimore.

Boyle J 1992 Motility of the upper gastrointestinal tract in the fetus and neonate. In: Polin R, Fox W (eds) Fetal and neonatal physiology. W B Saunders, Philadelphia: 1028–1033.

Boyle J T, Altschuler S M, Nixon T E et al 1985 Role of the diaphragm in the genesis of lower esophageal sphincter pressure in the cat. Gastroenterology 88(3): 723–730.

Burkitt D, Morley D, Walker A 1980 Dietary fibre in under- and overnutrition in childhood. Arch Dis Child 55(10): 803–807.

Canivet C, Jakobsson I, Hagander B 2000 Infantile colic. Follow-up at four years of age: still more "emotional". Acta Paediatr 89: 13–17.

Canivet C A, Ostergren P O, Rosen A S et al 2005 Infantile colic and the role of trait anxiety during pregnancy in relation to psychosocial and socioeconomic factors. Scand J Public Health 33: 26–34.

Canivet C A, Ostergren P O, Jakobsson I L et al 2008 Infantile colic, maternal smoking and infant feeding at 5 weeks of age. Scand J Public Health 36: 284–291.

Cashore W J 1992 Bilirubin metabolism and toxicity in the newborn. In: Polin R A, Fox W (eds) Fetal and neonatal physiology. W B Saunders, Philadelphia: 1160–1165.

Cavell B 1979 Gastric emptying in preterm infants. Acta Paediatr Scand 68(5): 725–730.

Cavell B 1981 Gastric emptying in infants fed human milk or infant formula. Acta Paediatr Scand 70(5): 639–641.

Connell A M, Hilton C, Irvine G et al 1965 Variation of bowel habit in two population samples. BMJ ii: 1095–1099.

Davidson M, Waserman R 1966 The irritable colon of childhood (chronic nonspecific diarrhea syndrome). J Pediatr 69(6): 1027–1038.

Davies G J, Crowder M, Reid B et al 1986 Bowel function measurements of individuals with different eating patterns. Gut 27(2): 164–169.

Dodds W J 1982 Joint report of the Subcommittees on Animal Models of Hemorrhagic and Thrombotic Diseases and on platelets. Thromb Haemostat 48(1): 106–107.

Dodds W J, Hogan W J, Helm J F et al 1981 Pathogenesis of reflux esophagitis. Gastroenterology 81(2): 376–394.

Drossman D A, Sandler R S, McKee D C et al 1982 Bowel patterns among subjects not seeking health care. Use of a questionnaire to identify a population with bowel dysfunction. Gastroenterology 83(3): 529–534.

Ennever J F 1992 Phototherapy for neonatal jaundice. In: Polin R A, Fox W (eds) Fetal and neonatal physiology. W B Saunders, Philadelphia: 1165–1173.

Euler A R, Ament M E 1977 Value of esophagus manometric studies in gastroesophageal reflux in infancy. Pediatrics 59: 58–61.

Field T, Ignatoff E, Stringer S et al 1982 Nonnutritive sucking during tube feedings: effects on preterm neonates in an intensive care unit. Pediatrics 70: 381–384.

Fielding J F 1977 The irritable bowel syndrome. Part I: clinical spectrum. Clin Gastroenterol 6(3): 607–622.

Forsyth B W 1989 Colic and the effect of changing formulas: a double-blind, multiple-crossover study. J Pediatr 115(4): 521–526.

Fraval M 1998 A pilot study: osteopathic treatment of infants with sucking dysfunction. American Academy of Osteopathy Journal Summer: 25–33.

Gourley G R 1992 Pathophysiology of breast-milk jaundice. In: Polin R A, Fox W (eds) Fetal and neonatal physiology. W B Saunders, Philadelphia: 1173–1181.

Gupta M, Brans Y W 1978 Gastric retention in neonates. Pediatrics 62(1): 26–29.

Guyton A C 1996 Textbook of medical physiology, 9th edn. W B Saunders, Philadelphia.

Harding R, Titchen D A 1981 Oesophageal and diaphragmatic activity during sucking in lambs. J Physiol 321: 317–329.

Hayden C, Mullinger B 2006 A preliminary assessment of the impact of cranial osteopathy for the relief of infantile colic. Compl Ther Clin Pract 12: 83–90.

Hendren W H 1978 Constipation caused by anterior location of the anus and its surgical correction. J Pediatr Surg 13(6): 505–512.

Herbst J J 2000 Gastroesophageal reflux. In: Behrman R E, Kliegman R M, Jenson H B (eds) Nelson's textbook of pediatrics. W B Saunders, Philadelphia.

Herbst J J, Book L S, Johnson D G et al 1979 The lower esophageal sphincter in gastroesophageal reflux in children. J Clin Gastroenterol 1(2): 119–123.

Holloway R H, Hongo M, Berger K et al 1985 Gastric distention: a mechanism for postprandial gastroesophageal reflux. Gastroenterology 89(4): 779–784.

Illingworth R S 1955 Crying in infants and children. BMJ i: 75–78.

Jensen R G, Hagerty M M, McMahon K E 1978 Lipids of human milk and infant formulas: a review. Am J Clin Nutr 31(6): 990–1016.

Kahn A, Rebuffat E, Sottiaux M et al 1992 Lack of temporal relation between acid reflux in proximal oesophagus and cardiorespiratory events in sleeping infants. Eur J Pediatr 151: 208–212.

Keating J P 1996 Jaundice. In: Walker W A, Durie P R, Hamilton J R et al (eds) Pediatric gastroenterology. Mosby, St Louis: 395–405.

Kelsay J L, Goering H K, Behall K M et al 1981 Effect of fiber from fruits and vegetables on metabolic responses of human subjects: fiber intakes, fecal excretions, and apparent digestibilities. Am J Clin Nutr 34(9): 1849–1852.

Kenigsberg K, Aiges H, Alperstein G 1981 A unique device to measure lower esophageal sphincter pressure in unsedated infants. J Pediatr Surg 16: 370–373.

Kerremans R P, Pennickx F M, Beckers J P 1974 Functional evaluation of ectopic anus and its surgical consequences. Am J Dis Child 128(6): 811–814.

Kiely E M, Chopra R, Corkery J J 1979 Delayed diagnosis of congenital anal stenosis. Arch Dis Child 54(1): 68–70.

Kivlahan C, James E J 1984 The natural history of neonatal jaundice. Pediatrics 74(3): 364–370.

Leape L L, Ramenofsky M L 1978 Anterior ectopic anus: a common cause of constipation in children. J Pediatr Surg 13(6D): 627–630.

Leung A K, Lemay J F 2004 Infantile colic: a review. J R Soc Health 124: 162–166.

Magoun H I S 1976 Osteopathy in the cranial field, 3rd edn. The Journal Printing Company, Kirksville, Missouri.

Maisels M J, Gifford K 1986 Normal serum bilirubin levels in the newborn and the effect of breast-feeding. Pediatrics 78(5): 837–843.

Measel C P, Anderson G C 1979 Non-nutritive sucking during tube feedings: effect upon clinical course in premature infants. J Obstet Gynecol Neonatal Nurs 8: 265.

Milla P J 1996 The ontogeny of intestinal motor activity. In: Walker W A, Durie P R, Hamilton J R et al (eds) Pediatric gastrointestinal disease. Mosby, St Louis: 31–43.

Miller-Loncar C, Bigsby R, High P et al 2004 Infant colic and feeding difficulties. Arch Dis Child 89: 908–912.

Mittal R K, McCallum R W 1988 Characteristics and frequency of transient relaxations of the lower esophageal sphincter in patients with reflux esophagitis. Gastroenterology 95(3): 593–599.

Mittal R K, Chiareli C, Liu J et al 1996 Characteristics of lower esophageal sphincter relaxation induced by pharyngeal stimulation with minute amounts of water. Gastroenterology 111(2): 378–384.

Murphy M S, Clayden G 1996 Constipation. In: Walker W A, Durie P R, Hamilton J R et al (eds) Pediatric gastrointestinal disease. Mosby, St Louis: 293–323.

Ogorek C P 1995 Gastroesophageal reflux disease. In: Haubrich W, Schaffner F, Berk J (eds) Bockus gastroenterology. W B Saunders, Philadelphia: 445–468.

Orenstein S R, Whitington P F 1983 Positioning for prevention of infant gastroesophageal reflux. J Pediatr 103: 534–537.

Orenstein S R, Magill L H, Brooks P 1987 Thickening of infant feedings as therapy of gastroesophageal reflux. J Pediatr 110: 181–186.

Orenstein S R, Shalaby T M, Putnam P E 1992 Thickened feedings as a cause of increased coughing when used as therapy for gastroesophageal reflux in infants. J Pediatr 121: 913–915.

Osborn L M, Reiff M I, Bolus R 1984 Jaundice in the full-term neonate. Pediatrics 73(4): 520–525.

Paterson W G, Rattan S, Goyal R K 1986 Experimental induction of isolated lower oesophageal sphincter relaxation in anesthetized opossums. J Clin Invest 77(4): 1187–1193.

Pelot D 1995 Anatomy, anomalies and physiology of the esophagus. In: Haubrich W, Schaffner F, Berk J (eds) Bockus gastroenterology. W B Saunders, Philadelphia: 397–411.

Reisner S H, Sivan Y, Nitzan M et al 1984 Determination of anterior displacement of the anus in newborn infants and children. Pediatrics 73(2): 216–217.

Reynolds J C 1995 Anatomy, anomalies and physiology of the esophagus. In: Haubrich W, Schaffner F, Berk J (eds) Bockus gastroenterology. W B Saunders, Philadelphia: 411–418.

Rosenthal P 1992 Bilirubin metabolism in the fetus and neonate. In: Polin R A, Fox W (eds) Fetal and neonatal physiology. W B Saunders, Philadelphia: 1154–1160.

Schneider A P 1986 Breast milk jaundice in the newborn. A real entity. JAMA 255(23): 3270–3274.

Sifter C A, Braungart J 1992 Infant colic: a transient condition with no apparent effects. J Appl Dev Psychol 13: 447–462.

Standring S (ed.) 2004 Gray's anatomy, 39th edn. Churchill Livingstone, New York.

Stevenson R D, Allaire J H 1991 The development of normal feeding and swallowing. Pediatr Clin North Am 38(6): 1438–1453.

Taitz L S, Wales J K, Urwin O M et al 1986 Factors associated with outcome in management of defecation disorders. Arch Dis Child 61(5): 472–477.

Titchen D A 1979 Diaphragmatic and oesophageal activity in regurgitation in sheep: an electromyographic study. J Physiol 292: 381–390.

Walker A R, Walker B F 1985 Bowel behaviour in young black and white children. Arch Dis Child 60(10): 967–970.

Weaver L T, Stevens H 1988 The bowel habit of young children. Arch Dis Child 59: 649–652.

Welch R W, Gray J E 1982 Influence of respiration on recordings of lower esophageal sphincter pressure in humans. Gastroenterology 83(3): 590–594.

Wessel M A, Cobb J C, Jackson E B et al 1954 Paroxysmal fussing in infancy, sometimes called 'colic'. Pediatrics 14: 421–434.

Williams T A 1989 Mechanisms of gastroesophageal reflux in recumbent neurologically impaired children. Gastroenterology 96: 547a.

Woodward D R, Rees B, Boon J A 1989 Human milk fat content: within-feed variation. Early Hum Dev 19(1): 39–46.

Further reading

Barr R G 1998 Reflections on measuring pain in infants: dissociation in responsive systems and 'honest signalling'. Arch Dis Child Fetal Neonatal Ed 79(2): F152–F156.

Barr R G 1998 Colic and crying syndromes in infants. Pediatrics 102(5 Suppl): E1282–E1286.

Barr R G, Chen S, Hopkins B et al 1996 Crying patterns in preterm infants. Dev Med Child Neurol 38(4): 345–355.

Field S K, Underwood M, Brant R et al 1996 Prevalence of gastroesophageal reflux symptoms in asthma. Chest 109(2): 316–322.

Field S K, Evans J A, Price L M 1998 The effects of acid perfusion of the esophagus on ventilation and respiratory sensation. Am J Respir Crit Care Med 57: 1058–1062.

Harding S M, Richter J E, Guzzo M R et al 1996 Asthma and gastroesophageal reflux: acid suppressive therapy improves asthma outcome. Am J Med 100(4): 395–405.

James-Roberts I, Hurry J, Bowyer J 1993 Objective confirmation of crying durations in infants referred for excessive crying. Arch Dis Child 68(1): 82–84.

Lúdvíksdóttir D, Björnsson E, Janson C et al 1996 Habitual coughing and its associations with asthma, anxiety, and gastroesophageal reflux. Chest 109(5): 1262–1268.

Mittal R K 1990 Current concepts of the antireflux barrier. Gastroenterol Clin North Am 19(3): 501–516.

Mittal R K 1993 The crural diaphragm, an external lower esophageal sphincter: a definitive study. Gastroenterology 105(5): 1565–1567.

Mittal R K 1993 The sphincter mechanism at the lower end of the esophagus: an overview. Dysphagia 8(4): 347–350.

Mittal R K, Balaban D H 1997 The esophagogastric junction. N Engl J Med 336(13): 924–932.

Mittal R K, Fisher M J 1990 Electrical and mechanical inhibition of the crural diaphragm during transient relaxation of the lower esophageal sphincter. Gastroenterology 99(5): 1265–1268.

Mittal R K, Fisher M, McCallum R W et al 1990 Human lower esophageal sphincter pressure response to increased intra-abdominal pressure. Am J Physiol 258(4 Pt 1): G624–630.

Mittal R K, Holloway R H, Penagini R et al 1995 Transient lower esophageal sphincter relaxation. Gastroenterology 109(2): 601–610.

Mittal R K, Shaffer H A, Parollisi S et al 1995 Influence of breathing pattern on the esophagogastric junction pressure and esophageal transit. Am J Physiol 269(4 Pt 1): G577–583.

Shaw A D, Davies G J 1999 Lactose intolerance: problems in diagnosis and treatment. J Clin Gastroenterol 28(3): 208–216.

Shimizu T, Mochizuki H, Tokuyama K et al 1996 Relationship between the acid-induced cough response and airway responsiveness and obstruction in children with asthma. Thorax 51(3): 284–287.

Standring S (ed.) 2004 Gray's anatomy, 39th edn. Churchill Livingstone, New York.

Weaver L T, Lucas A 1993 Development of bowel habit in preterm infants. Arch Dis Child 68(3 Spec No): 317–320.

Weaver L T, Steiner H 1984 The bowel habit of young children. Arch Dis Child 59(7): 649–652.

Chapter Fifteen

15

Orthopedics

CHAPTER CONTENTS

COMMON PROBLEMS IN THE HEAD AND NECK

Plagiocephaly/craniosynostosis

By definition, plagiocephaly is an abnormal shape or deformity of the skull. Craniosynostosis affects 3–5 infants per 10,000 (Kimonis et al 2007). Craniosynostosis may be syndromic or nonsyndromic. Syndromic craniosynostosis is a genetically linked defect associated with one of the more than 180 congenital syndromes (Kimonis et al 2007, Passos-Bueno et al 2008). Specific genes encoding the fibroblastic growth factor receptor (FGFR) have been identified as playing a role in some cases of syndromic craniosynostosis, while mutations in the Twist and muscle segment homeobox genes are associated with others (Bonaventure & El 2003). The mechanisms by which premature fusion occurs and the presentation vary with the genes involved. By contrast, nonsyndromic craniosynostosis appears to occur in response to mechanical forces (Hunenko et al 2001, Kirschner et al 2002, Smartt et al 2005). Osteopaths have long noted a relationship between cranial dysmorphology, including craniosynostosis, and abnormal patterns in the cranial base patterns, but other researchers have noticed this relationship as well. Hoyte (1991) contends that the cranial base morphology is most affected by the coronal suture ring, with the spheno-occipital synchondrosis being the next most influential area. Nonsyndromic craniosynostosis typically affects a single suture and may be associated with strabismus, astigmatism, speech–language and psychological dysfunction (Magge et al 2002, Becker et al 2005, Lehman 2006, Kapp-Simon et al 2007, Baranello et al 2007) but not mental retardation (Kapp-Simon et al 1993, 2007.)

Very often, clinicians view the problem as one of abnormal compressive forces across the suture area. Many osteopaths approach the problem as such, with the intention to resolve the compression in the sutural tissue. However, if we review the physiology of cranial development, we see that there is another possibility. Under normal conditions, the cranial vault begins to ossify in response to forces of stretch, not compression. Consequently, when evaluating children with craniosynostosis or plagiocephaly, we must recognize the potential for abnormal stretch forces across the sutures to stimulate premature ossification. Compressive forces in the cranial base will create abnormal stretch on the dural tissues in the vault.

Severe cases of craniosynostosis are evident at birth and characterized by significant skull deformity. Usually, a prominent bony ridge in the area of the suture can be palpated. This is different from the ridge produced by suture overlap, as may occur with some deliveries. Plain X-rays may show that the suture is fused. Surgery is the definitive treatment. Postsurgical osteopathic evaluation is helpful to resolve any concomitant strains. However, it is best to leave osteopathic evaluation and treatment until at least 8–12 weeks after surgery, unless the practitioner is well skilled in treating post-craniotomy heads. It takes many weeks for the osseous, membranous and fluid mechanisms of the post-craniotomy head to re-establish a functional relationship, and the findings can be very misleading. It may be useful for the practitioner to observe the process of resolution which the patient's mechanism chooses to take, but I would warn against interfering or assisting in any way. This may be an important opportunity for the perceptive osteopath to learn from nature.

Many cases of craniosynostosis do not present at birth. It develops later, and although associated with unresolved plagiocephaly, there may or may not be a causal relationship.

From a clinical standpoint plagiocephaly can be thought of in terms of primary or secondary strains. Primary strains may occur intrauterine, as the result of an abnormal lie, or during labor and delivery. In either case, the problem originates in the head. Left untreated, the child with primary plagiocephaly can develop torticollis and/or scoliosis. Primary plagiocephaly is usually noticed soon after birth. Secondary plagiocephaly develops in response to a strain somewhere else in the body and is often not noticed until the child is a few months old.

Primary plagiocephaly

Congenital or primary plagiocephaly develops as a result of uterine lie, or through the forces of labor and birth. It has a strong developmental component. Risk factors include primiparity, assisted delivery, long labor, cephalohematoma, twin gestation and intrauterine constraint (Dias & Klein 1996, Littlefield et al 1999, Peitsch et al 2002). Depending on the length of time it has been present, the child's body will adapt to the strain pattern. During times of growth, the distorted pattern can be exacerbated. For example, torticollis associated with plagiocephaly appears to develop subsequent to the head deformity (Peitsch et al 2002).

Plagiocephaly can be categorized by the shape of the infant's head. True plagiocephaly is a parallelogram-shaped head (Fig. 15.1) with prominence of one posterior quarter and the contralateral anterior quarter of the skull. The ears are not level and there is usually some facial asymmetry. The parallelogram head can develop secondary to torticollis but in most cases there is a lateral strain at the cranial base. The asymmetry is typically more pronounced in one quarter depending on the direction of rotation and whether the primary strain is in the sphenoid or the occiput. There is typically more facial asymmetry with primary sphenoid involvement. When the strain is primarily in the occiput there is more posterior deformation and adaptations at the craniocervical junction producing a torticollis appearance. The malpositioning of the head

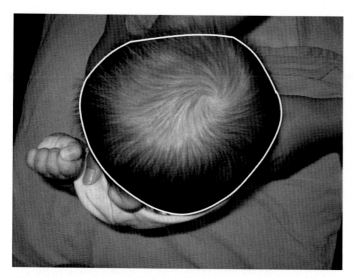

Fig. 15.1 • This 8-week-old infant has a parallelogram head, with prominence of the left frontal quarter and facial asymmetry. He had a lateral strain basisphenoid to the left, basiocciput to the right. *Used with permission of the Willard & Carreiro Collection.*

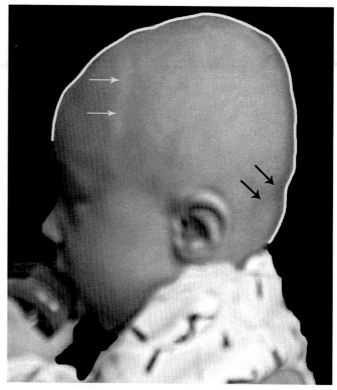

Fig. 15.2 • This 10-week-old boy has a brachycephalic head. There is no facial asymmetry. There is prominence of the junction between the supraocciput and intraparietal occiput (black arrows) and the sagittal suture has overlap of the frontal on the parietal (white arrows). This little boy had a vertical strain: basiocciput inferior, basisphenoid superior. *Used with permission of the Willard & Carreiro Collection.*

and neck may contribute to postural imbalances and delays in early milestones. Infants and toddlers with spastic torticollis or paroxysmal vertigo should be evaluated for lateral strain. Parallelogram deformity is rarely limited to the vault without cranial base involvement. The brachycephalic head is typically broader across the coronal and vertical planes and narrow at the anterior–posterior (AP) axis (Fig. 15.2). It may develop from lying supine or it may represent cranial base strain. A flexed cranial base pattern can produce a head that looks brachiocephalic; however, the posterior aspect is round and not flat. When the posterior skull is flat and the face symmetrical, one must consider vertical strain with basisphenoid superior. When the face is broad and flattened and the occiput round, the vertical strain may be basisphenoid inferior. The scaphocephalic head is narrow on the coronal plane and long on the AP axis. This appearance is most often associated with prematurity and extension patterns of the cranial base.

Timing of osteopathic treatments in these children is important. Resolving any membranous and fluid strains just prior to the growth spurt seems to allow the body to re-establish tissue balance in the distorted area. Therapeutic intervention should occur as early as possible to prevent adaptations in other areas of the body and worsening of the distortion. It becomes much more difficult for these strains to resolve once the osseous, membranous and fluid mechanics have established a more mature relationship. This seems to begin to happen towards the end of the first year. Although the plagiocephaly is a mechanical strain, it is still very different from what one would observe in an older child or adult. The components of the head are cartilaginous and the sutures are not developed in infants. As a result the tissue strain has both a membranous and osseous quality, and the fluid assumes the 'shape of the container', but there is

not a strain in the fluid per se. If the initial strain occurred in the cranial base, then the vault deformity is secondary and will only resolve with normalization of base mechanics. The only truly functional joint in the neonatal head is the occipital atlantal joint. Consequently, the condylar area is commonly involved in plagiocephaly that originates in the cranial base. Although true condylar compression may not be present more often than not, there will be some strain between the occiput and the atlas, which may or may not involve C2 and C3. Mechanically, C3 is a junctional area of the cervical spine, resolving the forces occurring in the upper complex – cranium, atlas, axis – with those of the lower. The other area not to be forgotten is the cerebellar falx extending inferiorly from the tentorium along the midline of the inner table of the supraocciput to anchor into the periosteum of the neural arch of C1 through C3. This area is often of concern in plagiocephaly originating in the base. If not addressed, there will be additional strain created through the tissues of the neck which may have two effects: first, the secondary strain in the cervical area will maintain the base pattern; and second, it may be sufficient to produce a torticollis in the neck. Primary plagiocephaly originating in the neonatal vault will be much more responsive to treatment in the first week or so. Unfortunately, these children are often not brought to the office until later, when the pattern has become exacerbated by the sleep habitus of the infant. Consequently, some behavioral modification has to occur to discourage the infant from 'lying on the flat spot' (see below).

Deformational plagiocephaly

Deformational plagiocephaly is thought to develop from a combination of abnormal tissue forces from a subtle cranial asymmetry and the supine sleeping position (Argenta et al 1996, Mulliken et al 1999, Peitsch et al 2002). Unless severe, the abnormal position is taken to be a position of comfort assumed by the neonate and ignored by the parents. Ironically, this is the case. Cranial flattening is slightly more common on the right than left (Turk et al 1996, Mulliken et al 1999, Peitsch et al 2002) and in males than females. Tissue strains in the neck and back may be transmitted through the cranial base and vault. This is most often the case in torticollis and scoliosis. However, sometimes the torticollis does not directly distort the cranium through mechanical influences. Instead, the torticollis creates an abnormal position of the head and neck which causes the infant to lie in an awkward position. The awkward lie can distort the cranial vault without creating a significant strain in the base. As previously mentioned, this type of plagiocephaly can be difficult to treat in the older infant. In addition to addressing the dysfunction contributing to vault distortion, the child needs to be encouraged to lie in a different position to prevent exacerbation of the deformity. This requires parental assistance. While awake or supervised, young infants should be placed on their stomach, a position these children often resist. They should be placed in the crib so that they will turn their head and not lie on the 'flat spot'. This can be accomplished by positioning babies to look towards the door and away from the affected side, and by placing toys and mobiles so they turn away from the affected side. Helmets or dynamic cranial orthotic devices can be appropriately integrated into the treatment plan so that they support the changes made with osteopathic manipulation. This requires clear communication and understanding between the osteopath and the orthotist, or preferably that the osteopath is trained to do the orthotic fittings. Cranial orthotic devices may prevent a child from exacerbating the deformity by stopping him from lying on a flattened aspect. Discussion with various colleagues suggests that when used correctly they do not create any new strain patterns or exacerbate the existing ones.

Differential diagnosis of plagiocephaly

Craniosynostosis must be considered and ruled out in every case of plagiocephaly. There are a few clinical clues that can help to determine if a child with plagiocephaly is developing craniosynostosis. Slowed or arrested growth of head circumference, worsening of the plagiocephaly, developmental delay, palpable bony prominence and abnormal pattern of hair growth are all associated with craniosynostosis. X-ray evaluation is valuable in spite of the cartilaginous nature of the infant skull. Head computed tomography (CT) scan or plain X-ray can be used to evaluate suture characteristics and the presence or absence of ossification. In cases of severe plagiocephaly, the child is at risk for development of craniosynostosis, and appropriate and timely evaluation must occur. Surgical correction is necessary to avoid restriction of vault growth and impediment of brain development.

Treatment of uncomplicated plagiocephaly

Treatment of plagiocephaly, especially secondary plagiocephaly, requires two things: resolution of any mechanical strains or abnormal tensions which are contributing to maintaining the distortion of the cranial bones, and, very importantly, somehow getting the child to stop lying on the flat spot. Plagiocephaly resulting from or concurrent with torticollis will not improve until the mechanical strains in the neck, craniocervical junction and cranial base are resolved. This is especially true in very young infants. At the same time, interventions must be taken to encourage the child to use the cervical muscles in a more balanced way and to alternate the sleeping position. Unfortunately, nagging, explaining and cajoling do not seem to work with 4-month-olds; the parents must be engaged in the process. Placing infants in the prone position when their caregiver is nearby and watchful will encourage them to try to lift their head, thus engaging the cervical extensors. If the parents are certain that they can be observant, a child may be allowed to nap in this position, although bedtime sleeping posture should not be prone. Having the child lie on the unaffected side can alter night-time sleeping position. This can be done by rolling a small towel or nappy into an infant-size pillowcase and placing the infant on her side with her back propped against it. The towel should be thin enough that the infant is almost supine but her head and body are slightly turned. The crib and the baby should be placed so that the doorway or direction from which family members approach the crib is on the unaffected side. The baby will have a tendency to look towards the direction from which her visitors arrive. If the child sleeps in the parental bed, the mother should lie next to the baby on the unaffected side. For example, if the right parietal-occipital area is affected, the mother should lie on the infant's left side. The baby will tend to turn towards the mother (and dinner). During feeding, infants can be held so that they need to turn their head away from the affected muscles, thereby lengthening them. This requires a little more creativity in the breastfed infant. For example, if we need to encourage the child to turn her head to the right, the muscles on the left are shortened. Feeding from the left breast is no problem; however, feeding from the right is a little trickier. Hold the child in the same position as was used on the left breast, the infant's right arm in against the mother. Maintaining that position, move the baby to the right breast. Prop the baby and mother's arms onto some pillows. Finally, mobiles, toys, pets and any other thing of interest should also be placed on the unaffected side.

Torticollis

Torticollis is a malposition of the neck whereby the head is side-bent in one direction and the chin is pointed towards the other. The most common cause is muscular. Rarely, torticollis may occur as a result of spinal cord and brain abnormalities. It may arise as a functional compensation for strabismus. Torticollis may be secondary to plagiocephaly or primary to its development (Clarren 1981, Peitsch et al 2002). Infantile torticollis has also been associated with thoracic scoliosis (Cheng & Au 1994). Magoun describes congenital torticollis as a sign of accessory nerve irritation secondary to strains of the cranial base (Magoun 1973). The most common cause of torticollis in older children is muscular strain, although it can develop with respiratory infections. Classically, torticollis is thought to be due to injury or spasm of the sternocleidomastoid muscle. However, in congenital torticollis the scalene muscles are often involved. The strain may occur during delivery or as a result of uterine lie. Often it is not diagnosed until the child is 4–6 weeks old, at which time the parent or physician notices an awkward positioning of the head or the early development of a flat spot due to the persistent position of the head. When the torticollis is due to scalene muscle spasm, there will be associated dysfunction of rib mechanics and palpable hypertonicity in the muscle. Palpation of the scalene muscles often makes the child irritable, while palpation of the sternocleidomastoid is well tolerated. There are associated strains in the cranial base and craniocervical junction that may be primary or secondary to the torticollis. Often, the cranial findings will not respond to treatment until the scalene dysfunction is resolved, which suggests that they may occur secondary to the torticollis. Conversely, the cranial findings can be primary and must be addressed prior to any improvement in the neck. It is sometimes difficult to determine which problem is primary; however, there are certain clues one can look for. When the primary problem is the cranial base the most significant findings of the cranial base pattern will be in the occiput and the condyles, although compensation at the sphenoid has occurred. There will be very little facial asymmetry present and the child is more likely to have asymmetry in the posterior aspect of the skull at birth or soon after. The mastoid portions are often not level and lie on different AP planes. The area of greatest restriction to motion testing is the cranial–cervical junction. The infant may have a more difficult time stabilizing his or her posture with head support because the occipitoatlantal muscles are under greater strain and the oculocephalic reflex may be disturbed. When the torticollis is cervical there is often palpable, frank, spasm in the sternocleidomastoid or scalene muscles. The upper ribs on the involved side are elevated and markedly restricted. The child is more likely to be able to engage postural reflexes when visual stimulation is provided as the head is supported. Asymmetry in the posterior skull usually develops later; most parents do not notice it until the eighth or ninth week of life.

Torticollis involving the sternocleidomastoid muscle may result from bleeding within the belly of the muscle secondary to trauma. When this is the case, a palpable swelling in the muscle and bruising may be visualized. Complications include fibrosis and shortening of the muscle. The mechanism of injury is related to labor and delivery. Large babies with long or difficult deliveries or shoulder dystocia are at risk. If suspected, a stretching program should be implemented to avoid contracture of the muscle. Surgical release is occasionally necessary in severely affected children.

Torticollis may be picked up early in infants through physical exam. Active rotation will be restricted and side-bending and rotation may be uncoupled. Passive head rotation away into the restrictive barrier will engage the shoulder (Fig. 15.3). The baby's response to infantile reflexes may also be affected. During the Moro reflex, the

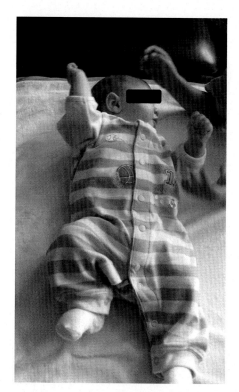

Fig. 15.3 • An 8-week-old boy with right-sided torticollis. With left head rotation there is early engagement of the right shoulder (it lifts from the table). The tonic neck reflex is impaired. This child has infantile postural asymmetry. *Used with permission of the Willard & Carreiro Collection.*

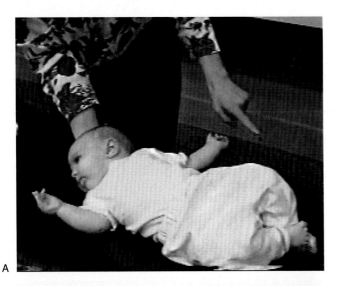

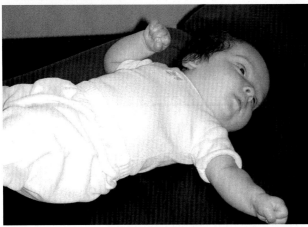

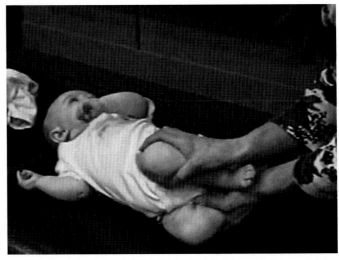

Fig. 15.5 • Demonstration of the rolling maneuver. The child's gaze is forward-fixed on a toy or the examiner as the hips are slowly rolled. The upper thorax, head and neck will log roll as a unit when the restrictive barrier is engaged. Likewise, the shoulder will usually rise as the neck and head rotate. *Used with permission of the Willard & Carreiro Collection.*

Fig. 15.4 • (A, B) The asymmetric tonic neck reflex demonstrated in two 12-week-old girls. As the head and neck are rotated, the ipsilateral arm and knee flex, while the contralateral limbs extend. In the presence of torticollis, the reflex will engage sooner as the head is rotated towards the restrictive barrier. Failure of the child to exhibit the correct posture suggests infantile postural asymmetry. *Used with permission of the Willard & Carreiro Collection.*

arm on the affected side will often remain more flexed than the contralateral arm. During the asymmetric tonic neck reflex, the child may not exhibit the appropriate postural response when turning into the restrictive barrier (Fig. 15.4). Head on body rotation may also be affected. This can be assessed by first attracting a child's attention so that her gaze is directed forwards. Then the physician slowly rotates the infant's hips. The rotation should proceed smoothly and symmetrically through the spine to the neck and head. Symmetry of head and neck movement in relation to the torso is assessed (Fig. 15.5). Restricted active cervical rotation in the supine position suggests dysfunction in the sternocleidomastoid or trapezius muscles, the upper cervical complex (C1–C2), or atlantal–axial junction, whereas restricted active rotation in the prone position indicates dysfunction of the lower cervical complex (C3–C7) (Pang & Veetai 2004, Philippi et al 2006a, b).

Treatment of the torticollis should focus on the primary strain within the complex. Various manual modalities are thought to be effective and are often used in combination. Balanced ligamentous techniques can be used to address the articular dysfunction of the cervical area. Myofascial or facilitated positional release can be helpful in treating the myofascial components. The occipital–atlas strain and cranial base strain may respond to balanced membranous techniques. Atlas impulse technique can be useful to address postural patterning that is being maintained at the cranial–cervical junction via the cervicospinal, cervicocollic and other reflexes.

Klippel–Feil syndrome

Klippel–Feil syndrome is a congenital malformation of the cervical spine in which two or more vertebrae are fused. It is most likely due to an abnormality in somatic segmentation. The term Klippel–Feil syndrome was originally used to describe the clinical triad of fused cervical vertebra, short neck and low posterior hairline; however, now the term is used more broadly for cervical fusion. Klippel–Feil syndrome can be classified into three types. Type 1 is an extensive fusion, involving many vertebrae and sometimes extending into the thoracic spine. Type 2 describes two fused vertebrae. Type 3 is either of the other types associated with anomalies in the thoracic or lumbar spine. The incidence of the condition is unclear. Clinical presentation and age depend on the extent and level of the fusion. In general, fusions involving

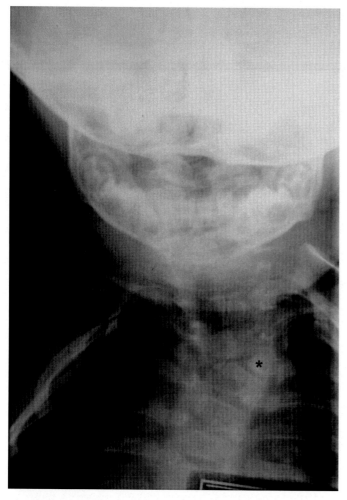

Fig. 15.6 • Plain X-ray of a 10-month-old infant with hemivertebrae at T4 (*) and partial formation of T5. *Used with permission of the Willard & Carreiro Collection.*

the cranial–cervical junction or extensive fusions present earlier due to cosmetic deformity, pain and delay in development milestones. Lower cervical fusion often does not present until later in life. Type 2 patterns may be asymptomatic and reported as incidental findings on X-ray examination. Klippel–Feil syndrome can be associated with fetal alcohol syndrome, congenital malformations in the urogenital system, hearing loss, webbed neck, abducens nerve palsy, cervical ribs and ventricular septal defect.

COMMON PROBLEMS OF THE SPINE AND PELVIS

Congenital scoliosis

In children scoliosis is usually congenital or idiopathic. There are cases of trauma-induced and iatrogenic scoliosis, but they usually occur in adults. Congenital scoliosis may be

due to hemivertebrae, failure of segmentation, or a combination of the two (Fig. 15.6). Unilateral unsegmented bars have the worst progression. Hemivertebrae may or may not cause significant deformity, but 75% will demonstrate curve progression. The spinal curves in congenital scoliosis are rigid, so orthotic treatment is of limited value. Combined anterior and posterior spinal fusion at the level of deformity is sometimes necessary, but quite often conservative management is all that is needed. Congenital scoliosis is associated with genitourinary and cardiac abnormalities, as well as other skeletal abnormalities, such as spina bifida occulta, spinal cord tethers and Klippel–Feil syndrome (described above). Congenital scoliosis may not be diagnosed until the child begins standing or walking. Depending on the level of the deformity, the number of segments affected, and the neurological involvement, congenital scoliosis can either be benign and asymptomatic or be of significant clinical import. Vertebral deformities associated with tethering of the spinal cord can be associated with neurological sequelae. In mild cases the child may have pain and or paresthesias; in more severe cases involvement may be associated with weakness, paralysis and organ dysfunction. Uncomplicated deformities in the upper thoracic and cervical areas may interfere with the attainment of early motor milestones. The child may present with a torticollis unresponsive to appropriate treatment. Hemivertebrae and fusions in the lower thoracic and lumbar area may present as an incidental finding on radiography or as pain exacerbated with activity. Deformities in the very distal lumbar spine may only become symptomatic when the child becomes involved in more demanding activities such as organized sports (Fig. 15.7).

Idiopathic scoliosis

Scoliosis is a lateral curvature of the spine. Scoliosis represents a rotational malalignment of one vertebra on another. Rotation and side-bending occur to opposite sides. Ribs are rotated posteriorly and are prominent on the convex side of the curve. The positional strain is exacerbated in forward flexion, producing a rib hump. Diagnosis is made by physical examination. Most clinicians can visually diagnose a curve of 10°. X-ray evaluation is used to establish a precise measurement of the angle.

Idiopathic scoliosis affects 17 in 1000 children in Western countries. It may develop in young children, preadolescents or adolescents. Adolescent idiopathic scoliosis is the most common form of idiopathic scoliosis. It occurs near or at puberty. There is a structural lateral curvature of the spine of at least 10° for which no cause can be established (Fig. 15.8). Children between 10 and 16 years are at greatest risk of development and progression of a curve. Girls are almost four times as likely to be affected than boys for mild curves. There are many and various hypotheses as to the etiology of the condition, ranging from vestibular dysfunction to cortical asymmetries to uneven

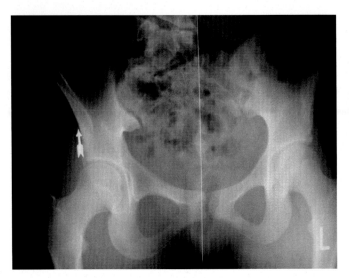

Fig. 15.7 • Standing AP X-ray (postural study) of a 14-year-old girl who complained of persistent low back pain after soccer practice. There is an incomplete hemivertebra at L4 and only a remnant of L5. The girl had no scoliosis on visual examination, but there was pelvic unleveling and leg length difference. Her symptoms resolved with a 10 mm lift in her right shoe. Neurosurgical and orthopedic consults were obtained to confirm appropriateness of using a lift. The patient has been followed for 4 years without recurrence of the complaint. *Used with permission of the Willard & Carreiro Collection.*

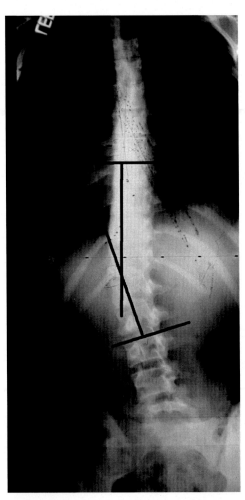

Fig. 15.8 • Plain X-ray of a 13-year-old girl with idiopathic scoliosis. This is a mild curve. *Used with permission of the Willard & Carreiro Collection.*

leg lengths. There is no definitive proof that idiopathic scoliosis is genetically linked; however, if it is hereditary, there appears to be a decreasing frequency from first-degree to third-degree relations. Significantly decreased levels of melatonin have been found in adolescents with progressive curves, whereas those with stable curves have normal levels (Machida et al 1996). However, age-matched comparison with normal children has not been done. Interestingly, the level of platelet calmodulin in skeletally immature patients with progressive curves is significantly higher than in those with stable curves (Kindsfater et al 1994). Patients with idiopathic scoliosis have a higher incidence of abnormal postural reflexes. These involve the righting reflex, drift reaction, optokinetic nystagmus, ocular reflex system, proprioceptive reactions and vestibular dysfunction. While the nature of the relationship is unclear, the degree of spinal curvature appears to correlate with the amount of equilibrium disturbance (Machida 1999). Furthermore, although these various factors may be present in children with idiopathic scoliosis, there is no evidence of a causal relationship. Consequently, we may need to view scoliosis as a symptom common to several pathologies.

Scoliosis can be induced experimentally in animals by damaging the posterior horn. The convexity of the scoliosis will develop ipsilateral to the damaged side of the spinal cord (Pincott & Taffs 1982). Resection of the dorsal spinal nerves in primates can create scoliosis with the convexity to the side of the resection (Pincott et al 1984). Yamada et al (1984) showed that virtually any disruption in the postural reflex system can result in scoliosis.

Within any scoliotic curve there is a structural component and a functional component. The structural component results from changes in the architecture of the vertebrae that distorts the normal articular relationships. This is true for congenital and developmental scoliosis. For example, the presence of a hemivertebra will result in side-bending of the vertebra above and below the affected side. A compression fracture may also produce side-bending of the adjacent vertebrae. In both cases the side-bending adaptation is a structural change in the curve. It will not alter with positional changes in the spine. In contrast, a functional curve is caused by mechanical and postural forces and will decrease or resolve in certain positions. Functional curves are mechanical adaptations. The curve will adapt to changes in position of the spine. Passively moving the involved vertebrae in a different plane reduces the curvature.

During the scoliosis screening examination, the child is asked to bend forward and the back is examined for any evidence of spinal malalignment or rib hump. This is called Adam's forward bending tests. The area involved is then motion tested by applying a side-bending force and observing the response of the curve. A functional curve will decrease or resolve. Virtually every child with idiopathic scoliosis has some functional component to the curve. This is extremely important, because if left untreated, functional curves will ultimately develop into a structural deformity as the spine grows.

Diagnosis

The most common screening examination is Adam's forward bending test (Fig. 15.9). It is used to detect asymmetry of the back or the presence of a rib hump. The amount of rib rotation does not always correlate with the scoliosis. It is important to note that trunk asymmetry in small children is common and not necessarily related to or predictive of scoliosis. The sensitivity and specificity of Adam's forward bending test is greater than 70% for curves less than 10°, and greater than 90% for curves greater than 20°. A scoliometer or inclinometer can be used to determine the angle of trunk

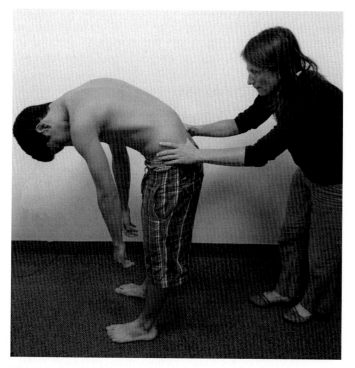

Fig. 15.9 • Adam's forward bending test. The child stands with feet hip width apart. He is asked to slowly bend forward, allowing the hands to dangle in front of his body. The physician observes the quality of motion of the spine during flexion for symmetry. If there is rotation of the spine or asymmetry in the appearance of the ribs the child is instructed to halt his flexion. The physician then introduces side-bending into the curve through the shoulders to test the flexibility of the asymmetry and determine the functional component of the curve. The curve is named for the side of the convexity, the side contralateral to the rib prominence or rib hump. *Used with permission of the Willard & Carreiro Collection.*

rotation. Radiographs are usually definitive, although even they show some variation in results. Two views, posterior–anterior (PA) and lateral, are obtained for measurement. The degree of curvature is measured from the two end vertebrae. The angle at the line of intersection is Cobb's angle. Curves measuring less than 25° are considered mild. Those measuring between 25° and 40° are considered moderate. Curves are named for the side of the convexity. Descriptions are based on the position of the apical vertebrae.

Idiopathic scoliosis is not uncommon; consequently, it is easy to assume the diagnosis without extensive work-up. Knowing the most common presentations of idiopathic scoliosis can help the physician to recognize an adolescent scoliosis that may be due to a more serious pathology. Left-sided thoracic curves and right-sided lumbar curves deserve further investigation, as do thoracic curves that extend into the cervical spine. Scoliosis with pain or significant stiffness is also unusual and may signify something more ominous. Tingling in the extremities or neurological symptoms may represent spinal cord involvement. Scoliosis in the thoracic area is over 90% convexity to the right with an average of six vertebrae involved. When the upper thorax is concerned, the apex is at T8 or T9. For lower thoracic scoliosis, the apex will be at T11 or T12. Seventy percent of scoliosis in the lumbar spine is convexity to the left. Five vertebrae are generally involved with the apex at L1 or L2. The upper end of the curve is usually T11 or T12, and the lower L3 or L4. Thoracolumbar curves average six to eight vertebrae and are usually convex to the right. The apex is at T11 or T12. Double major curves involve oppositional curves in the thoracic and lumbar areas. Ninety percent of the thoracic curves are convex to the right, with left convexity in the lumbar area. Generally, double major curves involve five thoracic and five lumbar vertebrae with the respective apices at T7 and L2.

Natural course of idiopathic scoliosis

The progression of scoliosis is primarily due to altered biomechanical forces, which, in turn, create structural changes (Wolff's law). The structural changes, in turn, alter the biomechanics. It is a vicious cycle. Regardless of the etiology, idiopathic scoliosis will eventually cause vertebral asymmetry in the child. The epiphyseal plates on the concave side of the curve will have decreased growth due to the chronic increased pressure, while on the convex side there is decreased pressure and accelerated growth. This results in a structural deformity of the vertebral body. Furthermore, most children compensate for the curve by exaggerating the lumbar lordosis. This creates increased pressure on the posterior aspect of the vertebral body and decreased pressure anteriorly, resulting in a growth differential. These structural and biomechanical forces cause wedging of the intervertebral disk as well as the vertebral body. Researchers have found decreased glycosaminoglycan and increased collagen in the disks of patients with scoliosis. This is probably due to the abnormal stress placed upon the disk (Zaleske et al 1980). Although the biomechanical changes associated with idiopathic scoliosis influence the progression of the curve, they are probably not causal.

Progression of the curve is influenced by the child's age and the severity of the curve. Young children with severe curvature have a greater chance for progression. Progression is usually most rapid during large growth spurts. Premenarchal girls with curves over 20° are at the greatest risk for progression. Almost 70% of these children will have worsening of their curves. Double curves appear to progress faster than single curves. The likelihood of progression increases with decreasing age of onset, presumably because the curve has to weather more growth spurts. Curves over 20° may be treated conservatively with observation and yearly X-ray or photography. Depending on the child's age, curves over 40° require bracing and follow-up X-rays every 6–12 months. Once the child completes puberty, progression of the curve slows significantly, although curves frequently progress throughout life as a result of the aforementioned biomechanical factors.

Bone age is an important factor in the assessment and management of idiopathic scoliosis. The earlier the curve presents, the greater the opportunity for deformation with subsequent growth. Bone age can be measured on X-ray. A common tool is the Riser scale. A PA view of the pelvis is taken. The iliac crest is then divided into four segments.

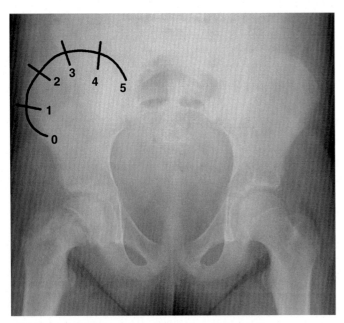

Fig. 15.10 • An AP X-ray of female pelvis with Riser scale superimposed in black. Each number equates with a grade. Grade 0 = no ossification; grade 1 = 25% ossification; grade 2 = 26–50% ossification; grade 3 = 51–75% ossification; grade 4 = 76–100% ossification; grade 5 = fusion of the apophysis. *Used with permission of the Willard & Carreiro Collection.*

Ossification of the iliac crest progresses from the anterior iliac spine towards the sacrum. The degree of ossification of the crest is measured against the four segments. No ossification is a '0' and complete fusion of the apophysis is a '5'. This tool allows the radiologist to estimate how much growth is left (Fig. 15.10).

Treatment

Conventional and osteopathic treatment of scoliosis should be initially focused on addressing any postural decompensation which has occurred, because of the potential for cardiopulmonary complications. If the curve is greater than 30°, orthotic bracing should be considered, and at 40°, bracing is highly recommended. Bracing will not correct the curve, but is meant to prevent further progression. Surgery needs to be considered when the curve passes 45°. The procedure consists of internal fixation of the involved vertebrae to prevent further progression of the curve. Segmental fixation has been shown to have similar efficacy to regional fixation in many patients. Fusion does not appear to increase the rate of success. Long-term complications of surgery appear to be few and far between. Untreated idiopathic scoliosis increases an individual's mortality by 10%. This is primarily due to the cardiopulmonary complications. A third of patients with scoliosis go on to have constant moderate-to-severe back pain. Approximately 14% have cardiopulmonary symptoms that affect their lifestyle.

Osteopathic manipulative treatment should address all compensatory biomechanical changes resulting from the curve. Careful evaluation of the functional component should be performed, because this component is biomechanical and will respond to manipulative treatment, exercise and reconditioning. Frequently, the lumbar component of the double major curve has a strong functional element. In almost every curve, there is a functional aspect. In addition to spinal mechanics, rib function on the concave side needs to be addressed. Normal respiratory movement of the ribs is usually restricted on the concave side when compared to the convex. It has been shown in experimental animals that the spine will grow away from the side of greater rib motion. Pelvic asymmetries, sacral base unleveling and leg length discrepancies need to be resolved to balance antigravity muscle tone in the pelvis and low back. Dysfunction in the neck and cranium may contribute to the curve through proprioceptive input affecting balance and posture (Fig. 15.11). Lumbar muscle tone is affected by cervical spine mechanics. In the older child, postural rebalancing exercises such as yoga, t'ai chi, and even some martial arts, can be useful in reconditioning postural muscles. It is paramount that the child and the curve be followed through growth, even if the curve resolves with osteopathic treatment. The growth spurts of puberty will often exacerbate a radiographically resolved curve.

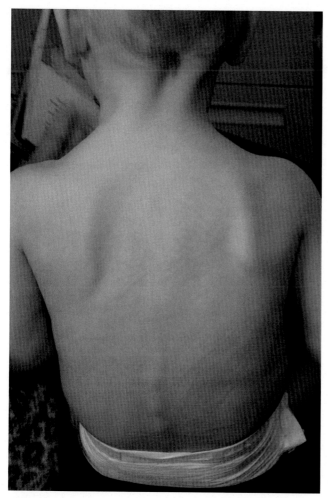

Fig. 15.11 • A 15-month-old boy with mild scoliosis secondary to persistent torticollis and plagiocephaly. Note the asymmetric scapulae. *Used with permission of the Willard & Carreiro Collection.*

Back pain

In the past, back pain in children was thought to be rare and only due to malignant organic pathology. Although it is still dismissed and underdiagnosed by some, many health-care professionals recognize that back pain is not an uncommon complaint in children and is probably underreported (Micheli & Wood 1995). Most authors describe five categories of back pain in children (Bunnell 1982, King 1999): mechanical, developmental, inflammatory, neoplastic and conversion (Table 15.1).

Spondylolysis and spondylolisthesis are reported to be the most common etiology of reported back pain in pediatric athletes. This seems to be especially true in adolescents engaging in repetitive hyperextension and rotation activities such as gymnastics, diving, dancing and contact sports (Micheli & Wood 1995, Herman et al 2003). The conditions may be congenital or traumatic. Repetitive microtrauma has been implicated by some authors. Spondylolysis

involves a defect or break at the pars interarticularis which may be congenital or developmental. Once the pars defect occurs, shearing stresses can causes anterior displacement or slippage of the vertebral body. Children with spondylolysis or slippage typically complain of back pain and muscle spasm that worsens with activity. There is usually an increased lumbar lordosis and lumbosacral angle with spasm of the erector spinae muscles, hip, and knee flexors. Acute spondylolysis responds best to conservative treatment, rest, anti-inflammatory medication and limited gentle manipulative techniques to address muscle spasm and abnormal posturing. Thrust techniques and indirect techniques should be avoided in the acute phase. Bracing may be required. Many children with acute defects will heal without intervention, so repetitive manipulation, even if gentle, may not be the best approach. Once the accentuated postural strain is addressed, the body can be left to heal on its own. In children with spondylolisthesis the degree of the displacement will determine clinical management. In children with less than 50% anterior displacement, treatment is similar to spondylolysis. When greater than 50% anterior displacement is present, and the child is still growing, surgery may be necessary.

While the literature reports spondylogenic pathologies as the most common cause of back pain in children it is also known that pediatric back pain is underreported, primarily because the children (or their parents) do not seek medical attention. One study determined that 36% of children over 15 years have low back pain yet only 2% seek medical attention (Balague et al 1998, Olsen et al 1992). Back pain appears to increase in adolescence, especially between 12 and 14 years of age (Leboeuf-Yde & Kyvik 1999). This is also a period of significant growth for most children. In general most back pain in children is mechanical; that is, it is the result of a mechanical or functional strain rather than another type of organic pathology. Recently, the effect of carrying a book-laden backpack or rucksack has come under scrutiny as a possible factor in pediatric back pain (Pascoe et al 1997, Negrini & Carabalona 2002, Cottalorda et al 2003, Sheir-Neiss et al 2003). Nevertheless, ascertaining the actual etiology of the pain, and finding a method to alleviate the patient's symptoms remains a challenge.

The etiology of mechanical back pain includes spinal nerve irritation, neurogenic pain, spondylosis, musculoskeletal strain and diskogenic pain. Whereas spinal nerve root irritation presents with motor and sensory signs, most mechanical back pain does not. The pain presentations without neurological signs are often the most difficult to precisely diagnose and successfully treat. There are primarily three axial pain patterns that present in the spine. They can be explained by the innervation patterns present in the vertebral column. The spine has a rather complex nerve supply which is best understood if we divide it into three parts: a posterior portion innervating the areas of the facet joints,

Table 15.1 Differential diagnosis of back pain in children

	Mechanical	Developmental	Inflammatory/ Infectious	Neoplastic	Conversion
Typical presentation	Focal	Focal	Focal or diffuse	Focal or diffuse ± fever and systemic signs	Diffuse
Conditions	Somatic dysfunction ± scoliosis	Spondylosis; spondylolisthesis; most common >10 years worse with activity	Rheumatological condition: ankylosing spondylitis, juvenile rheumatoid arthritis	Primary vertebral body	Diagnosis of exclusion, usually a history or emotional trauma or stress
	Overuse syndromes	Scheuermann's disease; low-grade pain in adolescents	Disk calcification	Spinal cord	
	Functional scoliosis/ other postural problem	Hemivertebrae/fusion; usually associated with scoliosis	Inflammatory diskitis; associated with fever, malaise, *Staphylococcus aureus*	Metastasis	
	Disk pathology ± radiculopathy; may be present at rest		Osteomyelitis	Primary muscle	

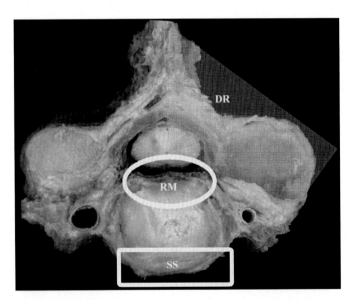

Fig. 15.12 • Superior view of a cross-section through a cervical vertebra. The three regions of innervation are depicted; the neural arch, articular process, and posterior elements of the vertebra via the dorsal ramus (DR), the posterior vertebral body and anterior meninges via the recurrent meningeal nerve (RM), and the anterior vertebral body and disk via the somatosympathetic nerve (SS). *Used with permission of the Willard & Carreiro Collection.*

spinous process and paravertebral musculature; an intermediary portion supplying the posterior aspect of the vertebral body and disk and the dura mater; and an anterior portion supplying the anterior and lateral portions of the vertebral body (Fig. 15.12). The three nerves servicing these portions are the dorsal ramus (DR), the recurrent meningeal (RM), and the somatosympathetic (SS) nerves (Groen et al 1990). Irritation to any of these nerves can result in clinical presentations that are often confusing and difficult to properly diagnose. In these cases the patient's history may conflict with physical examination and imaging studies, and the physician will have to rely on a thorough understanding of the anatomical relations involved to guide the treatment plan.

Radiating pain without sensory or motor changes

One of the most common presentations for patients with back pain involves radiation into the extremity. The pain may originate at the cervical thoracic junction and radiate down the arm, or it may be in the low back and radiate down a leg. Typically the pain follows a dermatomal distribution. It is often not accompanied by weakness or muscle atrophy of the associated limb. There may be some sensory changes, but they are subtle and can be attributed to the pain. Although the patient's symptom complex suggests nerve root irritation, no true neurological deficits are present in the affected extremity and imaging studies are usually normal without any evidence of nerve root pathology. Such a presentation suggests irritation to the dorsal ramus of the dorsal nerve. The dorsal ramus is a branch of the dorsal spinal root. It separates into three smaller branches to innervate the muscles of the back. Most laterally it innervates

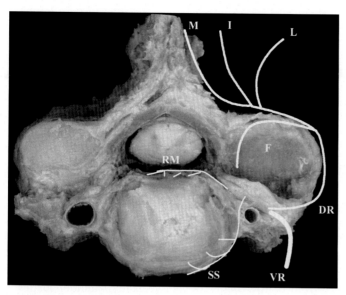

Fig. 15.13 • Superior view of a cross-section through a cervical vertebra. The dorsal ramus (DR) and its medial (M), intermediate (I) and lateral (L) branches, the ventral ramus (VR), the somatosympathetic (SS), and the recurrent meningeal (RM) nerves are labeled. *Used with permission of the Willard & Carreiro Collection.*

the iliocostalis muscle (Fig. 15.13; L), the intermediate division innervates the longissimus muscle (I) and the medial division sends fibers to the multifidus muscle (M). A small twig off the dorsal ramus penetrates the articular capsule of the facet joint. It also sends fibers to the interspinous and supraspinous ligaments. Strain or irritation to any of these tissues may present with radiating pain.

When the dorsal ramus is irritated the child will complain of radiating, burning pain that is well circumscribed, usually following a dermatome distribution. It is much like the pain pattern one sees with a nerve root irritation. Although there will not be any muscle atrophy in the extremity, there may be atrophy in the paraspinal muscles associated with the segment that is irritated. In the lumbar spine the multifidus muscle tends to be the easiest muscle in which to observe these changes. On magnetic resonance imaging (MRI) the muscle may have fatty invasion. Irritation of the dorsal ramus may result in atrophy or weakness of the muscle band associated with that neurological segment (Macintosh & Bogduk 1986). In some cases, muscle atrophy can be assessed by palpating the midline paravertebral muscles as the child hyperextends his spine while in a prone position.

With irritation of the dorsal ramus there may be tenderness to palpation over the interspinous ligaments of the associated segments. Flexion/extension injuries that stretch the interspinous and supraspinous ligaments may irritate the primary afferent fibers in these tissues. Inflammation in the ligaments can also activate these nociceptive fibers. The primary afferents of the interspinous ligaments are terminal branches of the dorsal ramus. Biomechanical strains

in the upper extremities or torso can affect intervertebral mechanics through the spinous insertion of the thoracolumbar fascia and cause irritation to the supraspinous ligaments.

The dorsal ramus provides nociceptive innervation to the vasculature and articular capsule of the facet joint. Anything that alters the weight load across the vertebral body and facet joint may activate these primary afferents. The maximum load on any articular surface is approximately $16 \text{kg}/\text{cm}^2$. Weight loads exceeding this value will create microfractures in the articular cartilage. This is the first step in joint degeneration. Under ideal circumstances the small muscles of posture surrounding a joint will interact to maintain the unit load within the appropriate parameters. However, biomechanical dysfunction may interfere with this process, resulting in abnormal weight loads across joint surfaces. Postural imbalances such as scoliosis, increased lumbar or cervical lordosis, or pes planus will shift the body's center of gravity and alter the weight line transmitted through the spine. This in turn changes the weight load across the facet joint, creating an imbalance in the weight distribution. With time and use the increased unit load on the facet's articular surface may cause damage. As the articular surface is damaged, surrounding vasculature and synovium attempt to participate in the repair process. An inflammatory response is mounted with release of proinflammatory substances. These substances activate nociceptive fibers running with the vasculature of the articular capsule and synovium. Nociceptive fibers in facet joints are branches of the dorsal ramus. Consequently, when they are activated, the pain is referred along the dermatome distribution of the associated dorsal root (Bowen & Cassidy 1981, Ahmed et al 1993, Jinkins 1993). The patient complains of radiating pain similar to that experienced with nerve root compression. When the primary afferent fibers associated with the facet joint are activated, they will fire into the spinal cord and facilitate the segment. This will alter the output to associated muscles, resulting in increased muscle tone. When the muscle spasms, its connective tissue sheath is irritated. This activates nociceptive fibers traveling within the sheath. Furthermore, the fibers innervating the muscle itself will be activated, 50% of which are nociceptive. Lactic acid builds up in the muscle fiber, altering the pH and further sensitizing nociceptive fibers. This cycle will sustain the segmental facilitation so that even if the initial stimulus is removed the symptoms may not resolve.

Pain that varies with position

When back pain varies with position or if the child describes pain that is contralateral to an area of injury one must consider irritation to the recurrent meningeal nerve, or sinu vertebral nerve as it is sometimes called. In these cases the quality of the pain will be similar to a nerve root irritation – burning and radiating – but the pain may also migrate. It can move from side to side. It may be aggravated by position.

It can be bilateral or contralateral to the pathology. Similar to irritation of the dorsal ramus, no motor or sensory changes are associated with the complaint.

The recurrent meningeal is a small delicate nerve which starts just distal to the dorsal root ganglion and turns back on itself to innervate the posterior aspect of the intervertebral disk, the posterior longitudinal ligament and the anterior surface of the dura (Pedersen et al 1956). Twigs from the recurrent meningeal nerve will penetrate a third of the way into the intervertebral disk and posterior longitudinal ligament (Groen et al 1990). The posterior longitudinal ligament has a scalloped appearance. As it passes along the posterior vertebral body it widens over the intervertebral disk and narrows over the vertebral body. It tends to be adhered closely to the disk and has a looser attachment to the vertebrae, thereby providing more support to the disk. The recurrent meningeal nerve lies over the posterior longitudinal ligament following its contours down the vertebral column. The fibers of the recurrent meningeal are not segmented; they cross the midline, entering the neural canal from one side and exiting on the other. They will travel up or down one to three segments before exiting. Each fiber has fine branches that travel up and down and side to side along the posterior longitudinal ligament. Consequently, irritation on the left side of the canal may activate a fiber that originated from the right side two segments below the pathology. The patient's pain presentation would be contralateral and distal to the site of irritation. If a pathology such as a bulging disk occurred at a location where two fibers crossed, the patient might experience pain which traveled from side to side as changes in position slightly altered the position of the disk.

Tiny twigs leave the recurrent meningeal nerve to penetrate the posterior longitudinal ligament and pierce into the posterior aspect of the intervertebral disk. These twigs will penetrate through the annulus fibrosis and a third of the way into the periphery of the disk. At birth the nucleus of the disk is composed of a gelatinous material; as we age it converts to fibrocartilage. (This process begins in the fourth decade for men and the fifth decade for women.) During the aging process the nucleus will develop little rents or tears (Ghosh 1990, Hutton 1990, Taylor 1990, Twomey & Taylor 1990, Ebara et al 1996, Iatridis et al 1996). Rents and tears can also occur with trauma, especially torsional injuries. Disk fluid located in the nucleus pulposus is immune privileged. In other words, because this fluid is isolated from our hematological system, our immune system views it as a 'foreign substance'. Disk fluid that leaks from the little rents or tears will come into contact with the primary afferent fibers piercing the annulus fibrosis. This results in an inflammatory reaction (Ashton & Eisenstein 1996, Olmarker et al 1996). Inflammatory and proinflammatory substances secreted in the immune response will activate the primary afferent fibers in the periphery of the disk. The disk fluid itself can also act as an irritant to the nociceptive fibers. The patient will feel pain in the distribution of the recurrent meningeal nerve: axial pain with burning and radiating along the associated dermatomes. Imaging studies will be negative for disk bulge or nerve root pathology. Occasionally, evidence of degenerative changes may be present; however, early on in the conversion process they may not be detectable.

Diffuse, boring pain at a junctional area

While most back pain is described as localized or burning with a definable radiation, patients will sometimes present with diffuse, vague pain patterns. Typically the pain is boring or aching, lacking the burning or electrical quality seen with nerve root irritation. The patient may describe the pain as 'across the middle of my back' or 'aching down the front of my thighs' or 'between my shoulder blades'. The pattern of distribution is not well defined. There are no sensory changes, paresthesias or weakness. Pain of this description is usually traveling through the fibers of the somatosympathetic nerve. The somatosympathetic nerve represents a series of nerves, which arise from the sympathetic trunk. The sympathetic trunk arises between T1 and L2 and runs along the sides of the anterior longitudinal ligament throughout the course of the spine from neck to pelvis. Tiny hair-like fibers branch off from the communicating rami between the sympathetic ganglion and the somatic nerves and turn medially onto the anterior longitudinal ligament. These branches carry small-calibre sensory fibers which innervate the anterior longitudinal ligament. They form a dense network that follows the course of the ligament from the cranial–cervical junction to the sacrum. The anterior longitudinal ligament is closely adhered to the vertebral body and has looser connection over the intervertebral disk. The anterior aspect of the disk does not enjoy the same reinforcement present posteriorly. Predictably, anterior disk bulges are more common than posterior disk bulges although they are less often symptomatic.

The somatosympathetic nerve provides innervation to the anterior longitudinal ligament, the anterior and lateral portion of the vertebral body and the anterior aspect of the intervertebral disk. Sensory information carried in the somatosympathetic fibers will enter the dorsal horn at the levels of T1 through L2, regardless of where the stimulus is applied. The receptor fields for these fibers are larger and less well defined than those of purely somatic nerves. This explains the diffuse boring nature of the pain (Hobbs et al 1992, Gillette et al 1994, Schott 1994). Changes in muscle tone triggered by the injury may also be referred. While injury to the posterior aspects of the vertebral column will fire into the spinal cord at the level associated with that nerve fiber, injury to the anterior tissues of the neck or lumbosacral areas will be referred to the dorsal horn cells between T1 and L2. Consequently, muscle spasm or tissue inflammation that occurs in response to the injury may manifest at the referred site. Injury to the anterior tissues of the cervical spine will produce changes in muscle tone at the cervical–thoracic junction and upper thoracic area. Injury to the lumbosacral area may manifest as changes in muscle tone at the thoracolumbar junction or upper lumbar area.

Primary afferent fibers innervating the longitudinal ligaments of the spine are able to adapt to slow gradually applied compressive or stretch forces. In fact, it has been demonstrated that nerve fibers can adapt to significantly higher levels of compression when applied gradually as compared to forces applied rapidly. However, when the force is rapid, as in a whiplash injury or a sudden disc herniation, the fibers cannot adapt. Neurochemical changes which occur will activate the nociceptive fiber, stimulate the release of proinflammatory substances and be interpreted by the child as pain.

Mechanism of injury and treatment

The differential diagnosis for back pain in children must include congenital, inflammatory, and metabolic processes as well as the more common mechanical and traumatic. A thorough history will help the physician to determine the mechanism of injury. The pain pattern reported will direct us towards the involved nerve. These two facts will help determine the choice of technique and the treatment plan. Rapid flexion injuries suggest stretch of the posterior longitudinal ligament. Conversely, rapid extension injuries will stress the anterior longitudinal ligament, and increase the compressive load on the facet articulation. During maximum flexion of the spine the annulus pulposus of the intervertebral disk is displaced posteriorly, increasing the strain on the posterior annulus fibrosis. With extension the opposite occurs. This can be a mechanism in annular tears and disk bulges. Complaints of pain exacerbated by hyperextension may represent inflammation or damage of the articular cartilage of the facet joint.

Back stiffness present in the morning on awakening that resolves with movement often indicates either a pathological increase in joint fluid or disk volume or limitation of the connective tissues to compensate for diurnal fluid volume changes. There is a diurnal pattern to the fluid volume present in the intervertebral disks and most joints. At night while we are asleep the fluid volume increases slightly (Fig. 15.14). This will stretch the connective tissue capsule surrounding the joint and annular ligament surrounding the disk. Under normal circumstances this is asymptomatic. However if the fluid volume of the joint is already increased due to inflammation, or the connective tissue is irritated because of inflammation in the joint or biomechanical stress, then the increased volume may be interpreted as a

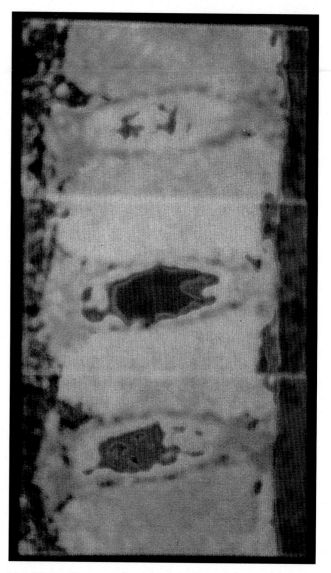

Fig. 15.14 • Three magnetic resonance (MR) images of intervertebral disks that were enhanced after image processing showing water contents. The pale green on top is flow water content at midnight. The bright blue is high water content after a night recumbent. The image in the middle is intermediate water content in the afternoon. *Used with permission from Williams P (ed.) 1995 Gray's anatomy, 38th edn. Churchill Livingstone, London.*

noxious stimulus. When the child awakens and gets out of bed, the loading and movement of the spine and joints acts to displace some of this fluid from the joint space or from the disk, and the discomfort and stiffness improves.

Compression injuries where a force is transmitted through the spine either by something falling on the patient's head, or if the patient has fallen from a height and landed on their feet or pelvis, may produce injury to the facet joints or compromise the integrity of the disks. The disk and the annular ligament appear to be most vulnerable to rotational forces when the parallel relationship of vertebral bodies is distorted. When the vertebrae are stacked upon each other such that the bodies lie in a parallel plane, the spine can be loaded to withstand a substantial amount of force without disruption of the integrity of the intervertebral disk. However, when the parallel orientation is altered, disruption of the disk will occur under a much lighter load.

In the face of injuries that may have stretched the posterior longitudinal ligament it is very important to normalize any rotational stress on the vertebra which can further stretch the ligament. The small paraspinal muscles should be specifically addressed, as they will exhibit the increased tone in response to the irritation. Exercises performed with the spine in a neutral position may be beneficial. Modified Kiegel exercises can reduce strain in the lumbar and sacral areas. Chin tucks will have a similar effect on the cervical tissue. If disk compression is involved, non-weightbearing exercises such as aquatic therapy can be very helpful in the acute phase. In athletes with acute or recent injury, rotational stress should be minimized. If a posterior disk bulge is thought to be the initiating event, postural rebalancing exercises may help to minimize posterior loading of the disk. Normally, the nucleus of the disk is more posterior, and spinal flexion may displace the disk further posterior.

Injuries or disruption of the interspinous and supraspinous ligaments are best approached using a similar rationale as that for posterior longitudinal ligament injuries. Special attention should be paid to biomechanical stress placed upon these ligaments by rotational, side-bending or extension strains. Abnormal or asymmetrical tension on the thoracolumbar fascia may also aggravate these midline structures due to its insertion on the supraspinous ligaments. As a result biomechanical stress originating in the shoulders or upper extremities must be addressed.

Rapid extension injuries will affect the anterior longitudinal ligament. As with the other structures of the spine, somatic dysfunction resulting in rotational, torsional or sagittal stress must be addressed. Exercises or positions that prevent postural hyperlordosis or hyperkyphosis may bring some symptomatic relief to the child. Supine lying with the knees flexed on a pillow decreases the lumbar lordosis, a small towel placed under the thoracic spine can flatten the kyphosis and a small pillow placed under the head so the chin is tucked may all be comfortable positions depending on the location of the injury. Diaphragmatic function should be evaluated. As the diaphragm contracts the crura 'pulls up' on its attachment to the anterior longitudinal ligament. This will increase stress in the ligament and may aggravate the patient's symptoms. Because of the vague, boring quality of the pain and the constancy of the stress, the patient may not recognize the connection. However, he or she may unconsciously splint their respirations, which may lead to other problems. If tension in the two leaves of the diaphragm is not balanced, different contractile forces will be generated through the crura. This may result in an asymmetrical tension on the anterior longitudinal ligament, creating a torsional stress. Normalizing diaphragmatic function so that the muscle is placing a uniform and balanced stress on the anterior longitudinal ligament may improve the patient's symptoms.

Hyperlordosis or restriction at the lumbosacral junction will affect the pattern of relaxation which occurs in the spinal curves in response to respiration. Normally, the lumbar and cervical lordosis decrease with respiratory inhalation. Inhibiting this pattern of change can place a tonic stretch on the anterior longitudinal ligament that may contribute to the patient's symptoms. Correcting biomechanical dysfunction at the junctional or transitional zones of the spine may facilitate normal respiratory mechanics and alleviate some of the factors contributing to the patient's symptoms.

COMMON PROBLEMS IN THE HIP

Infants and young children with hip dysfunction may present with delayed developmental milestones. Older children may experience a sudden change in activity level. They will walk with a limp or shuffle in an attempt to minimize motion and compensate for improper anatomical weightbearing. If old enough, the child may complain of pain in the area that may be localized, diffuse, constant or remitting. Alternatively, the pain may be referred to the knee or back. Another common symptom in older children is stiffness, decreased range of motion or cramping, especially at night. The pain may improve with activity and be exacerbated when the child rests. For example, adolescents may be physically active during the day, but at night they are kept awake by the pain. Other complaints include sensory changes such as numbness or tingling, weakness, fatigue and feeling unstable.

Observation of the general attitude of both lower extremities in the supine position may reveal valuable information about asymmetry in the hip area. Examination should include full orthopedic and neurological evaluation. Examining the unaffected leg prior to the affected one may provide valuable information concerning what is 'normal' for this child. Fullness or any increase in the girth of the thigh is an indication of disturbed chemistry and retained metabolites. Inguinal fullness, tautness, tenderness or lymphadenopathy are all important findings, because the superficial and deep lymphatic channels of the lower extremity drain into this area. Palpation of this tissue, as with palpation of any tissue, should be done in a layer-by-layer fashion. The physician should also evaluate the texture of the skin. Fascial tensions are usually present in hip dysfunction and may be evaluated along the tensor fascia lata and iliotibial tract. Evaluation of the knee and below also gives the physician valuable information concerning the hip function, since all nourishment to and byproducts from these areas must pass through the region of the hip. The relationships and stresses affecting the composite innominate bone need to be addressed. This will include the short and long restrictor muscles, fascial and ligamentous components. This can be done through a combination of passive range of motion, ligamentous and osseous springing, tissue loading, and gentle sensing.

Developmental dysplasia

Probably the best-known disease of the hip in children, developmental dysplasia is thought to occur as a result of three possible mechanisms: mechanical, ligamentous laxity, or primary acetabular dysplasia. A broad spectrum of instability is possible in developmental dysplasia. While the problem may be due to maldevelopment of the acetabulum, often the initial pathology is a laxity of the hip capsule or supportive tissues that allows the femoral head to be displaced from the acetabulum during movement. In severe cases, the femoral head may displace from the acetabulum in the resting position. In response to the displacement of the femoral head, the supporting ligamentous tissues may hypertrophy, preventing the femoral head from spontaneously establishing its normal position. With time, contractures of the short and long restrictors develop, further complicating the picture. These changes affect growth patterns in the hip and leg.

In the newborn and young infant, the first signs of developmental dysplasia are seen during the physical exam, with a positive click on Barlow's (Fig. 15.15) or Ortolani's reduction maneuver (Fig. 15.16). Definitive diagnosis is based on joint ultrasound. The parents may notice an asymmetrical range of motion in the hips, or difficulties with changing diapers. Movement of the hip does not usually produce pain in very young infants. Older infants may show delayed crawling, standing and walking. In toddlers, gait asymmetry is present.

Delayed motor milestones or positive Ortolani's or Barlow's without evidence of acetabular abnormality suggests a mechanical etiology. The functional relationships influencing the hip joint need to be evaluated. This includes the composite innominate – pubic, ilia and ischia. A change in the angle of the femoral neck or head alters rotational dynamics of the joint. This may occur as a result of structural changes or through the effects of muscular and somatic strains in the restrictor muscles of the hip and pelvis.

If signs of dysplasia persist, then appropriate treatment with bracing is indicated to prevent deformity, arthritis and septic necrosis. If there is any evidence of hip instability, i.e. the femur is dislocatable or dislocated, the hip must be stabilized, reduced and correctly positioned as soon as possible. In children younger than 6 months, Pavlik's harness, a dynamic brace that allows flexion and abduction of the hips while

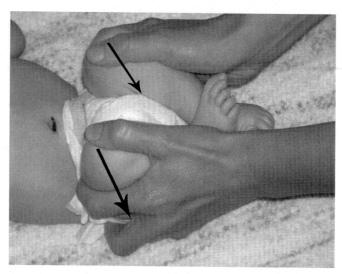

Fig. 15.15 • Barlow's maneuver demonstrated on a 3-day-old baby boy. The hips and knees are flexed. Then the hips are compressed directly posteriorly (black arrows). This is a provocative test. A 'clunk' or displacement of the femur signifies dysplasia. The diaper has been unfastened and is lying loosely over the infant's genitalia to prevent an unforeseen shower in the physician's face. *Used with permission of the Willard & Carreiro Collection.*

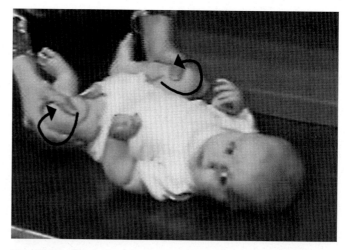

Fig. 15.16 • Ortolani's reduction maneuver demonstrated on a 2-month-old baby girl. The hips are compressed posteriorly as they are circumducted (black arrows). A click or skip in the arch of movement may indicate muscle or ligamentous laxity. Ortolani's maneuver can be used to reduce a dislocated hip. *Used with permission of the Willard & Carreiro Collection.*

supporting the hips in a reduced position, is used. Treatment usually lasts at least 6 weeks and has good results without complications. The child can be treated osteopathically during this time to address somatic dysfunction. This will support the effects of the brace. If the condition has persisted beyond 6 months, it is usually impossible to manually reduce the hips due to tissue contractures and closed reduction, and casting necessary. This procedure is done under general anesthesia. Frequently, traction may be applied prior to the procedure to stretch the shortened tissues. Osteopathic treatment prior to closed reduction may help to normalize some of the compensatory muscle spasm. When closed reduction fails, open surgical reduction is necessary. In children over 18 months, the morphological changes in the hip often necessitate surgical reduction with osteotomy. In older children, surgical reduction has a poor outcome and complications are more likely. Unfortunately, these children often go on to experience pain and disability throughout their life.

Slipped capital femoral epiphysis

Slipped capital femoral epiphysis (SCFE) is probably the most common hip pathology of adolescence. It is classified as an epiphyseal disorder. Although its cause is unknown, SCFE (Fig. 15.17) is most often seen in adolescents with skeletal growth delay and obesity or in those who are tall and thin and have had a recent growth spurt. SCFE is also associated with endocrine disorders. The pathology of SCFE involves initial widening of the physis that is thought to result form abnormal shearing forces. The subsequent forces of weightbearing result in a rotation of the femoral neck, while the capital femoral epiphysis remains in the acetabulum. This creates a slippage, a varus, and retroverted femoral neck and head. The degree of slippage is classified as mild (0–33%), moderate (34–50%) or severe (greater

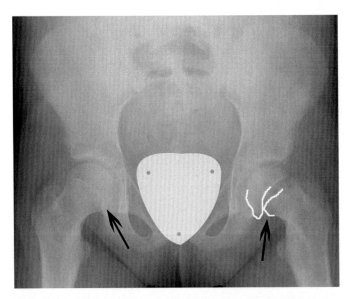

Fig. 15.17 • PA X-ray of adolescent girl with slipped capital femoral epiphysis. The black arrows indicate the epiphysis on each side. The deformity on the right is outlined in white. *Used with permission of the Willard & Carreiro Collection.*

than 50%). In most children the non-symptomatic hip will also show some degree of involvement although the extent of the damage may be less.

SCFE most often presents insidiously, developing over several months. Symptoms worsen as the slippage progresses. The condition is stable and the child is usually able to walk, although the gait is antalgic with the leg externally rotated. Passive movement is tolerated but uncomfortable. With the hip flexed internal rotation is limited. Children with chronic SCFE may experience acute exacerbations during which the joint is unstable and the child cannot stand. Occasionally SCFE may be acute and spontaneous without preceding trauma. It is usually painful and unstable, and the child cannot bear weight. Unlike the chronic condition, in acute slippage passive joint motion on physical examination movement is exquisitely painful. There is risk of avascular necrosis and malunion. A condition called pre-slippage involves widening of the epiphysis without rotation of the femoral neck or head. This is usually stable, and the child is able to walk, although there may be some discomfort present. Physical examination is usually normal.

Children with SCFE may present with knee pain rather than hip pain. Children with pre-slippage can be treated conservatively, and osteopathic evaluation and treatment form a part of that approach. Children with chronic SCFE may also benefit from osteopathic treatment, with a goal of minimizing contributing somatic strains, and improving vascular and lymphatic function in the area. Children with acute changes need immediate evaluation by an orthopedic surgeon; osteopathic manipulation may form a part of the overall treatment plan, but the severity of the problem and potential for complications must be clearly evaluated and addressed.

Complications of SCFE include necrosis of the femoral head and chondrolysis – degeneration of articular cartilage. Appropriate treatment involves stabilizing the epiphysis to prevent further slippage and correction of the displacement. Depending on the severity of the condition, open reduction and pinning or percutaneous pinning may be necessary.

Legg–Calvé–Perthes disease

Legg–Calvé–Perthes disease is an idiopathic condition affecting the growth of the capital femoral epiphysis. Unlike slipped capital femoral epiphysis, Legg–Calvé–Perthes disease usually presents between the ages of 5 and 8 years as a limp or pain in the extremity. It is associated with ischemia of the capital epiphysis and mild skeletal growth retardation in the femoral head not due to an infectious or inflammatory process. As such, Legg–Calvé–Perthes disease can be classified as an osteochondrosis, a disease of the epiphyses that coincides with the time of its greatest developmental activity. Boys are more likely to develop

Legg–Calvé–Perthes disease than girls. The condition initially presents as mild and intermittent limping lasting 2–4 weeks. This is followed by a short period of improvement or resolution after which the child has recurring episodes of stiffness and pain. Synovitis and arthritic changes occur and can lead to permanent damage of the joint. Physical exam reveals restricted motion to passive extension, abduction and internal rotation. Abductor and hamstring muscles may have atrophied from disuse and inhibition.

Prognosis is best in the youngest male patients (under 6 years) with sclerotic and degenerative changes in less than 50% of the femoral head. Goals of treatment are to prevent further deformation of the femoral head, reduce pain and improve mechanics. The synovitis often responds to restriction of activities, and non-weightbearing lymphatic and fluid techniques to improve vascular function may also help. In severe synovitis traction may be necessary to decompress the joint tissues. In older patients or those with deformation of more than 50% of the femoral head containment of the femoral head may be necessary. This can be done non-surgically through abduction casts, braces and therapy, or when that does not appear to be working, through surgical intervention via intratrochanteric osteotomy, innominate osteotomy or Chiari pelvic osteotomy. The goal is for a rim of new bone to form on the femoral head. The treatment process can last months to years, depending on the age of the child at the time of diagnosis and the extent of the damage to the femoral head.

Persistent femoral anteversion

As previously described the hip joint responds to weightbearing and ambulation by remolding and moving into a retroverted position. However, in some children the anteverted position of birth persists due to delayed walking, spasticity, hypotonia or congenital malformations. Mechanical dysfunction, persistent 'W' sitting and sleeping in a prone fetal position may also interfere with retroversion; however, the outcome is subtler than that found with organic conditions. Persistent intoeing accompanied by genu valgus in children over 4–5 years may be due to anteversion.

Femoral anteversion may be due to congenital malformation or functional mechanical influences. Most children respond to conservative treatment, although surgery may be necessary in severe cases. The success of the treatment depends on the age at which it is initiated. The normal retroversion process is a function of growth, as such treatment should begin when the child is still young and can benefit from the growth periods. Children with organic problems such as primary muscle disease or spasticity require long-term treatment plans, and ongoing therapy. Somatic dysfunction and mechanical imbalances in the associated musculature need to be addressed. Isometric and isotonic muscle energy techniques can be used in older children to address resting length, strength and firing patterns. Balanced ligamentous techniques can be used to correct fascial and ligamentous dysfunction. Isolytic muscle energy techniques, articular techniques and joint mobilization may be needed in young athletes to correct restricted joint motion. Children should be encouraged to avoid postures that reinforce the anteversion such as 'W' sitting and prone fetal positions. However, in most cases the child is choosing these postures because they are most comfortable. Correction of the mechanical dysfunction will often facilitate normal sitting and sleeping postures. Exercises and activities that reinforce core stabilization and postural mechanics need to be added to the treatment regimen in addition to normal play and sports. Activities should be chosen with input from the child and parents, and be appropriate to the child's interests and capabilities. The attitude and focus of the coach or instructor is the key to whether the activity can be used to enhance therapy or not. Some activities that deserve to be considered include martial arts, horseback riding, yoga and dance.

Miserable malalignment syndrome

Persistent femoral anteversion predisposes the child to develop a complex compensatory pattern called miserable malalignment syndrome or MMS. MMS is a cluster of adaptations developed in the leg and foot as a postural adaptation to the anteverted hip. Initially the child compensates with a genu valgus, a medial-placed patella and a pronated foot. With weightbearing, the external rotation of the tibia is exaggerated at the knee, and with time a compensatory intraosseous internal tibial torsion develops. When standing, the child's patella face each other, called 'kissing patella' (Fig. 15.18) and there is an acute angulation at the medial aspect of the knee or 'bayonet sign'. This abnormal posturing places significant stress on the patella, hip and foot, predisposing the child to Osgood–Schlatter disease, patella femoral syndrome and degenerative changes later in life. Miserable malalignment syndrome usually arises as an adaptation to femoral anteversion, but it may also develop secondary to subtalar pronation.

Functional changes in the hip

There is a significant difference between mechanical restriction of the hip due to functional muscle imbalance and mechanical restriction due to anteversion, although the two often exacerbate each other. Femoral anteversion can be seen on plain X-ray, functional malposition cannot. Infants normally have a greater degree of anteversion or internal rotation than adults. Slipped capital epiphysis (inferior and posterior slipping of the upper femoral epiphysis) usually results in a relative retroversion, limiting internal

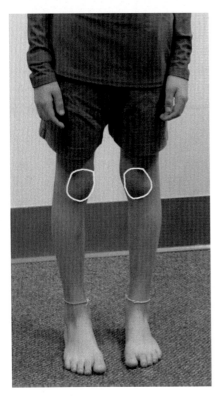

Fig. 15.18 • This child has medially positioned patella (kissing patella) but fortunately has not developed the other components of miserable malalignment syndrome. Mild femoral anteversion is apparent. *Used with permission of the Willard & Carreiro Collection.*

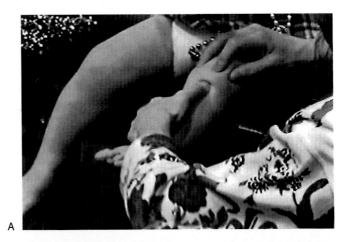

A

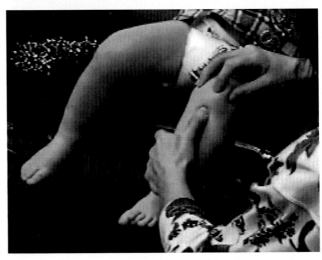

B

Fig. 15.19 • Evaluation of the screw-home mechanism between the tibia and femur. In (A), the child's knee is flexed and the tibial tubercle is in line with the middle of the patella. In (B), the child's knee is extended and the tibia tubercle moves laterally as compared to the same landmark on the patella. This is normal. *Used with permission of the Willard & Carreiro Collection.*

rotation. Abnormal uterine lie, multiple fetus gestation, uterine fibroids or morphological abnormality can all result in abnormal posturing of the extremities. Fascial and muscle shortening, strictures and altered tone may be present in the infant. In children and young athletes rapid growth and mechanical stress may account for functional changes. In either case the mechanical strain should be addressed so that normal growth and function can resume.

COMMON PROBLEMS IN THE KNEE

The knee is one of the most complicated and perhaps the most misunderstood joint in the body. Anatomically, it is very stable because of the strong ligaments and related myofascial tissues. The knee joint is most vulnerable to trauma when flexed and loaded. The knee is described as a ginglymus or hinge joint, but is really of a much more complicated character. *Gray's anatomy* (Standring 2004) describes it as three articulations in one, two condyloid joints and one joint between the patella and the femur.

In any knee complaint, the screw-home mechanism must be assessed for normal function (Fig. 15.19). Biomechanical dysfunction in the pelvis and lumbar spine may place an

abnormal weight load and stress on the knee, since each step imposes a torsional force upon the articulation. Also, rotation of the femur can put stress on the knee. A flat foot (pes planus) will cause a slight gapping of the knee joint and secondary strain of the medial and lateral ligaments through the abnormal leverage caused by the abducted foot. In the presence of an anatomically short leg, normal structural balance may be disrupted. This can also lead to dysfunction in the knee.

Pathophysiology of the hip will ultimately cause backpressure and congestion of veins and stagnation of lymphatic vessels and glands which drain the knee. The popliteal lymph nodes may be more indurated and congested behind the affected knee than on the unaffected side. Tenderness is often present. This subtle congestion surrounding the knee will hamper any attempts to correct somatic dysfunction until the tissues are prepared by restoring the thoraco-abdominopelvic pump to aspirate these fluids. Sometimes it is necessary to massage the tissues to facilitate fluid drainage before correcting articular strains.

Osgood–Schlatter disease

Osgood–Schlatter disease is a benign, self-limiting disease of adolescence and late childhood. It presents as knee pain exacerbated by exercise, accompanied by swelling and tenderness over the tibial tubercle. It occurs as a result of microfractures of the tibial tubercle. It most often resolves once the epiphysis of the tuberosity has closed. Associated findings include tibial torsion, abnormal tracking of the patella, and altered foot or hip mechanics. Abnormal strain or tensions on the patella tendon may create increased strain on the tuberosity, which is more susceptible during the rapid growth of adolescence and late childhood. Addressing the biomechanical dysfunctions and retraining the long restrictors of the knee and ankle will often rectify the problem. Children who overpronate may also benefit from a flexible orthotic.

Genu varum and genu valgum

Genu varum or bowlegs (Fig. 15.20), and genu valgum or knock-knees (Fig. 15.21), may be due to metabolic disease, skeletal dysplasia or asymmetric growth. Of the three, the last is most amenable to osteopathic treatment. In preambulatory infants, genu varum is often associated with external rotation of the hip on the involved side. This may be secondary to uterine position, and the relationships of the components of the innominate need to be addressed. Many children also have an external rotation of the tibia. Lumbar lordosis may be slightly decreased. These findings become more prominent as the child begins to stand and then walk. In the ambulatory infant, fascial strains in the foot will also be present. Genu valgum is usually associated with internal rotation of the hips, and the sacral base is nutated. With each of these conditions, the persistent biomechanical stress may lead to structural deformity. The goal of osteopathic treatment is to eliminate or minimize the abnormal biomechanical stress.

Tibial torsion

Tibial torsion is an intraosseous external or internal twisting of the tibia. In the very young child, this is due to uterine lie. Tibial torsion commonly develops in children with motor dysfunctions, such as cerebral palsy due to the abnormal muscle and fascial tensions. Distortion of normal tibial response during flexion–extension maneuvers can be observed. Distortion of the longitudinal plane of the bone can be assessed grossly through examining the orientation of the ankle mortis in relation to the tibial tubercle

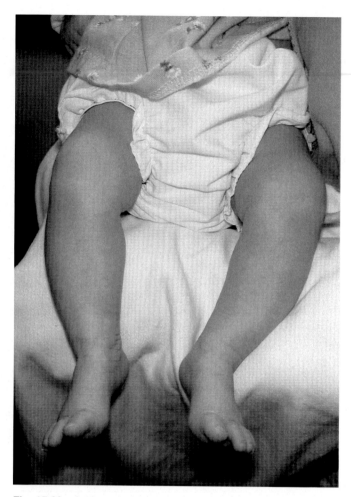

Fig. 15.20 • A 10-week-old infant with bowlegs or genu varum. The varum deformity is worse in the left leg. *Used with permission of the Willard & Carreiro Collection.*

(Fig. 15.22). Addressing this problem will frequently stop progression of the torsion. Foot mechanics also need to be evaluated, as a pes planus will exacerbate the problem. The goal of osteopathic treatment is to resolve these strain patterns to the point where minimal orthotic use is necessary. This is especially critical in those children in whom proprioceptive and balance mechanisms are already distorted by motor dysfunction.

Meniscal injuries

Meniscal injuries that develop gradually are typically the result of altered biomechanics in the hip, knee or foot, which create abnormal load and wear on the menisci. Restriction of external rotation of the tibia during knee extension may result in increased load on the medial meniscus. Genu valgus and varus also alter menisci loading. Overpronation of the foot may be associated with medial complaints. Injuries resulting from trauma are often associated with a lateral impact and

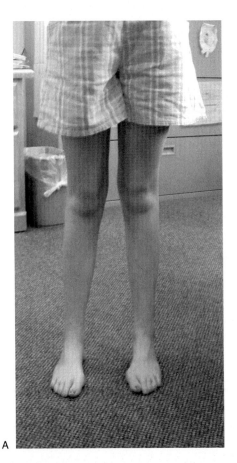
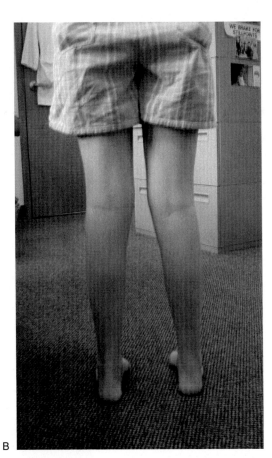

A   B

Fig. 15.21 • Anterior (A) and posterior (B) views of a 10-year-old girl with genu valgus, worse on the right than left. Note the hallus valgus on the left, and internal rotation of both legs although more exaggerated on the right. *Used with permission of the Willard & Carreiro Collection.*

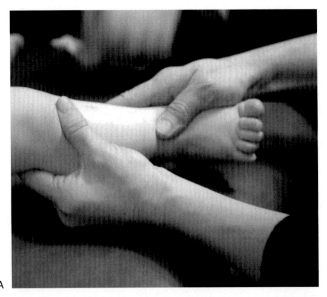
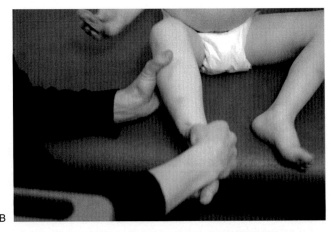

A   B

Fig. 15.22 • Assessing the tibia for torsional strain in a 14-month-old girl (A) and a 3-year-old boy (B). The midpoint of the ankle mortis is palpated and marked with the examiner's right thumb. The tibial tubercle is palpated and marked with the examiner's left thumb. The two points are compared. In the younger child it is normal to have a slight tibial torsion with the inferior aspect lateral to the tibial tubercle. The tibia should then be assessed for passive involuntary motion. *Used with permission of the Willard & Carreiro Collection.*

associated with strain to the ligaments. They may respond to conservative treatment, including osteopathic manipulation, but quite often require arthroscopic intervention.

Patellofemoral syndrome

Patellofemoral syndrome is usually associated with a biomechanical dysfunction in the extremity or hip. The vastus medialis muscle is often weaker than the lateral musculature, resulting in lateral tracking of the patella during knee extension and quadriceps contraction. This can be assessed by palpating the patella while asking a child to contract his quadriceps or raise an extended leg. The patella will move laterally with contraction of the quadriceps. Tibial mechanics during the screw-home mechanism should be assessed. Exercises which selectively strengthen the vastus medialis may be helpful. These include asking the child to sit with the legs extended out in front. The affected leg is rotated slightly laterally, and leg lifts are performed to strengthen the muscle. Externally rotating the extended leg isolates the vastus medialis. When conservative treatment and retraining prove ineffective, surgical release of the lateral tension may be necessary.

Compartment syndrome

Compartment syndromes occur when there is increased tissue pressure which compromises the circulation to the muscles and nerves within the space. The lower leg has four compartments (anterior, lateral, superficial and deep posterior). The most commonly involved is the anterior. This syndrome can be acute or chronic. Most cases are chronic. Stress fractures, tendonitis and other forms of 'shin splints' can be confused with this syndrome. In the anterior compartment of the leg, the anterior tibial, the extensor hallucis and extensor digitorum longus muscles arise from the sides of the tibia, fibula and interosseous membrane. They completely fill the anterior compartment. This compartment is tightly roofed by the anterior fascia of the leg. In the anterior tibial syndrome, for various reasons, there is rapid swelling of the muscles within this compartment. This condition may follow active exercise alone, and, in theory, is due to the fact that muscles which have not been previously conditioned are overused and respond with swelling and edema. It may also follow direct injury, localized infection or anything that causes intractable swelling.

Presenting signs and symptoms of compartment syndrome include severe pain due to the ischemia to nerve and muscle, paresthesia, puffiness, pallor and paralysis. There is increased compartment pressure, which can be directly measured. Treatment depends on the severity of this condition. In acute situations, early treatment should be ice, elevation and osteopathic manipulative treatment to the axial skeleton with lymphatic drainage techniques to the areas proximal to the injury. If the symptoms do not respond

within a short time (preferably less than 1h), treatment must be surgical. If the anterior fascia of the leg is promptly sectioned, complete relief is obtained from pain and other symptoms. There should be a low threshold for taking the patient to surgery. If the operation is postponed, necrosis of the muscles may occur. Fibrous replacement may produce irreparable damage to these muscles. In chronic presentations, the treatment regimen should include rest, heat before and ice after exercise along with ongoing osteopathic manipulative treatment to the axial skeleton with lymphatic drainage techniques, as well as appropriate treatment of the area, including the foot and pelvis; and proper footwear. If the response using the above is not adequate, further invasive procedures may be necessary.

Common peroneal nerve entrapment

The proximal tibiofibular joint is a common area for somatic dysfunction. Biomechanical strain of this joint may lead to a variety of circulatory, neurological and myofascial signs and symptoms. Often, the child will complain of pain in the lateral aspect of the distal leg subsequent to a mild ankle sprain. The symptoms are usually exacerbated with running or prolonged walks. The applied anatomy of the proximal tibiofibular joint involves the facet on the tibia that forms the articulation for the fibula. This facet faces posteriorly, laterally and inferiorly. The facet facing explains why, in the correction of the posterior fibular head lesion, we draw the fibular head anterolaterally and slightly superiorly. The fibers of the interosseous membrane, which attach the fibula to the tibia, provide the vehicle through which the anterior tibial vessels reach the popliteal space. The interosseous membrane also provides openings near its distal end for perforating vessels. The common peroneal nerve, after emerging from the popliteal fossa, winds around the head of the fibula. The nerve trunk is often palpable at this point when rolled under the fingers.

Compression of the common peroneal nerve can lead to neurological signs of foot drop, inability to dorsiflex the foot, and paresthesias or anesthesia on the lateral aspect of the foot. This condition may be caused by a contraction of the biceps femoris muscle that can lesion the fibular head posteriorly and cause entrapment of the common peroneal nerve and related vessels. Myofascial tension can lead to muscle cramping, pain, tenderness and circulatory disturbances due to overstretching of the interosseous membrane causing vessels to be impinged as they perforate and run along the membrane. Manual medicine and appropriate retraining are the key components of therapy.

Iliotibial band syndrome

Iliotibial band syndrome shares similarities with snapping hip syndrome in that there are altered forces across the iliotibial band and tensor fascia lata. The problem may arise due to leg length inequality, altered foot mechanics, innominate dysfunction, and tibial rotations. Calcaneal varus, tibial varus, cavus foot and iliotibial band tightness, when combined with chronic or repetitive forces, result in a reactive bursitis between the iliotibial band and the lateral epicondyle of the femur. This is most common in young athletes participating in sports requiring significant running, stopping and turning, such as soccer, lacrosse, football, and basketball. The patient usually presents with lateral knee pain extending from the lateral epicondyle of the femur to the insertion of the iliotibial band on the tibia. There may be tender points along the length of the band. Biomechanical realignment along with stretching exercises are among the mainstays of therapy for this syndrome.

COMMON PROBLEMS IN THE FOOT AND ANKLE

Sprained ankle (traumatic inversion of the foot)

Inversion injuries of the ankle are significantly more common than eversion injuries because of the stabilizing characteristics of the lateral malleoli. Strains describe injuries where the ligaments are stretched while sprains describe injuries resulting in ligamentous tear. Sprains are more likely to arise when the child is in a accelerated phase of gait due to the increased load on the ankle at ground contact. An inversion sprain typically occurs during running when the foot inverts with full weightbearing. A simple sprained ankle may produce minor ligamentous tears involving the fibulocalcaneal and anterior and posterior talofibular ligaments. Inversion ankle injuries like most soft tissue injuries can be classified into three categories. Grade 1 sprains occur when there is mild stretching of a ligament resulting in microtears. The patient can bear weight on the foot but passive and active movement is painful. There is generalized tenderness to palpation and minimal edema. Grade 2 describes incomplete tear of a ligament. It is usually painful with weightbearing and movement. There is marked swelling and some ecchymosis may be present. Grade 3 sprains occur when there is complete disruption of the ligament, and pain, swelling and ecchymosis are marked. The child is unable to bear weight on the extremity. Children presenting with this clinical picture need to be carefully evaluated to rule out avulsion fracture. The Ottawa rules for imaging are often invoked in ankle injuries (Auleley 1998). X-ray examination is warranted if the child has pain near the lateral malleolus that is accompanied by inability to bear weight or point tenderness on the malleoli. X-rays are also necessary if there is pain in the midfoot and the child is unable to bear weight or there is point tenderness at the navicular or fifth metatarsal.

In addition to the ligamentous damage other structures are often injured. During the inversion injury, the peroneus longus and brevis muscles are often overstretched, resulting in strain and spasm. The sudden stretch and spasm of the peroneus muscle often pulls the fibular head posteriorly. Fibular head dysfunctions may also occur secondary to the actual inversion of the ankle, which carries the distal fibula anterior and inferior. Inversion usually occurs between the tibia and talus with the tibia anterior on the talus. Dysfunction between the talus and calcaneus is also present. A concomitant posterior third rib lesion on the same side and a rotation of the third thoracic vertebra towards the injured side may be found, probably due to the traction transmitted through the thoracolumbar fascia. Rest, ice, compression and joint elevation are the hallmarks of acute care. Rehabilitation requires correction of the biomechanical dysfunctions, and improving flexibility and strength in the damaged structures.

Sever's disease (calcaneal apophysitis)

Sever's disease is an inflammation of the apophysis between the posterior epiphysis of the calcaneus and the main body of the bone. It usually presents as pain with weightbearing and moving from the flat foot to toe off phase of gait. Swelling may be present. There is tenderness to palpation at the insertion of Achilles' tendon or over the posterior inferior aspect of the calcaneus. Symptoms can be elicited or exacerbated by plantar flexion against resistance, or forced dorsiflexion. This condition is most common in athletes participating in sports involving running with frequent stops or turns. Children taking part in soccer, basketball and track sports are most at risk. The condition is more common in boys than girls and typically involves young athletes between 8 and 16 years. Treatment requires elimination of the offending trauma to allow healing to occur. Soft accommodating heel lifts may provide symptomatic relief. The lifts should be used in both shoes, whether or not the condition is bilateral.

Tarsal tunnel syndrome

The tarsal tunnel is located on the posterior inferior aspect of the tibia. It is roofed by the flexor retinaculum, which extends from the medial malleolus to the calcaneus. Through this tunnel pass several tendons and the posterior tibial nerve, as well as the tibial artery, veins and lymphatics. Compression of the posterior tibial nerve in this tarsal tunnel produces numbness, burning pain, or paresthesias in portions of the plantar surface of the foot. The diagnosis can be confirmed by measuring nerve conduction velocities. This syndrome may result from fracture or dislocation of the bones near the tunnel, overpronation, edema of the tunnel, tenosynovitis, or venous or lymphatic stasis. Tarsal tunnel syndrome is associated with hypothyroidism. Endocrinopathy can be ruled out through a thorough patient history and/or laboratory evaluation. Treatment of non-metabolic tarsal tunnel syndrome requires addressing biomechanical strains which may be contributing, along with postural correction of the foot, to alter pronation. It is sometimes necessary to inject a local anesthetic into the tarsal tunnel when symptoms are unresponsive to conservative treatment. Surgical decompression may be required to relieve the tarsal tunnel syndrome.

Metatarsalgia

Metatarsalgia is pain and tenderness of the plantar heads of the metatarsal bones. This occurs when the transverse arch becomes depressed and the middle metatarsal head bears a disproportionate amount of weight. Metatarsalgia can occur in athletes or runners wearing inappropriate footgear. The athlete's sports shoes should be examined for abnormal wear patterns. Typically, the foot pronates and the transverse arch becomes depressed. There will be excessive wear on the medial aspect of the heel and under the metatarsal arch. Osteopathic manipulative treatment helps to restore structure and function of the foot. Elevating the middle portion of the arch avoids pressure on the painful metatarsal heads. The pronated foot is treated by exercises to strengthen the intrinsic muscles, Achilles' tendon stretching, improvement of gait mechanics, and the use of orthotics such as an inner heel wedge, and various metatarsal pads placed behind the metatarsal heads. Localized injection of anesthetic to abort the pain cycle may be necessary in athletes with severe pain.

Pes planus (flat foot)

Pes planus is normal in infants and toddlers during weight-bearing activities (Fig. 15.23). However, in the older toddler there should be some arch visible in the non-weightbearing posture; this is functional pes planus. Although pes planus during weightbearing may or may not be symptomatic, it will create abnormal stresses and loads in the tissues of the lower extremity. In the early developmental phases of stance and ambulation, children are often flat-footed; however, if the arch is evaluated with the child sitting, a medial arch should be visualized. If absent, then the medial components of the foot should be evaluated for flexibility, alignment and range of motion. The aforementioned supporting structures of the arch also need to be addressed. Pes planus may result from abnormal structural relationships in

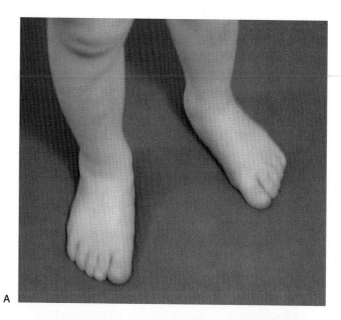

A

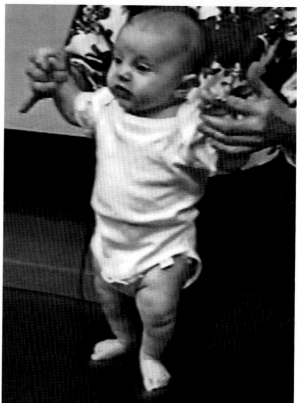

B

Fig. 15.23 • (A) A 3-year-old boy walking unsupported. The medial arch is slightly present. (B) Plantar arches are absent in the infant; however, the plantar grasp reflex still exists. *Used with permission of the Willard & Carreiro Collection.*

the foot, low muscle tone, or dysfunctional biomechanics in the extremity or hip. It may also be associated with neurological dysfunction, but in the absence of other findings, mechanical etiology is most likely. The lateral longitudinal and medial transverse arches develop later, some time after 6 years. Normalizing the arches of the foot will often rectify problems in the ankle, knee or hip.

Plantar fasciitis

The child with plantar fasciitis may present with pain under the heel, and tenderness of the plantar fascia. This is usually secondary to foot strain with a pronated foot, which can be exacerbated by excessive walking or standing. Biomechanical strains, which increase the distance between the proximal and distal aspects of the foot, may also cause irritation of the plantar fascias. This can occur when the calcaneus has shifted posteriorly, or if the articular relationships in the arches are distorted. The calcaneus may shift posteriorly as a result of ankle or knee injury. Osteopathic manipulative treatment and appropriate footwear are employed to re-establish function of the arches, normalize plantar fascia tensions, and balance weightbearing load.

Metatarsus adductus

Metatarsus adductus (Fig. 15.24) is a common congenital varus deformity of the metatarsals and phalanges which may be associated with intrauterine lie. There is often an asymmetry in tensions in the fascia and muscles of the distal lower extremity, external rotation of the femur and compensatory changes in the tibia. The condition is classified based upon the flexibility of the forefoot. Type I corrects actively with contraction of the peroneus. This can be done by stroking the lateral aspect of the child's foot. Type II can be corrected passively, but the child is unable to correct the position using muscle contraction. Type III is rigid and does not correct with passive motion testing. Type I usually resolves spontaneously, although osteopathic treatment can be beneficial. Type II responds to osteopathic manipulation, although treatment is prolonged and an at-home stretching program may need to be implemented. Children with Type I and II should be followed to ensure that the foot does not become rigid. Type III requires casting for correction, although a short course of osteopathic treatment may sometimes improve flexibility and response to passive correction.

COMMON PROBLEMS IN THE UPPER EXTREMITY

The upper extremity, suspended from one small articulation at the sternum and several myofascial structures surrounding the upper thorax, exhibits exquisitely fine movement patterns and extraordinary strength. It is rare for a problem

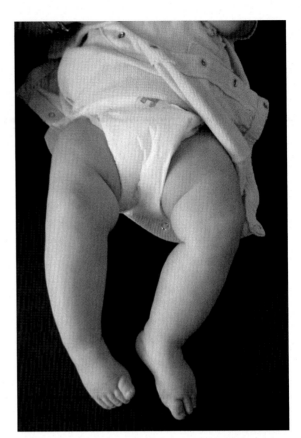

Fig. 15.24 • Metatarsus adductus deformity of the right foot in a 4-week-old newborn. Internal torsion of the right is also present. Both moding deformities are probably from uterine lie. *Used with permission of the Willard & Carreiro Collection.*

in the upper extremity to exist without dysfunctional changes at both ends: the scapulothoracic area and shoulder complex, and the wrist and fingers. Determining which is primary can be a bit of a chicken and egg exercise, but all components need to be addressed before the patient can return to normal functional capacity. Motor retraining should involve the entire arm, from the shoulder stabilizers to the fine movements of the hands. The osteopathic concept of functional integrity plays an important role in optimum function in this area.

Shoulder complex

Rotator cuff strains

The muscles of the rotator cuff are the dynamic stabilizers of the glenohumeral joint. The subscapularis, supraspinatus, infraspinatus and teres minor muscles act in concert to compress the humeral head into the glenoid fossa and counterbalance the translational forces of larger muscles acting on the joint. Rotator cuff strains may be acute and traumatic or chronic and due to overuse or improper training practices. In general, problems of the rotator cuff range from microtears to complete tears. Four categories of classification are used to describe the pathological progression. Stage 1 injury describes microtrauma with inflammation. Stage 2 refers to tendonitis with fibrotic changes. Stage 3 is a partial thickness tear, a degeneration of the tendon. Stage 4 is a full-thickness tear in the tendon. Stage 4 occurs rarely in young athletes as a result of overuse, but it can occur with trauma. Rotator cuff strains develop due to abnormal mechanics in the shoulder complex. Prior to retraining the muscles of the cuff, any biomechanical dysfunction needs to be resolved. Key areas include the scapulothoracic joint and the clavicle. Once this is accomplished, muscle energy techniques are helpful in retraining the rotator cuff muscles.

Impingement syndrome

Impingement syndrome is most common in young swimmers, although tennis players and pitchers are also at risk. The supraspinatus and biceps tendons are most commonly involved due to the repetitive overhead motions involved with these sports. The syndrome represents a continuum of injury, beginning with microtrauma and inflammation and culminating in partial and complete tears of the tendon. Impingement syndrome is an example of an overuse syndrome. Repetitive activity creates microtrauma and inflammation. There is a resultant change in biomechanics and joint use that further exacerbates the strain. Preexisting or concomitant somatic dysfunction will exacerbate the problem and accelerate the process. Early presentations often include pain alleviated with rest. As the condition progresses, pain and inflammation are persistent and eventually joint instability will develop. Impingement syndrome is often seen as an extension of rotator cuff strain and described with a classification process similar to that used for the rotator cuff injury. Treatment should focus on decreasing inflammation, improving functional mechanics and proper retraining, including flexibility and strengthening of antagonist muscle groups. Depending upon the severity of the symptoms, the athlete may be required to stop swimming for an indeterminate amount of time. Steroid injections can be used sparingly in the initial phases of treatment to break the inflammation–irritation cycle. Injectable anesthetics such as Marcaine (bupivacaine) or procaine can be used to address the trigger points which typically develop in athletes with significant symptoms.

The elbow

Nursemaid's elbow

Nursemaid's elbow or subluxation of the radial head is probably the most well-known disorder of the elbow in children. It typically occurs in toddlers and young children secondary to an episode where the child wanted to go in one direction and the care-giver prevented it by holding the child's

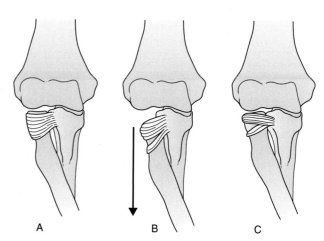

Fig. 15.25 • (A) Schematic diagram of the mechanism of nursemaid's elbow. As the radius is tractioned distally, the annular ligament slips over the head (B). The forces of tissue recoil pinch the ligament between the radial head and the humerus (C).

outstretched arm. The radial head of infants and small children is undeveloped and does not have the bulbous shape of the older child's. When the elbow is extended, longitudinal traction will pull the radius distally, and the annular ligament can slip over the top of the radial head. Tissue recoil through the interosseous membrane and somatic structures pulls the radius back towards the humerus, pinching the ligament between the two (Fig. 15.25). The mechanism of injury is usually a parent catching a falling child by an outstretched arm, or the care-giver trying to lift or pull the child by an outstretched arm. In either case the child presents with the elbow flexed and the hand held in a pronated position. This posture minimizes friction of the annular ligament. Treatment can be accomplished by gently but firmly stabilizing the humerus and radial head with one hand and supinating the hand and forearm while applying gentle traction. This usually reduces the annular ligament. Osteopathic treatment should then be directed at minimizing tissue congestion in the area and treating any associated findings. Depending on the severity and duration of the injury, the ligament may be inflamed and irritated following the reduction, so icing the area may be helpful. Proper instruction should be given to the care-givers to avoid future incidents. However, there is an increased risk for repeated injury once a nursemaid's elbow has occurred. This is probably due to the microdamage to the ligament.

Extensor tendonitis, tennis elbow and lateral epicondylitis

These conditions are similar in that they all involve the common extensor tendons or the wrist. They typically result from overuse due to overtraining, poor training practices, incorrect equipment, or poor form. As such all are more commonly seen in athletes and young adults, and are rare in young children. The common tendon of the wrist and finger extensors becomes inflamed and irritated as a result of repetitive wrist extension against resistance, but it may also occur as a result of forceful overloading of wrist flexors, or repetitive eccentric contraction of extensors against resistance. The activities most likely to increase a youth's risk for developing one of these lateral conditions are tennis and other racquet sports, bowling, batting (baseball, cricket) and weightlifting using wrist extensors. When severe, the pain may radiate into the distal arm along the radial side and tingling in the fourth and fifth digits is not uncommon. The condition can be categorized into three grades. Grade 1 is the mildest and presents as generalized ache over the lateral aspect of the elbow that is aggravated by the activity, but does not interfere with play. Symptoms resolve spontaneously once play is stopped. This represents the first stages of inflammation and tissue damage. If training practices and the mechanics of form are not addressed the condition will progress to grade 2 in which the pain becomes more localized at the tendon site with point tenderness to palpation. Edema often develops and the symptoms do not resolve when play is stopped. With continued progression, tingling in the digits and radiation of pain may occur. In grade 3 the persistent pain, inflammation and tissue damage result in weakness that interferes with normal activities. Inhibitory reflexes trigger compensatory adaptations in the shoulder, neck, and thorax, further aggravating the problem. Symptoms can be reproduced by active wrist extension against resistance, passive wrist flexion to stretch the extensor muscles, or active radial deviation against resistance. The differential diagnosis of severe or chronic lateral epicondylitis must include supinator syndrome (see below). The patient should be instructed to rest, and ice the area after activity. Treatment needs to include resolution of the biomechanical dysfunction that led to the irritation and retraining the involved muscles. Manipulation and retraining may be augmented by the use of injectable anesthetics in athletes with severe presentations.

Medial epicondylitis and flexor tendonitis

Inflammatory conditions of the medial elbow are less common than those of its lateral counterpart. They typically result from overloading or repetitive strain to the flexor muscles of the wrist and the pronator muscle. Irritation of the medial structures is more likely to occur with forceful or repetitive flexion and pronation against resistance. This can be seen in tennis players, golfers and pitchers (baseball, cricket), especially those working on perfecting their curve ball. Medial epicondylitis is characterized by three grades of injury, similar to lateral epicondylitis. In addition, if medial epicondylitis is left untreated the ulnar collateral ligament can also become inflamed, leading to joint instability. Treatment is similar to that for lateral epicondylitis.

Cubitus valgus and varus

Cubitus valgus exists if the 'carrying angle' is greater than the 5–15° described. This can be due to epiphyseal damage secondary to a lateral epicondylar fracture. It may cause delayed ulnar nerve palsy. Cubitus varus is a decrease in the carrying angle referred to as a 'gunstock deformity'. It is usually the result of trauma. A supracondylar fracture in a child which disturbs the distal humeral epiphyseal plate leads to this deformity.

Acute synovitis

Repeated small traumas or acute trauma may result in acute synovitis. This can occur with repeated falls backwards onto the flexed elbow. It is more likely to be seen in athletes playing contact sports. The joint cavity becomes distended with fluid. Owing to the posterior laxness of the capsule, the fluid bulges out around the olecranon. There may also be some swelling around the radial head, or the elbow may assume a fusiform shape secondary to the accumulated fluid. Treatment includes rest, ice, avoidance of trauma, and manual techniques aimed at improving venous and lymphatic drainage. There is a small risk that the synovial fluid may become infected; this requires immediate attention.

The wrist

The wrist is a complex system composed of many articulations which function as three articular segments: the distal carpal row, the proximal carpal row and the radioulnar articulation. These segments act as two articular complexes: the midcarpal joint and the radiocarpal joint. There are no direct muscular attachments to the proximal carpal row, so it acts as an intermediary between the radial articulation and the distal carpal row. The proximal row has been described as an intercalated segment, a relatively unattached middle segment of a three-segment linkage (Norkin & Levangie 1992).

Scapulolunate ligament strain

The scapulolunate ligament is the most frequently injured ligament in the wrist. It is intimately related to the position of the proximal capitate through its connections to the lunate and scaphoid. Movement of the lunate and scaphoid occurs around the capitate. The scapholunate ligament limits rotation of the scaphoid upon the radio-scaphocapitate ligament. The pain is usually deep and poorly localized to the radial side of the wrist. It is worse with pronation and supination while the fist is clenched or the hand is supporting something. The injury most commonly occurs in skiing due to forces transmitted through the ski poles, gymnastics and racquet sports. As with other ligamentous injuries, repetitive action will worsen the condition. Rest, correction of biomechanical dysfunction, and retraining in proper grip and forearm mechanics must be part of the treatment plan.

Scaphoid bone avascular necrosis

The scaphoid is the most frequently fractured carpal bone (70%). In a minority of individuals, the nutrient foramina are located in the distal portion of the bone, increasing the risk of non-union in a fracture along the 'waist' of the bone. The space of Poirier lies between the deltoid ligament and the insertions of the radiolunate and ulnolunate ligaments. There is a synovial outpouching overlying the capitolunate articulation. This area is inherently weak and susceptible to flexion- and extension-type injuries. Children suspected of having avascular necrosis of the scaphoid should be urgently referred to an orthopedic surgeon.

References

Ahmed M, Bjurholm A, Kreicbergs A et al 1993 Sensory and autonomic innervation of the facet joint in the rat lumbar spine. Spine 18: 2121–2126.

Argenta L C, David L R, Wilson J A et al 1996 An increase in infant cranial deformity with supine sleeping position. J Craniofac Surg 7: 5–11.

Ashton I K, Eisenstein S M 1996 The effect of substance P on proliferation and proteoglycan deposition of cells derived from rabbit intervertebral disc. Spine 21: 421–426.

Auleley G R 1998 Validation of Ottawa ankle rules. Ann Emerg Med 32(1): 14–18.

Balague F, Dutoit G, Waldburger M 1998 Low back pain in school children: an epidemiological study. Scand J Rehabil Med 20: 175–179.

Baranello G, Vasco G, Ricci D et al 2007 Visual function in nonsyndromic craniosynostosis: past, present, and future. Childs Nerv Syst 23: 1461–1465.

Becker D B, Petersen J D, Kane A A et al 2005 Speech, cognitive, and behavioral outcomes in nonsyndromic craniosynostosis. Plast Reconstr Surg 116: 400–407.

Bonaventure J, El G V 2003 Molecular and cellular bases of syndromic craniosynostoses. Expert Rev Mol Med 5: 1–17.

Bowen V, Cassidy J D 1981 Macroscopic and microscopic anatomy of the sacroiliac joint from embryonic life until the eighth decade. Spine 6: 620–628.

Bunnell W A 1982 Back pain in children. Orthop Clin North Am 13: 587–604.

Cheng J C, Au A W 1994 Infantile torticollis: a review of 624 cases. J Pediatr Orthop 14: 802–808.

Clarren S K 1981 Plagiocephaly and torticollis: etiology, natural history, and helmet treatment. J Pediatr 98: 92–95.

Cottalorda J, Rahmani A, Diop M et al 2003 Influence of school bag carrying on gait kinetics. J Pediatr Orthop B12: 357–364.

Dias M S, Klein D M 1996 Occipital plagiocephaly: deformation or lambdoid synostosis? II. A unifying theory regarding pathogenesis. Pediatr Neurosurg 24: 69–73.

Ebara S, Iatridis J C, Setton L A et al 1996 Tensile properties of nondegenerate human lumbar anulus fibrosus. Spine 21: 452–461.

Ghosh P 1990 Basic biochemistry of the intervertebral disc and its variation with ageing and degeneration. Journal of Manual Medicine 5: 48–51.

Gillette R G, Kramis R C, Roberts W J 1994 Sympathetic activation of cat spinal neurons responsive to noxious stimulation of deep tissues in the low back. Pain 56: 31–42.

Groen G J, Baljet B, Drukker J 1990 Nerves and nerves plexuses of the human vertebral column. Am J Anat 188: 282–296.

Herman M J, Pizzutillo P D, Cavalier R 2003 Spondylolysis and spondylolisthesis in the child and adolescent athlete. Orthop Clin North Am 34: 461–467.

Hobbs S F, Chandler M J, Bolser D C et al 1992 Segmental organization of visceral and somatic input onto C3-T6 spinothalamic tract cells of the monkey. J Neurophysiol 68: 1575–1588.

Hoyte D A 1991 The cranial base in normal and abnormal skull growth. Neurosurg Clin N Am 2: 515–537.

Hunenko O, Karmacharya J, Ong G et al 2001 Toward an understanding of nonsyndromic craniosynostosis: altered patterns of TGF-beta receptor and FGF receptor expression induced by intrauterine head constraint. Ann Plast Surg 46: 546–553.

Hutton W C 1990 The forces acting on a lumbar intervertebral joint. Journal of Manual Medicine 5: 66–67.

Iatridis J C, Weidenbaum M, Setton L A et al 1996 Is the nucleus pulposus a solid or a fluid? Mechanical behaviors of the nucleus pulposus of the human intervertebral disc. Spine 21: 1174–1184.

Jinkins J R 1993 The pathoanatomic basis of somatic and autonomic syndromes originating in the lumbosacral spine. Lumbosacral Spine 3(3): 443–463.

Kapp-Simon K A, Figueroa A, Jocher C A et al 1993 Longitudinal assessment of mental development in infants with nonsyndromic craniosynostosis with and without cranial release and reconstruction. Plast Reconstr Surg 92: 831–839.

Kapp-Simon K A, Speltz M L, Cunningham M L et al 2007 Neurodevelopment of children with single suture craniosynostosis: a review. Childs Nerv Syst 23: 269–281.

Kimonis V, Gold J A, Hoffman T L et al 2007 Genetics of craniosynostosis. Semin Pediatr Neurol 14: 150–161.

Kindsfater K, Lowe T, Lawellin D et al 1994 Levels of platelet calmodulin for the prediction of progression and severity of adolescent idiopathic scoliosis. J Bone Joint Surg [Am] 76(8): 1186–1192.

King H A 1999 Back pain in children. Orthop Clin North Am 30(3): 467–474.

Kirschner R E, Gannon F H, Xu J et al 2002 Craniosynostosis and altered patterns of fetal TGF-beta expression induced by intrauterine constraint. Plast Reconstr Surg 109: 2338–2346.

Leboeuf-Yde C, Kyvik K O 1999 Low back pain and lifestyle, II: obesity. Information from a population-based sample of 29,424 twin subjects. Spine 24: 779–784.

Lehman S 2006 Strabismus in craniosynostosis. Curr Opin Ophthalmol 17: 432–434.

Littlefield T R, Kelly K M, Pomatto J K et al 1999 Multiple-birth infants at higher risk for development of deformational plagiocephaly. Pediatrics 103: 565–569.

Machida M 1999 Cause of idiopathic scoliosis. Spine 24(24): 2576–2583.

Machida M, Dubousset J, Imamura Y et al 1996 Melatonin – a possible role in pathogenesis of adolescent idiopathic scoliosis. Spine 21(10): 1147–1152.

Macintosh J E, Bogduk N 1986 The biomechanics of the lumbar multifidus. Clin Biomech 1: 205–213.

Magge S N, Westerveld M, Pruzinsky T et al 2002 Long-term neuropsychological effects of sagittal craniosynostosis on child development. J Craniofac Surg 13: 99–104.

Magoun H I S 1973 Idiopathic adolescent spinal scoliosis. The DO 13(6).

Micheli L J, Wood R 1995 Back pain in the young athlete: significant differences from adults: causes and patterns. Arch Pediatr Adolesc Med 149: 15–18.

Mulliken J B, Vander Woude D L, Hansen M et al 1999 Analysis of posterior plagiocephaly: deformational versus synostotic. Plast Reconstr Surg 103: 371–380.

Negrini S, Carabalona R 2002 Backpacks on! Schoolchildren's perceptions of load, associations with back pain and factors determining the load. Spine 27: 187–195.

Norkin C C, Levangie P C 1992 Joint structure and function. F A Davis, Philadelphia.

Olmarker K, Nordborg C, Larsson K et al 1996 Ultrastructural changes in spinal nerve roots induced by autologous nucleus pulposus. Spine 21: 411–414.

Olsen T L, Anderson R L, Dearwater S R et al 1992 The epidemiology of low back pain in the adolescent population. Am J Public Health 82: 606–609.

Pang D, Veetai L 2004 Atlantoaxial rotatory fixation: part 1 – biomechanics of normal rotation at the atlantoaxial joint in children. Neurosurgery 55: 614–626.

Pascoe D D, Pascoe D E, Wang Y T et al 1997 Influence of carrying book bags on gait cycle and posture of youths. Ergonomics 40: 631–641.

Passos-Bueno M R, Serti Eacute A E, Jehee F S et al 2008 Genetics of craniosynostosis: genes, syndromes, mutations and genotype–phenotype correlations. Front Oral Biol 12: 107–143.

Pedersen H E, Blunck C F J, Gardner E 1956 The anatomy of lumbosacral posterior rami and meningeal branches of spinal nerves (sinu-vertebral nerves). J Bone Joint Surg [Am] 36: 377–391.

Peitsch W K, Keefere C H, LaBrie R A et al 2002 Incidence of cranial asymmetry in healthy newborns. Pediatrics 110(6): E72.

Philippi H, Faldum A, Jung T et al 2006a Patterns of postural asymmetry in infants: a standardized video-based analysis. Eur J Pediatr 165: 158–164.

Philippi H, Faldum A, Schleupen A et al 2006b Infantile postural asymmetry and osteopathic treatment: a randomized therapeutic trial. Dev Med Child Neurol 48: 5–9.

Pincott J R, Taffs L F 1982 Experimental scoliosis in primates: a neurological cause. J Bone Joint Surg [Br] 64(4): 503–507.

Pincott J R, Davies J S, Taffs L F 1984 Scoliosis caused by section of dorsal spinal nerve roots. J Bone Joint Surg [Br] 66(1): 27–29.

Schott G D 1994 Visceral afferents: their contribution to 'sympathetic dependent' pain. Brain 117: 397–413.

Sheir-Neiss G I, Kruse R W, Rahman T et al 2003 The association of backpack use and back pain in adolescents. Spine 28: 922–930.

Smartt J M Jr, Karmacharya J, Gannon F H 2005 Intrauterine fetal constraint induces chondrocyte apoptosis and premature ossification of the cranial base. Plast Reconstr Surg 116: 1363–1369.

Standring S 2004 Gray's anatomy, 39th edn. Churchill Livingstone, New York.

Taylor J R 1990 The development and structure of lumbar intervertebral discs. Journal of Manual Medicine 5: 43–47.

Twomey L, Taylor Jr 1990 Structural and mechanical disc changes with age. Journal of Manual Medicine 5: 58–61.

Turk A E, McCarthy J G, Thorne C H et al 1996 The 'back to sleep campaign' and deformational plagiocephaly: is there a cause for concern? J Craniofac Surg 7: 12–18.

Yamada K, Yamamoto H, Nakagawa Y et al 1984 Etiology of idiopathic scoliosis. Clin Orthop Relat Res 184: 50–57.

Zaleske D J, Ehrlich M G, Hall J E 1980 Association of glycosaminoglycan depletion and degradative enzyme activity in scoliosis. Clin Orthop Relat Res: 177–181.

Further reading

Adams M A, Dolan P 1995 Posture and spinal mechanisms during lifting. In: Vleeming A, Mooney V, Snijders C J et al (eds) The integrated function of the lumbar spine and sacroiliac joints. European Conference Organ, Rotterdam: 19–28.

Adams M A, Dolan P 1995 Recent advances in lumbar spinal mechanics and their clinical significance. Clin Biomech 10(1): 3–19.

Andrews J R, Whiteside J A 1993 Common elbow problems in the athlete. J Orthop Sports Phys Ther 17: 289–295.

Anetzberger H, Putz R 1996 The scapula: principles of construction and stress. Acta Anat (Basel) 156(1): 70–80.

Arbuckle J D, McGrouther D A 1995 Measurement of the arc of digital flexion and joint movement ranges. J Hand Surg [Br] 20B(6): 836–840.

Archer I A, Dickson R A 1985 Stature and idiopathic scoliosis. A prospective study. J Bone Joint Surg [Br] 67: 185–188.

Ash H E, Joyce T J, Unsworth A 1996 Biomechanics of the distal upper limb. Curr Orthop 10(1): 25–36.

Balague F, Dutoit G, Waldburger M 1998 Low back pain in school children: an epidemiological study. Scand J Rehabil Med 20: 175–179.

Beal M C 1982 The sacroiliac problem: review of anatomy, mechanics and diagnosis. J Am Osteopath Assoc 81: 667–679.

Beal M C, Dvorak J 1984 Palpatory examination of the spine: a comparison of the results of two methods and their relationship to visceral disease. Manual Medicine 1: 25–32.

Beard R W, Highman J H, Pearce S et al 1984 Diagnosis of pelvic varicosities in women with chronic pelvic pain. Lancet ii: 946–949.

Beard R W, Reginald P W, Wadsworth J 1988a Clinical features of women with chronic lower abdominal pain and pelvic congestion. BJOG 95: 153–161.

Beard R, Reginald P, Pearce S 1988b Psychological and somatic factors in women with pain due to pelvic congestion. Adv Exp Med Biol 245: 413–421.

Berthier N E, Clifton R K, McCall D D et al 1999 Proximodistal structure of early reaching in human infants. Exp Brain Res 127(3): 259–269.

Binder H, Eng G D, Gaiser J F et al 1987 Congenital muscular torticollis: results of conservative management with long-term follow-up in 85 cases. Arch Phys Med Rehabil 68: 222–225.

Britz G W, Haynor D R, Kuntz C et al 1996 Ulnar nerve entrapment at the elbow: correlation of magnetic resonance imaging, clinical, electrodiagnostic, and intraoperative findings. Neurosurgery 38(3): 458–465.

Browning J E 1990 Mechanically induced pelvic pain and organic dysfunction in a patient without low back pain. J Manipulative Physiol Ther 13: 406–411.

Burnett C, Johnson E 1971 Development of gait in childhood II. Dev Med Child Neurol 13(2): 207–215.

Canale S T, Griffin D W, Hubbard C N 1982 Congenital muscular torticollis. A long-term follow-up. J Bone Joint Surg [Am] 64: 810–816.

Cathie A 1974 Applied anatomy, the Angus Cathie Yearbook. AAO, Indianapolis.

Dandy D J 1996 Chronic patellofemoral instability. J Bone Joint Surg [Br] 78(2): 328–335.

Dorman T A, Vleeming A 1995 Self-locking of the sacroiliac articulation. Spine 9: 407–418.

Fernandez-Bermejo E, Garcia-Jimenez M A, Fernandez-Palomeque C et al 1993 Adolescent idiopathic scoliosis and joint laxity. Spine 18: 918–922.

Fuss F K, Wagner T F 1996 Biomechanical alterations in the carpal arch and hand muscles after carpal tunnel release: a further approach toward understanding the function of the flexor retinaculum and the cause of postoperative grip weakness. Clin Anat 9(2): 100–108.

Gordon A M, Soechting J F 1995 Use of tactile afferent information in sequential finger movements. Exp Brain Res 107(2): 281–292.

Greenman P E 1990 Clinical aspects of sacroiliac function in walking. Journal of Manual Medicine 5: 125–130.

Greenman P E 1991 Principles of manipulation of the cervical spine. Journal of Manual Medicine 6: 106–113.

Gwinnutt C L 1988 Injury to the axillary nerve. Anaesthesia 43(3): 205–206.

Haggard P, Hutchinson K, Stein J 1995 Patterns of coordinated multi-joint movement. Exp Brain Res 107(2): 254–266.

Hall J E 1996 Three-dimensional effect of the Boston brace on the thoracic spine and rib cage – point of view. Spine 21(1): 64.

Hamanishi C, Tanaka S 1994 Turned head-adducted hip truncal curvature syndrome. Arch Dis Child 70: 515–519.

Hay M C 1976 Anatomy of the lumbar spine. Med J Aust 1(23): 874–876.

Hollowell J P, Vollmer D G, Wilson C R et al 1996 Biomechanical analysis of thoracolumbar interbody constructs – how important is the endplate? Spine 21(9): 1032–1036.

Horton W C, Holt R T, Muldowny D S 1996 Controversy fusion of L5–S1 in adult scoliosis. Spine 21(21): 2520–2522.

Johnston R B, Seiler J G, Miller E J et al 1995 The intrinsic and extrinsic ligaments of the wrist. A correlation of collagen typing and histologic appearance. J Hand Surg [Br] 20(6): 750–754.

Kaigle A M, Holm S H, Hansson T H 1995 Experimental instability in the lumbar spine. Spine 20(4): 421–430.

Kalin P J, Hirsche B E 1987 The origins and function of the interosseous muscles of the foot. J Anat 152: 83–91.

Kapandji I A 1982 The physiology of the joints. Churchill Livingstone, Edinburgh.

Kissling R O 1995 The mobility of the sacro-iliac joint in healthy subjects. In: Vleeming A, Mooney V, Dorman T et al (eds) The integrated function of the lumbar spine and sacroiliac joint. ECO, Rotterdam: 411–422.

Klein P, Mattys S, Rooze M 1996 Moment arm length variations of selected muscles acting on talocrural and subtalar joints during movement: an in vitro study. J Biomech 29(1): 21–30.

Klein-Nulend J, van der Plas A, Semeins C M et al 1995 Sensitivity of osteocytes to biomechanical stress in vitro. FASEB J 9(5): 441–445.

Lehman G J, McGill S M 1999 The influence of a chiropractic manipulation on lumbar kinematics and electromyography during simple and complex tasks: a case study. J Manipulative Physiol Ther 22(9): 576–581.

McGregor A H, McCarthy I D, Hughes S P 1995 Motion characteristics of the lumbar spine in the normal population. Spine 20(22): 2421–2428.

Macintosh J E, Bogduk N 1986 The biomechanics of the lumbar multifidus. Clin Biomech 1: 205–213.

Machida M, Murai I, Miyashita Y et al 1999 Pathogenesis of idiopathic scoliosis. Experimental study in rats. Spine 24(19): 1985–1989.

Macintosh J E, Bogduk N 1990 Basic biomechanics pertinent to the study of the lumbar disc. Journal of Manual Medicine 5: 52–57.

Macintosh J E, Valencia F, Bogduk N et al 1986 The morphology of the human lumbar multifidus. Clin Biomech 1: 196–204.

Matsen F A, Harryman D T, Sidles J A 1991 Mechanics of glenohumeral instability. Clin Sports Med 10: 783–788.

Mitchell F L, Moran P S, Pruzzo N A 1979 An evaluation and treatment manual of osteopathic muscle energy procedures. Mitchell, Moran and Pruzzo, Valley Park, MO.

Morrey B F, An K N 1983 Articular and ligamentous contributions to the stability of the elbow joint. Am J Sports Med 11: 315–319.

Mosca V S 1995 Flexible flatfoot and skewfoot. J Bone Joint Surg [Am] 77(12): 1937–1945.

Moseley L, Smith R, Hunt A et al 1996 Three-dimensional kinematics of the rearfoot during the stance phase of walking in normal young adult males. Clin Biomech 11(1): 39–45.

Nordin M, Frankel V H 1989 Basic biomechanics of the musculoskeletal system. Lea & Febiger, Philadelphia.

Oda I, Abumi K, Lü D S et al 1996 Biomechanical role of the posterior elements, costovertebral joints, and rib cage in the stability of the thoracic spine. Spine 21(12): 1423–1429.

Ogon M, Haid C, Krismer M et al 1996 The possibility of creating lordosis and correcting scoliosis simultaneously after partial disc removal – balance lines of lumbar motion segments. Spine 21(21): 2458–2462.

Panjabi M M, White A 1990 Clinical biomechanics of the spine. J B Lippincott, Philadelphia.

Pappas A D, Goss T P, Kleinman P K 1983 Symptomatic shoulder instability due to lesions of the glenoid labrum. Am J Sports Med 11: 279–288.

Patwardhan A G, Rimkus A, Gavin T M et al 1996 Geometric analysis of coronal decompensation in idiopathic scoliosis. Spine 21(10): 1192–1200.

Perry J 1983 Anatomy and biomechanics of the hindfoot. Clin Orthop Relat Res 177: 9–15.

Prasad R, Vettivel S, Isaac B et al 1996 Angle of torsion of the femur and its correlates. Clin Anat 9(2): 109–117.

Raschke U, Chaffin D B 1996 Trunk and hip muscle recruitment in response to external anterior lumbosacral shear and moment loads. Clin Biomech 11(3): 145–152.

Reddy N P, Krouskop T A, Newell P H Jr 1975 Biomechanics of a lymphatic vessel. Blood Vessels 12: 261–278.

Regan W D, Korinek B F, An K N 1991 Biomechanical study of ligaments around the elbow joint. Clin Orthop Relat Res 271: 170–179.

Rodosky M W, Harner C D, Fu F H 1994 The role of the long head of the biceps muscle and superior glenoid labrum in anterior stability of the shoulder. Am J Sports Med 22: 121–130.

Rupp S, Berninger K, Hopf T 1995 Shoulder problems in high level swimmers – impingement, anterior instability, muscular imbalance? Int J Sports Med 16(8): 557–562.

Scholz J P, Millford J P, McMillan A G 1995 Neuromuscular coordination of squat lifting, I: effect of load magnitude. Phys Ther 75(2): 119–132.

Shekelle P G, Coulter I 1997 Cervical spine manipulation: summary report of a systematic review of the literature and a multidisciplinary expert panel. J Spinal Disord 10(3): 223–228.

Snijders C J, Vleeming A, Stoeckart R 1993 Transfer of the lumbarsacral load to iliac bones and legs. Clin Biomech 8: 285–294.

Soslowsky L J, An C H, Carpenter J E 1994 Geometric and mechanical properties or the coracoacromial ligament and their relationship to rotator cuff disease. Clin Orthop Relat Res 304: 10–17.

St John D, Mulliken J B, Kaban L B et al 2002 Anthropometric analysis of mandibular asymmetry in infants with deformational posterior plagiocephaly. J Oral Maxillofac Surg 60: 873–877.

Steinberg B G, Plancher K D 1995 Clinical anatomy of the wrist and elbow. Clin Sports Med 14: 299–313.

Stroyan M, Wilk K E 1993 The functional anatomy of the elbow complex. J Orthop Sports Phys Ther 17: 279–288.

Stubbs M, Harris M, Solomonow M et al 1998 Ligamento-muscular protective reflex in the lumbar spine of the feline. J Electromyogr Kinesiol 8(4): 197–204.

Sutherland D, Olsen R, Cooper L et al 1980 The development of mature gait. J Bone Joint Surg [Am] 62: 354–363.

Taylor J R, Slinger B S 1980 Scoliosis screening and growth in Western Australian students. Med J Aust 1: 475–478.

Thompson S K 1980 Prognosis in infantile idiopathic scoliosis. J Bone Joint Surg [Br] 62: 151–154.

Van Dieen J H, Boke B, Oosterhuis W et al 1996 The influence of torque and velocity on erector spinae muscle fatigue and its relationship to changes of electromyogram spectrum density. Eur J Appl Physiol 72(4): 310–315.

Vleeming A, Pool-Goudzwaard A L, Stoeckart R et al 1995 The posterior layer of the thoracolumbar fascia: its function in load transfer from spine to legs. Spine 20: 753–758.

Vleeming A, Snijders C J, Stoeckart R et al 1995 A new light on low back pain: the selflocking mechanism of the sacroiliac joints and its implication for sitting, standing and walking. In: Vleeming A, Mooney V, Snijders C J et al (eds) The integrated function of the lumbar spine and sacroiliac joints. European Conference Organ, Rotterdam: 149–168.

Walsh J J, Morrissy R T 1998 Torticollis and hip dislocation. J Pediatr Orthop 18: 219–221.

Willard F H, Carreiro J E, Manko W, 1998 The long posterior interosseous ligament and the sacrococcygeal plexus. Third interdisciplinary World Congress on Low Back and Pelvic Pain.

Wu P B, Date E S, Kingery W S 2000 The lumbar multifidus muscle is polysegmentally innervated. Electromyogr Clin Neurophysiol 40(8): 483–485.

Yahia L, Rhalmi S, Newman N et al 1992 Sensory innervation of human thoracolumbar fascia. An immunohistochemical study. Acta Orthop Scand 63(2): 195–197.

Chapter Sixteen

Neurology

CHAPTER CONTENTS

CLASSIFICATION OF NERVE INJURY

The pathophysiological changes occurring in injured nerves can be categorized into five groups or degrees of injury. Prognosis for recovery is related to the extent of the disruption of nerve morphology. First-degree injury occurs when nerve compression increases intraneural pressure, and conduction across the site of compression is blocked. This form of injury may result from swelling of adjacent tissues. There is no disruption of axonal anatomy, and once the compression is relieved, recovery is complete. If the compression is not relieved, second-degree involvement occurs. There is obstruction of neural veins and arteries, resulting in interruption of axoplasmic and nutrient flow. Pathological changes and degeneration occur in the myelin sheath and axons. Like first-degree injury, these changes are reversible if the compression is relieved. The axon and myelin are capable of regenerating, and although recovery may take 8 or more weeks, it is complete. Third-degree involvement occurs with prolonged or intense compression. There is venous congestion, obstruction of axoplasmic flow, myelin degeneration and disruption of the endoneural tubes. Unlike the axon and myelin, the endoneural tubes have poor regenerative capabilities. Consequently, recovery is incomplete in third-degree injuries. Partial or complete transection of the nerve disrupts the perineurium and requires surgical repair. Recovery is poor.

BRACHIAL PLEXUS OR ERB'S PALSY

The brachial plexus may be damaged during labor or delivery. The mechanism of injury is usually stretching of the involved nerve roots, or compression of the neurovascular bundle. The latter has a better prognosis. The most severe form of injury involves damage to the nerve from traction. The birth history is usually complicated, and the baby

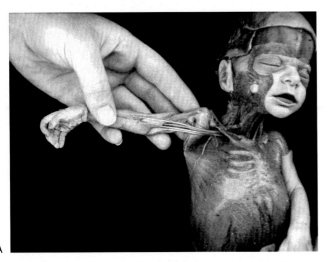 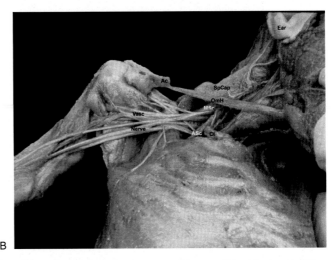

Fig. 16.1 • (A) Dissection of a 36-week gestation specimen. The pectoralis major and minor have been removed to reveal the neurovascular bundle in the right axillary fossa. Considerable connective tissue and fat needed to be removed from this space in order to clearly see the neurovascular structures. (B) A close-up of the axillary fossa. The clavicle (Cl) has been cut and removed. The omohyoid (OmH), anterior and middle scalene (ASc, MSc) muscles, splenius capitis (SpCap) and acromion process (Ac) are labeled. *Used with permission of the Willard & Carreiro Collection.*

large for gestational age. The nerve roots may be damaged when the head has delivered and there is shoulder dystocia. Hyperextension of the head may stretch the nerve roots in the cervical spine. In this scenario the roots of C5 and C6 are most commonly damaged. Confirmation can be made by electromyographic (EMG) studies.

The less severe form of brachial plexus palsy results from compression of the neurovascular bundle. This may occur from musculoskeletal forces or edema, as in severe torticollis, shoulder dislocation or clavicle fracture. In either case, active and immediate rehabilitation needs to be implemented to prevent the development of contractures and adhesions.

Diagnosis

The shoulder on the involved side will be limp, but the hand and wrist are typically flexed if C5 and C6 have been damaged by stretch. Conversely, if the problem is due to compression of the neurovascular bundle, the entire arm and hand may be affected, with weakness but not necessarily flaccidity; pulses will be weak and the extremity slightly cool to the touch when compared with the other. Swelling and color changes may or may not be present, depending upon the extent of the injury. In both cases, the Moro response is asymmetrical, as is the grasp reflex.

Pathophysiology of neurovascular compression

The neurovascular bundle to the upper extremity passes between the clavicle and first rib as it leaves the torso to

enter the axilla. The subclavian artery rides over the clavicle and joins the neural bundle to pass between the anterior and middle scalenes. These muscles are primary muscles of inspiration and are particularly active in the newborn. Joining the subclavian vein, these structures travel between the first rib and clavicle just deep to the subclavius muscle. This is a very narrow space filled with connective tissue and fat (Fig. 16.1). The scalene muscles are often involved in torticollis in the newborn. Abnormal tension in these muscles will raise the ribs, narrowing the infraclavicular space and potentially compressing its neural contents. The bundle then passes under the pectoralis minor muscle; although this is a small muscle, it forms the anterior wall of the tunnel. Edema within the axilla or infraclavicular space may compress the neural structures and impede normal function. A history of torticollis or clavicular fracture suggests neural entrapment or compression.

Osteopathic examination

Osteopathic findings associated with compression of the brachial plexus include scalene spasm or restricted clavicular motion on the involved side. There is palpable edema in the axilla or paraclavicular area. Internal rotation of the humerus or depression of the scapula may be a result of pectoralis involvement. Scalene spasm lifts the ribs and may shift the position of the scapula, narrowing the brachial passageway by affecting clavicle position. When signs of neural and/or vascular entrapment or compression are present, tissue strains should be addressed to promote vascular and lymphatic flow. Passive movement therapy should be instituted as soon as possible to ensure complete return of normal extremity function.

FACIAL NERVE PALSY

Facial muscle paralysis may result from damage or irritation to the facial nerve, its radiations or nucleus. When presentation is unilateral, involving both upper and lower aspects of the face, one can be confident that the etiology is a peripheral neuropathy involving the nerve after it exits the brainstem as opposed to a central process. Insults occurring within the brain do not present with involvement of the frontalis or orbicular muscles. Evaluating these muscles in the infant or toddler can be quite challenging. Engaging the child in playful enterprise with the modus of generating exaggerated facial expression will often work in the toddler and older child. Corneal testing may be used to elicit contraction of the orbicularis oculi muscle. Gently touching the cornea with the tip of a cotton swab should result in closure of the eyelid if the motor function is intact.

Evaluation of the infant may require stimulating a crying episode to observe facial muscle activity. This is often more difficult to do than one might expect. Facial nerve palsy may also result in decreased or absent tears in the involved eye, and loss of taste and salivary gland function, depending upon the location of the insult. Assessing the presence of tears may be challenging in very young infants whose tear production is still immature. Evaluating chorda tympani involvement can also be a trial in very young children, although examination of the papillae of the tongue may show atrophy on the involved side.

Neurological damage to the peripheral nerve (after it exits the brainstem) may occur secondary to direct mechanical injury or infectious/inflammatory process. The most common etiology for facial nerve palsy is injury or irritation from physical or chemical insult along the nerve, either after it exits the styloid foramen or within the facial canal. It is most often deemed idiopathic and given the diagnosis of Bell's palsy. Facial nerve palsy is less common in toddlers and children than in adolescents and newborns. In the newborn, injury to the peripheral nerve may result from forceps delivery; in the adolescent, it most often occurs secondary to facial or cervical trauma or viral illness.

Functional anatomy

The facial nerve leaves the brainstem and traverses through the facial canal located in the petrous portion of the temporal bone to exit at the stylomastoid foramen. Along the way, it gives off three branches. Most proximally, at the level of the geniculate ganglion, the greater superficial petrosal nerve exits the canal, carrying parasympathetic fibers to the lacrimal, palatal and nasal glands and the sphenopalatine ganglion. The second branch to be given off is the nerve to the stapedius muscle. The chorda tympani is the third branch, which leaves the facial nerve while it is still in

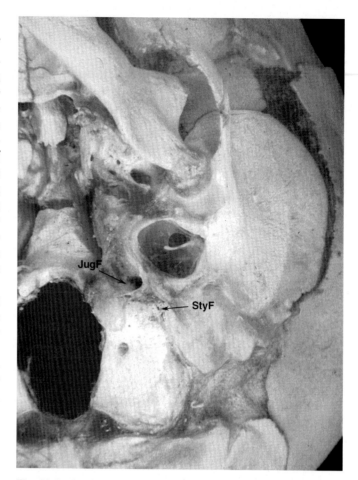

Fig. 16.2 • Inferior view of a fetal skull. Note the position of the stylomastoid foramen (StyF) and jugular foramen (JugF). The mastoid process has not yet developed. *Used with permission of the Willard & Carreiro Collection.*

the facial canal. At the terminal end of the canal, the facial nerve passes through the stylomastoid foramen, a small aperture around which many muscles and connective tissue structures of the neck make their attachments. In the adult, this foramen is protected to some extent by the mastoid process. However, newborns and young infants do not have mastoid processes (Fig. 16.2). There is a mastoid portion out of which the process will develop in response to the forces of the neck lengthening and the attachment of the sternocleidomastoid muscle. Air cells of the middle ear will expand into the resulting prominence, producing the mastoid air cells. This process will occur over the first 6 or 7 years of life, in concert with changes in the cranial base.

Accompanying the nerve through the facial canal is an extensive venous complex (Fig. 16.3). The proximal third of this complex drains back towards the cranium into the lesser petrosal sinus, and the distal two-thirds drain into the deep venous plexus of the lateral neck. This extracranial plexus is surrounded by the connective tissue and muscles of the cervical area. Fascial or muscular strains in this

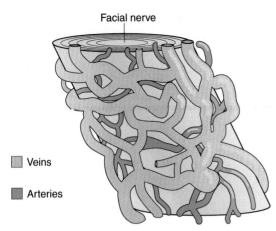

Facial nerve

■ Veins

■ Arteries

Fig. 16.3 • Schematic diagram depicting the facial nerve and the dense venous plexus which accompanies it through the facial canal. *Adapted from reconstruction of actual histological sections.*

area may produce venous congestion within the plexus. The resulting increased pressure within the canal will compromise function of the microscopic vasculature of the nerve itself, i.e. the vasa nervorum. Alterations in arterial or venous function of the facial nerve have the potential to affect conduction times and stimulate the release of proinflammatory substances by nociceptors traveling with the vascular structures. This could lead to first- or second-degree injury. This same mechanism is probably responsible for many cases of idiopathic facial nerve palsy in adults.

The facial nerve may be injured anywhere along its course, from the brainstem through the internal auditory meatus, along the facial canal, out of the stylomastoid foramen and over the facial muscles. Presenting signs and symptoms will reflect the location of the insult. The course of the facial nerve can be divided into five compartments: internal auditory canal, labyrinthine segment, tympanic segment, mastoid segment and extracranial portion. As the facial nerve leaves the brainstem, it is joined by the vestibulocochlear nerve. Damage occurring intracranially or at the internal auditory meatus is associated with auditory and vestibular signs and symptoms. The seventh and eighth cranial nerves part at the entrance to the facial canal. The first part of the canal passes between the cochlea and vestibular labyrinth and is referred to as the labyrinthine segment. This is the narrowest section of the canal. Consequently, the nerve is quite vulnerable to compression from inflammation or vascular congestion as it traverses this area. Furthermore, the arterial supply to the nerve is compromised, because this is the only area along the length of the nerve without collateral blood supply. The rest of the facial nerve is supplied by arterial arcades. If this segment of the nerve is damaged, everything distal to it will be affected. In addition to the hemifacial palsy, the motor fibers to the lacrimal and parotid glands will be affected, as will those to the stapedius

and chorda tympani. There will be absence of tears along with the other expected signs of facial nerve palsy.

Once past the narrow labyrinthine portion of the canal, the facial nerve makes a U-shaped turn and enters the tympanic segment. The wall of this segment is very thin compared to the rest of the canal, and fenestrations may be present. Chronic infection of the middle ear may lead to abscess or granulomatous formation, which can affect the nerve. The nerve to the stapedius muscle exits from the labyrinthine segment. Injury to the facial nerve in this portion of the canal results in hyperacusis, loss of taste and facial nerve palsy without loss of tears. The mastoid segment lies in the fourth portion of the canal. This segment travels inferiorly to the stylomastoid foramen. Insult to the nerve along the mastoid portion presents as loss of taste and ipsilateral facial paralysis. As the facial nerve exits the stylomastoid foramen, it passes through fascial tissue. In infants and young children, the nerve lies directly under the skin and subcutaneous tissues. As the mastoid process develops, this bony structure provides some protection to the nerve. However, injury to the extracranial portion may result from direct trauma or mechanical compression. It presents as unilateral facial paralysis without hyperacusis, decreased tearing or loss of taste.

Diagnosis and treatment

Congenital facial palsy occurs in fewer than two births per 10 000. It may result from trauma during the birthing process, compression from the intrauterine position, or embryological anomaly. Facial paralysis which is developmental is permanent. It is often associated with congenital anomaly of the face or another part of the body. Facial paralysis which arises from compression or trauma will often resolve spontaneously (Shapiro et al 1996), although, depending upon the extent of involvement, traumatic injury may require surgical intervention. Evidence of ecchymosis, swelling or hemotympanum warrants evaluation to rule out underlying fracture.

Bell's palsy is the most common neuropathy diagnosis in older infants and children (Shapiro et al 1996). It is often associated with tingling, pain or sensory changes on the involved side. Bell's palsy is sometimes called idiopathic facial palsy and is thought to involve the nerve after it leaves the stylomastoid foramen. However, many patients diagnosed with Bell's palsy also present with hyperacusis, decreased tearing and/or changes in taste. Rather than being a polyneuropathy, as has been proposed by some authors (Shapiro et al 1996), these symptoms point to involvement of the branches exiting in the facial canal and suggest compression in the canal, perhaps at the labyrinthine segment, as opposed to outside the foramen. First-degree or second-degree injury within the canal may arise from inflammation of the nerve in response to viral infection or from distention of the vascular plexus surrounding the nerve. The latter hypothesis is supported by the associated osteopathic findings of muscle spasm and fascial strain at the craniocervical junction and the cervical tissues on the involved side. Furthermore, resolution of these strain patterns is often followed by improvement in the patient's symptoms over the following few days. As would be expected, this response is predicated on the duration and extent of the nerve injury. The chances of recovery are markedly decreased when symptoms have persisted for over 4 months (chart review), regardless of the etiology or whether or not the somatic component is contributory.

Facial palsy occurring with acute otitis media is not uncommon in children and may be due to direct extension of the inflammation or infection into the canal. Treatment includes myringotomy, culture and sensitivity and appropriate antibiotics. Surgical drainage and debridement of the area may be warranted in severe cases. However, even if the infection is treated appropriately, complete recovery of nerve function occurs in fewer than half of the children (Shapiro et al 1996). The osteopath should evaluate and address any tissue strains which might impede lymphatic and vascular clearance of the area, to facilitate optimum recovery. Chronic otitis media may lead to the development of cholesteatoma, which can directly compress the nerve. Or, less often, the gradual accumulation of the granulomatous tissue may erode through the wall of the canal. In both cases, surgical decompression is usually curative (Shapiro et al 1996).

Osteopathic findings associated with uncomplicated facial nerve palsy include significant myofascial and muscular strains at the craniocervical junction and cervical tissues on the ipsilateral side. Osseous restrictions are often present in the cranial base and upper cervical complex and may present on either side. Frequently, there are associated findings at the cervicothoracic junction and dysfunction in the upper ribs, which is usually ipsilateral. Occasionally, intercranial membranous strains involving the ipsilateral petrosphenoid area are found; however, more often, the cranial findings are occipitomastoid. In older children and adults, a corticosteroid bolus with a 5–7 day wean is very useful in decreasing inflammation of the nerve, especially when the symptoms have been present for more than 2–3 days but less than 1 month. However, amelioration of the strain pattern needs to occur to ensure a return of function.

Differential diagnosis of facial palsy

Unilateral facial palsy may also occur as a result of Lyme disease, a systemic illness resulting from an infection with a spirochete, *Borrelia burgdorferi*, acquired through tic bite. An erythematous area with central clearing is the characteristic response to inoculation but it is often missed. After 10–14 days, the patient develops arthralgia, myalgia and chronic fatigue, which are signs of infection. Facial palsy may develop at this time, but more often develops after chronic infection. Treatment with appropriate medications in the early phases gives an excellent response; however, response to treatment in the chronic stages is less predictable. An accurate history and *Borrelia* titers will confirm the diagnosis. In severe cases, facial palsy can be a complication of herpes zoster infection involving the ear, which may progress to the facial nerve. On physical examination, the characteristic vesicles can be seen over the pinna and in the ear canal.

COMMON NERVE COMPRESSION SYNDROMES

Median nerve

Pronator syndrome

In 80% of individuals, the median nerve passes between the heads of the pronator teres. It may also pass deep to both heads or pierce either head. The patient usually presents with pain in the forearm which may or may not radiate into the wrist. Tingling and paresthesias are common. Weakness may be present in severe cases. This condition is more common in young athletes whose activities involve repetitive elbow flexion with the forearm in supination or pronation, or pronation against resistance. The sites of compression can often be determined on physical examination. When compression occurs at the distal third of the humerus beneath the supracondylar process, the symptoms are aggravated by flexion between 120° and 130° against resistance (compression at ligament of Struthers). If the nerve is compressed by the bicipital aponeurosis, active flexion of the elbow with the forearm in pronation will reproduce the symptoms. If the problem is due to hypertrophy of the aponeurosis, resistance to pronation with the wrist in neutral will produce symptoms. Finally, if the nerve is compressed by the arch of the flexor digitorum superficialis, the symptoms will reduce with resisted flexion of the isolated flexor superficialis muscle of the middle finger.

Anterior interosseous syndrome

This syndrome involves irritation to the anterior interosseous nerve, a branch of the median nerve. It is characterized by non-specific pain in the proximal forearm occasionally radiating into the hand. In severe cases there may be weakness of the finger flexors. Because this nerve also innervates the carpal ligament, its compression can mimic carpal tunnel syndrome, albeit without the muscle wasting or sensory changes in the hand. The symptoms of nerve irritation worsen with exercise, especially motions involving repetitive forearm supination and pronation, as might be seen with throwing a ball, ping-pong or fencing. In addition, repetitive finger movements such as occur with prolonged computer activity (game playing) or piano playing may aggravate symptoms.

Carpal tunnel syndrome

The carpal tunnel lies deep to the palmaris longus. Its proximal border is the pisiform and the tubercle of the scaphoid. The distal border is defined by the hook of the hamate and the tubercle of the trapezium. The transverse carpal ligament runs between these four prominences and forms the anterior border. Traveling through the carpal tunnel is the median nerve, the flexor digitorum profundus tendon, the tendon of the flexor pollicis longus, and the tendon of the flexor digitorum superficialis. Impingement, compression or irritation of the median nerve will result in paresthesias of the lateral aspect of the palm, middle and index fingers, and thumb. There may be associated weakness of the thumb abductors. Phalen's and Tinel's tests will be positive. The tunnel of Guyon lies between the pisiform and the hook of the hamate. The pisohamate ligament acts as the anterior wall. The ulnar nerve and artery pass through this fibro-osseous tunnel and may become compressed or irritated, resulting in symptoms in the hypothenar eminence and fifth digit. There will be tenderness to deep palpation of the ulnar nerve; however, it will be mild if the nerve is not inflamed. More often, ulnar nerve compression will occur at the level of the cubital tunnel.

Ulnar nerve

Cubital tunnel syndrome

Ulnar nerve irritation can occur in young athletes performing repetitive elbow flexion with resistance. As with many other conditions, the risk is increased with poor training practices, overtraining, or excessive load. Weightlifting training is one of the more common activities associated with this condition, especially biceps curls, bench presses, and squat lifts. Unconditioned athletes are at greater risk due to muscle hypertrophy and edema. The ulnar nerve passes through the intramuscular septum between the biceps and brachialis muscles. It runs in a groove on the medial head of the triceps. In 70% of individuals, it is crossed by the arcade of Struthers. The ulnar nerve descends in a groove posterior to the medial condyle of the humerus, and then passes through a fibrous cubital tunnel between the humeral and ulnar heads of the flexor carpi radialis. During flexion, the distance between the ulna and humerus increases and the aponeurosis is stretched, decreasing the tunnel by 55%. This increases the likelihood of neural irritation or compression with repetitive movements. When the ulnar nerve becomes compressed within the ulnar tunnel, symptoms are aggravated by flexion of the elbow and/or shoulder abduction.

There is paresthesia of the fourth and fifth digits and dysthesia of the medial forearm and ulnar digits. Sensory dysfunction usually predates motor involvement. Ulnar compression can be categorized as follows:
- Grade I – no motor weakness
- Grade II – weakness of the ulnar muscles
- Grade III – paralysis and wasting of the intrinsic muscles of the hand.

Radial nerve

Supinator syndrome

The radial nerve passes between the fibrous arch of the supinator muscle and the superior border of the extensor carpi radialis brevis. The nerve can become compressed between the two structures during elbow extension with forearm pronation and wrist flexion, such as one might use in a tennis serve. This can occur in young athletes due to overtraining or poor form. Young athletes will present with posterior elbow pain associated with tenderness at the radial head and the common extensor tendon. The differential diagnosis needs to include extensor tendonitis; however, in the presence of weakened extensor muscles of the thumb and metacarpophalangeal joints, nerve compression is the more likely diagnosis. Key findings differentiating supinator syndrome from lateral epicondylitis include the presence of weakness of the extensor digitorum muscles, reproducing the pain by active pronation against resistance, point tenderness that is greatest distal to the lateral epicondyle, and exacerbation of paresthesias with compression over the radial nerve tunnel.

SPASTICITY

Spasticity occurs when the cortical control of spinal reflexes is removed or decreased. Under normal conditions, the spinal reflex arc is down-modulated by descending input from the brain. As a result, when a tendon is stretched, the associated muscle contracts in a relatively controlled manner. This represents a normal stretch reflex or deep tendon reflex. When the cortical or spinal pathways involved with down-modulation of reflexive muscle contraction are damaged, the muscle reaction to tendon stretch is exaggerated. The stretch reflex is said to be brisk or elevated. When the stretch reflex is elevated, normal movements will trigger an exaggerated muscle response. For example, passive extension of a joint may meet with involuntary resistance. This is a sign of hyperreflexia or spasticity. Active movement may also be met with muscle resistance. Extending the knee during the swing phase of gait will slightly stretch the tendons of the hamstrings and gastric muscles. Under normal conditions, this input serves a proprioceptive function and contributes to stabilizing motor patterns of gait. However, if a child has hyperreflexia or spasticity of the hamstrings or gastric muscles, extending the knee will trigger an exaggerated muscle response. The muscles will contract, limiting knee extension. With the next step, the muscle shortens a little bit more. Taken separately, each contraction may be barely perceptible, but they are cumulative. This additive effect is going to influence the child's ability to execute an effective gait pattern. The contraction of the knee flexors alters joint position and proprioceptive patterning, both of which influence posture and balance. Each time the child attempts to use the affected extremity, muscle tone increases a bit, joint mobility decreases a bit, motor patterning is altered a bit and the ability of the child to properly execute the function is impaired. Over time this snowballs, so that the altered muscle tone alters joint mechanics, which impairs the way the child executes the movement, which places more stress on the myofascial tissues, and triggers an exaggerated response from the muscle. Somewhere buried under all these layers is the actual baseline muscle tone that has resulted from the neural injury. The goal of management in children with spasticity is to peel away the layers and find that baseline level of tone.

Osteopathic approaches which influence proprioception and joint position can be helpful. It must be remembered that any attempt to move the joint has the potential to trigger an elevated reflex and undermine the treatment goal. Slow, gentle techniques which rely on activating forces in the patient appear to be most effective. Counterstrain, Sutherland's approach, balancing techniques, and facilitated positional release tend to be helpful in younger children. In older children who can follow directions, muscle energy techniques using isotonic eccentric contraction and reciprocal inhibition may also effective and can be taught to parents as part of an at-home therapy program. Because the down-regulation of the stretch reflex is permanently altered, the process of 'winding up' the hyperreflexia is ongoing. Treatment must also be an ongoing process. This is especially true during times of growth or motor development when the child's tone often increases precipitously in response to the sudden lengthening of a bone or the new movement pattern in a joint. This increased tone needs to be addressed aggressively because it has the potential to distort long bone growth or impair motor development.

TICS

Tics are spontaneous, uncoordinated, involuntary movements involving multiple muscle groups. They occur sporadically and are exacerbated by stress. The underlying pathophysiology is not well understood. The three most common forms of motor tics in children are transient tic disorder, chronic motor tic disorder, and Tourette's syndrome. Transient tic disorder is a self-limiting movement disorder

which resolves within 1 year of onset. It is more common in boys than in girls and usually presents as eye movements, throat clearing or facial movements. Chronic motor tic disorder involves muscle groups in the extremities as well as those in the face. It initially presents in childhood but persists throughout life.

Tourette's syndrome is a cluster of symptoms including motor tics, vocal tics, obsessive compulsive disorder and attention deficit hyperactivity disorder (ADHD). Most children meet at least three of the four criteria. Tourette's syndrome may present in infancy or just after adolescence and last throughout life. There is a broad spectrum of involvement, ranging from focal frequent motor tics, accompanied by sighs, to almost constant multifocal ballisms associated with uncontrollable verbalizations and ADHD.

Conventional treatment of motor tic disorders is dependent on the extent and intensity of involvement. Children with transient tic disorder are typically not treated with pharmaceutical medications. Those with chronic motor tics or Tourette's syndrome may be treated if the movement disorder becomes severe or interferes with normal life activities. Children with Tourette's syndrome may be treated for the behavioral component of the syndrome. Unfortunately, many of the pharmaceuticals used in the treatment of ADHD and obsessive compulsive disorder will unmask or exacerbate the motor disorder.

From an osteopathic perspective, we need to remember that tics are exacerbated by stress. This includes emotional, psychological, physical and somatic stress. Biomechanical stress will contribute to the cumulative stress load carried by the child. Osteopathic manipulative treatment can be a means of decreasing the cumulative stress load, by addressing nociceptive input from biomechanical or tissue strains and balancing proprioceptive influences from the involved structures. In addition, most older children experience a general state of relaxation following osteopathic manipulative treatment, and this may also have a role in their response. Based on clinical reports and experience, children with milder forms of Tourette's syndrome appear to respond well to osteopathic manipulative treatment, although ongoing treatment is necessary. Once somatic findings have reached a baseline or background level, treatment usually needs to be repeated every 4–8 weeks, depending on the severity of the child's symptoms. Children with severe Tourette's syndrome seem to have a better response to osteopathic manipulation if their symptoms involve more motor tics than when the behavioral (obsessive compulsive) component is prevalent.

CEPHALGIA

A complete discussion of headache, its various forms, pathogenesis and etiologies would encompass a very large textbook and is well beyond the scope of this section. Therefore, we will limit this presentation to the rather poorly understood but surprisingly common phenomenon of cervicogenic cephalgia. Except for the pain and its interference with life activities, cervicogenic cephalgia is a benign headache unrelated to increased intracranial pressure, infection, hemorrhage or infarct. It usually begins as a vague ache in the occipital area, base of the head or top of the neck. Within hours, it progresses over the top of the head to involve the entire head. The patient may complain of pain behind the eyes. Because of this latter presentation, the child is often sent for optometric evaluation, with little improvement in symptoms. The headaches usually worsen as the day goes on and improve with sleep. When severe, they may trigger 'migraine-type' symptoms of nausea, photophobia and even vomiting, but one must remember that these signs can be present in any very painful headache, including cervicogenic, sinus and meningeal.

The patient with cervicogenic cephalgia often complains of chronic low-grade headache, pressure or ache and stiffness at the base of the head or upper neck, which then develops into the severe headache. Children may have several episodes per week which require them to see the school nurse or miss class. There may or may not be a history of headache or migraine in the family. Frequently, there is no predisposing history or precipitating event, although cervicogenic headache may arise after acceleration/deceleration-type injury. This headache pattern may be exacerbated by stress, sitting at a desk or computer for a prolonged period of time, or activities which require prolonged extension and shortening of the craniocervical tissues. Studies have shown that cervicogenic cephalgia can be generated by irritation to musculoskeletal components of the cervical spine and craniocervical area; hence the name (Bogduk 1992).

Obtaining a description of the headache from a child can be challenging, if not impossible. Much of the necessary information needs to be inferred from the parent's observations. Irritability, squinting eyes on voluntarily lowering the volume on the stereo may be signs of the early phase. Other signs include going to bed early, complaining of the intensity of light or sound, poor appetite and seeking out sedentary activities. Although the relationship is not well understood, children with headaches will sometimes complain of stomach pain, but not nausea.

Functional anatomy

The innervation of the head can be viewed in two ways: peripheral nerve innervation and mapping in the brainstem. This is akin to the way in which we view innervation in the upper extremity. The tissues of the arm are innervated by the radial, medial and ulnar nerves. These are peripheral nerves. Each nerve carries sensory fibers from the spinal segments C4 through C8. We can map the areas of innervation

from these spinal segments as dermatomes, myotomes or sclerotomes (see Ch. 1). Most people know the dermatome map (Fig. 16.4A). However, the peripheral nerves can also be mapped (Fig. 16.4B). The same arrangement exists in the head. There are three peripheral nerves, the ophthalmic, maxillary and mandibular, which can be mapped to the head (Fig. 16.5A). Each of these peripheral nerves carries fibers from the 'segments' of the brainstem. These segments can be viewed as a stacked column of cells, similar to the way in which we can view the segments of the spinal cord as a stacked column of cells. The ophthalmic division of the trigeminal nerve carries fibers from cells located at the very top of the trigeminal column and from cells at the very bottom, just as the median nerve of the arm carries fibers from cells located in C6, C7 and C8. In both the arm and the head (and everywhere else), the peripheral nerves carry fibers from a range of cells in the central nervous system. Just as there is an overlap between the radial, median and ulnar nerves and the mapping from C4 to C8 (see Fig. 16.4B), there is an overlap between the ophthalmic, maxillary and mandibular nerves and the mapping from the brainstem (Fig. 16.5B).

Headache or head pain is generated through the trigeminal system of the brain. It is called a system, because it is rather complicated. Cells in the trigeminal ganglion send fibers to the structures of the head such as the tissues of the face, sinuses, teeth, periosteum of the anterior cranial fossa and cranial vasculature. These fibers have receptors which respond to nociception and temperature. When stimulated, the signal travels to the trigeminal ganglion and on to the column of the cells in the brainstem. The column of cells in the brainstem is composed of the trigeminal nuclei. These cells receive information about pain and temperature and relay that information to the cortex. The column of cells in the brainstem is organized into a map. Fibers coming from the lips will synapse on cells at the top of the column; fibers coming from the top of the head will synapse on cells at the bottom of the column (Fig. 16.6). However, this column of cells receives sensory information from all types of tissue: bone, muscle, connective tissue, blood vessels and skin. Consequently, in addition to the dermatome map, we need to consider myotome and sclerotome maps. These maps can be visualized as a cross-section taken right through the head. Every tissue in that section is included in the sensory map.

The column of trigeminal cells is a continuation of the column of cells in the spinal cord which are also concerned with pain and temperature, the anterolateral system (ALS). There is some overlap between the two columns. The cells receiving pain and temperature information from the top of the neck are scattered among the cells receiving pain and temperature from the top of the head. When there is chronic constant irritation to the structures of the upper neck or craniocervical junction, the cells at the top of the ALS become excited or facilitated; this can lower the

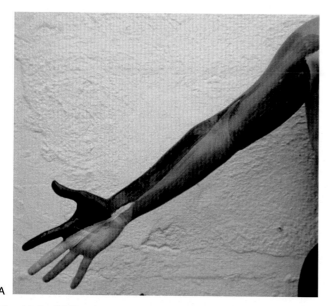

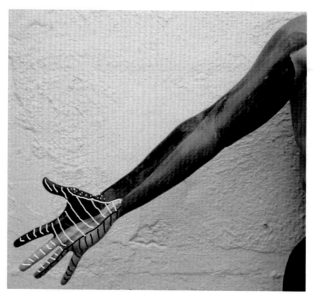

Fig. 16.4 • (A) The dermatomes of the upper extremity are depicted from the anterior surface. (B) The map of the peripheral nerves has been laid over the dermatome map. The territory of the ulnar nerve is most medial and is outlined by the black stripes. The territory of the median nerve is outlined by the white stripes. The territory of the radial nerve is outlined by the white dots. *Used with permission of the Willard & Carreiro Collection.*

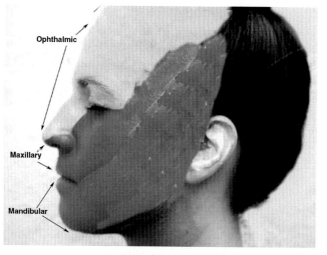

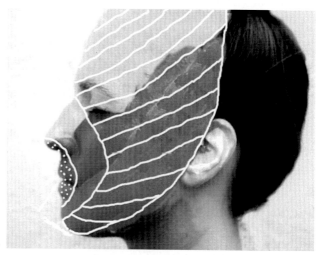

Fig. 16.5 • (A) The familiar mapping of the peripheral nerve innervation patterns in the face and head are depicted. The territory of the ophthalmic branch of the trigeminal nerve, that of the maxillary and that of the mandibular are marked and shaded. (B) The territory of the segments of the trigeminal nucleus have been laid over the peripheral nerve map. Each of the three 'segments' of the column of trigeminal cells will receive sensory information from all the tissues located in the depicted area. *Used with permission of the Willard & Carreiro Collection.*

threshold for activation or actually stimulate the adjacent trigeminal cells. Because they are trigeminal cells, when they are activated the brain will interpret the pain as coming from the head, i.e. a headache. This is a form of referred pain. The mapping of the trigeminal cells results in the patient perceiving the pain over the head, or behind the eyes, or in the temporal area. The prodrome of pressure, ache and stiffness occurs while the cervical neurons are being stimulated but before the trigeminal system is activated.

Palpatory examination

Cervicogenic cephalgia is generated by irritation to structures in the upper cervical or craniocervical areas. On physical examination, there is usually extension of the occiput on the atlas and significant restriction of mechanics at the craniocervical junction. There may or may not be trigger points in the short deep extensors of the head, but tender points are commonly present. There is marked

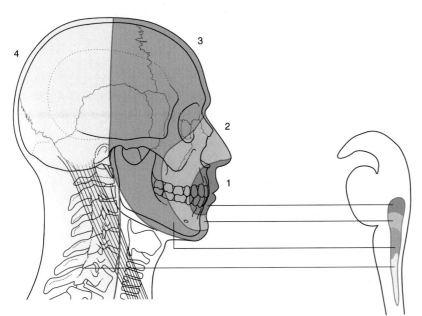

Fig. 16.6 • Schematic diagram depicting all of the tissues which share innervation from the trigeminal 'segments' in the brainstem. Area 1 maps onto the most caudal cells, 2 onto the middle cells, and 3 onto those cells in the cephalad portion. Note the overlap between cells receiving input from the upper cervical tissues (4) and those receiving input from the posterior aspect of the head (1). *Adapted from the Willard & Carreiro Collection.*

compression and restriction of normal mechanics in the cranial base, with apparent secondary restriction in the vault. In some children, tender points over the lambdoidal and occipitomastoid sutures will reproduce the pain pattern and a feeling of lightheadedness. SBS compression is frequently palpated and may be primary or secondary to the strain. Fascial restriction throughout the cervical and upper thoracic area is present. In those patients in whom the headache has a tendency to evolve into a migraine, there is often paraspinal muscle spasm in the area of T4.

POSTCONCUSSION SYNDROME

Postconcussion syndrome (PCS) is a collection of signs and symptoms associated with closed head injury. The *Diagnostic and Statistical Manual of Mental Disorders* (DSM)-IV defines the diagnostic criteria for PCS as a history of traumatic brain injury (TBI) with at least three of the following: headache, dizziness, fatigue, impulsiveness, irritability, impaired memory, impaired concentration, insomnia, hyperacusis and photophobia. The signs and symptoms may present immediately at the time of injury or may develop over several hours. Unfortunately PCS is a common sequela of mild closed head trauma. The risk is increased in young athletes compared with children due to the nature of the activities in which they engage. Helmets and other protective devices have a role in mitigating the severity of the injury, but are not foolproof. Children and young athletes are active and frequently bang their heads. Most of the time it is insignificant and the child will not develop PCS, but there are certain clues in the trauma history that increase the likelihood that cerebral concussion occurred.

Children who experience any loss of consciousness (even seconds) following head trauma or acceleration–deceleration injury have experienced cerebral concussion. Loss of memory concerning specific events occurring within 24 hours before or after an injury can be indicative of concussion and increases the risk of PCS (Hessen et al 2008). As long as the amnesia resolves within 24 h of the injury, there is no correlation with the severity of the PCS. Amnesia that is dense or lasts longer than 24 h warrants work-up for ischemic injury. A history of post-traumatic acute mental status change such as confusion that does not progress and lasts less than 12 h is associated with mild concussion, whereas mental status change which progresses over time, develops several hours after the injury, and/or deteriorates is a sign of increased intracranial pressure, or cerebral hemorrhage. Cerebral concussion can also be associated with mild, stable, and focal neurological deficit that presents acutely following the injury. Patients with a score of 13–15 on the Glasgow Coma Scale at 30 min have a higher probability of concussion injury and are at risk for PCS.

The Glasgow Coma Scale evaluates the injured child for three things: eye opening, verbal response and motor response. The child is scored based on the level of his or her response to the examiner (Table 16.1). A score of 13–15 correlates with mild head trauma, a score between 9 and 12 defines moderate head trauma and a score below 8 is indicative of severe head trauma. The Glasgow Coma Scale is often performed on athletes at the time of injury. However, if the patient is presenting with a history of injury, the examiner can often estimate the Glasgow Coma Scale score during the history taking. For example, one might ask a parent: 'Were his eyes open when you (they) found him?' 'Did he answer to his name?' 'Could he tell you (them) where it

Table 16.1 Glasgow Coma Scale

Eye opening		Verbal response		Motor response	
Spontaneous	4 points	Oriented	5 points	Obeys directions	6 points
To speech	3 points	Confused conversation	4 points	Localizes area	5 points
To pain	2 points	Inappropriate word	3 points	Withdraws from pain	4 points
Unresponsive	1 point	Incomprehensible	2 points	Abnormal flexion	3 points
		Unresponsive	1 point	Decerebrate posture	2 points
				Unresponsive	1 point
Total score		Total score		Total score	

Table 16.2 Summary chart of postconcussion severity (PCS) types

Severity of PCS	Clusters	Other
Type I	Mild signs and symptoms from all	Likelihood LOC and potential for underlying psychiatric diagnosis
Type II	Moderate-severe cognitive *and* affective; mild sensory; mild/absent somatic	
Type III	Moderate-severe cognitive *and* affective; moderate sensory *or* somatic	
Type IV	Severe global complaints; no depression	Decreased likelihood of LOC

LOC = loss of consciousness

hurt?'. Although the Glasgow Coma Scale was developed for use with older children and adults, it can be adapted somewhat for younger patients. For example it is important to note whether or not the child responded appropriately to comforting, would he look when his name was spoken, and was his level of receptive language skills appropriate.

The most common sequelae of PCS are headache and dizziness. These symptoms may present in combination with others to form a clinical cluster. Each clinical cluster has a primary sign and/or symptom, and one or more associated signs and symptoms. The literature describes four clinical cluster presentations of PCS (Cicerone 1995): a somatic, a sensory, a cognitive and an affective cluster. The somatic cluster is one of the most common presentations of PCS. In addition to headache, these patients present primarily with complaints of loss of balance, clumsiness, and feeling lightheaded or unsteady. They also complain of one or more of the following associated symptoms: visual changes, nausea, loss of appetite and, less frequently, insomnia. Another common presentation of PCS is the cognitive cluster. Patients with this clinical cluster experience slowed thinking, poor concentration, forgetfulness and difficulty making decisions

(Wozniak et al 2007). They typically have headaches and sleeping difficulties. The cognitive cluster appears to be the more common presentation in young athletes playing sports that allow head contact such as football (soccer), rugby, and American style football. One study of Australian-rules football players reported deterioration of cognitive function and an exacerbation of cognitive cluster symptoms in players with head injury (Maddocks 1996). These changes occurred over a relatively short period of time – the length of time they were in the game. Patients presenting with the sensory cluster of PCS experience hyperacusis and photophobia, with or without headache. They may also have multifocal paresthesias and changes in taste or smell. The fourth cluster, the affective cluster, describes the patient who presents with irritability, anxiety, depression and frustration. These patients often have headaches as well.

Patients may present with signs or symptoms from more than one clinical cluster. The more clusters involved, the more severe the condition, and probably the more severe the initial concussion. Patients with mild symptoms from all the clusters but primarily cognitive and affective symptoms fall into type 1 severity (Table 16.2). Reportedly, virtually all of these patients had some loss of consciousness at the time of injury and, more importantly, half of them may have an underlying depression (Cicerone 1995). Patients with moderate to severe cognitive and affective symptoms, mild sensory symptoms, and absent or mild somatic symptoms are classified as type II. Most patients with PCS fall into this category. Type III patients present with moderate to severe cognitive and affective changes and moderate sensory or somatic complaints. Patients with severe global complaints who also manifest depression are considered type IV.

A child who has had a mild traumatic brain injury is at risk for developing more severe symptoms with each new injury. A young athlete exhibiting mild postconcussion symptoms should be removed from play until those symptoms resolve (Kissick & Johnston 2005, Kirkwood et al 2006). The prognosis for PCS is not well reported (Lee 2007, Rees & Belton 2007). In general, patients who fall into the type II and III categories appear to have a good long-term prognosis although in some cases it may take several months for the symptoms to resolve, and with repeated injury the prognosis worsens. Patients with symptoms falling into the type 1 and IV categories have a more guarded prognosis and often need treatment for their psychiatric symptoms.

From an osteopathic perspective, treatment of patients with PCS is directed at normalizing biomechanical stresses and strains resulting from the injury and facilitating optimal function of areas, which may be indirectly contributing to the patient's symptoms. For example, an athlete who has had a head contact injury in a football game may experience symptoms from the cognitive, somatic and sensory clusters. While these symptoms may be due directly to the TBI, they also represent symptoms associated with biomechanical strains. The headache may be a combination of the brain injury and somatic dysfunction at the craniocervical junction and upper cervical spine. Eustachian tube dysfunction may contribute to the hyperacusis. Restriction at the thoracic inlet may impede movement of fluids through the low-pressure circulatory system in the extremities and contribute to swelling, stiffness and paresthesia. The experience of these symptoms will summate and influence the child's perception of well-being and coping strategies, which in turn contributes to his or her irritability, fatigue and frustration. All of the aforementioned factors barrage the locus ceruleus and hypothalamus altering the hypothalamic–pituitary–adrenal system, increasing cortisol levels, and creating a cycle of depression.

References

Bogduk N 1992 The anatomical basis for cervicogenic headache. J Manipulative Physiol Ther 15(1): 67–70.

Cicerone K D 1995 Persistent post-concussion syndrome: the structure of subjective complaints after mild traumatic brain injury. J Head Trauma Rehabil 10(3): 1–17.

Hessen E, Anderson V, Nestvold K 2008 MMPI-2 profiles 23 years after paediatric mild traumatic brain injury. Brain Inj 22: 39–50.

Kirkwood M W, Yeates K O, Wilson P E 2006 Pediatric sport-related concussion: a review of the clinical management of an oft-neglected population. Pediatrics 117: 1359–1371.

Kissick J, Johnston K M 2005 Return to play after concussion: principles and practice. Clin J Sport Med 15: 426–431.

Lee L K 2007 Controversies in the sequelae of pediatric mild traumatic brain injury. Pediatr Emerg Care 23: 580–583.

Maddocks D 1996 Neuropsychological deficits following concussion. Brain Injury 10(2): 99–103.

Rees R J, Bellon M L 2007 Post concussion syndrome ebb and flow: longitudinal effects and management. Neuro Rehabilitation 22: 229–242.

Shapiro A M, Schaitken B M, May M 1996 Facial paralysis in children. In: Bluestone C D, Sylvan S E, Kenna M A (eds) Pediatric otolaryngology. W B Saunders, Philadelphia.

Wozniak J R, Krach L, Ward E et al 2007 Neurocognitive and neuroimaging correlates of pediatric traumatic brain injury: a diffusion tensor imaging (DTI) study. Arch Clin Neuropsychol 22: 555–568.

Further reading

Adams R D, Victor M 1993 Principles of neurology, 5th edn. McGraw-Hill, New York.

Andermann E, Andermann F, Silver K et al 1994 Benign familial nocturnal alternating hemiplegia of childhood. Neurology 44(10): 1812–1814.

Binder H, Eng G D, Gaiser J F et al 1987 Congenital muscular torticollis: results of conservative management with long-term follow-up in 85 cases. Arch Phys Med Rehabil 68: 222–225.

Boere-Boonekamp M M, van der Linden-Kuiper A T, 2001 Positional preference: prevalence in infants and follow-up after two years. Pediatrics 107: 339–343.

Bogduk N, Marsland A 1986 On the concept of third occipital headache. J Neural Neurosurg Psychiatry 49: 775–780.

Bogduk N, Windsor M, Inglis A 1988 The innervation of the cervical intervertebral discs. Spine 13(1): 2–8.

Brown J K, Rodda J, Walsh E G et al 1991 Neurophysiology of lower-limb function in hemiplegic children. Dev Med Child Neurol 33(12): 1037–1047.

Canale S T, Griffin D W, Hubbard C N 1982 Congenital muscular torticollis. A long-term follow-up. J Bone Joint Surg [Am] 64: 810–816.

Dubowitz L M S, Cowan F, Rutherford M et al 1995 Neonatal neurology, past present and future – a window on the brain. Brain Dev 17: 22–30.

Hamanishi C, Tanaka S 1994 Turned head-adducted hip truncal curvature syndrome. Arch Dis Child 70: 515–519.

Menkes J H, Sarant H B 2000 Child neurology, 6th edn. Lippincott, Williams & Wilkins, Philadelphia.

Phillippi H, Faldum A, Jung T et al 2006 Patterns of postural asymmetry in infants: a standardized video-based analysis. Eur J Pediatr 165: 58–164.

Phillippi H, Faldum A, Schleupen A et al 2006 Infantile postural asymmetry and osteopathic treatment: a randomized therapeutic trial. Dev Med Child Neurol 48: 5–9.

Roberts W J, Kramis R C 1990 Sympathetic nervous system influence on acute and chronic pain. In: Fields H (ed.) Pain syndromes in neurology. Butterworth Heineman, Oxford: 85–105.

St John D, Mulliken J B, Kaban L B et al 2002 Anthropometric analysis of mandibular asymmetry in infants with deformational posterior plagiocephaly. J Oral Maxillofac Surg 60: 873–877.

Standring S (ed.) 2004 Gray's anatomy, 39th edn. Churchill Livingstone, New York.

Thompson S K 1980 Prognosis in infantile idiopathic scoliosis. J Bone Joint Surg [Am] 62: B151–154.

Volpe J J 1995 Neurology of the newborn, 3rd edn. W B Saunders, Philadelphia.

Wall P D, Melzack R 1990 Textbook of pain, 2nd edn. Churchill Livingstone, Edinburgh.

Walsh J J, Morrissy R T 1998 Torticollis and hip dislocation. J Pediatr Orthop 18: 219–221.

Willard F H 1997 The autonomic nervous system. In: Ward R (ed.) Foundations for osteopathic medicine. Williams & Wilkins, Baltimore.

Woolsey R M, Young R R 1991 The clinical diagnosis of disorders of the spinal cord. Neurol Clin 9(3): 573–583.

Wyke B 1981 The neurology of joints: a review of general principles. Clin Rheum Dis 7(1): 223–239.

Chapter Seventeen

17

Cerebral palsy

CHAPTER CONTENTS

OVERVIEW

Cerebral palsy (CP) is a condition that consists of non-progressive, but changing motor dysfunction resulting from brain damage acquired during development (Menkes & Sarant 2000). The key points are that it is non-progressing, changing and involves the motor system. The pathological process in the central nervous system is stable, but as the child develops, the manner in which it manifests changes. This happens because the insult to the brain occurs very early in the child's life, usually during gestation or birth. As the child's motor and sensory systems mature, the expression of new motor skills is altered because of the cortical damage. Consequently, the clinical presentation changes as the child gets older. For example, if a child with CP is at the stage where she should be creeping (crawling on all fours), but she has sustained a cerebral insult which resulted in weakness of the hip flexors, then she may not be able to creep. However, upper extremity milestones may be appropriate. When it comes time for this same child to walk, she may be delayed, needing assistance to stand and then cruising rather than engaging in independent walking.

During development, children learn, refine and integrate new movement strategies to interact with their environment. The ability of the child with CP to incorporate and express new strategies will depend on the extent and location of the injury. Some new motor strategies can be incorporated, some can only partially be incorporated and some cannot be incorporated at all. Consequently, the child's presentation keeps changing, making it very difficult to make the diagnosis during the first year or two of life, unless there are overt signs. Nelson and Ellenberg (1996) showed that of 229 children diagnosed with cerebral palsy at 1 year of age, half no longer had the diagnosis by the age of 7.

PATHOGENESIS

The types of injury to the brain which can result in CP are many and varied, ranging from genetic to infectious to traumatic processes. The most common, however, are perinatal asphyxia and the complications of prematurity. Perinatal asphyxia is a condition in which the brain is subjected to hypoxia, ischemia and hypercarbia, resulting in cerebral edema and metabolic changes (Volpe 1995). Studies indicate that the injury occurs during the antepartum period in 40–50% of cases, in the intrapartum period in 30–40% of cases, and postpartum in approximately 10% of cases (Brown et al 1974, Low et al 1989, Volpe 1995). Asphyxial brain damage may result from hypoperfusion, focal ischemia or asphyxia (Menkes & Sarant 2000). According to Volpe (1995), the primary problem in each of these events is a loss in the autoregulatory mechanisms of cerebral blood flow such that there is necrosis and edema in the affected tissues, resulting in a condition called hypoxic–ischemic encephalopathy. A thorough discussion of the pathogenesis can be found in Menkes and Sarant (2000) and Volpe (1995). The area of the brain affected by hypoxic–ischaemic encephalopathy is dependent on the duration of the insult and the gestational age of the fetus. During gestation, the vulnerability of particular areas changes as the vascular pattern of the brain develops.

TERMINOLOGY

In the past, children with CP were classified based on the suspected anatomical area of the infarct. Terms such as cortical palsy, cerebellar palsy and vestibular palsy were used. More recently, there has been a push to describe the functional problem and categorize CP in terms of the motor dysfunction. There are basically six forms of CP: spastic, extrapyramidal, atonic, cerebellar, ataxic and combined. These terms describe the functional characteristics of the child. The distribution, i.e. unilateral or bilateral, depends on the laterality of the injury.

SPASTIC CEREBRAL PALSY

Spasticity is the most common form of CP, affecting 70–80% of all cases (Dormans & Pellegrino 1998). It occurs when there is damage to the descending control systems, which modulate interneuron, α motor neuron and γ motor neuron activity (Pearson & Gordon 2000). A spinal reflex involves increased deep tendon reflexes and resistance to stretch (see Ch. 16). A spinal or stretch reflex is a monosynaptic reflex involving sensory input via dorsal ganglion cells and motor output from ventral horn cells. Under normal conditions, descending pathways from the cortex inhibit or down-regulate the ventral horn response. However, when the efferent control is removed, there is a heightened muscle response to the tendon stretch (Fig. 17.1). For example, if the connection in the brain and the spinal cord is intact, then when the patellar tendon is stretched, the quadriceps muscle response will be modulated; that is, contraction of the muscle is regulated by the intensity of the stretch. If the brain is not modulating the spinal cord cells, then the quadratus muscle contraction is not down-regulated. Regardless of the intensity of the stretching of the tendon, the muscle

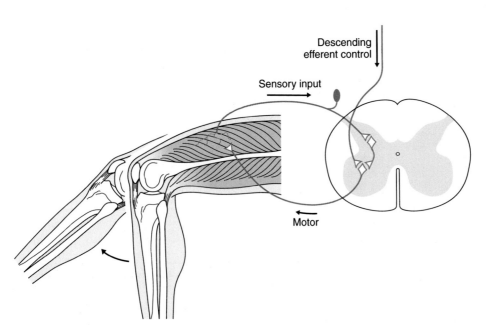

Descending efferent control

Sensory input

Motor

Fig. 17.1 • Schematic diagram of the tendon stretch response in the knee. Under normal conditions, the descending control dampens the motor response. However, when this is lost due to spinal cord or brain damage, the response becomes heightened, resulting in an increased deep tendon reflex, i.e. spasticity.

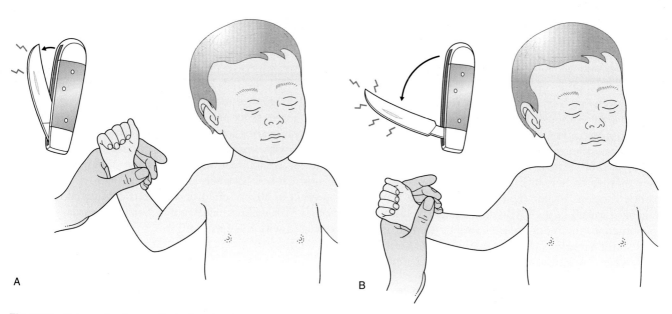

Fig. 17.2 • Schematic diagram illustrating the clasped knife response. In (A), the examiner attempts to extend the patient's arm but is met with resistance. (B) Suddenly the arm gives way.

will respond with a very rapid and forceful contraction, an elevated deep tendon reflex (DTR). When an area of the brain involved with the descending modulating pathways is injured, the child will have an exaggerated stretch reflex. In certain conditions, the inhibitory control can be so affected that even passive stretching will activate the spinal reflex. This is a form of rigidity.

A DTR does not necessarily give any clues concerning the muscle's strength. It is a measurement of the spinal or primary reflex – the response of a muscle to the stretching of its tendon. Spasticity, by definition, describes the DTR, although it is often used to describe a tight or rigid muscle. Voluntary control of the muscle may or may not still be present. A child may be able to control his muscle use but has spasticity because cortical regulation of the spinal reflex is absent. Strength is often present but coordinated movements are difficult, because of the increased stretch reflex. Many children with spasticity also have hypertonic muscles or rigidity. However, rigidity and spasticity are different phenomena and do not necessarily appear in the same child. Rigidity is usually more prominent in flexor muscles than extensor muscles, although it affects both (Adams & Victor 1993). There is increased resistance to passive muscle stretch that may present as a slightly increased resistance, as frank rigidity, or as anything in between. Rigidity represents a lowered threshold for α and γ motor neuron excitation (Adams & Victor 1993); however, DTRs are not elevated. Electromyographic analysis has shown that the elevated activity of the motor unit, the many hundreds of skeletal muscle fibers innervated by the affected α motor neuron, persists even after apparent relaxation (Adams & Victor 1993). A special form of rigidity or hypertonia is

called clasped knife rigidity. Passive movement of the joint feels like opening and closing a pocketknife. The muscle will initially resist passive stretch. If the stretch is maintained, the muscle will suddenly 'give way' over a short distance. For example, if one attempts to gently extend the elbow of a child with clasped knife rigidity, the joint is initially quite resistant to movement; the muscle stays contracted against the applied force (Fig. 17.2). Then suddenly the muscle gives way, allowing some movement of the joint. The same response happens if the examiner attempts to flex the elbow. The movement of the arm feels like a pocketknife. You have to pull on the blade and suddenly it partially opens. Then, to close the knife, you push on it and suddenly it closes. This is clasped knife reflex or rigidity. Another form of rigidity is called cogwheel rigidity. In this situation, the arm will also resist movement, except instead of the muscle giving way and allowing large degrees of motion, the muscle only gives way in short bursts over a very small distance, resulting in a rhythmic ratchet-like movement (Adams & Victor 1993). Thus, it feels to the examiner as though he is moving a cog in a wheel. In both of these cases, the tone in the muscle is abnormally high, primarily because the response to passive stretch is heightened.

EXTRAPYRAMIDAL CEREBRAL PALSY

Another form of CP involves dyskinesias or abnormal involuntary movements and is called extrapyramidal CP. Most often these children will have athetosis or chorea, but other forms of dyskinesia, such as hemiballism, dystonia, myoclonus and ataxic tremor, also occur. Athetosis is an involuntary, slow, writhing, snake-like movement, usually of the extremities, but it can involve the torso. Like other dyskinesias, athetosis represents a distortion in the scaling of movement, a process normally regulated through the basal ganglia. Although it is involuntary, athetosis can often be suppressed. For example, Sonia is a small 5-year-old girl who has athetosis involving the right upper extremity. Often, as she is sitting on the treatment table talking with her mother or her doctor, she will begin to exhibit very subtle motions in her right hand, wrist and arm. If she remains engaged in the discussion and distracted from the phenomenon, the motions will continue to increase in amplitude until her arm is writhing by the side of her head. However, when Sonia realizes that the motion is happening, she can stop it. The athetosis began when she was almost 3 years old and she grew up calling it 'Righty'. When her arm starts to exhibit the athetotic movements, Sonia will say, 'Get down Righty. Get down.' Sonia's arm will slowly come down as she keeps scolding it.

Dyskinesias may begin very subtly. When it first manifested in Sonia at the age of 3, it looked as though she had a little nervous twitch in a mildly spastic right arm. Sonia had a diagnosis of CP but she started developing athetosis. Does she have CP or something else? Is that a change or is that a progression?

It is not uncommon for dyskinesias to remain dormant during the first 2 years of life. According to Menkes and Sarant (2000), the delayed presentation of dyskinesias is probably due to immature function of the nervous system. Athetosis arises when there is damage to structures of the extrapyramidal system. Frequently, these children have experienced one or more risk factors for cerebral damage, including maternal pre-eclampsia, low birthweight or perinatal asphyxia (Menkes & Sarant 2000). Clinically, children with extrapyramidal CP usually present with a generalized hypotonia with increased DTRs in infancy which progresses to dyskinesias in childhood (Menkes & Sarant 2000). In very mild forms, dyskinesias such as athetosis may be confused with tics or fidgeting (Adams & Victor 1993). In more severe cases, the dyskinesia can be quite dramatic, interfering with normal movements. When it is quite severe, athetosis may be accompanied by chorea, which is a jerky motion. Often, athetotic movements in young children will evolve into larger, more complex patterns of movement called choreoathetosis.

Other forms of dyskinesia include hemiballism – large sudden movements involving an entire limb or the head. The presence of dyskinesia will interfere with normal development of both gross and fine motor tasks (Menkes & Sarant 2000). The severity of the motor impairment is related to the severity of the dyskinesia. Hemiballism will significantly impede a child's ability to master most motor skills and may prevent the child from learning to stand or walk independently, whereas the child with an ataxic tremor or athetosis can reach most motor milestones, although they are delayed. Dyskinesias may also affect the lips and tongue, resulting in speech delay, although receptive language skills are usually age-appropriate, providing there is no hearing loss. In addition to the dyskinesia, many children with extrapyramidal CP have other problems (Menkes & Sarant 2000). One of two children with this form of CP will have sensorineural hearing loss. Strabismus is present in 30% of children with extrapyramidal CP, while another 30% will have nystagmus. Seizure disorders are also associated with this form of CP.

ATONIC CEREBRAL PALSY

Atonic or hypotonic CP is also fairly common. It is characterized by persistent generalized hypotonia. Often, the flaccidity occurs in the presence of elevated DTRs. The flaccidity is not due to problems of peripheral nerve or muscle, but its etiology is unclear (Menkes & Sarant 2000). These children often develop cerebellar signs or extrapyramidal signs, or are profoundly mentally retarded. Muscle biopsy suggests a delay in muscle fiber maturation, although, again, its cause is unclear (Menkes & Sarant 2000).

CEREBELLAR CEREBRAL PALSY

Cerebellar CP is less common than the other forms. It results from damage to the cerebellum. The child's signs of cerebellar deficit are usually masked until the child begins to exhibit posture-dependent activity such as sitting, standing or walking (Adams & Victor 1993). Unsteadiness with these activities persists beyond the expected time. Titubations of the head often accompany truncal ataxia (Adams & Victor 1993). Once established, the child's gait is usually wide-based, with lateral veering, arrhythmic limb movements are awkward, with endpoint correction for past pointing, and speech may be slow and poorly articulated. Cerebellar signs are usually associated with spasticity and most often involve the lower extremities and trunk, although other areas are common. The cerebellum is most susceptible to injury at term.

ATAXIA IN CHILDREN WITH CEREBRAL PALSY

A child with CP may also present with ataxia, an abnormality of the timing of movement. All voluntary movement requires coordination between agonist and antagonist muscle groups. Proper timing or meter between muscle groups creates a smooth, uniform motion. When the timing or the meter of the movement is disturbed, the motion becomes clumsy and disjointed, and the child will overshoot the target he is reaching towards and have to correct. The agonist muscle may be overcontracted, so the antagonist muscle tries to correct, and overshoots, and so on. Meter is coordinated through the cerebellum. Feedback information from joint and muscle proprioceptors guides the cerebellum. Distorted feedback may further compromise the process. The whole process is happening in the cerebellum. A child with ataxia may walk with a wide-based gait and have trouble maintaining balance. Some children have ataxia of speech, which may make it sound as though they are stuttering, but it is a problem with coordination of the tongue and laryngeal muscles. Ataxia can present in any part of the motor system: the extremities or the torso, or speech.

DISTRIBUTION OF INJURY

To understand the distribution of CP, we need to briefly review the morphology of the brain. The vasculature of the brain travels from the periphery towards the midline, and the collateral circulation is less well developed in the newborn than in the adult. This creates a watershed area wherever the small end vessels meet. The location and distribution of the watershed areas change as the brain enlarges and the vascular tree expands. In a term infant, at 40 weeks of gestation, the most vulnerable area is the cerebellum. Injuries that occur in a term infant tend to present with cerebellar signs. In the premature infant, the periventricular area tends to be susceptible to hypoxic–ischemic insult. Consequently, cortical fibers passing through the internal capsule may be affected. When the cortical fibers or the motor system are damaged, the child will present with involvement of the limbs or torso associated with that area.

The most common locations for hypoxic–ischemic injury in children with CP are the periventricular areas, resulting in spastic diplegia (McDonald 1963, Grether et al 1992). The condition involves bilateral spasticity with greater involvement in the legs than arms (Menkes & Sarant 2000). The most common finding in evaluation of premature infants with spastic diplegia with magnetic resonance imaging (MRI) is the presence of periventricular leukomalacia (Krageloh-Mann et al 1995a, b, Okumura et al 1997a, b, Olsen et al 1997), a condition resulting from cystic formation, gliosis and microcalcification in response to hypoxic–ischemic insult. MRI shows damage extending into the internal capsule where cortical fibers for lower extremity control are located. This explains the tendency for children with spastic diplegia to have greater tone in the lower extremities than in the upper. The degree of spasticity varies from child to child. When spasticity is severe, the child may develop contractures. These most often affect the ankle and foot, but other joints may become involved. Locked flexion at the ankle, knee or hip will significantly limit mobility. If untreated, the contractures can affect limb growth and development. Seizure disorders, frequently grand mal, are present in 27% of children with spastic diplegia (Menkes & Sarant 2000). Moreover, untreated seizure disorder may contribute to increased tone.

The relationship between spasticity and cognition remains unclear. It is often mistakenly assumed that the child with CP has a severe cognitive dysfunction, when many children have normal or only slightly below average intelligence. Older studies done in the early 1960s showed a strong association between lower IQ scores and upper extremity spasticity (Ingram 1964). This may have been more reflective of test-taking abilities, i.e. communication skills, than actual cognitive processing. Some of the more recent studies give conflicting information; Krageloh-Mann et al (1995a, b) reported abnormal visual motor and visual–perceptual function in preterm infants, with MRI documenting periventricular leukomalacia, whereas another study, also using MRI, showed grossly normal intelligence (Olsen et al 1998). Ultimately, the functional capabilities – physical, emotional, cognitive, etc. – cannot be predicted by the MRI scan. All too often, individuals err on the side of underestimating the potential of the child with CP. When a physician or healthcare provider sets limits on the potential of a newborn or infant, it only hurts the child and family. As we have discussed in earlier chapters, development is highly dependent on stimulation and experience. Telling a family that their baby will be bedridden, or is mentally retarded, or will never function independently, forever changes the family's perception of their child. The very things that the child needs to maximize his potential may now be denied to him. Conservative advice regarding the child's prognosis is most prudent. Explain the findings clearly, but do not take away the family's hope. Ultimately, no one knows what the future holds for this child or his family. To paint a dire picture focusing on the child's anticipated limitations, shortcomings, dependencies, etc., is to focus on the disease. It sets up an expectation for failure. We focus on the health within the child when we can intelligently acknowledge the pathology and, with just as much intelligence, recognize the nervous system's amazing plasticity and potential for compensation.

Spastic hemiparesis presents as unilateral spasticity with involvement of the arm greater than that of the leg. Typically, the involved arm is held at the child's side with the elbow and wrist flexed (Fig. 17.3). Research suggests that the inciting event occurs during gestation (Michaelis et al 1980, Molteni et al 1987). Intrauterine insults, resulting from anomalies in fetal circulation, fetal transfusion, twin pregnancies, embolic phenomena and alterations in maternal hemodynamics, have been implicated in the pathogenesis of spastic hemiparesis (Larroche 1986). Vascular infarcts involving the middle cerebral artery are the most common cause of hemiparesis in term infants (Fig. 17.4), with the left side more often involved than the right. In general, these occur in children after 35 weeks of gestation (Bouza et al 1994a, de Vries et al 1997). Potential causes include perinatal asphyxia, embolism, polycythemia, dehydration and cocaine misuse. The child with spastic hemiparesis will present with a flexed posture in the involved arm. Fine movements of the hand and wrist are commonly affected. Lower extremity tone is increased and there is a tendency to hold the leg with the knee flexed and the foot dorsiflexed and everted. Power in the shoulder girdle and hip muscles is usually preserved, but coordination is affected. Gross motor milestones are usually late but generally achieved (Brown et al 1991). Approximately 10% of children with spastic hemiparesis will develop movement disorders that primarily involve the fingers and hand (Menkes & Sarant 2000). Two-point discrimination and stereognosis may be impaired in the affected limb, and neglect may be present as well if the non-dominant cortex was involved. Interestingly, the presence of language or perceptual skills is not related to the laterality of the injury (Menkes & Sarant 2000), and nor is the extent of the injury predictive of function (Bouza et al 1994b). This suggests that the newborn brain has the functional plasticity needed to compensate for damaged areas.

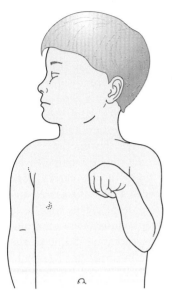

Fig. 17.3 • Schematic diagram depicting typical posturing of the arm in a spastic hemiparesis.

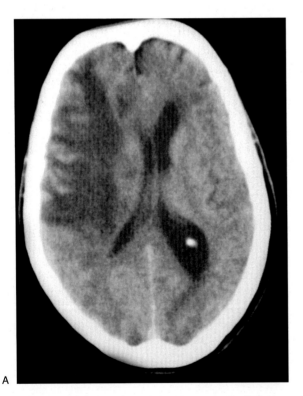

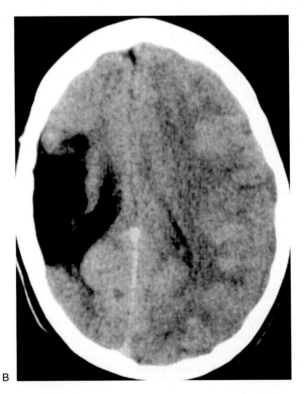

Fig. 17.4 • (A, B) Axial view computed tomography (CT) scans showing area of infarct in middle cerebral artery in a boy with spastic hemiparesis. (A) is a more cephalad cut. *Used with permission of the Willard & Carreiro Collection.*

Spastic quadriparesis is the third form of CP and the most devastating. In one study, it was present in 22% of children with CP (Grether et al 1992). It presents as a generalized hypertonicity with rigidity in all extremities. One side may be more severely affected than the other, with arms more affected than legs (Menkes & Sarant 2000). Motor impairment can be complete, with little permissible voluntary movement. These children will often assume a rigid decerebrate posture. Appropriate adaptive equipment can be most beneficial, affording the child and family a level of independence which would otherwise not exist. It is important to remember that even small changes can make huge differences for children and families struggling with the day-to-day demands of dealing with a motor handicap. Adaptive devices that allow the child to sit up unattended, or which simplify toileting tasks, are often the springboard to broader experiences. Being able to sit up gives a child a different perspective of his world, and other people a different perspective of the child.

CLINICAL PRESENTATION

The end result of asphyxial brain injury in children is hypoxic–ischemic encephalopathy. These children will present with generalized hypotonia and normal or slightly increased tendon reflexes in the postnatal period. There is often an associated abnormality of suck, swallowing, alertness and/or breathing (Adams & Victor 1993, Menkes & Sarant 2000). Seizure activity is not always present in hypoxic–ischemic encephalopathy and, when present, correlation with the severity of the damage is unclear.

The earliest signs of spasticity usually involve resistance to passive movement, especially flexion (Adams & Victor 1993, Menkes & Sarant 2000). The initial site of presentation will depend on the site of injury. Spastic diplegia first presents as resistance to abduction of the hips or movement of the ankles. Hemiplegia is first apparent in the arms, with subsequent expression in the legs. The pattern of progression is related to maturation of the nervous system. Various authors describe the pattern of expression of the initial hypotonia as lasting from 6 weeks to 3 years, depending on the severity of the damage (Menkes & Sarant 2000).

Widespread injury will often complicate the picture. For example, if a child has a hemiplegia (one side of the body) and his thoracic muscles are involved, his ability to maintain balance will be affected. His ability to control his posture may be compromised due to weakness as well as abnormal proprioceptive feedback. Often, the child will sway and correct. Compare this with a second child who has damage to cells of the basal ganglia affecting the trunk. How will trunk control be affected in the second child? What will happen when this child is asked to sit upright? The clinical picture for these two children may look very similar: swaying back and forth in a slow, jerky fashion. However, while both

the children may be swaying, the first child does not have athetosis – he is trying to maintain his balance. If you stabilize the first child's head and neck, the swaying will stop. As described in earlier chapters, postural stability in a young child is influenced by the eyes, ears and neck musculature. As the child sways, he is responding to information from these three systems. Supporting the head and neck may help the child stabilize; this has been demonstrated in very young infants who have not yet established strategies for sitting (Shumway-Cook & Woollacott 2000). If the child's sway during unsupported sitting is due to a postural problem, stabilizing the head and neck will decrease the sway. However, if the sway is athetotic it will continue despite the examiner's intervention.

CONSEQUENCES OF SPASTICITY

When a child has increased tone in a muscle group, the postural and cortical function is affected. As discussed in previous chapters, biomechanical strains have been shown to influence cortical mapping of somatosensory input (Merzenich & Jenkins 1993, Merzenich et al 1993) (see Chs 9 and 10). Furthermore, the biomechanics of a joint influence the proprioception coming from it. Increased muscle tone alters joint mechanics and proprioception. Thus, spasticity can influence primary somatosensory mapping, muscle coupling and movement strategies. Woollacott et al (1998) have suggested that the abnormal postural control in children with some forms of spasticity is due to biomechanical rather than neurological factors.

In children with spasticity, the baseline tone due to the neurological insult is often much lower than the tone that they are functioning with every day. This happens because each and every movement they make has the potential to increase the existing muscle contraction through the unmodulated spinal reflex. For example, suppose a child has increased tone in the hamstring muscle group. The antagonist muscle group, the quadratus, will often contract to compensate for the postural instability created by the contracted hamstring. This increases the stretch on the already hypertonic hamstring muscle, causing a reflexive contraction. A reflex loop is created, facilitating the spinal reflex. The hypertonia of the involved muscle, the hamstring, worsens. Thus, even a child with a mild spasticity is at risk for developing severe muscle contraction and even losing function of a limb if appropriate therapies are started too late or discontinued too early.

Billy is a 13-year-old boy with severe flexion contractures of the right arm. He has a diagnosis of CP involving the right arm and leg. As a young child, he received physical therapy and had fairly good use of his arm, hand and fingers. He could manipulate thick crayons and would color pictures. When he reached 9 years of age, the therapy to his arm was discontinued, although he continued to wear a splint on his leg. The contractures in his arm developed over the next 3 years, and he lost function of the arm, hand and fingers. He cannot hold a thick crayon or marker. He is unable to write or type. He cannot turn the door handle or push the elevator button. Yet these are all activities that he had previously done effectively. It is very important to begin treating children with suspected spasticity as early as possible and to continue appropriate treatment to maintain function.

In a child with CP, somatic dysfunction in the neck and torso may alter the proprioceptive input from these areas and further compromise stability and posture. Alleviating biomechanical stresses with osteopathic manipulation may help the child by normalizing input to joint afferents and balancing agonist–antagonist muscle tone. Appropriate orthotic devices and exercises may also be used for this purpose. The head and neck stabilizing maneuver described above can also be used to reinforce postural control mechanisms in the child. The parents can be taught to gently hold the head and the neck in good alignment while the child attempts some other task such as looking at a book or playing with a toy. In older children, well-developed compensatory mechanisms for stability may be compromised by increased muscle tone or other biomechanical stresses. Occasionally, an older child can be seen propping himself up against something or holding his head and neck. If these postures are associated with attention difficulties or behavior problems, the child should be evaluated for biomechanical imbalances that may be affecting postural mechanisms. Frequent postural adjustments can be misinterpreted as inattentiveness and distractibility. Yet in the child with CP, this movement may be necessary to maintain stability or relieve muscle ache and fatigue. Children prone to fidgeting or frequent postural correction (with or without attention difficulties) should also receive a complete functional optometry evaluation to ensure that they are not using their posture to compensate for visual stresses.

A child's center of gravity tends to be up at the thoracolumbar junction, but some time before puberty it will settle into the pelvis. Muscle weakness or poor motor control of the hip flexors and pelvic musculature may compromise a child's ability to do unsupported sitting. He or she may accommodate by attempting to use muscles of the torso. Complete evaluation of agonist–antagonist muscle relationships in the rotator cuff of the hip and muscles of the pelvis and extremities needs to be done periodically. Coordinated activity and appropriate muscle tone levels can be addressed with osteopathic manipulation. In older children, reconditioning activities, which reinforce postural mechanics, can be added. Activities which are often beneficial include dance, gymnastics, martial arts, yoga, swimming, horseback riding and trampoline activities. Of course, the activity needs to be geared towards the child's capabilities. Frequently, groups will welcome the addition of a challenged child to a group.

There is increased tone in the hamstrings in spastic hemiplegic and diplegic CP. The increased tone will cause posterior rotation of the ipsilateral innominate bone, often resulting in loss of the lumbar lordosis. When upright, the child will compensate by extending at the thoracolumbar junction, flattening the thoracic kyphosis, and extending the occiput on the atlas. This shifts the center of gravity forward and superiorly, alters respiratory mechanics, and creates much restriction and compression at the craniocervical junction and cranial base. When sitting, the child will flex the hips and knees. The increased hamstring tone rotates the innominates posteriorly and tips the pelvis backwards. The child will often lean forwards to counteract the position of the innominates. Maintaining a balanced seat in this position consumes energy and attention. How can a child pay attention to the teacher when she is trying to stay upright? As the child gets older, these postural adaptations will alter mechanical forces on the growing and developing joints, frequently creating a different set of problems.

Hypertonicity in the lower extremity will alter the mechanics at the hip, sometimes placing excessive forces on the acetabulum. A child's acetabulum is relatively flat, and the neck of the femur oriented more inferiorly than in the adult. The femoral head and neck have three ossification centers. As the child grows, the biomechanics and vascular pattern of the hip joint change, reaching an adult position towards the end of puberty. Displaced postural forces and ligament laxity may result in true hip displacement or slipped capital femoral epiphysis, a posteromedial slippage of the femoral epiphysis associated with extension and external rotation of the femoral neck. Hip displacement needs to be evaluated by an orthopedic surgeon and often requires pinning or casting. Addressing the changes in hip and gait mechanics as the child grows needs to be a part of every osteopathic evaluation. Abnormal stresses on the ligaments or articular surfaces of the hip may originate in the foot and distal extremity, or may be the result of altered mechanics in the pelvis, sacrum and lumbar spine. The innominate bone is in three parts: pubic bone, ischium and ilium. These three bones join at the center of the acetabulum, which is primarily cartilaginous until mid-adolescence. Growth occurs within the acetabulum as well as at the peripheral growth centers. Chronic muscle spasm of biceps femoris will increase inferior tension on the ischial component and may potentially affect the shape of the acetabular space, compromising the joint relationships. Evaluation of the three components of the innominate bone and their relationship to each other and the femoral head is important. Comparison between the two hip mechanisms may shed light on distortions in relationships (see Ch. 15).

GOALS OF OSTEOPATHIC TREATMENT

Ultimately, the goal of osteopathic treatment is to facilitate and nurture health within the child and within the family.

In general, the physical goals of osteopathic treatment of the child with CP are to decrease pain, limit or prevent contractures, hip dislocations and scoliosis, and improve functional capabilities. The first goal is to decrease pain. Chronic muscle spasm can cause pain and discomfort, disrupting normal activities, including sleep. Osteopathic techniques aimed at passive or isometric muscle stretch, such as muscle energy techniques, are effective in the older child who can follow directions, as are strain–counterstrain techniques, especially in the shoulder and hip girdle. If the clinician can monitor tissue texture changes and need not rely on verbal reporting from the child, strain–counterstrain techniques can be used in the toddler and young child, and are usually well tolerated. Balanced ligamentous and other 'indirect' techniques are appropriate, well tolerated and useful in all age groups, especially very young children or children unable to follow commands.

Another goal of osteopathic manipulative treatment in a child with CP is to effect changes in proprioceptive input from joints, connective tissues and muscle, which may be compromising posture, balance and movement. Furthermore, joint contractures, scoliosis and hip dislocation may all be complications of chronic muscle spasm, abnormal postural forces and altered joint mechanics. Children with CP are creating, refining and incorporating movement strategies to interact with their environment. The child with a right-sided spastic hemiplegia will develop strategies to accommodate the hemiplegia. That same child will also develop compensatory changes in his musculoskeletal system in response to the hemiplegia. For example, if the hemiplegia involves hypertonicity of the hamstrings, the right innominate bone will rotate posteriorly on its horizontal axis. This will create a relative nutation of the sacrum and potential flattening in the lumbar lordosis as well as a left rotation and right-side bending of the lumbar spine. Flexion in the upper thoracic area may occur to accommodate the postural changes in the pelvis. The child's center of gravity will shift forwards. He may extend his head and flatten the cervical lordosis. All these areas provide proprioceptive input to maintain balance. Now we have a child with a right-sided hemiplegia who also has to accommodate all the postural changes that have occurred. Osteopathic treatment should be directed towards alleviating some of these abnormal or stressful inputs resulting from the compensatory changes. This will allow the child to create motor strategies that are unencumbered by these compensatory changes. In other words, although one may not be able to change the original spasticity or hypertonia, appropriate osteopathic treatment will be able to influence any muscle spasm or somatic dysfunction which has developed secondarily and is now contributing to the overall level of tone in the child, improving the child's ability to perform motor planning and execute movement.

Let us consider an 18-month-old child with a mild spastic hemiplegia on the left side who is learning to walk. The left leg is a little bit shorter than the right, because of the muscle tone, and the left elbow and wrist are slightly flexed. To keep his balance, he has to shift his weight slightly. The child's sense of midline is going to be shifted as well. Part of his compensatory adaptations include side-bending his lumbar spine slightly and correcting for it in the cervicothoracic and craniocervical junctions. This is the beginning of a scoliosis. Meanwhile, the child needs to orient his eyes to the horizon, so he cocks his head a bit. Years pass and now the child is 5 years old. He has constructed spatial maps in his cortex based on this cockeyed posture. He wants to pick up a pen and write his name. In order to write, one needs to have depth perception to interpret the spaces between the letters and the spatial shape of the letter. The spatial shape of that letter is also associated with a sound. But this child's spatial maps are different from those of most other children. He has to work very hard to interpret the shapes he sees written. He is 5 years old, going to school, and the teacher is writing on the board. His spatial map did not develop around a balanced midline. He is trying to watch the teacher write on the board and interpret these shapes with eyes that are stuck in a head that is a little tilted. His eyes get tired, he gets tired and he stops paying attention. Everyone thinks he has attention deficit disorder and should be given methylphenidate (Ritalin).

Many children with mild forms of CP are first brought in for osteopathic evaluation when the parents are faced with this type of scenario. Although the child may be receiving various therapies, each tends to focus upon a different part of the patient. Someone needs to step back and look at the big picture. It will all continue to snowball until someone starts to gently untangle the threads of this child's tapestry.

Children with CP need consistent osteopathic treatment to keep the afferent drive turned down. Most children will need to be treated fairly regularly, at least as often as every growth spurt, providing there is good follow-up at home or in school. For example, increased tone in the knee and hip flexors lead to toe walking. The toe walking is often addressed with an orthotic which holds the ankle in dorsiflexion. All too often, these orthotics are rigid and force the foot into a slightly everted position. The navicular is internally rotated and the medial plantar arch is compromised. This will internally rotate the tibia (see Ch. 15). Very often, the tibial torsion becomes exacerbated and the bone will twist as the child grows. Early intervention is very important. Always evaluate the child's gait with and without the orthotic. Initially, the pes planus will be functional; however, with continued use of the orthotic and worsening of the tibial torsion, the pes planus may be present even when not weightbearing. Nevertheless, rebalancing the joint relations of the forefoot and hindfoot with attention to the talonavicular, navicular–cuneiform and fibular positions will often correct the dropped arch. Correction of the tibial torsion is a longer process, and if the tibia has twisted as opposed to rotated, manual correction may be impossible in the older child. Compensatory changes in the hip, pelvis and lumbosacral mechanism will arise in response to the position of the tibia and the dropped arch. These all need to be addressed if the arch is to stay functional. Sometimes the child may still need an orthotic that provides maximum stability with minimum disruption of balance mechanisms.

Sarah is an 8-year-old girl with spastic CP involving both lower extremities. Another osteopathic physician who had been treating her since the age of 3, but only saw her occasionally, referred her. When she first presented, she was in a wheelchair because her gait was quite ataxic and unbalanced. Sarah had been using bilateral ankle, knee and hip braces to stabilize her balance. In the orthotics, her gait was very wide-based and she exhibited a lot of flaying about her arms, torso and head, which had worsened over the past 2 years. She was being evaluated at a large children's hospital for suspected cerebellar involvement, although the MRI did not show any cerebellar changes. After a careful history, Sarah's parents reported that at the age of 6 she had entered the local school system, and her gait and balance began to deteriorate. At that time, she was wearing an orthotic which locked her ankle in dorsiflexion. Over the next 2 years, Sarah's physical therapist and orthotist had attempted to stabilize her balance by extending the orthotic to her knees and then her hips. But, according to her parents, 'things just seemed to get worse' and now she was becoming dependent on a wheelchair to get around school. Sarah's family was concerned, she was losing function, and she had become depressed and reluctant to interact with people. We asked Sarah to walk down the office hallway wearing her orthotics. She often brushed her fingers against the wall but there was no awkward arm or torso movement. Next, we took her into the foyer of the building, a bustling cavernous room. Here, Sarah began flaying about, jerking her torso one way and then the other, losing her balance until one of us caught her and placed her in the wheelchair. Comparing the two demonstrations, it seemed that in the foyer Sarah appeared to be using torso and arm strategies to maintain her center of balance, i.e. to counteract the sway, whereas in the hallway, Sarah was using the wall to get some spatial bearings. It seemed that the orthotics had removed much of the proprioceptive input Sarah needed to maintain balance. In a controlled environment, such as a quiet office hallway, she was able to garner clues from touching the wall. But when she was put in an uncontrolled environment where multiple sensory stimuli converged, she could not compensate. Palpatory evaluation revealed tremendous fascial and biomechanical dysfunction throughout the feet, legs, hips, pelvis and back, including the cranium. The severity of the findings was much greater than I would have expected for the level of spasticity, and suggested another factor. After appropriate osteopathic treatment,

I suggested that the family return with the old ankle orthotics for re-evaluation the next day. We repeated the two exercises and noted that Sarah's arm movements and balance were no worse with the smaller orthotics. I instructed her to continue with the ankle orthotics and we continued osteopathic treatment. Over several weeks, Sarah's function improved to the point where she was maneuvering in the school hallways and playground safely and effectively. After discussing the case with an orthotist responsive to the osteopathic approach, we were able to put Sarah into a small orthotic consisting only of an arch support to correct for her oversupination. At the age of 13, Sarah began attending classes in the regional high school, a very large single-level complex. She was required to do much more walking, and once again found the chaotic environment a little too much to handle. Her balance and gait began to suffer. Rather than try to increase stability by locking out movement, we chose a different path. Sarah now has a working dog that is trained to counterbalance her weight whenever she begins to lose stability. Not only has she adapted nicely to being a high school student, but she recently started volunteer work at the hospital, delivering patient mail using a cart that the dog helps her push. This is a long story but the moral is that we need to seek maximum stability with minimum restriction. Frequently, one of your best allies will be an experienced and communicative orthotist, who can sculpt orthotic devices which support the body's inherent capabilities. This often requires educating everyone involved about osteopathic principles and practice.

Many children with CP will have associated problems in other systems. These need to be diagnosed and addressed as early as possible to avoid further compromising the child's development. Approximately 40% of children with CP will have visual problems, but a minority of those visual problems result from something anatomical that you can measure. Most of the visual problems that they have are visual processing problems – problems with interpreting the stimulus. This may be a result of altered somatosensory influences (see Ch. 10). Evaluation by a functional optometrist in conjunction with osteopathic management is very important.

Finally, one must remember that the child is part of a family. Many issues will arise which may be addressed by the osteopathic physician, especially one with a good rapport with the entire family. Family resources are often stretched, financially, physically and emotionally. Parents may be struggling with feelings of guilt. Often, there is an underlying fear concerning what will happen to the child when the parents are no longer there. Sisters and brothers are also dealing with feelings of guilt, fear, resentment, concern, love, etc. For some families, counseling can offer support and guidance. Other families will work it out themselves. Ultimately, the family needs to be a family, not a household of people focusing on this one child with a cerebral injury. And, as with each individual, each family is different. A good clinician must be able to step back and see the whole picture, not just the child's increased muscle tone.

CONCLUSION

CP is very complicated. There are many issues which need to be addressed, and the issues will change as the child matures and develops. The health of the child's family needs to be supported and nurtured as well. The team approach is important in the treatment of children with CP. The goal is to communicate so that everyone has a good idea of all the things to which this child is being exposed. There are probably going to be times when disagreement occurs. Two clinicians will look at the same thing from different perspectives and disagree on the best treatment. Sometimes there are two different issues, and the treatment prescribed for one issue may have adverse effects on the other. Ultimately, communication between all the concerned parties is essential. And the easiest and most efficient means for this to happen is through a well-informed, involved and supported parent who understands their child as a whole person.

References

Adams R D, Victor M 1993 Principles of neurology, 5th edn. McGraw-Hill, New York.

Bouza H, Dubowitz L M, Rutherford M et al 1994a Late magnetic resonance imaging and clinical findings in neonates with unilateral lesions on cranial ultrasound. Dev Med Child Neurol 36(11): 951–964.

Bouza H, Rutherford M, Acolet D et al 1994b Evolution of early hemiplegic signs in full-term infants with unilateral brain lesions in the neonatal period: a prospective study. Neuropediatrics 25(4): 201–207.

Brown J K, Purvis R J, Forfar J O et al 1974 Neurological aspects of perinatal asphyxia. Dev Med Child Neurol 16(5): 567–580.

Brown J K, Rodda J, Walsh E G et al 1991 Neurophysiology of lower-limb function in hemiplegic children. Dev Med Child Neurol 33(12): 1037–1047.

de Vries L S, Groenendaal F, Eken P et al 1997 Infarcts in the vascular distribution of the middle cerebral artery in preterm and fullterm infants. Neuropediatrics 28(2): 88–96.

Dormans J P, Pellegrino L 1998 Definitions, etiology and epidemiology of cerebral palsy. In: Dormans J P, Pellegrino L (eds) Caring for children with cerebral palsy. Paul H Brookes, Baltimore: 31–33.

Grether J K, Cummins S K, Nelson K B 1992 The California Cerebral Palsy Project. Paediatr Perinat Epidemiol 6(3): 339–351.

Ingram T T 1964 Child care in general practice. Cerebral palsy. I. BMJ ii: 1638–1640.

Krageloh-Mann I, Hagberg G, Meisner C et al 1995a Bilateral spastic cerebral palsy – a collaborative study between southwest Germany and western Sweden – III: Aetiology. Dev Med Child Neurol 37(3): 191–203.

Krageloh-Mann I, Petersen D, Hagberg G et al 1995b Bilateral spastic cerebral palsy – MRI pathology and origin. Analysis from a representative series of 56 cases. Dev Med Child Neurol 37(5): 379–397.

Larroche J C 1986 Fetal encephalopathies of circulatory origin. Biol Neonate 50(2): 61–74.

Low J A, Robertson D M, Simpson L L 1989 Temporal relationships of neuropathologic conditions caused by perinatal asphyxia. Am J Obstet Gynecol 160(3): 608–614.

McDonald A D 1963 Cerebral palsy in children of very low birth weight. Arch Dis Child 38: 579–588.

Menkes J H, Sarant H B 2000 Child neurology, 6th edn. Lippincott, Williams & Wilkins, Philadelphia.

Merzenich M M, Jenkins W M 1993 Reorganization of cortical representations of the hand following alterations of skin inputs induced by nerve injury, skin island transfers, and experience. J Hand Ther 6: 89–104.

Merzenich M M, Schreiner C, Jenkins W et al 1993 Neural mechanisms underlying temporal integration, segmentation, and input sequence representation: some implications for the origin of learning disabilities. Ann N Y Acad Sci 682: 1–22.

Michaelis R, Rooschuz B, Dopper R 1980 Prenatal origin of congenital spastic hemiparesis. Early Hum Dev 4(3): 243–255.

Molteni B, Oleari G, Fedrizzi E et al 1987 Relation between CT patterns, clinical findings and etiological factors in children born at term, affected by congenital hemiparesis. Neuropediatrics 18(2): 75–80.

Nelson K B, Ellenberg J H 1996 Antecedents of cerebral palsy. Multivariate analysis of risk. N Engl J Med 315(2): 81–86.

Okumura A, Hayakawa F, Kato T et al 1997a MRI findings in patients with spastic cerebral palsy. I: Correlation with gestational age at birth. Dev Med Child Neurol 39(6): 363–368.

Okumura A, Kato T, Kuno K et al 1997b MRI findings in patients with spastic cerebral palsy. II: Correlation with type of cerebral palsy. Dev Med Child Neurol 39(6): 369–372.

Olsen P, Paakko E, Vainionpaa L et al 1997 Magnetic resonance imaging of periventricular leukomalacia and its clinical correlation in children. Ann Neurol 41(6): 754–761.

Olsen P, Vainionpaa L, Paakko E et al 1998 Psychological findings in preterm children related to neurologic status and magnetic resonance imaging. Pediatrics 102(2 Pt 1): 329–336.

Pearson K, Gordon J 2000 Spinal reflexes. In: Kandel E R, Schwartz J H, Jessell T M (eds) Principles of neural science. McGraw-Hill, Philadelphia.

Shumway-Cook A & Woollacott M H 2000 Motor control: theory and practical applications. Williams & Wilkins, Philadelphia.

Volpe J J 1995 Neurology of the newborn, 3rd edn. W B Saunders, Philadelphia.

Woollacott M H, Burtner P, Jensen J et al 1998 Development of postural responses during standing in healthy children and children with spastic diplegia. Neurosci Biobehav Rev 22(4): 583–589.

Further reading

Kandel E R, Schwartz J H, Jessell T M (eds) 2000 Principles of neural science. McGraw-Hill, Philadelphia.

Merzenich M M, Nelson R J, Kaas J H et al 1987 Variability in hand surface representations in areas 3b and 1 in adult owl and squirrel monkeys. J Compr Neurol 258: 281–296.

van der Weel F R, van der Meer A L, Lee D N 1991 Effect of task on movement control in cerebral palsy: implications for assessment and therapy. Dev Med Child Neurol 33(5): 419–426.

Volpe J J 1992 Brain injury in the premature infant – current concepts of pathogenesis and prevention. Biol Neonate 62: 231–242.

Volpe J J 1995 Neurology of the newborn, 3rd edn. W B Saunders, Philadelphia.

Note: Page numbers in **bold** refer to figures.

suspensory ligament of the eye, 204, **204**
sustentaculum tali, **37**
Sutherland's cranial strain patterns, 133, 137, **138**
Sutherland's model of facial bone mechanics, 192–3
Sutures, cranial *see* cranial sutures
swallowing, 109, 229
    difficulty, 229
    esophageal phase, 229
    mechanics, 229
    oral phase, 229
    painful, 229
    pharyngolaryngeal phase, 229
Swan-Ganz catheter, 78
sway, 152, 160, 163, 295
    during postural adjustments, 150
sympathetic nervous system
    gastrointestinal system, 110
    mucociliary transport system, 194
synapses, 170
synaptogenesis, 170
synclitism, 132, **132**
synovitis, acute, 270
syntax problems, 177

T

tachycardia, 11–12, 81
taeniae coli, 109
t'ai chi, 164, 252
talocrural joint, **37**, 37–8
talus, **37**
    ossification, 37
    weight transmission, 41
tamponade, cardiac, 75
tarsal tunnel syndrome, 266–7
taste, loss of, 277, 278
tears, 200
    absent, 277, 278
temporal bone, 65
    at birth, 187
    development, **67–9**, 67–70
    postnatal changes/development, 63, 188–9
    remodeling, 69
temporal lobe, 59
temporal sequencing, 155
temporomandibular joint, **67**, 69
tenderness, 8
tendons, foot arches, 40, **40**
tennis elbow, 269–70, 280
tensor veli palatini muscle, 70, 188, **189**, 191
TENS (transcutaneous nerve stimulation), 125
tentorium cerebelli, 54, **55**, 59, 60, 61
teres minor, 42, 45, 268–9
term infants, definition, 137
testes, neonatal, 139, **140**
tetralogy of Fallot, 78–9
texture perception, 175

thermodilution method, 78
thoracic fulcrum, 88
thoracic spine development, 17, **17**
thoracoabdominal pump, 32–3
thoracolumbar fascia, 21, **22**, **23**, 25
    tension on, 258
thorax, anatomical relationships of, 95, **95**
tibia
    anatomy, 37
    condyles, 34
    development, 33
    distal, onset and closure of ossification, 20
    facet, 265
    knee biomechanics, 36
    plateau, onset and closure of ossification, 20
    torsion, 263, **264**
        in cerebral palsy, 297–8
    tubercle microfracture, 263
tibial arteries, 32, 38
tibialis anterior, 36, 40, **40**
tibialis posterior, 40, **40**
tibiocalcaneal ligament, **37**
tibiofibular joint, proximal, 265
tics, 281
T lymphocytes, 97, 116
toe walking, 161
toilet training, 183, 236
tongue, 72
    muscles, 226, **226**
    suckling, 226, **226**
tonic contractions, gut, 109
tonic neck reflex, 155–6, **156**, 180
tonsillar adenopathy, 218
torticollis
    brachial plexus palsy, 276
    causes, 142
    deformational plagiocephaly, 246
    strabismus, 209, **247**, 247–8, **248**
    treatment, 248
touch
    afferent fibers, 6
    afferent load, 8
    perception, 175
Tourette's syndrome, 281
trachea
    congenital deformity, 102, **102**
    development, 85
    embryological development, 102
tracheoesophageal fistula, 102, **102**
transcutaneous nerve stimulation (TENS), 125
transforming growth factor (TGF), 111
transient tachypnea of the newborn (TNN), 86, 217–18
transient tic disorder, 281
transposition of the great vessels, 78, 79
transverse abdominis muscle, 95
transverse humeral ligament, 44
transverse ligament, 37
transverse processes, **22**

transverse sinus, 59, **59**
transversus thoracic muscles, 90
traumatic brain injury, 284
triangular fibrocartilage complex, 49
triceps, 48
tricuspid valve atresia, 78, 79
trigeminal nerve, **207**
    ophthalmic division, 282, **283**
trigeminal system of the brain, 282
triglycerides, 115
triquetrum, 49
triradiate cartilage, 23, 24, 29
trisomy, 21, 143
trochlear nerve, 205, 207, **207**
trophis, 209
truncus arteriosus, 79
    persistent, 78
trypsin, 113, 115
tumour necrosis factor-alpha (TNF-α), 128
tunnel of Guyon, 280
tympanic membrane, 186
tympanic ring, 67, 68, **68**, 69
tympanic segment of facial nerve, 278
tympanograms, 191, **191**
tympanostomy tubes, 187

U

ulna, 46
ulnar collateral ligament, 47, 49, 270
ulnar nerve, 282
    compression, 280
ulnar trochanter, onset and closure of ossification, 20
ulnocarpal ligament, 49
ulnolunate ligament, 49
umbilical cord, cutting, 113
unimodal association areas, 171
upper airway obstruction, apnea, 218
upper extremities, 41–50
    common orthopedic problems, 268–71
    innervation, 282, **283**
    neurovascular bundle, 276 *see also specific area*
upper respiratory tract congestion, 220
utricle, 178
uvula, 142, 219

V

vacuum extraction, 135, 136, 213
vagus nerve, 97
    colic, 234–5
    effect on lower esophageal sphincter, 231
    gastroesophageal reflux, 233
    palsy, 227
    suckling, 227
valvulae conniventes, 102, 103
vascular resistance, 76, 78, 86

Printed in the United States
By Bookmasters